NURSING LEADERSHIP AND MANAGEMENT

Second Canadian Edition

Patricia Kelly

University of Texas, Austin

Heather Crawford

Vice President Clinical Services and Chief Nursing Executive

Brockville General Hospital

Brockville, Ontario

NELSON / EDUCATION

NELSON / EDUCATION

Nursing Leadership and Management, Second Canadian Edition
by Patricia Kelly and Heather Crawford

Vice President, Editorial Higher Education:
Anne Williams

Executive Editor:
Jackie Wood

Marketing Manager:
Alexis Hood

Developmental Editor:
Leah Blain

Photo Researcher:
Sandra Mark

Permissions Coordinator:
Sandra Mark

Content Production Manager:
Jennifer Hare

Production Service:
Integra Software Services

Copy Editor:
Carolyn Jongeward

Proofreader:
Integra Software Services

Indexer:
Integra Software Services

Manufacturing Manager:
Joanne McNeil

Design Director:
Ken Phipps

Managing Designer:
Franca Amore

Cover Design:
Martyn Schmoll

Cover Image:
Ryan McVay/Getty Images

Compositor:
Integra Software Services

Printer:
Edwards Brothers Malloy

Library and Archives Canada Cataloguing in Publication Data

Kelly, Patricia, 1941-Nursing leadership and management/Patricia Kelly, Heather Crawford. —2nd Canadian ed.

Includes bibliographical references and index.
ISBN 978-0-17-650460-1

1. Nursing services—Administration—Textbooks. 2. Nursing services—Canada—Administration—Textbooks. I. Crawford, Heather, 1950– II. Title.

RT89.K45 2012
362.17'3068   C2011-908018-4

ISBN-13: 978-0-17-650460-1
ISBN-10: 0-17-650460-5

CONTENTS

CONTRIBUTORS XVII

PREFACE XIX

Organization xix
Features xx
Acknowledgments xxi
About the Author xxii
How To Use this Book xxii

UNIT I
INTRODUCTION

CHAPTER 1

Canada's Health Care Environment 1

Organization of Health Care 4
   Types of Health Care Services 5
   Health Care Professionals in Canada 5
Health Care Spending 6
Approaches to Health Care in Canada 8
   Population Health 8
   Public Health 12
   Primary Health Care 13
   Integrated Health Care Delivery Systems 14
   Horizontal and Vertical Integration 21
   Disease Management 21
Accreditation 21
Health Care Variation and Evidence-Based Practice 23
   Variation in Client Outcomes 23
   Canadian Health Services Research Foundation 24
   Accreditation Canada's Patient Safety Goals 24
   Institute of Medicine Committee on Health Care
      Quality Reports 25
   Canadian Adverse Events Study 27
Quality Health Care 28
   Structure, Process, Outcome 28
   The 3M Health Care Quality Team Awards 30
   Outcome Measurements 30
Recent Changes in Health Care 30
   Privacy Legislation in Canada 30
   Canadian College of Health Leaders 30

Other Forces Influencing Trends in Health Care   33
 Nursing Role   34
 Interprofessional Nursing Practice   35

CHAPTER 2

Basic Clinical Health Care Economics   43

Traditional Perspective on the Cost of Health Care:
 Health Care as Altruism   45
 Need for Health Care Determined by Provider   45
 The Right to Health Care at Any Cost   45
 Federal and Provincial Reports   48
 Accountability   48
 Functions of the Health Care System   50
 Health Care Finance Reform   51
 Funding Health Reform   52
 Delivery Health Reform   56
Future Perspective on the Cost of Health Care   57

UNIT II

A NEW HEALTH CARE MODEL

CHAPTER 3

Evidence-Based Practice   62

History of Evidence-Based Practice   63
Importance of Evidence-Based Practice   64
Attributes of Evidence-Based Practice   66
Misconceptions about Evidence-Based Practice   67
Evidence: Sources, Types, and Evaluation   67
Levels of Evidence   76
Knowledge Transfer and Evidence-Based Decisions in Policy   78

CHAPTER 4

Nursing and Health Care Informatics   85

What Is Nursing Informatics?   87
 The Specialty of Nursing Informatics   87
  Education in Informatics   88
  Certification   89
  Career Opportunities   90
Clinical Information   90
 Clinical Information Systems   90
 Electronic Health Record   90
  Data Capture   91
  Storage   92

Information Processing   92
Information Communication   92
Security   92
Information Presentation   93
Canada Health Infoway   93
Interface between the Informatics Nurse and the Clinical
   Information System   93
Trends in Computing   94
Development of Modern Computing   94
Ubiquitous Computing   95
Virtual Reality   95
The Internet   97
Using the Internet for Clinical Practice   97
The P-F-A Assessment   97
Quick and Dirty Searching   98
Brute Force   98
Links and Bookmarks   98
Resources for Professionals and Consumers   98
Literature Resources   99
Evaluation of Information Found on the Internet   99

CHAPTER 5

Population-Based Health Care Practice   106

Population Health   107
Population-Based Nursing Practice   113
Nursing in Nontraditional Settings   113
Program Planning and Evaluation   117
Assessment   117
Planning and Implementation   117
Evaluation   118

CHAPTER 6

Personal and Interprofessional Communication   125

Trends in Society that Affect Communication   126
Elements of the Communication Process   127
Sender   127
Message   127
Receiver   127
Feedback   127
Channels of Communication   127
The Visual Channel   127
The Auditory Channel   127
The Kinesthetic Channel   128
Modes of Communication   128

Verbal Communication   128
Nonverbal Communication   128
Electronic Communication   128
Social Media   129
Level of Communication   130
Public Communication   130
Intrapersonal Communication   130
Interpersonal Communication   130
Organizational Communication   131
Communication Skills   131
Attending   132
Responding   132
Clarifying   132
Confronting   132
Barriers to Communication   133
Gender   133
Culture   133
Anger   133
Incongruent Responses   134
Conflict   135
Workplace Communication   136
Superiors   136
Co-workers   136
Subordinates   136
Physicians and Other Health Care Professionals   136
Clients and Their Families   137
Mentor and Prodigy   138

CHAPTER 7

Politics and Consumer Partnerships   143

Stakeholders and Health Care   144
The Politics and Economics of Human Services   147
Cultural Dimensions of Partnerships and Consumerism   148
Politics and Demographic Changes   148
Nurse as Political Activist   150
Politics and Advocacy   151
Advocacy and Consumer Alliances   151
Consumer Demands   152
Turning a Consumer-Oriented Vision into Reality   153
The Consumer Demand for Accountability   154
Credibility and Politics   154

UNIT III

PLANNING CARE

CHAPTER 8

Nursing Leadership and Management   159

Definition of Management   161
The Management Process   161
Management Theories   162
    Classical Viewpoint   163
    Scientific Management   163
    Bureaucratic Theory   163
    Administrative Principles   164
Human Relations   165
Motivation Theories   165
    Maslow's Hierarchy of Needs   166
    Herzberg's Two-Factor Theory   166
    McGregor's Theory X and Theory Y   167
    Ouchi's Theory Z   168
The Changing Nature of Managerial Work   168
Definition of Leadership   168
    Leadership Characteristics   169
    Factors that Influence the Quality of Nursing Leadership   171
    Leadership Theories   172
        Behavioural Approaches   173
        Contingency Approaches   175
        Contemporary Approaches   176
Kouzes and Posner's Five Leadership Practices   178
Nursing Leadership and Outcomes   178
Future Directions   179
    The New Leadership   180
    Generational Leadership Issues   181
    Nursing Leadership and Management: The Link   182

CHAPTER 9

Effective Team Building   191

Defining Teams and Committees   192
Stages of Team Process   193
    Group Roles   194
        Functional versus Dysfunctional Members   194
Key Concepts of Effective Groups   195
    Great Team Guidelines   196
Creating an Environment Conducive to Team Building   198
    Teamwork on a Client Care Unit   199
    Effective Team Meetings   200

Interprofessional Healthcare Teams   201
Developing Decision-Making and Problem-Solving Skills   202
Successful Team Membership   203

CHAPTER 10

Budget Concepts for Client Care   207

Types of Budgets   208
    Operating Budget   208
    Capital Budget   208
    Construction Budget   209
Budget Overview   209
Budget Preparation   212
    Demographic Information   212
    Regulatory Influences   212
    Strategic Plans   213
Scope of Service and Goals   213
    History   214
Budget Development   214
    Revenue   214
    Expenses   214
        Supplies   215
        Human Resources   215
        Staffing   216
Budget Approval and Monitoring   217

CHAPTER 11

Effective Staffing   221

Determination of Staffing Needs   222
    Core Concepts   222
    Resource and FTE Requirements   222
        FTEs   222
        Nursing Hours per Patient Day   223
    Workload Measurement Systems   223
        Factor System   224
        Prototype System   224
        Utilization of Classification System Data   225
    Considerations in Developing a Staffing Pattern   225
        Benchmarking   225
        Regulatory Requirements   225
        Skill Mix   226
        Staff Support   226
        Historical Information   226
    Establishing a Staffing Pattern   226
        Inpatient Unit   227

Determining the Number of FTEs Needed to Meet
  the Staffing Pattern   227
Determining the FTEs Needed to Staff an
  Episodic Care Unit   227
Scheduling   230
  Client Needs   230
  Experience and Scheduling of Staff   230
    New Options in Staffing Patterns   231
    Impact on Client Care   232
    Financial Implications   232
    Cyclical Scheduling   232
    Self-Scheduling   232
Evaluation of Staffing Effectiveness   233
  Client Outcomes and Nurse Staffing   233
  Nurse Staffing and Nurse Outcomes   233
Models of Care Delivery   235
  Total Patient Care   235
    Advantages and Disadvantages   235
  Functional Nursing   236
    Advantages and Disadvantages   236
  Team Nursing   236
    Advantages and Disadvantages   236
  Primary Nursing   237
    Advantages and Disadvantages   238
  Emerging Models of Care: Client-Centred Collaborative
    Practice   238
Care Delivery Management Tools   238
  Clinical Pathways (Care Maps)   240
    Advantages and Disadvantages   240
  Case Management   240

CHAPTER 12

Delegation of Nursing Care   246

Perspectives on Delegation   247
Delegation Defined   248
Accountability and Responsibility   248
Authority   249
Assignment Making   249
Responsibilities of Health Team Members   249
  The Nurse Manager's Responsibilities   250
  The New Graduate's Responsibilities   250
  The Registered Nurse's Responsibilities   250
  The UCP's Responsibilities   251
  The Licensed Practical Nurse's Responsibilities   251
Direct Delegation versus Indirect Delegation   251
  Underdelegation   252

Inappropriate Delegation   253
Transcultural Delegation   255
   Communication   256
   Space   256
   Social Organization   256
   Time   256
   Environmental Control   257
   Biological Variations   257

UNIT IV

MANAGING CARE

CHAPTER 13

Strategic Planning and Organizing Client Care   260

Strategic Planning   261
   Strategic Planning Definition   262
   The Purpose of Strategic Planning   262
   Steps in the Strategic Planning Process   262
   Assessment of External and Internal Environment   262
   Community and Stakeholder Assessment   263
   Other Methods of Assessment   263
      Surveys and Questionnaires   263
      Focus Groups and Interviews   263
      Advisory Panel   263
      Review of Literature Related to Identified Programs   267
   Relationship of Strategic Planning to the Organization's
      Mission   267
      Planning Goals and Objectives   268
      Developing a Marketing Plan   268
Organizational Purpose, Mission, Philosophy, Values   269
   Mission Statement   269
   Philosophy   269
   Vision   270
   Values   270
   Organizational Structure   271
   Types of Organizational Structures   272
      Matrix Structure   272
      Flat versus Tall Structure   272
      Decentralized versus Centralized Structure   272
   Division of Labour   273
   Roles and Responsibilities   275
      Reporting Relationships   275
      Division of Labour by Geographic Area   276
      Division of Labour by Program   276
      Primary Nursing   276
The Structure of Professional Practice   278

Shared Governance   278
Clinical Practice Council   278
Quality Council   278
Education Council   278
Research Council   278
Management Council   279
Coordinating Council   279
Ensuring Competency and Professional Staff Development   280
Benner's Novice to Expert   280
The Process of Professional Practice   282
Situational Leadership   282
Accountability-Based Care Delivery   284
Measurable Quality Outcomes   284
Unit-Based Performance Improvement   284

CHAPTER 14

Change and Conflict Resolution   291

Change   292
Traditional Change Theories   294
Emerging Theories of Change   294
The Change Process   296
Steps in the Change Process   296
Assessment   296
Planning   296
Implementation of Change Strategies   297
Evaluation of Change   297
Stabilization of Change   297
Responses to Change   298
The Change Agent   299
Change Agent Strategies   300
Conflict   301
Sources of Conflict   301
Types of Conflict   301
The Conflict Process   302
Conflict Resolution   302
Strategies to Facilitate Conflict Resolution   304
Leadership and Management Roles   305
Conflict Management and Change   307

CHAPTER 15

Power   311

Definitions of Power   312
Power and Accountability   314
Sources of Power   314

Personal Orientation and the Internet   316
Empowerment and Disempowerment   316
   Role of the Media   317
A Plan for Personal Empowerment   317
Power and the Limits of Information   317
   Machiavelli on Power   319

UNIT V
EVALUATION

CHAPTER 16

Managing Performance and Outcomes Using an Organizational Quality Improvement Model   324

History of Quality Assurance   325
   Total Quality Management   326
General Principles of Quality Improvement   328
   Customers in Health Care   329
   Participation of Everyone in the Organization   329
   Focus on Improvement of the Health Care Work Process   330
      Improvement of the System   330
      A Continuous Process   330
      Improvement Based on Data   330
Implications for Client Care   331
Methodologies for Quality Improvement   331
   The Plan-Do-Study-Act Cycle   331
   The Focus Methodology   331
   Other Improvement Strategies   335
      Benchmarking   335
      Regulatory Requirements   335
      Sentinel Events   335
      Balanced Scorecard   335
      Storyboard: How to Share Your Story   337
      Client Satisfaction Data   337
  Using Data   338
      Time Series Data   338
      Charts: Pareto, Histogram, Flowcharts, Fishbone Diagrams,
         Pie Charts, and Check Sheets   338
Principles in Action in an Organization   338
   Organizational Structure   342
Outcomes Monitoring   343
Enterprise Risk Management   343

CHAPTER 17

Decision Making   348

Critical Thinking   349
Reflective Thinking   350
Problem Solving   351
Decision Making   351
    An Introduction   351
      Nature of Decision Making in Nursing   352
      Factors Influencing Decision Making   353
        Personal Perception and Preference   354
        Knowledge and Experience   354
        Competence   355
        Self-confidence   355
        Stress   356
        Extrinsic Factors   356
      Steps in the Decision-Making Process   357
        Clinical Application   358
        Management Application   359
        Decision Tree   359
        Gantt Chart   359
Group Decision Making   360
    Techniques of Group Decision Making   364
      Nominal Group Technique   364
      Delphi Group Technique   364
      Consensus Building   364
      Groupthink   364
Limitations to Effective Decision Making   365
Use of Technology in Decision Making   366
Nurses' Role in Client Decision Making   366
Strategies to Improve Decision Making   366

UNIT VI

OTHER PROFESSIONAL CONSIDERATIONS

CHAPTER 18

Legal Aspects of Client Care   372

Sources of Law   373
Public Law   373
    Constitutional Law   373
    Criminal Law   374
    Statutory Law   374
Civil Law   375
    Contract Law   375
    Tort Law   376

Non-Intentional Torts   376
Intentional Torts   377
Informed Consent   377
Do Not Resuscitate (DNR) Orders   378
False Imprisonment   379
Right to Privacy   380
Legal Protections in Nursing Practice   380
Government Inquiries   380
Good Samaritan Laws   382
Skillful Communication   382
Following Doctors' Orders   382
Enterprise Risk Management Programs   385
Malpractice and Professional Liability Insurance   386

CHAPTER 19

Spirituality and the Profession of Nursing   390

Spirituality and Nursing   391
Leadership: Learning and Growing   392
Holistic Care   394
Models of Spirituality   394
Hierarchy of Care   395
History of Compassionate Care   395
Assessment Education   395
Religious Needs   397
What Health Professionals Need to Know   397
What about Sharing My Faith?   398
Cultural Care Theories   399
Multiculturalism in Canada   399
Needs   399
Spiritual Distress   400
Spiritual Distressors   400
Experiences of Loss   400
Spiritual Abuse   401
Working with a Spiritual Care Team   402
Leadership Roles for Modelling Spiritual and Cultural Care   402
Nursing Leadership   403
Spiritual Practices Every Nurse can Adopt   403
Spiritual Care at the End of Life   404
Ethical Concerns   405

CHAPTER 20

Ethics and the Profession of Nursing   410

Ethics and Morality   411
Nursing Ethics   412

Ethical Theories   413
   Principlism   414
   Feminist Ethics   414
Foundations for Ethical Care in Canada   415
Codes of Ethics in Nursing   415
Professional Dilemmas   417
   Consent and Autonomy   417
   Resource Allocation   418
   End-of-Life Issues   421
   Truth Telling   423
Leadership Roles and Challenges in Ethics   424
Two Models for Ethical Decision Making   425

CHAPTER 21

Collective Bargaining   430

History of Nursing Unionization in Canada   431
Collective Action Models   432
   Workplace Advocacy   432
   Collective Bargaining   432
      Factors Influencing Nurses to Unionize   432
      Unions   433
Whistle-Blowing   435
The Process of Unionization   435
   The Manager's Role   436
   The Employee's Role   436
   Striking   437
Nursing Associations   437
Professionalism and Unionization   439
   Physician Unionization   439
   Unionization of University Professors   439
Managing in a Union Environment   440
   Grievances   440
Pros and Cons of Collective Bargaining   440

UNIT VII

PREPARATION FOR ENTRY-LEVEL NURSING PRACTICE

CHAPTER 22

Career Planning and Development: Creating Your Path to the Future   444

Creating your Career Vision   446
Your Self-Assessment and Reality Check   447
Scanning Your Environment   448
Creating Your Strategic Career Plan   449

Marketing Yourself   449
   Personal Resources   451
   Written Resources   453
   Electronic Résumés   454
   Business Cards   458
Preparing for an Interview   458
   A Note about References   459

APPENDIX   462

ABBREVIATIONS   465

GLOSSARY   468

INDEX   482

CONTRIBUTORS

John P. Angkaw, RN, BScN, MEd, MBA(c)
Director, Hospital Operations
St. Michael's Hospital
Toronto, Ontario
Adjunct Lecturer
Lawrence S. Bloomberg Faculty of Nursing
University of Toronto
Toronto, Ontario
Chapter 6: Personal and Interprofessional Communication
Chapter 8: Nursing Leadership and Management
Chapter 11: Effective Staffing
Chapter 12: Delegation of Nursing Care
Chapter 17: Decision Making

Jeanne Besner, RN, PhD
Director, JFB Workforce Consulting Ltd
Calgary, Alberta
Chapter 11: Effective Staffing

Heather Crawford, BScN, MEd, CHE
Vice President Clinical Services and Chief Nursing Executive
Brockville General Hospital
Brockville, Ontario
Chapter 1: Canada's Health Care Environment
Chapter 2: Basic Clinical Health Care Economics
Chapter 4: Nursing and Health Care Informatics
Chapter 6: Personal and Interprofessional Communication
Chapter 7: Politics and Consumer Partnerships
Chapter 8: Nursing Leadership and Management
Chapter 9: Effective Team Building
Chapter 10: Budget Concepts for Client Care
Chapter 11: Effective Staffing
Chapter 13: Strategic Planning and Organizing Client Care
Chapter 14: Change and Conflict Resolution
Chapter 16: Managing Performance and Outcomes Using an Organizational Quality
         Improvement Model
Chapter 18: Legal Aspects of Client Care
Chapter 21: Collective Bargaining

Amy Curzon
The Sheridan Institute of Technology and Advanced Learning
Brampton, Ontario
Chapter 6: Personal and Interprofessional Communication

Eric Doucette, RN
Professional Practice Leader
Brant Community Healthcare System
Brantford, Ontario
Chapter 8: Nursing Leadership and Management
Chapter 17: Decision Making

Pat Frederickson
Former Executive Director/Registrar
College of Licensed Practical Nurses of Alberta
Chapter 7: Politics and Consumer Partnerships

Rita McGregor
Former Director of Professional Practice
College of Licensed Practical Nurses of Alberta
Chapter 7: Politics and Consumer Partnerships

Ined Parmar, RN, MHSc
Professor
The Sheridan Institute of Technology and Advanced Learning
Brampton, Ontario
Chapter 17: Decision Making

Victoria E Pennick, RN, MHSc
Senior Clinical Research Project Manager
Managing Editor, Cochrane Back Group
Institute for Work & Health
Toronto, Ontario
Chapter 3: Evidence-Based Practice
Chapter 5: Population-Based Health Care Practice

Janet Stark
Spiritual Care Director
Brockville General Hospital,
Brockville, Ontario
Certified Multi-faith Chaplain
Certified Health Administrator
Certified Adult Educator
Care Clown
Chapter 19: Spirituality and the Nursing Profession

Sandra Trubyk, MSA, BN, BA, CAE
Director of Care
Amica at Windsor
Windsor, Ontario
Chapter 15: Power

Janice Waddell, RN, PhD
Associate Professor
Associate Director, School of Nursing
Ryerson University
Toronto, Ontario
Chapter 22: Career Planning and Development: Creating Your Path to the Future

Nancy Walton, PhD
Associate Professor, School of Nursing, Faculty of Community Services
Chair, Research Ethics Board
Ryerson University
Toronto, Ontario
Chapter 20: Ethics and the Profession of Nursing

PREFACE

Nursing Leadership and Management, Second Canadian Edition, is designed to help students and beginning nurses develop the knowledge and skills to lead and manage nursing care delivery in the 21st century. Every nurse today must lead and manage nursing care delivery, and the need for nurse leaders and nurse managers has never been greater. The nursing shortage is pressuring health care organizations to require nurses to do more with less and to adapt quickly to change.

Today's nurses need to have the competencies required for the 21st century, which calls for changes to nursing, medical, and other health care curricula. Some recommendations for the health care profession highlight the need for nurses to be educated in a broader way, including education in the areas of interprofessional teamwork, population-based health care, evidence-based practice, informatics, ethics, quality improvement, culture, spirituality and change, to name just a few.

This text addresses many of these topics, along with others, to prepare the beginning nurse leader and manager to successfully function in the modern health care system. Many of the chapters are written by nursing faculty. Others are written by clinical nurses who are specialists in their fields. These contributors are from various areas of Canada, thus providing a broad view of nursing leadership and management.

ORGANIZATION

Nursing Leadership and Management consists of 22 chapters grouped into seven units. These seven units will provide beginning nurse leaders and managers with the expertise needed to succeed in today's health care environment. They are arranged as follows:

- Unit I presents the changing health care environment and basic clinical economics.
- Unit II outlines a new health care model, emphasizing the role of evidence-based health care, nursing and health care informatics, population-based health care practice, interprofessional and personal communication, and politics and consumer partnerships in health care today.
- Unit III discusses planning care through leadership and management, effective team building, budget concepts for client care, the allocation of human resources for effective staffing, and delegation of client care.
- Unit IV discusses organizing and coordinating care. It presents strategic planning and organizing client care, change and conflict resolution, and power.
- Unit V covers evaluation of care, including managing outcomes using an organizational performance improvement model, enterprise risk management, and decision making.
- Unit VI presents other professional considerations, such as legal aspects of client care, spirituality, ethical dimensions of client care, and collective bargaining.
- Unit VII presents preparation for entry-level nursing practice. It discusses career planning, your first job, and integrating personal and professional needs.

An appendix outlines how to prepare for the Canadian Registered Nurse Examinations (CRNE) and the Canadian Practical Nurse Registration Examinations (CPRNE). The textbook uses graphics and photographs to engage readers and enhance their learning. Photographs provide visual reinforcement of concepts such as teamwork and the changes occurring in health care settings today while adding visual interest. Figures and tables depict concepts and activities described in the text.

FEATURES

Each chapter includes several pedagogical features that provide the reader with a consistent format for learning and an assortment of resources for understanding and applying the knowledge presented. These features and their functions include the following:

- Objectives state each chapter's learning goals.
- An introduction to each chapter briefly describes the purpose and scope of the chapter.
- A bulleted list of key concepts at the end of each chapter assists the reader in remembering and using the material presented.
- Review questions and review activities encourage students to think critically by applying chapter content to real-world situations and reinforcing key leadership and management skills. Exercises are numbered in each chapter to facilitate using them as assignments or activities.
- Key terms appear in bold type in each chapter and are designed to encourage the understanding of new terms presented in the chapter.
- References are the key to finding the sources of the material presented in each chapter.
- Suggested readings help the reader to find additional information concerning the topics covered in each chapter.

Special features are used throughout the text to emphasize key points and to provide specific types of information:

- An opening quote by a nursing or health care theorist provides a professional perspective on the chapter's topic.
- An opening scenario with thought-provoking questions introduces each chapter and establishes the background for the reader's approach to the chapter.
- Critical Thinking sections encourage serious consideration and personal reflection on important topics.
- Interviews with staff nurses, nurse practitioners, nursing managers and leaders, nursing administrators, nursing risk managers, nursing faculty, doctors, clients, and a hospital administrator are sprinkled throughout the chapters to illustrate various points of view. Interviews with Dr. Ginette L. Rodger, Dr. Lynn Nagle, Dr. Tim Porter-O'Grady, and other nursing leaders are included in some chapters.
- Literature applications illustrate the applicability of current literature for practice.
- Case studies provide real-world illustrations of the chapter's topic.
- Web exercises guide the reader to the Internet and provide Internet addresses for the latest and most reliable information related to the chapter content.

INSTRUCTOR SUPPORT

neta The **Nelson Education Teaching Advantage (NETA)** program delivers research-based instructor resources that promote student engagement and higher-order thinking to enable the success of Canadian students and educators.

Instructors today face many challenges. Resources are limited, time is scarce, and a new kind of student has emerged: one who is juggling school with work, has gaps in his or her basic knowledge, and is immersed in technology in a way that has led to a completely new style of learning. In response, Nelson Education has gathered a group of dedicated instructors to advise us on the creation of richer and more flexible ancillaries that respond to the needs of today's teaching environments.

In consultation with the editorial advisory board, Nelson Education has completely rethought the structure, approaches, and formats of our key textbook ancillaries. We've also increased our investment in editorial support for our ancillary authors. The result is the Nelson Education Teaching Advantage, which includes a *NETA Assessment* component designed to improve Nelson's testing materials. Under *NETA Assessment*, Nelson's authors create multiple-choice questions that reflect research-based best practices for constructing effective questions and testing not just recall but also higher-order thinking. Our guidelines were developed by David DiBattista, a 3M National Teaching Fellow whose recent research as a professor of psychology at Brock University has focused on multiple-choice testing. All Test Bank authors receive training at workshops conducted by Prof. DiBattista, as do the copyeditors assigned to each Test Bank. A copy of *Multiple Choice Tests: Getting Beyond Remembering*, Prof. DiBattista's guide to writing effective tests, is included with every Nelson Test Bank/Computerized Test Bank package. (Information about the NETA Test Bank prepared for *Nursing Leadership and Management* is included in the description of the *Instructor's Resource CD* below.)

INSTRUCTOR'S RESOURCE CD

Key instructor ancillaries are provided on the *Instructor's Resource CD* (ISBN 0176646167), giving instructors the ultimate tool for customizing lectures and presentations. (Downloadable web versions are also available at www.nursingleadershipmanagement2.com) The IRCD includes the following materials:

- **NETA Assessment**. The Test Bank was written by Sandra Gessler, University of Manitoba. It includes over 450 multiple-choice questions written according to NETA guidelines for effective construction and development of higher-order questions. Test Bank files are provided in Word format for easy editing and in PDF format for convenient printing whatever your system.

  The Computerized Test Bank by ExamView® includes all the questions from the Test Bank. The easy-to-use ExamView software is compatible with Microsoft® Windows and MacOS. Create tests by selecting questions from the question bank, modifying these questions as desired, and adding new questions you write yourself. You can administer quizzes online and export tests to WebCT, Blackboard, and other formats.
- **Instructor's Manual.** The Instructor's Manual to accompany *Nursing Leadership and Management* has been prepared by Beth Perry of Athabasca University. This manual contains answers to review questions and activities found throughout the textbook.
- **Microsoft PowerPoint.®** Key concepts from *Nursing Leadership & Management* are presented in PowerPoint format, with generous use of figures, photographs, and short tables from the text. The PowerPoint presentation was created by Jennie Miron, Humber College.

ACKNOWLEDGMENTS

Many people must work together to produce any book. A comprehensive book such as this requires even greater effort and the coordination of many people with various areas of expertise. I would like to thank all the contributors for their time and effort and for sharing their knowledge gained through years of experience in both the clinical and academic setting. I thank them all for being responsive, making the necessary revisions, and sounding happy to hear from me whenever I emailed or called them. I also thank the reviewers for their time spent critically reviewing the manuscript and providing the valuable comments that have added to this text. These reviewers include Stephanie Buckingham (Vancouver Island University), Andrea Deakin (Mohawk-McMaster Institute for Applied Health), Judith Finlay (John Abbott College), Heather Kilty (Brock University), and Judith Wells (Sir Wilfred Grenfell College).

I would like to acknowledge and sincerely thank the team at Nelson Education Ltd. that has worked to make this second Canadian edition a reality: Jackie Wood, Executive Editor; Leah Blain, Developmental Editor; Jennifer Hare, Content Production Manager; Vicki Gould, Director, Asset Management Services; Sandra Mark, Permission Editor; and Carolyn Jongeward, Copyeditor.

A special huge thank you goes to my husband and best friend, Maurice, supporting me through each stage of the project. I could not have completed this project without his help—cleaning the house, preparing meals, and encouraging me all the way!

—*Heather Crawford*

ABOUT THE AUTHOR

Heather Crawford earned a bachelor of science degree in nursing from the University of Toronto School of Nursing; a master's degree in education from Brock University in St. Catharines, Ontario; and a Certified Health Executive (CHE) designation from the Canadian College of Health Leaders. She completed the compulsory coursework related to doctoral studies in nursing at McMaster University; however, she withdrew from the program when she moved to the West! Heather has held progressively responsible positions as a health care administrator in both community hospitals and academic tertiary/quaternary acute care institutions. She was director of surgical, obstetrical, and gynecological nursing at the Wellesley Hospital in Toronto; vice president of St. Joseph's Hospital in Brantford, Ontario; nursing director of critical care, cardiac sciences, and internal medicine at the Royal Alexandra Hospital in Edmonton, Alberta; vice president and chief nursing officer of the Health Sciences Centre in Winnipeg, Manitoba; and Executive Director, Rural and Community Hospitals (provincial position) for Alberta Health Services, Alberta. In addition, she has held the position of director of practice and policy at the College of Nurses of Ontario.

Heather has taught at The Mack Centre, School of Nursing, Niagara College; George Brown College of Applied Arts and Technology; Mohawk College, Hamilton, Ontario; Ryerson University, Toronto; University of Alberta; and the Sheridan College Institute of Technology and Advanced Learning. Heather has taught fundamentals of nursing, adult medical-surgical nursing, obstetrical nursing, nursing leadership and management, nursing issues and trends, and legal aspects of nursing. She has taught nursing conferences on quality improvement and scope of practice in Alberta, Manitoba, and Nova Scotia. Heather reviews articles for Healthcare Management Forum, and is an item writer for the Canadian College of Health Leaders certified health executive examination. Heather is a member of the College of Nurses of Ontario, the Registered Nurses Association of Ontario, the Canadian Nurses Association, and the Canadian College of Health Leaders. She is registered with the College of Nurses of Ontario.

Heather has served on the board of directors of Mount Carmel Clinic, Winnipeg, Manitoba, and Cancer Care Manitoba. She also was a member of the board of directors at St. Joseph's Hospital and the St. Joseph's Hospital Foundation in Brantford, Ontario.

Over the course of her career, Heather has been registered as an RN in three provinces: Ontario, Alberta, and Manitoba. Heather can be reached at hcmq@bell.net.

HOW TO USE THIS BOOK

Quote A nursing or health care theorist quote presents a professional's perspective regarding the topic at hand; read this quote as you begin each new chapter and see whether your opinion matches or differs, or whether you are in need of further information.

Chapter Objectives These goals indicate the performance-based, measurable objectives that are targeted for mastery upon completion of the chapter.

Opening Scenario This mini case study with related critical thinking questions should be read prior to delving into the chapter; it sets the tone for the material to come and helps you identify your knowledge base and perspective.

Case Study These short cases with related questions present a beginning clinical nursing management situation calling for judgment, decision making, or analysis in solving an open-ended problem. Familiarize yourself with the types of situations and settings you will later encounter in practice, and challenge yourself to devise solutions that will result in the best outcomes for all parties, within the boundaries of legal and ethical nursing practice.

Literature Application Study these key findings from nursing and health care research, theory, and literature, and ask yourself how they will influence your practice. Do you see ways in which your nursing could be affected by these literature findings and research results? Do you agree with the conclusions drawn by the author?

Critical Thinking Ethical, legal, delegation, and performance improvement considerations are highlighted in these boxes. Before beginning a new chapter, page through and read the Critical Thinking sections and jot down your comments or reactions; then see whether your perspective changes after you complete the chapter.

Real World Interviews Real world interviews with well-known nursing leaders such as Dr. Ginette L. Rodger, Dr. Lynn Nagle, Dr. Tim Porter O'Grady are included as well as interviews with nurses, doctors, hospital administrators, staff, clients, and family members. As you read these, ask yourself whether you had ever considered that individual's point of view on the given topic. How would knowing another person's perspective affect the care you deliver?

Key Concepts This bulleted list serves as a review and study tool for you as you complete each chapter.

Key Terms Study this list prior to reading the chapter, then again as you complete a chapter, to test your true understanding of the terms and concepts covered. Make a study list of terms you need to focus on to thoroughly appreciate the material of the chapter.

Review Questions These questions will challenge your comprehension of objectives and concepts presented in the chapter and will demonstrate your mastery of the chapter content, build critical thinking skills, and achieve integration of the concepts.

Review Activities These thought-provoking activities at the close of a chapter invite you to approach a problem or scenario critically and apply the knowledge you have gained.

Exploring the Web Internet activities encourage you to use your computer and reasoning skills to search the Web for additional information on quality and nursing leadership and management.

References Evidence-based research, theory, and general literature, as well as nursing, medical, and health care sources, are included in these lists; refer to them as you read the chapter and verify your research.

Suggested Readings These entries invite you to pursue additional topics, articles, and information in related resources.

Photos, Tables, and Figures These items illustrate key concepts.

CHAPTER 1

Canada's Health Care Environment

Patricia Kelly, RN, MSN
Adapted by Heather Crawford, BScN, MEd, CHE

Our health care system defines us as communities, as a society, and as a nation. What Canadians are prepared to do, and more importantly, what we are not prepared to do for each other when we are sick, vulnerable, and most in need, says a great deal about Canada, our basic values, and the values that we want to hand on to future generations of Canadians. (Margaret Somerville, Founding Director, McGill Centre for Medicine, Ethics, and Law)*

OBJECTIVES

The purpose of this chapter is to enable the reader to

■ identify how health care is organized and funded in Canada;

■ review the movement toward population health and disease management;

■ discuss health care variation and evidence-based practice;

■ review the Canadian Adverse Events Study and the Institute of Medicine's Committee on Health Care Reports; and

■ identify recent changes and current forces and trends influencing the development of caring, interprofessional practice and health care delivery in Canada.

*Margaret Somerville, AM, FRSC, DCL Founding Director, McGill Centre for Medicine, Ethics and Law McGill University, Montreal, Quebec.

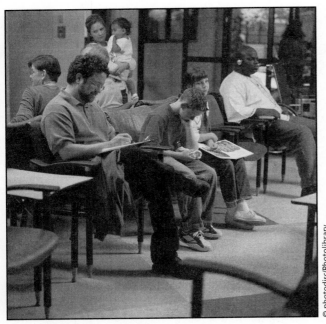

© photodisc/Photolibrary

We've been here almost four hours already!

You have just moved back to the province, and have seen a couple of old friends. They tell you they had to take their four-year-old son to the Emergency Department three days ago because he had a cut on his forehead. Although their son is all right now, they are worried about the length of time they waited in the Emergency Department before being treated, their lack of a family physician, and the attitude of the health professionals they met. This scene occurs over and over again in today's health care environment as Canadians struggle to find a way to ensure access to cost-effective, quality care for themselves and their families.

What are your thoughts about this situation?

What advice do you have for the family?

How can you contribute to improving access to health care for your friends and for the community?

To manage and lead effectively, every health care professional must have a working knowledge and understanding of Canada's health care system. Although many nurses comment on the system, few know its history.

Health care delivery in Canada is a combination of public and private initiatives organized to provide citizens with access to cost-effective, quality health care. Canadians are living longer and are generally in better health than previous generations. However, challenges in the health sector remain, including the reform of our health care system. Recent surveys indicate that most Canadians believe that they are in very good to excellent health. Life expectancy and health-adjusted life expectancy have increased, the infant death rate has dropped, many infectious diseases have been practically eliminated, and

medical techniques have continued to evolve (Statistics Canada, 2010, p. 209).

Although Canadians are healthier today than they were in the past, problems persist. Heart disease, cancer, mental health problems, HIV/AIDS, asthma, obesity, and diabetes continue to affect many Canadians. New infectious disease strains, such as H1N1 influenza, pose ongoing threats to public health. National newspapers and other publications regularly report on health problems in Aboriginal communities. First Nations adults, depending on their age group, are two to eight times more likely to have diabetes than the general Canadian population (Statistics Canada, 2010, p. 1). The incidence of diabetes is also increasing among First Nations children and adolescents. The Aboriginal Diabetes Initiative (ADI) Phase 1 was established in 1999, and subsequent phases were added. The ADI Phase 3 (2010–12) focuses on the following concerns: initiatives for children, youth, parents, and families; diabetes in pre-pregnancy and pregnancy; community-led food security plans to improve access to healthy foods, including traditional foods; and enhanced education for home and community care nurses on clinical practice guidelines and chronic disease management strategies. These initiatives have delivered a range of primary prevention, screening, and treatment programs in partnership with Tribal Councils, First Nations organizations, Inuit community groups, and provincial and territorial governments.[1]

The role of present-day, quality health care nursing began to develop in Canada following the efforts of Florence Nightingale in London, England. Although familiar practices today, her emphasis on cleanliness, fresh air, regular client observation, and monitoring of mortality rates was radical in the management of client care at that time. Nightingale illustrated mortality rates with a coxcomb diagram (see Figure 1-1).

Nightingale used these coxcomb diagrams to dramatize the number of preventable deaths in the Crimean War campaign. The light blue wedges on the coxcomb, measured from the centre of the circle, represent deaths from preventable diseases. Although Nightingale managed clients and their environment closely, she also emphasized health promotion and disease prevention. She paid close attention to physicians and government policymakers, recognizing their influence on her freedom to practise (Simms, Price, & Ervin, 2000). Nightingale's ideas spread from England to Canada in the 1870s. The Nightingale model of nursing reflected the social environment of the era. Today, nurses can improve the quality of client care by understanding and dealing with many of these same issues affecting today's health care system and the nursing profession. However, today's nurses practice within an information model in a global context.

This chapter describes how Canadian health care is organized, funded, and accredited. The topics of

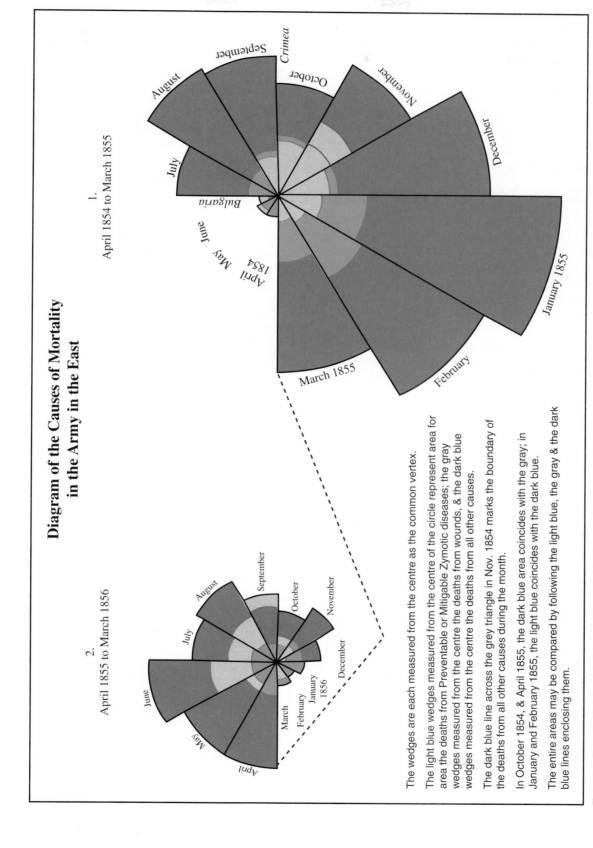

Diagram of the Causes of Mortality in the Army in the East

The wedges are each measured from the centre as the common vertex.

The light blue wedges measured from the centre of the circle represent area for area the deaths from Preventable or Mitigable Zymotic diseases; the gray wedges measured from the centre the deaths from wounds, & the dark blue wedges measured from the centre the deaths from all other causes.

The dark blue line across the grey triangle in Nov. 1854 marks the boundary of the deaths from all other causes during the month.

In October 1854, & April 1855, the dark blue area coincides with the gray; in January and February 1855, the light blue coincides with the dark blue.

The entire areas may be compared by following the light blue, the gray & the dark blue lines enclosing them.

Figure 1-1 Florence Nightingale's Coxcomb Diagram of the Causes of Mortality in the Army in the East
Source: Houghton Library, Harvard University. EC85.N5647,858n.

population health and disease management are introduced, and clinical variation and malpractice are explored. The chapter includes a review of the Canadian Adverse Events Study and two Institute of Medicine Committee on Health Care reports from the United States, which address the important issue of client safety. Finally, recent changes and current trends and forces affecting health care and the development of caring, interprofessional nursing practice are discussed.

ORGANIZATION OF HEALTH CARE

The Canadian health care system has evolved over the past five decades, and is based on a combination of political, social, and economic influences. The goal of the health care system is to provide Canadians with reasonable access to medically necessary insured services, without the need to pay. The Canadian provinces are constitutionally responsible for the administration and delivery of health services (Constitution Act, 1867). In other words, the provinces decide how much money to spend on health services, where to deliver these services, where to locate hospitals, and how many doctors are needed. Under the Canadian Constitution, the federal government has responsibility for health care in Yukon, Nunavut, and the Northwest Territories. It is also responsible for the health care of Aboriginal people who live on reserve, members of the armed forces and veterans, the Royal Canadian Mounted Police (RCMP), and inmates of federal institutions. Yukon, Nunavut, and the Northwest Territories assume responsibility for health care, even though they do not have the status of a province and, therefore, do not have formal constitutional powers over health care. This system, which gives all Canadians access to health care, has undergone many changes since universal health care was implemented in 1968 (Statistics Canada, 2006, p. 160).

In 1947 Saskatchewan was the first province to introduce public, universal *hospital* insurance. By 1957 the Government of Canada introduced legislation to share in the cost of these services. By 1961 all provinces and two territories had public insurance that provided access to hospital services. In 1962 Saskatchewan again led the way by providing insurance for *physician* services, in addition to the hospital services previously provided. The federal government again shared the cost of physician services in 1968. By 1972 all provinces and territories had extended their insurance plans to include both physician and hospital services.

Under the Federal-Provincial Fiscal Arrangements and Established Programs Financing (EPF) Act of 1977, block funding replaced cost sharing. This funding mechanism was a combination of cash payments and tax points, and provincial and territorial governments had the flexibility to invest in health care according to their needs and priorities. The EPF transfer from the federal government included funding for medical and hospital services and also for postsecondary education.

The federal legislation known as the Canada Health Act was passed in 1984. The Canada Health Act was based on five principles:

1. *Universality.* All residents of Canada must be entitled to public health insurance coverage.
2. *Comprehensiveness.* All medically necessary services provided by hospitals and doctors must be covered.
3. *Accessibility.* Reasonable access to medically necessary hospital and physician services must be unimpeded by financial or other barriers.
4. *Portability.* People must remain covered while temporarily absent from their province.
5. *Public administration.* Health plans must be administered by a nonprofit, public authority.

Two provisions in the Canada Health Act covered cost sharing. The first provision stipulated that there could not be extra billing for medical services by doctors who work under the particular terms of the health insurance plan of a province or territory. The second provision stated that no user charges would be required for insured health services by hospitals or other providers under a provincial or territorial health care plan.[2]

In 1995 new legislation revised the federal cash and tax transfers that supported health care and postsecondary education. These transfers became combined with transfers that supported social services and social assistance. As a result, a single block-funding mechanism was formed: the Canada Health and Social Transfer (CHST). Although passed in 1995, the legislation did not come into force until the beginning of fiscal year 1996–97. Since then, some provinces receive equalization payments from the federal government, and these provinces can provide reasonably comparable levels of service at reasonably comparable levels of taxation. In addition, Canada's three territories receive federal financial support, through the Territorial Formula Financing program, to assist them in providing public services.[3]

In 2003 the first ministers—that is, the prime minister of Canada and the provincial and territorial premiers—agreed on the Accord on Health Care Renewal. This agreement provided for changes to support access, quality, and long-term sustainability of the health care system. The reforms targeted the following needs: primary health care renewal, coverage for both short-term acute home care and the cost of prescribed drugs that reach high or catastrophic levels, enhanced access to diagnostic and medical equipment, and better accountability from governments. Under the Accord, the federal government increased cash transfers in support of health care and, effective April 2004, the CHST cash and tax transfers were split into the Canada Health Transfer for health, and the Canada Social Transfer for postsecondary education, social services, and social assistance.[4]

In 2004 further reforms were announced by the first ministers in "A 10-Year Plan to Strengthen Health Care." This plan focused on improving access to quality care and reducing wait times. Other key reforms included the following: health human resources; Aboriginal health; home care; primary health care; prescription drug coverage and elements of a national pharmaceutical strategy; health care services in the North; medical equipment; prevention, promotion, and public health; and enhanced reporting on progress made on these reforms. To support this plan, the federal government budget restructured the Canada Social Transfer (CST) to provide equal per capita cash support to provinces and territories effective 2007–08. Similar changes will be made to the Canada Health Transfer (CHT) effective 2014–15, when the current legislation is renewed. The CST was extended to 2013–14, and has grown 3 percent annually as a result of an automatic escalator, effective 2009–10. The CHT cash levels have grown annually by 6 percent as a result of the automatic escalator, and will continue until 2013–14. In addition, the 2007 federal budget provided $300 million for the immunization of girls and women against cancer of the cervix and $612 million to accelerate the implementation of wait time guarantees.[5]

TYPES OF HEALTH CARE SERVICES

Health care can be categorized according to four levels (Table 1-1): health promotion; disease and injury prevention (protection); diagnosis and treatment of existing health problems (i.e., primary, secondary, and tertiary care); and rehabilitation.

HEALTH CARE PROFESSIONALS IN CANADA

Health care professionals in Canada include a wide range of regulated and unregulated care providers. Regulated providers include, but are not limited to, physicians, nurses, physiotherapists, occupational therapists, and dentists. Family members, friends, community volunteers, and non-regulated workers make up the second category. Following is a description of the regulated health care workforce in Canada according to statistics for 2009, published by the Canadian Institute for Health Information (CIHI) in 2010(b).

The largest group of regulated health care professionals was nurses. The total regulated nursing workforce comprised 348,499 nurses. This included 266,253 registered nurses (RNs) (76.4 percent); 77,018 licensed practical nurses (LPNs) (22.1 percent); and 5,227 registered psychiatric nurses (RPNs) (1.5 percent).

Of the RN workforce, 8.3 percent graduated from an international RN program; this represented the highest proportion of international graduates among the Canadian nursing professions. Of the internationally educated RN graduates, 31.6 percent were educated in the Philippines and 17.6 percent were educated in the United Kingdom.

The number of licensed nurse practitioners (NPs) in the workforce was 1,990—which is more than double the number in 2005. Since 2007 all territories and provinces, except Yukon, had licensed NP programs (CIHI, 2010, p. xii). Most registered nurses and licensed practical nurses worked in hospitals, and, increasingly, they worked in community health. From 2005 to 2009 the number of regulated nurses increased by 8.5 percent.[6]

The average age of regulated nurses in 2009 was 45.2 years, which represents a slight increase—less than one year—over the average age in 2005. The largest group was nurses aged 40 to 59. This age group accounted for 57.1 percent of the RN workforce, 54.1 percent of the LPN workforce, and 62.1 percent of the RPN workforce (CIHI, 2010(c), p. xi).

Physicians were the second largest group of regulated health care professionals. More than 68,101 physicians worked in clinical and non-clinical practices. An increase of 4.1 percent between 2008 and 2009, this represents the largest annual growth rate in the supply of Canada's physicians since the late 1980s. Canadian faculties of medicine awarded a record number of medical degrees in 2009 (2,344): an increase of 33.5 percent over 2004, and 47.1 percent over 1999 (CIHI, 2010(d), p. 2).

The average age of physicians in 2009 was 49.7. The average age of a family medicine physician was 49.1, and that of a specialist was 50.3. Between 2008 and 2009, the average age of physicians decreased by 0.1 years. This decrease, related to an increase in graduates and younger physicians, suggests that physicians' average age might be stabilizing (CIHI, 2010(d), p. 3).

Byers (1997) identified certain subcultures of health professionals, including nursing, medicine, and health care administration. The general characteristics of three of these subcultures are outlined in Table 1-2. These dynamic characteristics constantly change the culture of the health care organization and the way these groups of health professionals work together to provide quality health care. Ultimately, the health profession subcultures affect the delivery of client care in different settings.

TABLE 1-1   TYPES OF HEALTH CARE SERVICES

Type of Care	Description	Examples
Health Promotion	*Goal:* To improve or maintain health status *Explanation:* General health promotion and protection against specific illnesses or disability	Lifestyle modification for health (e.g., smoking cessation, nutrition counselling) Promotion of a safe environment (e.g., sanitation, protection from toxic agents) Population health
Disease and Injury Prevention	*Goal:* To protect from the spread of disease, to alleviate disease, and to prevent further disability through early intervention *Explanation:* Early detection and intervention	Screening and immunization
Diagnosis and Treatment of Existing Health Problems	*Goal:* To maintain or improve a client's level of health functioning *Explanation:* Includes primary, secondary, and tertiary care (i.e., first, second, and third levels of encounter with the health system)	*Primary care:* the first contact entry to the health care system (e.g., a physician or a nurse practitioner who provides health promotion, illness prevention) *Secondary care:* a specialized medical service or hospital to which a client is referred by the primary care physician (e.g., for detection and early intervention) *Tertiary care:* A specialized, highly technical care related to diagnosing and treating complicated or unusual health problems (e.g., regional or provincial hospitals equipped with high-tech equipment and services)
Rehabilitation	*Goal:* To minimize effects and to prevent permanent disability from a chronic or irreversible condition *Explanation:* Restorative and rehabilitative activities to obtain a client's optimal level of functioning	Education and retraining Provision of direct care Environmental modifications (e.g., advising on necessity of wheelchair accessibility for a person who has experienced a cardiovascular accident [i.e., a stroke]) Continuing care

HEALTH CARE SPENDING

Canada spent approximately $191.6 billion on health care in 2010. This is an average of $5,614 per person. Of the provinces, Québec had the lowest spending per person ($5,096), and Alberta had the highest ($6,266). In the territories, Yukon had the lowest spending per person ($7,977), and Nunavut had the highest ($12,356).[7]

Of the total health care expenditure in Canada, provincial and territorial governments contributed 65.3 percent, the federal government contributed 3.5 percent, municipal governments provided 0.5 percent, and social security funds provided 1.3 percent. The rest of the funding, approximately 30 percent of total health care spending ($56.6 billion), came from the private sector, which generally funded services such as dental care, vision care, chiropractic care, and medication.[8] Private health care services are paid for either directly by the client or through private insurance plans or employee benefit plans.

Of the total health care expenditures, hospital spending accounted for 28.9 percent, retail drug sales accounted for 16.3 percent, and physician services, 13.7 percent.[9] The proportion of Canada's gross domestic product (GDP) dedicated to health care spending was approximately 11.7 percent. According to the most recent international data, from 2008, Canada was one among six

TABLE 1-2	GENERALIZED CHARACTERISTICS OF THREE SUBCULTURES OF HEALTH PROFESSIONALS		
Characteristics	**Nursing**	**Medicine**	**Health Care Administration**
Major task	Client care; client safety	Diagnosis and treatment of disease; client safety	Organizational continuity; quality of care; quality of worklife; client safety; managing change and stability
Membership	Historically female, white, middle-class; humanistic	Historically male, white, middle- and upper-class; scientific	Historically male-dominant;* rational
Leading role strength	Comforter; nurturer; health educator	Lifesaver and problem-solver; miracle worker	Keeper of the house; protector
Role centrality	Coordinator of health services	Gatekeeper of health services	Proprietor of health services; holder of the purse strings
Relationships with other professional groups	Collaborative ethic	Autonomy; directing the team	Negotiating; seeks cooperation
Model of authority within profession	Hierarchy	Collegiality; equality	Hierarchy
Perspective	Client-centred; clinical unit/area	Client- and practice-centred	Hospital's business and government relations
Conflict management	Interpersonal approach	Use leverage available (e.g., resources and authority) to maintain control	Structural and rational approach
Core dilemmas in era of health care reform	Degree of proactivity within context of high uncertainty; traditional vs. new role initiatives	Choice of organizational and network affiliations, and the conditions and extent of affiliation; the future destiny of medical specialists	Options for investing strategic resources during an era of high future uncertainty
Major threats (current)	Decrease in job security; constraints on staffing levels and other resources; (undesirable) changes in role; nursing shortage	Health economics; changes in role; losses in authority and income; malpractice	Organizational survival; job security (restructuring; regionalization; rationalization)

*The management of Catholic hospitals, typically run by orders of Catholic sisters, is a notable exception to the generalizations about health care administrators.

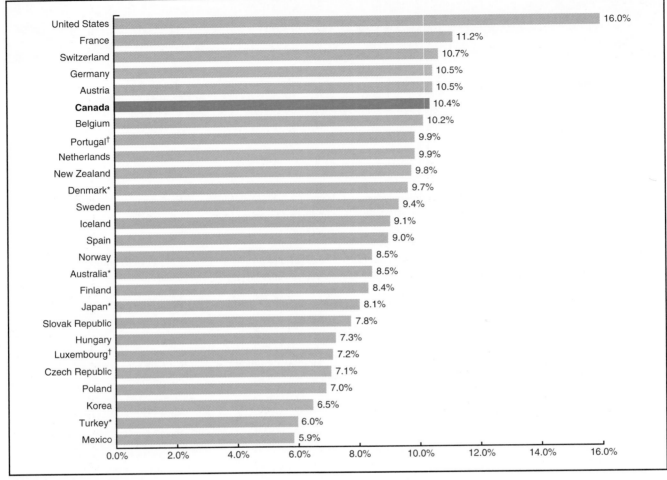

Figure 1-2 Total Health Expenditure as a Percentage of GDP, 26 Selected Countries, 2008
Notes:
* Data for 2007.
† Data for 2006.
Source: Organization for Economic Co-operation and Development, *OECD Health Data* 2010 (June Edition) (Paris, France: OECD, 2010). Reprinted with Permission.

countries that have the highest ratio of total health expenditure to GDP (see Figure 1-2). In 2008 the United States had the highest ratio of total health expenditure to GDP at 16 percent, while Canada was at 10.4 percent.[10]

APPROACHES TO HEALTH CARE IN CANADA

Population health, integrated health care delivery, and disease management are the key approaches to health care in Canada.

POPULATION HEALTH

Population health is a broad approach that examines health not only of individuals but also of distinctive population groups. It examines factors that affect health overall and trends in the health of different groups within society. Population health focuses on the social determinants of health with the aim to reduce the inequities among different population groups, particularly those that are most vulnerable. The determinants of health include a range of factors that explain why a person is or is not healthy. Such factors include income, social status, education, employment and working conditions, healthy child development, and nutrition (Raphael, 2008). The ultimate goal of this approach is to improve the health of the entire population (see Figure 1-3 and Figure 1-4).

In 1974 the Canadian minister of health, Marc Lalonde, published a seminal report on the determinants of health. In the decades since the Lalonde Report, Canadians have continued to focus on population health, as demonstrated by such reports as *Achieving Health for All: A Framework for Health Promotion*, in 1986, by then federal

This deceptively simple story speaks to the complex set of factors or conditions that determine the level of health of every Canadian.

Why is Jason in the hospital?

Because he has a bad infection in his leg.

But why does he have an infection?

Because he has a cut on his leg and it got infected.

But why does he have a cut on his leg?

Because he was playing in the junk yard next to his apartment building, and there was some sharp, jagged steel there that he fell on.

But why was he playing in a junk yard?

Because his neighbourhood is kind of run down. A lot of kids play there, and there is no one to supervise them.

But why does he live in that neighbourhood?

Because his parents can't afford a nicer place to live.

But why can't his parents afford a nicer place to live?

Because his Dad is unemployed, and his Mom is sick.

But why is his Dad unemployed?

Because he doesn't have much education, and he can't find a job.

But why ...?

— from Toward a Healthy Future: Second Report on the Health of Canadians

Figure 1-3 Determinants of Health: What Makes Canadians Healthy or Unhealthy?

Source: Toward a Healthy Future: Second Report on the Health of Canadians. Health Canada, 1999. Reproduced with the permission of the Minister of Health, 2011.

minister of health Jake Epp (known as the Epp Report); *Early Years Study* by the Ontario government in 1999; and the work conducted by the Canadian Institute for Advanced Research. The population health approach has been endorsed in the recommendations of all recent Canadian health care reports, including the following:

- *Canada Health Action: Building on the Legacy* (National Forum on Health, 1997)
- Québec's *Emerging Solutions,* known as the Clair Report (Commission d'étude sur les services de santé et les services sociaux, 2000)
- Saskatchewan's *Caring for Medicare: Sustaining a Quality System,* known as the Fyke Report (Commission on Medicare, 2001)
- Alberta's *Framework for Reform,* known as the Mazankowski Report (Premier's Advisory Council on Health, 2001)
- *Reforming Health Protection and Promotion in Canada,* known as the Kirby Report (Standing Committee on Social Affairs, Science and Technology, 2002)
- *Building on Values: The Future of Health Care in Canada* (Commission on the Future of Health Care in Canada, 2002).

In 1999 the Canadian Institute for Health Information launched the Canadian Population Health Initiative (CPHI) to expand the public's knowledge of population health. From 2007 to 2010, CPHI focused on four key areas: healthy weight, place and health, determinants

of mental health and resilience, and reducing gaps in health. This initiative increases the public understanding of population health in these areas by concentrating on the following four complementary functions:

1. building an improved understanding of the factors affecting population health (knowledge generation and synthesis)
2. improving the health of Canadians through new policy development (policy synthesis and analysis)
3. forming collaborative networks with groups and individuals to improve understanding of the determinants of health (knowledge exchange)
4. disseminating information on population health issues (knowledge transfer and reporting)[11]

The social determinants of health contribute significantly to whether individuals stay healthy or become ill. They also determine whether a person possesses the physical, social, and personal resources to identify and achieve personal aspirations, satisfy needs, and cope with the environment (Raphael, 2008). Table 1-3 summarizes some of the findings from evidence-based studies. Table 1-4 identifies some of the features of the new role of health care management in a population health system.

Populations do not become healthier as the result of large investments in clinical care after illness has begun. Populations become healthier when investments are made in preventing illness and keeping people healthy. To measure and assess the overall health of Canadians, a

Health Indicator Framework

Health Status

How healthy are Canadians?

Health status can be measured in a variety of ways.
Including well-being health conditions disability of death.

Well-being	Health conditions	Human function	Death

Non-Medical Determinants of Health

Non-medical determinants of health are known
to affect our health and, in some cases, when
and how we use health care.

Health behaviours	Living and working conditions	Personal resources	Environmental factors

Health System Performance

How healthy is the health system?
These indicators measure various aspects
of the quality of health care.

Acceptability	Accessibility	Appropriateness	Competence
Continuity	Effectiveness	Efficiency	Safety

Community and Health System Characteristics

These measures provide useful contextual
information, but are not direct measures of
health status or the quality of health care.

Community	Health system	Resources

Equity

Figure 1-4 Health Indicator Framework

Source: CIHI. (2010). *Health Indicators*. Retrieved from <www.cihi.ca/CIHI-ext-portal/pdf/internet/DEFINITIONS_052010_EN>, Feb.28, 2011.

TABLE 1-3	EVIDENCE-BASED STUDIES: WHAT THEY SHOW

- Positive association between income, air pollution, and mortality (Finkelstein et al., 2003)
- Relationship between job strain and coronary heart disease (CHD), especially among blue-collar workers and men (Theorell, 2001)
- Study about International Innovations in Public Sector External Service Delivery to help inform the Canadian experience (Kernaghan, 2010)
- Barrier to medication reconciliation in ambulatory care due to limited health literacy (Persell et al., 2007)
- Relationship between limited literacy and occupational injuries, degree of awareness of dangers in the workplace, and installation of home safety features (Health Canada, 2003)
- Relationship between homelessness and health: An Overview of Research in Canada (Frankish et al., 2009)

TABLE 1-4	FEATURES OF THE NEW ROLE OF HEALTH CARE MANAGEMENT IN A POPULATION HEALTH SYSTEM

- Emphasis is on the continuum of care.
- Emphasis is on maintaining and promoting wellness.
- Accountability is required for the health of defined populations.
- Differentiation is based on ability to add value.
- Success is achieved by increasing the number of individuals served and keeping people healthy.
- Goal is to provide care at the most appropriate level.
- Health delivery system is integrated.
- Managers operate service areas across organizational borders.
- Managers actively pursue quality and continuous improvement.

number of population health indicators must be taken into consideration. These indicators allow the key determinants of health to be measured and the health of Canada's populations to be compared with other populations around the world. According to the United Nations Human Development Index, Canada scores very high on measures of income per capita, literacy, and life expectancy. However, the United Nation's Human Poverty Index (HPI) shows a different picture. The HPI measures relative deprivation in terms of standard of living, education, and longevity. According to this measure, Canada is in 11th place behind the Scandinavian countries, Germany, France, Japan, and Spain. On this index, Canada is not doing as well as it should (Commission on the Future of Health Care in Canada, 2002, p. 10).

Life expectancy at birth is one of the most established and widely available summary measures of health status. In 2003 the life expectancy at birth in Canada was 79.9 years,

almost two years higher than the OECD average, and fifth among all OECD countries. Canada's infant mortality rate decreased from a rate of 27.3 deaths per 1,000 live births in 1960 to 5.3 deaths per 1,000 in 2003 (Commission on the Future of Health Care in Canada, 2002, p. 11). In 2005 Canadian life expectancy at birth was 80.4 years: 78.0 years for men and 82.7 years for women (Human Resources and Skills Development Canada, 2010).

Another key consideration in addressing the performance of any health care system is equity. Equity addresses questions such as whether some groups in our society have better access to health care or better health outcomes than others (Goddard & Smith, 2001). Significant disparities exist between people who live in Atlantic Canada and the rest of the country, and between those who live in the northern part of Canada versus the south. For example, one study demonstrated that inhabitants of the Nunavik region in Québec live an average of 15.8 years less than those who live in Richmond, British Columbia (Commission on the Future of Health Care in Canada, 2002, p. 16).

If our society really wants to increase the health of Canadians, perhaps it would be better to direct resources toward strengthening the following determinants of health:

- health care system influences (e.g., access to medical care and health care costs)
- individual influences (e.g., the impact of lifestyle and genetics)
- interpersonal, social, and work influences (e.g., job satisfaction and social supports)
- community influences (e.g., the availability of services and programs)
- environmental influences (e.g., air quality and water quality) (Donatelle & Davis, 1998).

A society that spends so much on medical care that it cannot or will not spend adequately on other health-enhancing activities may actually be reducing the health of its population (Evans & Stoddard, 1990).

PUBLIC HEALTH

The **public health system** is responsible for helping protect Canadians from injury and disease and for helping Canadians stay healthy. Experts in the field of public health suggest that there are three responsibilities of a public health system:

1. Health emergencies—to prevent, discover, and respond to outbreaks of infectious disease, such as SARS or H1N1 influenza; to work with national security agencies to respond to disasters, bioterrorism, and other threats to Canada's health security
2. Chronic disease and injury prevention—to help to prevent and manage chronic diseases, such as diabetes, cancer, and mental illness; to help prevent injuries
3. Health promotion—to promote good health; to contribute to government policies that affect our health, such as policies on poverty, housing, and the environment[12]

See Table 1-5 for a list of the many individuals involved in public health services.

The Public Health Agency of Canada (PHAC) was created in 2004 in response to concern about the capacity of Canada's public health system to anticipate and respond effectively to public health threats. Its mandate was to focus on emergency preparedness and response, infectious and chronic disease prevention and control, and injury prevention, supported by a collaborative, national network.[13]

The National Collaborating Centre for Healthy Public Policy provides national focal points for key priority areas in public health, building on established regional expertise. The centre will speed up the development and implementation of new research findings and best practices in public health practice. See Table 1-6 for the six centres that have been identified.

In addition to the six National Collaborating Centres for Public Health, the Pan-Canadian Public Health Network was established in 2005 by the federal, provincial and territorial health ministers. The mandate of the

TABLE 1-5	WHO DELIVERS PUBLIC HEALTH SERVICES?

The public health system, like the health care system, involves doctors, nurses and a wide range of health professionals. But it involves many more people too, including:

Provincial and territorial chief medical officers of health
Local chief public health officers
Community leaders
Teachers and school principals
Families
Employers
Aboriginal communities
Multicultural communities
Social organizations
Sports and recreation clubs

Source: Who delivers public health services? Public Health Agency of Canada. Reproduced with the permission of the Minister of Health, 2011.

TABLE 1-6	SIX NATIONAL COLLABORATING CENTRES FOR PUBLIC HEALTH

1. National Collaborating Centre for Aboriginal Health (British Columbia)
2. National Collaborating Centre for Determinants of Health (Nova Scotia)
3. National Collaborating Centre for Environmental Health (British Columbia)
4. The National Collaborating Centre for Healthy Public Policy (Québec)
5. The National Collaborating Centre for Infectious Diseases (Manitoba)
6. The National Collaborating Centre for Methods and Tools (Ontario)

Source: Reproduced with the permission of the National Collaborating Centre Program (NCCP).

Network includes a range of activities: facilitating the sharing of information among all jurisdictions in Canada, working with and providing policy and technical advice to the deputy ministers of health on public health matters, and supporting the public health challenges that jurisdictions may face during emergencies or crises. The development of the Canadian Pandemic Influenza Plan for the Health Sector, a Pan-Canadian Pandemic Vaccine Strategy, and recommendations concerning the use of antivirals for prophylaxis are a few examples of the Public Health Network's achievements to date.[14]

The Canadian Public Health Association (CPHA) is a national, independent, not-for-profit, voluntary association that represents public health in Canada and provides linkages to the international public health community. The mission of CPHA is to advocate for the improvement and maintenance of personal and community health according to the public health principles of disease prevention, health promotion and protection, and healthy public policy.[15] See Table 1-7 to learn the goals of the CPHA.

PRIMARY HEALTH CARE

Primary health care refers to basic, everyday health care: visiting a family doctor or nurse practitioner, talking to a dietician or pharmacist, or calling a toll-free health advice line to talk to a health professional. It is usually the client's first encounter with a health care provider. Primary health care is concerned with preventing people from becoming ill or being injured, managing chronic conditions, and using health provider expertise most effectively. In addition, primary health care relates to improving both the quality of health care and access to health care services. Primary health care has five guiding principles:

1. equitable access to health and health services
2. public participation
3. appropriate technology

4. intersectoral collaboration
5. reorientation of the health system to promote health and prevent disease and injury

For example, in Ontario, the Sault Ste. Marie Group Health Centre's congestive heart failure program reduced hospital re-admissions by 44 percent in two years. Primary health care is not a new concept. A number of well-established primary health care centres across Canada have been in operation for many years—for example, the North East Community Health Centre in Edmonton, Alberta.

Countries around the world agreed to the importance of primary health care in 1978, when the World Health Organization (WHO) held an international conference on primary health care. This conference concluded with the Alma Ata Declaration, the first international declaration underlining the importance of primary health care. This approach was accepted by member countries of the WHO as the key to achieving the goal of "Health for All by the Year 2000." Since Alma Ata, four international conferences have been held in different countries: Adelaide, Australia (1988); Sundsvall, Sweden (1991); Jakarta, Indonesia (1997); and Mexico City, Mexico (1999). The theme of the most recent conference was on bridging the equity gap and strengthening the "art and science" of health promotion and the political skills and actions needed for health promotion to ensure healthy public policy. Although none of the 13 institutes of the Canadian Institute for Health Research (CIHR) has been dedicated to health promotion research per se, one is called the Institute for Population and Public Health.

When the first ministers of Canada met in 2000, they agreed that improving primary health care was crucial to the renewal and long-term sustainability of the health care system. As a result, the federal government invested $800 million in the Primary Health Care Transition Fund to support the provinces and territories in their plans

TABLE 1-7   GOALS OF THE CPHA

CPHA achieves its mission through the following nine goals:

- Acting in partnership with a range of disciplines including health, environment, agriculture, transportation, other health-oriented groups and individuals in developing and expressing a public health viewpoint on personal and community health issues;
- Providing an effective liaison and partnership between CPHA's Provincial and Territorial Public Health Associations;
- Providing an effective liaison and network both nationally and internationally in collaboration with various disciplines, agencies, and organizations;
- Encouraging and facilitating measures for disease prevention, health promotion and protection, and healthy public policy;
- Initiating, encouraging, and participating in research directed at the fields of disease prevention, health promotion, and healthy public policy;
- Designing, developing, and implementing public health policies, programs, and activities;
- Facilitating the development of public health goals for Canada;
- Identifying public health issues and advocating for policy change;
- Identifying literacy as a major factor in achieving equitable access to health services.

Source: Canadian Public Health Association. *About CPHA: Goals*. Retrieved from http://www.cpha.ca//en/about.aspx, March 5, 2011. Copyright CPHA. All rights reserved.

to improve and expand primary health care delivery in Canada. Following the release of the Romanow Report in 2002, the first ministers continued their focus on primary health care. The 2003 Health Care Renewal Accord identified primary health care as a priority and placed particular focus on increasing access and building primary health care teams. In 2004 the First Minister's Meeting on the Future of Health Care announced a 10-year plan to strengthen health care by focusing on the following issues: a reduction in wait times, improved access, strategic health human resource action plans, home care, primary care reform, access to care in the North, a national pharmaceuticals strategy, disease prevention, health promotion and public health, health innovation, accountability and reporting to citizens, and dispute avoidance and resolution (Health Canada, 2004).

INTEGRATED HEALTH CARE DELIVERY SYSTEMS

An **integrated delivery system** is a network of health care organizations that provides or arranges to provide a coordinated continuum of services to a defined population. This network is willing to be held clinically and fiscally accountable for the outcomes and the health status of the population served (Shortell, 1996).

A coordinated continuum of health care services includes prevention, wellness, and health promotion services. It also includes acute, restorative, and maintenance care to serve the needs of a population of clients in a specific geographic area. These services are delivered by a network of organized, community-oriented health and social service systems focused on broad aspects of health care and chronic disease management. This network can include hospitals and nursing homes, as well as schools, public health departments, and social and community health organizations that provide service and education programs to address smoking cessation, exercise, and other illness prevention and health promotion initiatives.

A type of integrated delivery system used in Canada is called **regionalization**. Nine provinces have some form of regionalization in place. There are four main features in Canadian regionalization:

1. The regions are predominantly defined by geography; that is, they occupy specific areas within the province and receive their mandate and authority from the provincial government.
2. The authority, which had previously been held by individual organizations or agencies, is consolidated at the regional level into one authority.

3. The regions are now responsible for a full range of health services, from community health to mental health to long-term care to acute care to health promotion (Lewis & Kouri, 2004).
4. The provincial governments transferred their health care responsibility to the regional health authorities.

Regionalization is different in Ontario. There is a regional cancer care network, regions are in place for such clinical services as obstetrics, and planning bodies are geographically defined (i.e., Local Health Integration Networks).

Regionalization was recommended by the provincial task forces and commissions of the 1980s, which were charged with creating a new direction for health care. Because fragmentation was a concern, the solution was thought to be the consolidation of organizations and boards, and their integration into a more responsive and participatory system. The Health Services Restructuring Commission, chaired by Duncan Sinclair, was established in

1996 for a period of four years. Its mandate was to find solutions to such issues as rising costs, resistance to change, and lack of accountability (Sinclair, Rochon, & Leatt, 2005). The expected results were fewer "turf" battles, increased collaboration, and rationalization of services. The outcomes would include cost savings, increased efficiency, equity, increased consumer participation, increased accountability, and an emphasis on health promotion and prevention (Lewis & Kouri, 2004). See Table 1-8 for a summary of the potential impact of regionalization on attaining health system goals.

Regionalization in Canada's health care delivery has seen little stability. Most regions have restructured at least once since they were originally formed. See Table 1-9 for the changes in regionalization, by province, from the time of implementation to 2010.

In September of 2004 the Ontario minister of health announced the government's three-year health transformation agenda, which included the formation of Local Health Integration Networks (LHINs). The intent of these LHINs was to ensure that health care in Ontario

TABLE 1-8	POTENTIAL IMPACT OF REGIONALIZATION ON HEALTH SYSTEM GOAL ATTAINMENT

1a GOAL: Aligning Needs and Resources; Potential Impact of Regionalization: High

Factors Increasing Potential Impact	Factors Decreasing Potential Impact	Current Canadian Circumstances
Province genuinely committed to needs-based resource allocation and population health mandate	Province only rhetorically committed to needs-based and population health approach and more traditional in practice	Restrictions on reallocation vary from some to significant
RHA supports and prioritizes population health mandate	RHA uncommitted to mandate	Provinces struggling with population health mandate and accountability
RHA has authority to reallocate resources	Provincial funding rules rigid	RHAs struggling with population health mandate and accountability
Good needs-assessment protocols	Constrained RHA autonomy to reallocate resources	Needs assessments generally done but of varying quality
Good performance measurement and reporting mechanisms	Province focuses on utilization targets, not impact or distribution	Information systems still developing
Disadvantaged populations have effective voice and influence	Provincial government allows interest groups to end-run regions and have directions and decisions reversed	Performance measurement and reporting in early stages
Elites support a needs-based allocation of resources	RHAs responsive to interest groups and agenda derailed	Some provincial governments more prone to end-runs and intervention in RHA affairs than others
Evidence-based policy and practice	Provider resistance	
Adequate information base re: interventions as well as needs	Poor needs-assessment protocols	
	Poor performance measurement and reporting mechanisms	

(*Continued*)

TABLE 1-8	POTENTIAL IMPACT OF REGIONALIZATION ON HEALTH SYSTEM GOAL ATTAINMENT (CONTINUED)

1b GOAL: Integration of Services; Potential Impact of Regionalization: High

Factors Increasing Potential Impact	Factors Decreasing Potential Impact	Current Canadian Circumstances
Wide scope of services falling within RHA mandate	Important services (MDs, drugs) outside purview of RHAs	Generally wide range of services under RHA authority
Consolidation of authority over various programs and sectors	Vestigial program autonomy (affiliation agreements, competitive and narrowly focused program boards)	MDs and drugs not included in RHA mandates
Provincial funding formulae aligned with goal	Provincial funding formulae misaligned with goal	Regions have privately owned facilities and affiliation agreements
RHA autonomy to reallocate resources	Constrained RHA autonomy to reallocate resources	Provincial funding often comes with conditions such as utilization targets
Organizational charts that promote integrated planning and management	Organizational charts that promote "silo" thinking	Issues with provider contracts and morale
	Historical program territoriality	
	Resistance of providers	

1c GOAL: Service Quality and Evidence-Based Practice; Potential Impact of Regionalization: Low

Factors Increasing Potential Impact	Factors Decreasing Potential Impact	Current Canadian Circumstances
Rewarded by provincial funding and payment mechanisms	Perverse incentives in provincial funding and payment mechanisms	Payment mechanisms generally indifferent to evidence-based performance
Provincial health quality (HQ) and evidence-based practice (EBP) activities/resources	Absence of provincial HQ and EBP leadership	Three provinces (Sask, ON and AB) have established a quality council; others, e.g., Manitoba, planning to do so
An academic community committed to EBP	Lack of emphasis in academic programs	Several provinces have centres that promote EBP but impact limited
Good information and performance measurement systems	Lack of interest in HQ and EBP among opinion leaders and providers	Academic programs vary in commitment to EBP
Provider culture well-disposed to HQ and EBP	Poorly developed information and performance measurement systems	Provider culture ambivalent toward HQ and EBP
RHA authority to allocate resources	Provincially set utilization targets as a condition of funding	Some RHAs have invested considerably in EBP, and QI initiatives
RHA control over number and distribution of MDs	Excess capacity in some sectors	Information systems in early stages
	Excess funding that papers over substandard practice	Fee-for-service generally rewards volume over efficiency
	Public opposition to changes in access, service configuration	Generally restricted ability to reallocate resources at RHA level
	Provider opposition	RHAs have limited authority to create or close programs and facilities
		RHAs generally have little control over number and distribution of MDs, though increasing in some provinces

(Continued)

TABLE 1-8	POTENTIAL IMPACT OF REGIONALIZATION ON HEALTH SYSTEM GOAL ATTAINMENT (CONTINUED)

1d GOAL: Health Promotion and Prevention; Potential Impact of Regionalization: Moderate

Factors Increasing Potential Impact	Factors Decreasing Potential Impact	Current Canadian Circumstances
Provincial and RHA commitment to these activities	Public preoccupation with acute and medical care	Public health on radar screen because of SARS, West Nile, flu epidemics
Explicit and high-profile mandate to pursue these activities	Weak provincial commitment	Some RHAs very active in community development
Strong RHA leadership and buy-in from significant provider constituencies	Weak RHA commitment	Many RHAs have pursued intersectoral partnerships and programs
Accountability for performance in these areas	Lack of provider interest	
Mechanisms to ensure voices of the dispossessed are heard	Impatience with long-term time frame for achievement of goals	
	Lack of public and media interest	

1e GOAL: Improved Accountability; Potential Impact of Regionalization: Moderate

Factors Increasing Potential Impact	Factors Decreasing Potential Impact	Current Canadian Circumstances
Substantial authority and autonomy truly devolved to RHA	RHA has little authority and autonomy	Devolution to RHAs incomplete and some power has been reconsolidated at the provincial level in recent years
Sufficient RHA authority over the programs under its jurisdiction (i.e., clear and widespread consolidation of authority)	Public regards only provincial government as accountable	Government assumes ownership of major decisions even if RHA initiates them
Non-partisan board structures and behaviour	RHA boards partisan in nature	Consolidation of authority from local to the regional level has been partial
Public confident in RHA and views it as legitimate decision-making body with a mandate to change	Provincial government responds to end-runs and overrules RHA decisions	Elections terminated in Sask, AB, Québec; exist in PEI since 1999 and initiated in NB in 2004
Provincial government resistance to end-runs	RHAs attempt to offload tough decisions on government	Performance reporting to public still in embryo
RHAs willing to make and take responsibility for tough decisions	Opposition makes RHA-level decisions a constant political issue	Health remains a high-profile political issue among public
Opposition recognizes the devolution and legislative debate is altered	Poor information and reporting mechanisms	Public holds provincial government accountable to greater extent than RHA
Media create sense of legitimacy of RHA as decision-maker		Legislative debate for the most part traditional, partisan
Good information used and available for prioritizing		Media focuses on government behaviour more than RHAs
Good reporting mechanisms in place		

(Continued)

TABLE 1-8 — POTENTIAL IMPACT OF REGIONALIZATION ON HEALTH SYSTEM GOAL ATTAINMENT (CONTINUED)

1f GOAL: Increased Public Participation; Potential Impact of Regionalization: Moderate

Factors Increasing Potential Impact	Factors Decreasing Potential Impact	Current Canadian Circumstances
Explicit and high-profile mandate to pursue these activities	Weak RHA commitment	Some RHAs very active in experimenting with public participation
Tradition of civic engagement in various sectors	Lack of public and media interest	Does not appear in most performance agreements and indicator sets
Public believes its participation will be valued and valuable	Not included in performance agreements and indicator sets	
Included in performance agreements and indicators as important measure		

Source: Lewis, S., Kouri, S. (2004) *Healthcare Papers* 5(1): 17–19. Reprinted with Permission.

would be more client-focused, results-driven, integrated, and sustainable (Sunnak, 2005). The LHINs are responsible for planning, integrating, and funding local health services, including hospitals, community care access centres, home care, long-term care, mental health, community health centres, and addiction and community support services. In Ontario, 16 district health councils were disbanded in March 2005 to make way for 14 LHINs. In June 2005 the province announced the appointment of 14 new chief executive officers, nine of whom were registered nurses, and 42 board members, including chairs and directors (Sunnak, 2005). April 1, 2008 was the completion of the first full year of LHIN authority in Ontario's health care system. At the time of writing this edition, the future of the LHIN's is questionable because of the upcoming October 2011 provincial election in Ontario.

Suter et al. (2009) identified ten key principles for successful health systems integration. (See Table 1-10.)

REAL WORLD INTERVIEW

The Champlain Local Health Integration Network is moving forward with its plans to develop a blueprint to streamline clinical services distribution in the eastern counties. The LHIN has announced the next steps in its clinical services distribution project for the eastern counties, which include working with partners to draft a blueprint of a better way to organize and distribute health services across the entire LHIN.

According to Lisa Sullivan, senior planner with the Champlain LHIN, the blueprint will identify the best locations and sizes of health services and the best way to manage and co-ordinate those services.

"The blueprint will include services needed by the francophone and First Nations populations in the area." she explained. "It will also identify optimal health service delivery models and areas where health savings may be found to address current gaps."

Sullivan said the blueprint will be based on statistics, research and evidence-based practice. She said it is hoped the blueprint will be completed by the spring of 2011.

Source: Lahaie, L. (2010). Champlain LHIN working on draft blueprint for clinical services in eastern Ontario. *The Review*. Retrieved from http://thereview.ca/story/champlain-lhin-working-draft-blueprint-clinical-services-eastern-counties, December 30, 2010.

TABLE 1-9	CHANGES IN REGIONALIZATION FROM TIME OF IMPLEMENTATION TO 2010, BY PROVINCE		
Province	**Established**	**Restructured**	**Selected Changes**
British Columbia	1997	2001	There are now five RHAs (covering 16 Health Service Delivery Areas) and one Provincial Health Service Authority. Board members are appointed. Before restructuring, there were 11 Regional Health Boards, 34 Community Health Councils and seven Community Health Services Societies.
Alberta	1994	2002, 2003 and 2008	As of May 2008, there is one organization: Alberta Health Services, with one "superboard." This replaced nine RHAs, created in April 2003, and with all members appointed. Before 2003 there were 17 RHAs. In 2002 Alberta moved from an all-appointed board member structure to one that was two-thirds elected and one-third appointed. It reverted to an entirely appointed structure in 2003.
Saskatchewan	1992	2002	There are 13 regional health authorities, and board members are appointed. Before 2002 there were 32 health districts whose boards were initially all appointed. From 1995 to 2002, two-thirds of board members were elected and one-third appointed.
Manitoba	1997–1998	2002	There are 11 RHAs with appointed board members. Before restructuring, there were 12 RHAs.
Québec	1989–1992	2001, 2003–04	There are 18 RHAs whose roles have been in transition since November 2003. Before 2001 board members were elected by a representative caucus of stakeholders, and CEOs were appointed by the RHA board. Since then board members and regional CEOs have been appointed by the province, and CEOs are accountable jointly to the deputy minister and the regional board. In 2003 Québec initiated a reorganization of its regional structures, which is currently in progress.
Nova Scotia	1996	2001	There are nine District Health Authorities, with appointed boards. Before restructuring, there were four RHAs.
New Brunswick	1992	2002 2004 2010	By 2010 the previous eight RHAs had been amalgamated into two new health authorities: Vitalité Health Network and Horizon Health Network. The eight previous RHAs had been hospital corporations and board members were appointed. Since 2004 boards consisted of eight elected and seven appointed members.
Prince Edward Island	1993–1994	2002 2010	By 2010 the entire province was administered by a single health service authority called Health PEI. Previously, there were four RHAs, with mixed elected and appointed members, and a Provincial Health Services Authority that is responsible for secondary and tertiary acute care services. Before restructuring, there were five RHAs.
Newfoundland	1994	2010	By 2010 there were the Grenfell Regional Health Services Board, four Health and Community Services representing four regions, and the Health Labrador Corporation. Previously, there were six institutional health boards, four health and community services boards, two integrated boards, a nursing home board, and a cancer treatment and research board. Board members were appointed.

Source: Lewis, S., Kouri, S. (2004) Regionalization: Making Sense of the Canadian Experience. *Healthcare Papers* 5(1): 17–21. Reprinted with Permission.

TABLE 1-10   TEN KEY PRINCIPLES FOR INTEGRATION

1. Comprehensive services across the care continuum
   - Cooperation between health and social care organizations
   - Access to care continuum with multiple points of access
   - Emphasis on wellness, health promotion, and primary care

2. Patient focus
   - Patient-centred philosophy, focusing on patients' needs
   - Patient engagement and participation
   - Population-based needs assessment, with a focus on defined populations

3. Geographic coverage and rostering
   - Maximize patient accessibility and minimize duplication of services
   - Roster: responsibility for identified population; right of patient to choose and exit

4. Standardized care delivery through interprofessional teams
   - Interprofessional teams across the continuum of care
   - Provider-developed, evidence-based care guidelines and protocols to enforce one standard of care, regardless of where patients are treated

5. Performance management
   - Committed to quality of services, evaluation and continuous care improvement
   - Diagnosis, treatment and care interventions linked to clinical outcomes

6. Information systems
   - State of the art information systems to collect, track and report activities
   - Efficient information systems that enhance communication and information flow across the continuum of care

7. Organizational culture and leadership
   - Organizational support with demonstration of commitment
   - Leaders with vision who are able to instill a strong, cohesive culture

8. Physician integration
   - Physicians are the gateway to integrated healthcare delivery systems
   - Pivotal in the creation and maintenance of the single-point-of-entry or universal electronic patient record
   - Engage physicians in leading role, participation on Board to promote buy-in

9. Governance structure
   - Strong, focused, diverse governance represented by a comprehensive membership from all stakeholder groups
   - Organizational structure that promotes coordination across settings and levels of care

10. Financial management
    - Aligning service funding to ensure equitable funding distribution for different services or levels of services
    - Funding mechanisms must promote interprofessional teamwork and health promotion
    - Sufficient funding to ensure adequate resources for sustainable change

Source: Suter, E., Oelke, N.D., Adair, C.E., & Armitage, G.D. (2009). Ten Key Principles for Successful Health Systems Integration. *Healthcare Quarterly*, Volume 13 Special Issue. Reprinted with Permission.

HORIZONTAL AND VERTICAL INTEGRATION

Health care networks can be horizontally or vertically integrated. **Horizontal integration** occurs when a health care system contains several organizations of one type, such as hospitals. Health care networks can also be vertically integrated. **Vertical integration** occurs when different stages of health care are linked and delivered by one agency.

DISEASE MANAGEMENT

Disease management is a cost-effective approach both to improve service quality and integration and to promote consumer empowerment and quality of life. A number of disease management programs and research studies are conducted across Canada.

The Chronic Disease Self-Management Program (CDSMP) was developed at the Stanford Patient Education Research Center under the direction of Kate Lorig, RN; Virginia Gonzalez, MPH; and Diana Laurent, MPH. The CDSMP is based on the assumption that people living with chronic conditions have similar problems and concerns, and they have to deal with their disease and the impact it has on their lives and their psychological health. People who have no health care background in chronic conditions, but have been instructed about those conditions, can teach the chronic disease self-management program more effectively than health professionals.

How the content is taught is more important than what subject matter is taught. A five-year research project evaluated the CDSMP using a randomized study that included more than 1,000 subjects. The research showed that the people who took part in the program improved their healthful behaviours and their health status and decreased their stays in hospital.[16]

In Canada, the Chronic Disease Self-Management Program was implemented by the University of Victoria's Centre on Aging as a pilot program in Yukon in 1998 and, subsequently, became a permanent government-funded program. In 2000 the Centre on Aging implemented the program in the Vancouver and Richmond health regions, where it became a permanent program. In 2001 Health Canada provided a grant to the Centre on Aging to implement a 28-month project, the Diabetes Self-Management Program. From 2003 to 2006, the Centre on Aging received a grant from the British Columbia Ministry of Health to implement the program in British Columbia. In March 2006 the Centre on Aging received funds to implement the program at the same level for the next three years.[17]

Other disease management programs in Canada include, but are not limited to, the Cardiovascular Program in Nova Scotia; the Northern Diabetes Health Network in Ontario; arthritis, falls, fractures, and osteoporosis programs in various locations; and the Western GTA (Greater Toronto Area) Stroke Network.

The Western GTA Stroke Network includes a consortium of hospitals and Community Care Access Centres that work with the Heart and Stroke Foundation of Ontario, the Ministry of Health and Long-Term Care, and LHINs to implement a coordinated approach to stroke care throughout the western GTA. As a result of the collaboration, it is anticipated that stroke outcomes will improve and quality of life will be enhanced through awareness, education, and prevention measures.

The Kahnawake Schools Diabetes Prevention Program, in a First Nations community near Montréal, has reduced incidence rates of diabetes to almost the Canadian average (Health Council of Canada [HCC], 2007).

The Island Lake Regional Renal Health Program in northern Manitoba has been a catalyst for change in the prevention of diabetes and other chronic health conditions. This innovative program brought care to the community avoided disruption caused by long periods away from home, and allowed the community to focus its efforts on managing the disease and keeping healthy (HCC, 2007).

ACCREDITATION

Accreditation Canada (AC) is the current national organization that assists health service organizations across Canada to examine and improve the quality of care and service they provide to clients. Accreditation Canada introduced a new accreditation program in 2009 called Qmentum. This program emphasizes health system performance, client safety, risk prevention planning, performance measurement, and governance. A number of system-wide factors were assessed during accreditation, including governance, leadership and management, infection prevention and control, and medication management. At the same time, population-specific and service excellence standards address specific sectors, services, conditions, and populations, such as mental health, maternal and child health, populations with chronic conditions, and public health services. In Qmentum, there are 35 Required Organizational Practices (ROPs) that have been identified in six patient safety areas. These include safety culture, communication, medication use, worklife and workforce, infection control, and risk assessment. A new ROP on preventing workplace violence came into effect in January 2010.

Effective 2011, the organizations being assessed had to comply with the ROP and its eight tests for compliance. Three instruments—questionnaires—are currently used to collect information on critical aspects of health services: the Governance Functioning Tool completed by board members, and the Patient Safety Culture Tool and the Worklife Pulse Tool completed by staff members. Certain indicators are used to specify what data is collected related to various aspects of client care and services. These are available for Patient Safety and Hospice Palliative Care.[18]

The accreditation program is based on national standards that are developed and updated by experts in the field through peer review and knowledge exchange.

Following the accreditation process, initial findings from the assessment questionnaires are presented to the organization verbally. Within a few months, the organization receives a formal written evaluation report. The focus of the report is the organization's strengths and the areas requiring improvement. Recommendations are also made to assist the organization in developing plans for improvement or to maintain its strengths. See Table 1-11 for a list of the standards included in the AC accreditation program.

In 2011 AC introduced new Independent Medical/Surgical Facilities Standards to meet the needs of non-hospital-based surgical facilities across Canada. Emergency Department Standards were released in 2008, and Emergency Medical Services (EMS) Standards were released in 2009. Primary Care Services Standards were used by organizations for the first time in 2011. Three new sets of standards related to organ and tissue donation and transplant have also been released.[19]

Accreditation Canada International is the international department that promotes accreditation worldwide. The accreditation program is customized to meet the need

---

TABLE 1-11	ACCREDITATION CANADA QMENTUM STANDARDS

Accreditation Canada's Qmentum Standards include standards for system-wide, population-based, and service excellence areas.

System-wide
- Effective Organization
- Effective Organization for Assisted Reproductive Technology
- Effective Organization for Primary Care
- Infection Prevention and Control
- Managing Medications
- Sustainable Governance

Population-based
- Cancer Populations
- Child and Youth Populations
- Maternal/Child Populations
- Mental Health Populations
- Populations with Chronic Conditions
- Public Health Services

Service Excellence
- Acquired Brain Injury Services
- Ambulatory Care Services
- Assisted Reproductive Technology Standards for Clinical Services
- Assisted Reproductive Technology Standards for Laboratory Services
- Assisted Reproductive Technology Standards for Working with Third Party Donors
- Biomedical Laboratory Services
- Blood Banks and Transfusion Services
- Cancer Care and Oncology Services
- Case Management Services
- Child Welfare Services
- Community Health Services
- Critical Care Services
- Developmental Disabilities Services
- Diagnostic Imaging Services
- Emergency Department Services
- Emergency Medical Services
- Health Care Staffing Services

(Continued)

TABLE 1-11	ACCREDITATION CANADA QMENTUM STANDARDS (CONTINUED)

- Home Care Services
- Home Support Services
- Hospice Palliative and End-Of-Life Services
- Laboratory and Blood Services
- Long Term Care Services
- Medicine Services
- Mental Health Services
- Obstetrics/Perinatal Care Services
- Operating Rooms
- Organ and Tissue Donation Standards for Deceased Donors
- Organ and Tissue Transplant
- Organ Donation Standards for Living Donors
- Point-of-Care Testing
- Primary Care Services
- Providing an Integrated System of Services to People with Stroke
- Rehabilitation Services
- Reprocessing and Sterilization of Reusable Medical Devices
- Substance Abuse and Problem Gambling Services
- Surgical Care Services
- Telehealth Services

Distinction
- Acute Stroke Services
- Distinction Standards Audit Tool for Reprocessing and Sterilization of Reusable Medical Devices
- Inpatient Stroke Rehabilitation Services
- Providing an Integrated System of Services to People with Stroke

Source: Accreditation Canada. (2011). *Access to Standards*. Retrieved June 14, 2011 from <http://www.accreditation.ca/Shop-for-Standards>. © Accreditation Canada.

of the client. Accreditation Canada has been fully accredited three times since it served as a pilot for the International Society for Quality in Health Care (ISQua) in 1995.[20]

HEALTH CARE VARIATION AND EVIDENCE-BASED PRACTICE

Research on variation in medical care practice first began to be reported in the 1970s (Wennberg & Gittelsohn, 1973). Depending on what part of the country you lived in, client outcomes and costs varied significantly for the same health care condition. Studies on unnecessary surgery (Leape, 1987) and the occurrence of preventable complications in clients (Adams, Fraser, & Abrams, 1973)

led to more research into variations in physician practice patterns. Nursing and physician clinicians, as well as clients, began to consider which health care practices led to good health care outcomes. Previously, few studies had addressed the effect of various interventions on client outcomes. In 1992 the Institute for Clinical Evaluative Sciences started to guide decision making and suggest future research in Ontario by providing unbiased, evidence-based knowledge and recommendations related to care delivery, drug therapy, treatment modalities, health technology, and patterns of service utilization.[21]

VARIATION IN CLIENT OUTCOMES

Many variables affect client outcomes, including the severity of the client's illness. As mentioned earlier, health care outcome findings must be adjusted to allow for these variables. The process of statistically altering client data to reflect significant client variables is called **risk adjustment**.

Among the difficulties of using data on client outcomes is the variable condition of different clients in a group, even for clients admitted with the same diagnosis. For example, the particular conditions of two diabetic clients can be very different. One can be a new diabetic client with few complications. The other can be a seriously ill diabetic client with many complications. When all clients are grouped and compared, these variations between clients make it very difficult to identify the impact of a health care treatment on a single client's outcomes. Add to this situation the difficulties in gathering data based on valid and reliable client-record reviews by trained reviewers. Then the difficulties in using risk adjustment on data become clear (Wolper, 1999). If, after reviewing client records, all client record reviewers do not extract identical data, the data compilation figures from the record reviewers will be quite different. This will significantly affect the accuracy of measuring client outcomes.

CANADIAN HEALTH SERVICES RESEARCH FOUNDATION

The Canadian Health Services Research Foundation (CHSRF) is an independent, not-for-profit corporation established with funds from the federal government and its agencies. It promotes and funds management and policy research in health services and nursing. Its aim is to increase the quality, relevance, and usefulness of this research for health system policymakers and managers. The CHSRF also collaborates with these health system decision-makers to support and enhance their use of research evidence when addressing health management and policy challenges. CHSRF projects always involve researchers, managers, and policymakers from academia and Canada's health system.

In 2009 CHSRF adopted a new five-year strategic plan and introduced three key strategic priorities: engaging and supporting citizens, accelerating evidence-informed change, and promoting policy dialogue.[22]

In 2003 the CHSRF received $25 million, a 13-year grant for the Executive Training for Research Application (EXTRA) program, to develop the capacity of health service executives and their organizations to use research.[23] EXTRA is an intensive training program designed to assist health leaders to become better decision-makers by teaching them how to find, assess, and interpret research-based evidence.[24]

In 2009 EXTRA accepted 28 new fellows from across Canada into the program, and delivered and evaluated six education modules. This program included the following new projects:

- Reducing hospital use through early management of high-risk clients (Interior Health Authority, B.C.)
- Improving Aboriginal patient outcomes through pre- and post-hospital communication (Winnipeg Regional Health Authority)
- Improving patient outcomes through computer order entry by physicians (St. Joseph's Healthcare, Hamilton)
- Redesigning of outpatient services (Princess Margaret Hospital)
- Generating an innovative integrated health care delivery model (McGill University Health Centre)
- Realigning primary and secondary health services in a rural setting (Central Regional Health Authority, Newfoundland and Labrador)[25]

CHSRF identified three priority topics in 2009, including health care financing and transformation, Canada's aging population, and primary health care.[26]

ACCREDITATION CANADA'S PATIENT SAFETY GOALS

Accreditation Canada has always focused on client safety, and has developed nine Patient Safety Goals within the patient safety areas of culture, communication, medication use, worklife/workforce, infection control, falls prevention, and risk assessment. In 2008 six patient safety performance measures were introduced into the Qmentum accreditation program in the areas of patient safety culture survey, medication reconciliation admission, health care associated infection, and surgical site infection. Half of the adverse events in Canadian hospitals occur during or after surgery, as noted in the Canadian Adverse Events Study (2004). The Safe Surgery Saves Lives (SSSL) initiative was established by the World Alliance for Patient Safety as part of the World Health Organization's efforts to reduce the number of surgical deaths around the world. One of the initiatives was the establishment of a set of safety checks that could be carried out in any operating room in any country. These safety checks are combined in a surgical safety checklist for use at three critical points during surgery: before the patient receives any form of anaesthetic, before the incision is made, and at the end of the operation. Accreditation Canada participated in the working group led by the Canadian Patient Safety Institute (CPSI) that adapted the Checklist for the Canadian context.[27] Components of the Checklist are present in AC's standards. A full listing of Accreditation Canada's Patient Safety Goals and all Required Organizational Practices can be found on the AC website at www.accreditationcanada.ca. The Canadian College of Health Leaders (formerly Canadian College of Health Service Executives) has also written a position statement on the health executive's role in client safety. Examples of national efforts related to client safety can be found in Table 1-12.

LITERATURE APPLICATION

Citation: Priest, A. (2006). What's ailing our nurses? A discussion of the major issues affecting nursing human resources in Canada. Ottawa: Canadian Health Services Research Foundation.

Discussion: In 2005 the Canadian Health Services Research Foundation commissioned a review of six major research documents on Canadian nursing human resource issues. The following research documents were included in the review:

1. Nursing Sector Study Corporation. (2005). *Building the future: An integrated strategy for nursing human resources in Canada.* Ottawa: Nursing Sector Study Corporation.

2. Canadian Medical Association/Canadian Nursing Association. (2005). *Toward a Pan-Canadian framing network for health human resources.* Ottawa: Canadian Medical Association/Canadian Nursing Association.

3. El-Jardali, F., & Fooks, C. (2005). *An environmental scan of current views on health human resources in Canada: Identified problems, proposed solutions, and gap Analysis.* Toronto: Health Council of Canada.

4. Maslove, L. (2005). *Key and current health policy issues in Canada.* Ottawa: Canadian Policy Research Networks.

5. Maslove, L., & Fooks, C. (2004). *Our health, our future: Creating quality workplaces for Canadian nurses: A progress report on implementing the final report of the Canadian Nursing Advisory Committee.* Ottawa: Canadian Policy Research Network.

6. Baumann, A., O'Brien-Pallas, L., Armstrong-Stassen, M., Blythe, J., Bourbonnais, R., Cameron, S., Irvine Doran, D., Kerr, M., McGillis Hall, L., Vézina, M., Butt, M., & Ryan, L. (2001). *Commitment and care: The benefits of a healthy workplace for nurses, their patients and the system.*

The key messages included the following: the nursing shortage demands immediate action; clients' and nurses' welfares are closely aligned; the main focus needs to be the retention of existing nurses rather than boosting the number of education seats available; an improved work environment is key to retaining and attracting new nurses; of the many ways to address the crisis, practical policy and practice solutions have been identified, but few have been implemented; and overcoming barriers requires cooperation between professional associations and different levels of government with a dedicated political will.[28]

Implications for Practice: Nurses need to be cognizant of current research initiatives and evidence in order to be part of the solution.

Source: Priest, A. (2006). *What's ailing our nurses? A discussion of the major issues affecting nursing human resources in Canada.* Ottawa: Canadian Health Services Research Foundation. Reprinted with Permission.

INSTITUTE OF MEDICINE COMMITTEE ON HEALTH CARE QUALITY REPORTS

In 1999 the Institute of Medicine (IOM) released a report titled *To Err Is Human: Building a Safer Health System.* The report concluded that more people die annually from medication mistakes than from highway accidents, breast cancer, or AIDS (Kohn, Corrigan, & Donaldson, 1999). A second IOM committee report released in 2001, *Crossing the Quality Chasm: A New Health System for the 21st Century*, recommends that "all health care organizations, professional groups, and private and public purchasers should adopt as their own the explicit purpose of reducing the burden of illness, injury, and disability, and improving the health and functioning of the people of the United States" (Kohn, Corrigan, & Donaldson, 2001, p. 5). Health providers should pursue six major areas for improvement of health care (Maddox, 2001) (see Table 1-13).

The second IOM report identified four major areas to target for change in the health care environment: information technology, payment, clinical knowledge, and the professional workforce (Kohn, Corrigan, & Donaldson, 2001).

TABLE 1-12	NATIONAL EFFORTS RELATED TO CLIENT SAFETY

1. Policy statements related to client safety from the Canadian Nurses Association, the Canadian Healthcare Association and the Canadian College of Health Leaders

2. Saskatchewan client safety initiatives built upon the recommendations from the Fyke Report (2001)

3. Canada's first Health Quality Council (2002)

4. Saskatchewan has Quality Care Coordinators for each regional health authority.

5. Manitoba Health implemented a policy mandating reporting of critical incidents and other events in Manitoba health care organizations (2003).

6. Manitoba Institute for Patient Safety and Quality Care and a Provincial Patient Safety Council created in 2003.

7. Health Services Utilization and Outcomes Commission in Alberta assumed responsibility for assessing client safety in the province.

8. Calgary Health Region created the Quality Improvement Health Information portfolio to provide leadership, infrastructure, and support to clinical and non-clinical teams throughout the Region.

9. Alberta government supported the development of an electronic health record that will contribute to improved safety and quality of care.

10. Nova Scotia government established a formal provincial Health Care Safety Working Group to create a comprehensive plan to support districts with their safety initiatives.

11. Ontario government announced two client safety initiatives: the development of a province-wide Patient Safety Team and a Safe Medication Support Service (2002).

Source: Bonney, E., & Baker, G. R. (2004). Current strategies to improve patient safety in Canada: An overview of federal and provincial initiatives. *Healthcare Quarterly,* 7(2), 36–41. Reprinted with Permission.

TABLE 1-13	MAJOR AREAS TO BE PURSUED IN HEALTH CARE—THE SECOND IOM REPORT

Health care needs to be

■ Effective—providing services based on scientific knowledge to all who could benefit and refraining from providing services to those not likely to benefit (avoiding overuse and under use)

■ Client-centred—providing care that is respectful of and responsive to individual client preferences, needs, and values and ensuring that client values guide all clinical decisions

■ Timely—reducing waits and sometimes harmful delays for both those who receive and those who give care

■ Efficient—avoiding waste, in particular waste of equipment, supplies, ideas, and energy

■ Safe—avoiding injuries to clients from care intended to help them

■ Equitable—providing care that does not vary in quality because of personal characteristics, such as gender, ethnicity, geographic location, and socioeconomic data

CANADIAN ADVERSE EVENTS STUDY

International jurisdictions, such as the United States, the United Kingdom, and Australia, recognize that health care safety concerns are real and that their systems are prone to error. The 1999 U.S. Institute of Medicine report *To Err is Human* was an important stimulus for action, when it estimated that between 44,000 and 98,000 U.S. citizens die each year as a result of medical errors. This study and similar studies in Australia and the United Kingdom have provided the evidence base that is key to maintaining the momentum in addressing the issue of client safety. Canada recently completed its first national study on adverse events in acute care hospitals. The study found that in 2000, of approximately 2.5 million adult hospital admissions, nearly 7.5 percent (185,000) resulted in an adverse event. Of these, approximately 38 percent (70,000) were considered to be preventable. In total, the researchers estimated that, in 2000, between 9,000 and 24,000 clients experienced an adverse event that was preventable and later died. These results indicate that the incidence of health system error in Canada is comparable with other industrialized countries (Baker, Norton, Flintoft, Blais, Brown, Cox, J., et al., 2004).

As a result of the increased focus on client safety in Canada, the Canadian government budgeted $50 million from 2002 to 2007 for the creation of the Canadian Patient Safety Institute. CPSI currently focuses on four areas, including education, research, interventions and programs, and tools and resources. In addition, many health care organizations have initiated efforts to improve client safety (Baker et al., 2004). Safer Healthcare Now is a patient safety initiative aimed at reducing preventable adverse events and deaths in Canadian hospitals. It is patterned after the 100K lives campaign, which is led by the Institute for Healthcare Improvement in the United States. Safer Healthcare Now focuses on 10 targeted interventions that are known to reduce avoidable adverse events, such as deployment of rapid response teams, preventing surgical site infections, and medication reconciliation.

LITERATURE APPLICATION

Citation: Baker, G. R., Norton, P. G., Flintoft, V., Blais, R., Brown, A., Cox, J., Etchells, E., Ghali, W. A., Hébert, P., Majumdar, S. R., O'Beirne, M., Palacios-Derflingher, L., Reid, R. J., Sheps, S., & Tamblyn, R. The Canadian Adverse Events Study: The incidence of adverse events among hospital patients in Canada. *Canadian Medical Association Journal,* 170(11), 1678–1686.

Background: Research into adverse events (AEs) has highlighted the need to improve client safety. AEs are unintended injuries or complications that arise from health care management and result in death, disability, or a prolonged hospital stay. The incidence of AEs among clients in Canadian acute care hospitals was estimated by the authors.

Methods: One teaching hospital, one large community hospital, and two small community hospitals in each of five provinces (British Columbia, Alberta, Ontario, Québec, and Nova Scotia) were randomly selected. From each hospital, for the fiscal year 2000, a random sample of charts was reviewed for non-psychiatric, non-obstetric adult clients. Trained reviewers screened all eligible charts, and physicians reviewed the positively screened charts to identify AEs and determine their preventability.

Results: At least one screening criterion was identified in 1,527 (40.8 percent) of 3,745 charts. The physician reviewers identified AEs in 255 charts. After adjustment for the sampling strategy, the AE rate was 7.5 per 100 hospital admissions (95% confidence interval [CI] 5.7– 9.3). Among the clients with AEs, events judged to be preventable occurred in 36.9 percent (95% CI 32.0%–41.8%), and death occurred in 20.8 percent (95% CI 7.8%–33.8%). Physician reviewers estimated that 1,521 additional hospital days were associated with AEs. Although men and women experienced equal rates of AEs, clients who had AEs were significantly older than those who did not (mean age [and standard deviation] 64.9 [16.7] v. 62.0 [18.4] years; $p = 0.016$).

Interpretation: The overall incidence rate of AEs of 7.5 percent in this study suggests that, of the almost 2.5 million annual hospital admissions in Canada similar to the type studied, about 185,000 are associated with an AE, and close to 70,000 of these are potentially preventable.

An independent, national, non-profit agency, the Institute for Safe Medication Practices Canada (ISMP Canada), is committed to promoting medication safety in all health care settings.

QUALITY HEALTH CARE

It is useful to consider a basic framework for quality health care. Donabedian (1966) conceptualized such a framework (Bull, 1997). This framework is composed of the elements of structure, process, and outcome.

STRUCTURE, PROCESS, OUTCOME

Using Donabedian's framework, a health care organization that wishes to develop quality will organize or structure itself for quality. Quality client care does not just happen. It must be planned. Quality is the result of assessing client needs and delivering care to meet those needs. Donabedian's framework has three elements: structure, process, and outcome.

Structure elements of quality lay a foundation for quality in a health care system by identifying which structures must be in place to deliver quality. Structure elements consist of such things as a well-constructed hospital, quality client care standards, quality staffing policies, and environmental standards.

Process is the next element of the quality framework. **Process elements of quality** build on the structure elements and take quality a step further. Process elements identify which nursing and health care interventions must be in place to deliver quality. Process elements are such things as managing the health care process, utilizing clinical practice guidelines and standards for nursing and medical interventions, and administering medications.

Finally, an outcome element completes the quality framework. **Outcome elements of quality** are the end results of quality care. Outcome elements review the status of clients after health care has been delivered. Outcomes reflect the presence of structure and process elements of quality. Outcomes elements refer to whether the client is better as a result of health care. If a quality hospital (structure) and quality standards (process) are in place, clients should experience good health (outcome). See Table 1-14 for examples of quality performance measures based on structure, process, and outcome elements in three domains of activity: clinical care, financial management, and human resources management.

For quality to occur, the monitoring of all three elements of Donabedian's framework—structure, process, and outcome—should be in place. Today, many people who review quality focus initially on outcome evaluation. Quality outcomes are at least partially reflective of having quality structures and quality processes in place. For example, if a client is breathing better after health care interventions for an asthma attack, this quality outcome may be a reflection of quality structures (e.g., good equipment and medications) and quality processes (e.g., nursing and medical interventions). Of course, the client's overall initial health status and other factors also affect the outcome. When outcomes are not good, nurses and other health care leaders must examine the structure and process elements critically. Change in these elements may be needed to improve health care quality. See Chapter 16 for examples of other indicators of the quality of nursing care.

CRITICAL THINKING

Nurses who work in large health care settings can sometimes feel lost and may wonder how they and their system can deliver quality in the midst of rapid change. What can nurses do to ensure safe, high-quality care? Thinking about the following may be useful:

What can I do at my level to manage care and support and to contribute to the quality of health care in my organization and community? How can I work well with other people in my nursing unit, in the organization, and in the community? Where can I find "best evidence" clinical practice guidelines to apply to client care in my organization and community? How much do I control care or anything else at a beginning level? I want to be optimistic, yet realistic!

TABLE 1-14	EXAMPLES OF PERFORMANCE MEASURES BY CATEGORY

	Domain of Activity		
	Clinical Care	**Financial Management**	**Human Resources Management**
Structure	*Effectiveness* ■ Percentage of active physicians who have credentials ■ Accreditation Canada ■ Number of residencies and filled positions ■ Presence of council for quality improvement planning	*Effectiveness* ■ Qualifications of administrators in finance department ■ Use of pre-admission criteria ■ Presence of an integrated financial and clinical information system	*Effectiveness* ■ Ability to attract desired registered nurses and other health professionals ■ Size (or growth) of active physician staff ■ Salary and benefits compared to other organizations ■ Quality of in-house staff education
Process	*Effectiveness* ■ Rate of medication error ■ Rate of nosocomial infection ■ Rate of post-surgical wound infection ■ Rate of normal tissue removed *Productivity* ■ Ratio of total client days to total full-time equivalent (FTE) nurses ■ Ratio of total admissions to total FTE staff ■ Ratio of physician visits to total FTE physicians *Efficiency* ■ Average cost per client day ■ Total cost per client day	*Effectiveness* ■ Days in accounts receivable ■ Use of generic drugs and drug formulary ■ Market share ■ Size (or growth) of shared service arrangements *Productivity* ■ Ratio of collection to bad debt ■ Ratio of total admissions to FTE in finance department ■ Ratio of new capital to fundraising staff *Efficiency* ■ Cost per collection ■ Debt/equity ratio	*Effectiveness* ■ Grievances ■ Promotions ■ Organizational climate *Productivity* ■ Ratio of line staff to managers *Efficiency* ■ Cost of recruiting
Outcome	*Effectiveness* ■ Case-severity-adjusted mortality ■ Client satisfaction ■ Client functional health status	*Effectiveness* ■ Return on investments ■ Operating margins ■ Size (or growth) of government grants for teaching and research ■ Bond rating	*Effectiveness* ■ Turnover rate ■ Absenteeism ■ Staff satisfaction

THE 3M HEALTH CARE QUALITY TEAM AWARDS

In 1994 the Canadian College of Health Service Executives and 3M Health Care launched the 3M Health Care Quality Team Awards to recognize innovation in health services by linking the concepts of quality and teams. These awards are presented annually to recognize teams who are using quality frameworks to create measurable outcomes within their programs and services, in addition to demonstrating enhancements in client care. In 2010 the recipients of the 3M Health Care Quality Team Awards included IWK Health Centre for the "Twenty-four Hour Dial for Dining Program," Sunnybrook's Holland Orthopaedic and Arthritic Centre for "A Team-based Approach to Chronic Disease Management that Improves Patient Access and Care." You can read more about these programs online, at www.cchse.org/assets/awardsprogram/3M_Awards_2010_E.pdf.

OUTCOME MEASUREMENTS

Outcomes can be measured to indicate an individual's clinical state, such as the severity of an illness, the course of an illness, and the effect of interventions on the individual's clinical state. Outcome measures involving a client's functional status evaluate a client's ability to perform activities of daily living (ADLs). These measures assess physical health in terms of function, mental and social health, the cost of care, health care access, and general health perceptions. The measures distinguish the concepts of physical and mental health. They also identify five indicator categories of clinical status: functioning, physical symptoms, emotional status, client and family evaluation, and perceptions about quality of life. Selected quality-of-life measures include quality-adjusted life years (QALY), quality-adjusted life expectancy (QALE), and quality-adjusted healthy life years (QUALY) (Drummond, Stoddart, & Torrance, 1994).

A 2001 study by McGillis Hall et al. suggests that a higher proportion of registered nurses and registered practical nurses on inpatient medical surgical and obstetrical units in Ontario teaching hospitals is associated with better health and quality outcomes for clients at the time of hospital discharges, and with lower rates of medication errors and wound infections.[29]

RECENT CHANGES IN HEALTH CARE

Several recent changes have taken place in health care. A major current issue in Canada is how to balance the demands of rights under the Canadian Charter of Rights and Freedoms (in the first part of Constitution Act, 1982) and the realities of economic pressure and public demands. One of the most recent reports commissioned to examine these issues was *Building on Values: The Future of Health Care in Canada*. This report of the Commission on the Future of Health Care in Canada was prompted by increased public dissatisfaction, escalating health care costs, and evidence of systems failure (e.g., access and quality of care issues). The report contained 47 costed recommendations. See Table 1-15 for 11 critical focus areas from these recommendations. See Table 1-16 for a summary of the federal commissions related to health care.

PRIVACY LEGISLATION IN CANADA

Canada has two federal privacy laws: the Privacy Act and the Personal Information Protection and Electronic Documents Act. Through the Privacy Act, which took effect in 1983, individuals have the right to access and request correction of their personal information that is held by federal government organizations.

Individuals are protected by the Personal Information Protection and Electronic Documents Act (PIPEDA), which sets out ground rules for how private sector organizations collect, use, or disclose personal information. Individuals have the right to access and request correction of their personal information that organizations may have collected. This right not only applies to private sector organizations but also to personal information collected, used, or disclosed by the service industry.

Each province and territory has privacy legislation governing the collection, use, and disclosure of personal information held by government agencies. These acts provide individuals with a general right to access and correct their own personal information.[30]

CANADIAN COLLEGE OF HEALTH LEADERS

The Canadian College of Health Leaders (previously known as the Canadian College of Health Service Executives) is a national, non-profit, professional association dedicated to developing, promoting, advancing, and recognizing excellence in health leadership. Health care executives and managers in Canada face many challenges in today's health care environment, including the need for accountability, health human resource shortages, increasing consumer demands, and balancing budgets. To successfully manage these areas, health care executives need to master a variety of managerial and leadership capabilities. The Canadian College of Health Leaders has

TABLE 1-15	ELEVEN CRITICAL AREAS OF FOCUS

1. Sustaining service, needs and resources, new governance

2. Sustaining Medicare; expanding the Canada Health Act to include accountability

3. More comprehensive use of information management and technology

4. Investing in health care providers—role changes and supply, demand, and distribution of health personnel

5. Primary health care and prevention—focus on wellness and health promotion

6. Improving access and ensuring quality—reducing waiting times and improving access to local and global resources, multicultural services

7. Rural and remote communities—again, access to quality care services

8. Home care services—home care, community mental health and palliative care services under the jurisdiction of Canada Health Act to ensure funding

9. Prescription drugs—a national drug agency to monitor costs and safety

10. Aboriginal health—health disparities, consolidate funding

11. Globalization—international alliances

Source: *Commission on the Future of Health Care in Canada: The Romanow Commission*. Health Canada, 2001. Reproduced with the permission of the Minister of Health, 2011.

TABLE 1-16	FEDERAL COMMISSIONS ON HEALTH CARE

Commission on the Future of Health Care in Canada (Romanow Commission, 2001 to 2002)

Standing Senate Committee on Social Affairs, Science and Technology Study on the State of the Health Care System in Canada (Kirby Committee, 1999 to 2002)

National Forum on Health (1994 to 1997)

Health Services Review '79 (1979 to 1980)

A New Perspective on the Health of Canadians (Lalonde Report, 1973 to 1974)

Royal Commission on Health Services (Hall Commission, 1961 to 1964)

Source: *Federal Commission on Health Care*. Health Canada, 2009. Reproduced with the permission of the Minister of Health, 2011.

developed the **LEADS in a Caring Environment** capabilities framework, which defines the knowledge, skills, and attitudes a leader needs to exhibit in order to successfully contribute to an effective and efficient Canadian health system.[31] This framework is a foundational element for health leadership development in Canada. See Table 1-17 for the five general categories of these capabilities.

TABLE 1-17	CCHL LEADS IN A CARING ENVIRONMENT CAPABILITIES FRAMEWORK

LEADS in a Caring Environment

Lead self
- be self-aware
- manage oneself
- develop oneself
- demonstrate character

Engage others
- foster development of others
- contribute to the creation of healthy organizations
- communicate effectively
- build teams

Achieve results
- set direction
- strategically align decisions with vision, values, and evidence
- take action to implement decisions
- assess and evaluate

Develop coalitions
- purposefully build partnerships and networks to create results
- demonstrate a commitment to customers and service
- mobilize knowledge
- navigate socio-political environments

Transform Systems
- demonstrate systems- and critical thinking
- encourage and support innovation
- orient oneself strategically to the future
- champion and orchestrate change

These capabilities apply to all leaders, regardless of role or formal position. All leaders must be able to lead themselves, engage others, achieve results, develop coalitions, and conduct systems transformation in order to create the Canadian health system of the future.

Source: Adapted from: Canadian College of Health Leaders. "Leaders for Life" Brochure. Retrieved from http://www.cchl-ccls.ca/assets/LEADS/LEADS_Print_Brochure_EN.pdf. February 27, 2011; and "The LEADS in a Caring Environment Leadership Capability Framework: Building Leadership Capacity In Canada to Lead Systems Transformation in Health" *February 2010 Communique*. Retrieved from http://www.cchl-ccls.ca July 11, 2011.

CRITICAL THINKING

You work in a large health care organization. One of your clients is not following her health care regime. You wonder what thought processes this client is using to justify continuing an activity that presents risks to her health.

How can you best assist this client in your health care organization and community? What kinds of structures, processes, and outcomes will your organization want to develop to improve care to this client and to the population of clients that your organization serves? How can you work in the community to enhance this population's choices for diet, exercise, or lifestyle?

OTHER FORCES INFLUENCING TRENDS IN HEALTH CARE

Shortell and Kaluzny (2000) identify nine major forces that will continue to shape health care in the new millennium (see Table 1-18). These include capitation, payment of clinicians based on performance using clinical practice guidelines, new technology, the aging population, genetic engineering, increasing cultural diversity, new diseases, information management, and the globalization of the world economy. These changes, as well as the emergence of terrorism and bioterrorism, call for ongoing changes in the education of health care professionals.

Canadians' needs for health care quality and access continue to develop. Nurses who work in health care today continue the tradition of nursing caring and excellence that began with Florence Nightingale, who served clients in her time by meeting their needs. Today

TABLE 1-18	NINE FORCES INFLUENCING HEALTH CARE DELIVERY AND THEIR IMPLICATIONS FOR MANAGEMENT
External Force	**Management Implication**
1. Capitated payments, expenditure targets, or global budgets for providing care to defined populations	■ Need for increased efficiency and productivity ■ Redesign of client care delivery ■ Development of strategic alliances that add value ■ Increased growth of networks, systems, and physician groups
2. Increased accountability for performance	■ Information systems that link financial and clinical data across episodes of illness and "pathways of wellness" ■ Effective implementation of clinical practice guidelines ■ Ability to demonstrate continuous improvements of all functions and processes
3. Technological advances in the biological and clinical sciences	■ Expansion of the continuum of care ■ Need for new treatment sites to accommodate new treatment modalities ■ Increased capacity to manage care across organizational boundaries ■ Need to confront new ethical dilemmas
4. Aging of the population	■ Increased demand for primary care, wellness, and health promotion services among the 65- to 75-year-old age group ■ Increased demand for chronic care management among those older than age 75 ■ Challenge of managing ethical issues associated with prolongation of life
5. Increased ethnic or cultural diversity of the population	■ Greater difficulty in understanding and meeting client expectations ■ Challenge of managing an increasingly diverse health services workforce
6. Changes in the supply and education of health professionals	■ Need for creative approaches in meeting the population's need for disease prevention, health promotion, and chronic care management services ■ Need to compensate for shortages in some categories of health professionals (i.e., physical therapy, pharmacy, and some areas of nursing) ■ Need to develop effective teams of caregivers across multiple treatment sites

(Continued)

TABLE 1-18	NINE FORCES INFLUENCING HEALTH CARE DELIVERY AND THEIR IMPLICATIONS FOR MANAGEMENT (CONTINUED)
External Force	**Management Implication**
7. Social morbidity (e.g., AIDS, drugs, violence, "new surprises")	■ Ability to deal with unpredictable increases in demand ■ Need for increased social support systems and chronic care management ■ Need to work effectively with community agencies
8. Information technology	■ Training the health care workforce in new information technologies ■ Increased ability to coordinate care across sites ■ Challenge of managing an increased pace of change due to more rapid information transfer ■ Challenge of dealing with confidentiality issues associated with new information technologies
9. Globalization and expansion of the world economy	■ Need to manage cross-national and cross-cultural tertiary and quaternary client care referrals ■ Increasing the productivity of the Canadian labour force ■ Managing global strategic alliances, particularly in the areas of biotechnology and new technology development

nurses will prosper by continuing this commitment to a personal ethic of social responsibility, service, and caring. Caring is the core of nursing practice because it renders technical, curative procedures tolerable and safe; it also helps clients and families weather illnesses and sustain or regain familiar life worlds (Benner, 2000).

NURSING ROLE

Nursing has come a long way in the past 100 years. The following six characteristics are commonly used to assess whether a job is considered a profession: maintaining quality education of the practitioner,

LITERATURE APPLICATION

Citation: Soukup, S.M. (2000). Evidence-based Nursing Practice. *Nursing Clinics of North America*, 35(2), xvii–xviii. Copyright © Elsevier, Inc. 2000.

Discussion: Author discusses a nurse's response to queries as to whether she has integrated evidence-based practice. The nurse responds, "Yes, I practise state-of-the-art nursing. My education and professional practice experiences have prepared me to care for more than 700 chronically ill clients annually, in the past five years. These clients have an average reported expected pain rating of 6.9 (using a scale of 1 to 10, with 10 being severe pain), and my pain management interventions have kept these clients, during my hours of care, at a reported actual pain rating of 4. Also, as a team member, these clients have not had any known pressure ulcers, skin tears, or catheter-related infections. On two occasions—for clients who were dying—I created a humanizing environment for the clients and their families when these clients were rapidly transferred from the critical care unit. My documentation has met organizational standards during monthly peer reviews; I have provided leadership for emergencies with positive outcomes; and physician and client satisfaction rating for clinical practice on our unit is 9.5 on a scale of 10, with 10 being the highest. Our unit-based team has not had a needle-stick-related or back-related injury during the past two years."

improves (Baggs & Ryan, 1990). Medical associations in most provinces have clearly articulated guidelines for disruptive physician behaviour.

INTERPROFESSIONAL NURSING PRACTICE

Fooks (2005) suggests that one of the future challenges for nursing will be an interprofessional care environment. This challenge arose as a result of the reorganization and expansion of the ways primary health care is delivered to Canadians. Teamwork with many different professionals will be required for the client to have a seamless process within the integrated continuum of care. Education needs to change so that in future health professionals will recognize and understand each other's roles and collaborate effectively. The future demands inter- and intra-professional education. The health needs will require a professional nurse who can demonstrate caring and competency and can practice in an interprofessional fashion, planning for the changing health care delivery system.

Interprofessional practice brings nurses to the table with a more equal footing and diminishes the notion that the team needs a captain to function. When each discipline brings its unique talents to the job of providing care for a client and the client's family, interprofessional practice removes the gatekeeper and allows clients access to all caregivers based on the expertise needed. Success in interprofessional practice will depend on each profession maintaining the highest standards, including expectations of advanced education, a certification process, and requirements for continuing education to maintain competency (Carroll-Johnson, 2001).

Interprofessional practice models have shown promise for optimizing the use of staff expertise and skills and improving quality of care and worklife satisfaction

CRITICAL THINKING

Are hospitals in your area rated? What kinds of ratings are given to hospitals? Review the criteria and evaluation system used to rate the hospitals. Is it valid and reliable? Are the criteria important to quality and client satisfaction? Will you choose a hospital for your own family's care using a rating system like this?

following a code of ethics, receiving compensation commensurate with the work, being organized to promote a needed service, having autonomy in practice, and being recognized by the government with licensure (Pinkerton, 2001). Nursing is recognized as a profession in most circles today, though nurse–physician work relationships continue to evolve. In the late 1990s some nurses still reported "knowing the right thing to do and having no support or authority to carry it out" (Aroskar, 1998). Anecdotally, nurses continue to suggest that they know the right thing to do, but they have no support to carry it out, or will be affected by reprisal. Workplace violence and harassment have also received much attention and some governments have introduced legislation to help curb these events, for example, Ontario's Bill 168. It is imperative that these events be dealt with promptly regardless of who the "offenders" might be. Development of the nurse–physician relationship must be part of improving the health care delivery system, particularly because when nurses and physicians work together, client care

CASE STUDY 1–1

Mrs. Williams comes to your unit from the emergency department (ED). Her admitting diagnosis is asthma. Her husband tells you she was really frightened and could not breathe when she came to the ED. They ask you how long she will be in the hospital and what will happen next. You give them a copy of your unit's asthma clinical practice guideline and review it with them.

How can you try to ensure a smooth transition home?

How will you work with your health care organization and the community you serve to ensure that Mrs. Williams and other asthma clients in the community are not admitted with asthma again soon? What kind of teaching will Mrs. Williams need to prevent future attacks?

(Suter et al., 2007). Fostering interprofessional practice is one of the three areas under Health Canada's Pan-Canadian Health Human Resource Strategy (Suter et al., 2007). Interprofessional practice describes a cohesive, coordinated approach to client care, involving providers from different disciplines and having the client be an important member of the team. In the future health care will be more client-centred, outcome-focused, evidence-based, wellness-oriented, population-based, technology-intensive, and highly cost-aware. Nursing must be ready to meet this challenge.

CRITICAL THINKING

Go to the website for the Integrated Pan-Canadian Healthy Living Strategy, 2005 (http://www.phac-aspc.gc.ca/hl-vs-strat/pdf/hls_e.pdf) and the Integrated Strategy on Healthy Living and Chronic Disease (http://www.phac-aspc.gc.ca/media/nr-rp/2005/2005_37bk1-eng.php).

What did you find?

How is your province doing on the Healthy Living Strategy indicators?

How could you work with leaders in your community and province to improve your province's performance?

KEY CONCEPTS

- The Canadian system of health care has developed within a political context. Our health care system may be highly sophisticated, but it does not deliver the same level of health care, access, and cost-effective quality to all its citizens.

- Various groups deliver Canadian health care in a variety of settings.

- Canadian health care is paid for by the public and private sectors.

- Health care can be categorized into four levels: health promotion, disease and injury prevention (protection), diagnosis and treatment of existing health problems (including primary, secondary, and tertiary care), and rehabilitation.

- Accreditation Canada is the national organization that accredits health care organizations.

- Donabedian developed a framework for quality. He identified structure, process, and outcome elements of quality. When outcomes are not good, nurses must review the structure and process of health care.

- The Canadian College of Health Leaders and the 3M Health Care Quality Team Awards provide a framework for the delivery of quality health care.

- Efforts to improve health care must address the multiple determinants of health in Canada.

- Canadian College of Health Leaders identified five capabilities for the 21st century for health care practitioners, regardless of their role or formal position. Nursing and other health care professions will have to adapt to a fast-changing environment in the future.

- Various forces are affecting health care in the new millennium.

- Caring, interprofessional practice promises to be an important part of nursing's future role in health care.

KEY TERMS

disease management	primary health care
horizontal integration	process elements of quality
integrated delivery system	public health system
LEADS in a Caring	regionalization
Environment framework	risk adjustment
outcome elements of quality	structure elements of quality
process elements of quality	vertical integration

REVIEW QUESTIONS

1. Which of the following is the national organization that accredits health care organizations?
   A. Canadian Nurses Association
   B. Canadian College of Health Leaders
   C. Canadian Institutes of Health Research
   D. Accreditation Canada

2. Which of the following is the largest expenditure related to health care in Canada?
   A. hospitals and institutions
   B. physicians
   C. pharmaceuticals
   D. nurses

3. Who identified a structure, process, and outcome framework for quality health care?
   A. Titler
   B. Elazar
   C. Wennberg
   D. Donabedian

4. Which of the following is the name of a national award for quality health care?
   A. Hill Burton
   B. 3M Health Care Quality Team Award
   C. Foundation for Accountability
   D. National Committee on Quality Assurance

REVIEW ACTIVITIES

1. You have just graduated from your nursing education program and have begun working on a new client care unit. Your nurse manager asks you to serve on the team to develop and improve the unit. Give examples of the three elements of quality that you will consider. Consider structure, process, and outcome examples in your answer. How will you monitor the effects of your improvements?

2. Your uncle is a director of quality improvement at a local manufacturing company. He comments on some of his company's activities to improve quality. What can you tell him about the quality improvement activities in the client care unit on which you have recently provided clinical care?

3. Review the Canadian College of Health Leaders LEADS in a Caring Environment capability framework. Consider how you can improve your own knowledge level in any of the competency areas in which you do not feel comfortable.

EXPLORING THE WEB

What sites would you recommend to clients and families seeking information about self-help, hospital accreditation, research, and clinical practice guidelines: for example, the Accreditation Canada, the Canadian Institutes for Health Research, and the Quality Healthcare Network?

■ *http://www.accreditation.ca*

■ *http://www.cihr.ca*

■ *http://www.cmaj.ca/cgi/collection/clinical_practice_guidelines*

Go to the sites for the CCHL and 3M Health Care Quality Team Awards and the Canadian Adverse Events Study. What information did you find there?

■ *http://www.cchl-ccls.ca/default_awards.asp?active_page_id=931*

■ *http://www.cmaj.ca/cgi/reprint/170/11/1678.pdf*

Where can you find statistics on health care spending?

■ *http://www.cihi.ca/CIHI-ext-portal/internet/EN/Home/honme/cihi000001*

Search the Internet and check these websites: Medicare, Canadian Institute for Health Information, Canadian Nurses Association, Canadian Cancer Society, Heart and Stroke Foundation, and Canadian Diabetes Association. What did you find?

■ *http://www.hc-sc.gc.ca/hcs-sss/medi-assur/index-eng.php*

■ *http://www.cihi.ca/CIHI-ext-portal/internet/EN/Home/home/cihi000001*

■ *http://www.cna-nurses.ca/cna/default_e.aspx*

■ *http://www.cancer.ca*

■ *http://www.heartandstroke.com/site/c.iklQLcMWJtE/b.2796497/k.BF8B/Home.htm*

■ *http://www.diabetes.ca*

Where can you find information related to diabetes in the Canadian population?

■ *http://www.healthcouncilcanada.ca/docs/rpts/2007/HCC_DiabetesRpt.pdf*

■ *http://www.phac-aspc.gc.ca/publicat/dic-dac99/d02-eng.php*

Go to PubMed. What did you find there? Can you access nursing and medical journals? Would you recommend this site to clients?

■ *http://www.ncbi.nlm.nih.gov/entrez/query.fcgi?DB=pubmed*

What are some helpful sites for nurses?

■ *http://www.nurse.ca/*

■ *http://www.anac.on.ca*

■ *http://www.cna-nurses.ca/cna*

Where could you go for information on the eHealth Internet Code of Ethics?

■ *http://www.ihealthcoalition.org/ethics/ethics.html*

■ *What are some sites to check on the Personal Information Protection and Electronic Documents Act?*

■ *http://laws-lois.justice.gc.ca/eng/*

REFERENCES

Accreditation Canada. (2010). Accreditation Canada Strategic Plan 2010 to 2013. Retrieved from http://www.accreditation.ca/uploadedFiles/About_Us/Strategic_Plan/Accreditation%20Canada%20Strategic%20Plan%202010%20to%202013.pdf

Accreditation Canada. (2011). Access to Standards. Retrieved from http://www.accreditation.ca/Shop-for-Standards

Adams, D. F., Fraser, D. B., & Abrams, H. L. (1973). The complications of coronary arteriography. Circulation, 48(3), 609–618.

Aroskar, M. (1998). Ethical working relationships in patient care. Nursing Clinics of North America, 33(2), 313–323.

Baggs, J. G., & Ryan, S. A. (1990). ICU nurse-physician collaboration and nursing satisfaction. Nursing Economics, 8(6), 386–392.

Baker, R., Norton, P., Flintoft, V., Blais, R., Brown, A., Cox, J., et al. (2004). The Canadian adverse events study: The incidence of adverse events among hospital patients in Canada. Canadian Medical Association Journal, 170(11), 1678–1686.

Benner, P. (2000). The wisdom of our practice. American Journal of Nursing, 100(10), 99–103.

Bonney, E., & Baker, G. R. (2004). Current strategies to improve patient safety in Canada: An overview of federal and provincial initiatives. Healthcare Quarterly, 7(2), 36–41.

Bull, M. J. (1997). Lessons from the past: Visions for the future of quality care. In C. G. Meisenheimer, Improving quality (2nd ed., pp. 3–16). Gaithersburg, MD: Aspen.

Byers, S. A. (1997). The executive nurse—leadership for new health care transitions. Clifton Park, NY: Delmar Learning.

Canadian College of Health Leaders. (2010). Leaders for Life.(Brochure). Retrieved from http://www.cchl-ccls.ca/assets/LEADS/LEADS_Print_Brochure_EN.pdf

Canadian Health Services Research Foundation. (2008). Summary report on the Aboriginal Health Human Resources Initiative Knowledge Exchange Workshop – QWQHC Summit March 18, 2008. Retrieved from http://www.f2fe.com/qwqhc/2008/Final_Report_E.pdf

Canadian Institute for Health Information. (2010a). Health Indicators. Retrieved from http://www.secure.cihi.ca/cihiweb/products/Healthindicators2010_en.pdf

Canadian Institute for Health Information. (2010b). National Health Expenditure Trends, 1975 to 2010. Ottawa: Author.

Canadian Institute for Health Information. (2010c). Regulated Nurses: Canadian Trends, 2005 to 2009. Ottawa: Author.

Canadian Institute for Health Information. (2010d). Supply, Distribution and Migration of Canadian Physicians, 2009. Ottawa: Author.

Carroll-Johnson, R. (2001). Redefining interdisciplinary practice. Oncology Nursing Forum, 28(4), 619.

Commission d'étude sur les services de santé et les services sociaux. (2000). Emerging solutions: Report and recommendations. Québec: Author. Chair: Michel Clair.

Commission on the Future of Health Care in Canada. (2002). Building on values: The future of health care in Canada. Saskatoon: Author. Commissioner: Roy J. Romanow.

Constitution Act (1867). Formerly the British North America Act (1867). Retrieved from http://www.solon.org/Constitutions/Canada/English/ca_1867.html

Donabedian, A. (1966). Evaluating the quality of medical care. Milbank Memorial Fund Quarterly, 44, 194–196.

Donatelle, R., & Davis, L. G. (1998). Access to health (8th ed.). Needham Heights, MA: Allyn & Bacon.

Drummond, M. F., Stoddart, F. L., & Torrance, G. W. (1994). Methods for the economic evaluation of health care programmes. Oxford: Oxford University Press.

Esmail, N., & Walker, M. (2005). How good is Canadian health care? 2005 report: An international comparison of health care systems (2005 Critical Issues Bulletin). Vancouver: The Fraser Institute.

Evans, R., & Stoddard, G. (1990). Consuming health care, producing health. Social Science and Medicine, 31(12), 1347–1363.

Finkelstein, M. M., Jerrett, M., DeLuca, P., Finkelstein, N., Verma., D. K., Chapman, K. & Sears, M. R. (2003). Canadian Medical Association Journal, 169(5), 397–402.

Fooks, C. (2005). Health human resources planning in an interdisciplinary health care environment: To dream the impossible dream? Canadian Journal of Nursing Leadership, 18(3), 26–29.

Frankish, C. J., Hwang, S. W., & Quantz, D. (2009). The Relationship between homelessness and health: An overview of research in Canada. In J. David Hulchanski, Philippa Campsie, Shirley Chau, Stephen Hwang, & Emily Paradis (Eds.), Finding home: Policy options for addressing homelessness in Canada. (E-book), Ch. 2.1. Toronto: Cities Centre, University of Toronto. Retrieved from http://www.homelesshub.ca/FindingHome

Goddard, M., & Smith, P. (2001). Equity of access to health care services: Theory and evidence from the UK. Social Science & Medicine, 53, 1149–1162.

Health Canada. (2000). Part one introduction: Challenges. Quest for quality in Canadian health care, continuous quality improvement. Retrieved from http://hc-sc.gc.ca/hcs-sss/pubs/qual/2000-qual/index-eng.php

Health Canada. (2003). How does literacy affect the health of Canadians? Retrieved from http://www.phac-aspc.gc.ca/ph-sp/literacy-alphabetisme/literacy2-eng.php

Health Canada. (2004). A 10-year plan to strengthen health care. Retrieved from http://hc-sc.gc.ca/hcs-sss/delivery-prestation/fptcollab/2004-fmm-rpm/bg-fi-eng.php

Health Council of Canada. (2007). Why health care renewal matters: Lessons from diabetes. Retrieved from www.healthcouncilcanada.ca

Kernaghan, K. (2010). International Innovations in Public Sector External Service Delivery. Retrieved from http://www.iccs-isac.org/en/pubs/FinalReport-June7-2010-FrontSection.pdf

Kohn, L., Corrigan, J., & Donaldson, M. (Eds.). (1999). To err is human: Building a safer health system. Report of the Committee on Quality of Care in America, Institute of Medicine. Washington, DC: National Academy Press.

Kohn, L., Corrigan, J., & Donaldson, M. (Eds.). (2001). Crossing the quality chasm: A new health system for the 21st century. Report of the Committee on Quality of Care in America, Institute of Medicine. Washington, DC: National Academy Press.

Lahaie, L. (2010). Champlain LHIN working on draft blueprint for clinical services in eastern Ontario. The Review. Retrieved from http://thereview.ca/story/champlain-lhin-working-draft-blueprint-clinical-services-eastern-counties.

Leape, L. (1987). Unnecessary surgery. *Health Services Research,* 24(3), 351–407.

Lewis, S., & Kouri, D. (2004). Regionalization: Making sense of the Canadian experience. *Healthcare Papers,* 5(1), 12–31.

Maddox, P. (2001). Update on national quality of care initiatives. *Nursing Economics,* 19(3), 121–124.

Murphy, T., & Greco, P. (2004). Leadership's role in patient/client safety: Are we doing enough? An accreditation perspective. *Healthcare Management Forum,* 17(14), 34–35.

National Forum on Health. (1997). *Canada health action: Building on the legacy.* Ottawa: Author.

Persell, S. D., Osborn, C. Y., Richard, R., Skripkauskas, S., & Wolf, M. S. (2007). Limited health literacy is a barrier to medication reconciliation in ambulatory care. *Journal of General Internal Medicine,* 22(11), 1523–1526.

Pinkerton, S. (2001). The future of professionalism in nursing. *Nursing Economics,* 18(3), 130–131.

Premier's Advisory Council on Health. (2001). *A framework for reform: Report of the premier's advisory council on health.* Edmonton: Author. Chair: Donald Mazankowski.

Priest, A. (2006). What's ailing our nurses? A discussion of the major issues affecting nursing human resources in Canada. Ottawa: Canadian Health Services Research Foundation.

Raphael, D. (2008). Social Determinants of Health: Canadian Perspectives. 2nd Edition. Canadian Scholars' Press. Toronto.

Saskatchewan Standing Committee on Health Care. (2001). *Caring for Medicare: Sustaining a quality system: Final report of the Commission on Medicare.* Regina: Author. Chair: Ken Fyke.

Shortell, S. M. (1996). *Remaking health care in America: Building organized delivery systems.* San Francisco: Jossey-Bass.

Shortell, S. M., & Kaluzny, A. D. (2000). *Health care management* (4th ed.). Clifton Park, NY: Delmar Learning.

Simms, L. M., Price, S. A., & Ervin, N. E. (2000). *Professional practice of nursing administration* (3rd ed.). Clifton Park, NY: Delmar Learning.

Sinclair, D., Rochon, M., & Leatt, P. (2005). *Riding the third rail: The story of Ontario's health services restructuring commission 1996–2000.* Montréal: Institute for Research on Public Policy.

Soukup, S. M. (2000). The Center for Advanced Nursing Practice evidence-based practice model: Promoting the scholarship of practice. *Nursing Clinics of North America,* 35(2), 301–309.

Standing Committee on Social Affairs, Science and Technology. (2002). *Reforming health protection and promotion in Canada: Time to act.* Ottawa: Author. Chair: Michael Kirby.

Statistics Canada. (2006). *Canada year book 2006.* Ottawa: Author.

Statistics Canada. (2010). *Canada year book 2010.* Ottawa: Author.

Sunnak, A. (2005). LHINs: Bringing it all back home: Ontario's shift to integrated health services. *Registered Nurse Journal,* 17(4), 13–16.

Suter, E., Oelke, N. D., Adair, C. E., & Armitage, G. D. (2009). Ten key principles for successful health systems integration. *Healthcare Quarterly,* 13(Special issue), 16–23.

Theorell, T. (2001). Stress and health: From a work perspective. In J. Dunham (Ed.), *Stress in the workplace: Past, present and future.* London: WHURR Publishers.

Wennberg, J., & Gittelsohn, A. (1973). Small area variations in health care delivery. *Science* 182 (4117): 1102–8.

Wolper, I. F. (1999). *Health care administration: Planning, implementing, and managing organized delivery systems* (3rd ed.). Gaithersburg, MD: Aspen.

SUGGESTED READINGS

Agency for Healthcare Research and Quality. (2003). The effect of health care working conditions on patient safety. Retrieved from ww.ahrq.gov/clinic/epcsums/worksum.htm

Alidina, S., Ardal, S., Lee, P., Raskin, L., Shennan, A., Young, L. M. (2006). Regionalization reigns—but is care being delivered accordingly? An evaluation of perinatal care delivery in a regionalized child health network. *Healthcare Management Forum,* 19(2), 22–26.

American Nurses Association. (1995). *Nursing's social policy statement.* Washington, DC: Author.

Baldridge National Quality Program. (2000). *Health care criteria for performance excellence.* Gaithersburg, MD: Baldridge National Quality Program.

Beach, C. M., Chaykowski, R. P., & Sweetman, A. (Eds.). (2006). *Health services restructuring in Canada: New evidence and new directions.* Montréal: Institute for Research on Public Policy.

Bellack, J. P., & O'Neil, E. H. (2000). Recreating nursing practice for a new century: Recommendations and implications of the Pew Health Professions Commission's final report. *Nursing and Health Care Perspectives,* 21(1), 14–21.

Berman, S. (2000). The AMA clinical quality improvement focus on addressing patient safety. *Joint Commission Journal on Quality Improvement,* 26(7), 428–433.

Berwick, D. M. (1994). Eleven worthy aims for clinical leadership of health system reform. *Journal of the American Medical Association,* 272, 797–802.

Browne, G., Roberts, J., Burne, C., Gafni, A., Weir, R., & Majumdar, B. (2001). The costs and effects of addressing the needs of vulnerable populations: Results of 10 years of research. *Canadian Journal of Nursing Research,* 33, 65–76.

Canadian Institute for Health Information. (2004). *Health care in Canada.* Ottawa: Author.

Casebeer, A., Reay, T., Golden-Biddle, K., Pablo, A., Wiebe, E., & Hinings, B. (2006). Experiences of regionalization: Assessing multiple stakeholder perspectives across time. *Healthcare Quarterly,* 9(2), 32–43.

Chodos, H., & MacLeod, J. J. (2004). Romanow and Kirby on the public/private divide in healthcare: Demystifying the debate. *Healthcare Papers,* 4(4), 10–25.

Davidson, A. (2005). Advancing the population health agenda. *Healthcare Management Forum,* 18(4), 17–21.

Dienemann, J. A. (Ed.). (1998). *Nursing administration: Managing patient care* (2nd ed.). Upper Saddle River, NJ: Prentice Hall Health.

Drummond, H., & Stoddart, G. (1995). Assessment of health producing measures across different sectors. *Health Policy,* 33, 219–231.

Ellwood, P. M. (1998). Outcomes management: A technology of patient experience. *New England Journal of Medicine,* 318, 1549–1556.

Ferguson, S. L. (1999). Institute for Nursing Leadership: A new program to enhance the leadership capacity of all nurses. *Nursing Outlook, 47*(2), 91–92.

Fos, P. J., & Fine, D. J. (2000). *Designing health care for populations.* San Francisco: Jossey-Bass.

Ginsberg, E. (1996). *Tomorrow's hospital: A look to the twenty-first century.* New Haven, CT: Yale University Press.

Gosfield, A. G., & Reinertsen, J. L. (2006). The 100,000 lives campaign: Crystallizing standards of care for hospitals. *Healthcare Quarterly, 9*(3), 1–7.

Grol, R., & Grimshaw, J. (1999). Evidence-based implementation of evidence-based medicine. *Joint Commission Journal on Quality Improvement, 25*(10), 503–513.

Guadagnoli, E., Epstein, A. M., Zaslavsky, A., Shaul, J. A., Veroff, D., Fowler, F. J., Jr. et al. (2000). Providing consumers with information about the quality of health plans: The consumer assessment of health plans demonstration in Washington State. *Joint Commission Journal on Quality Improvement, 26*(7), 410–420.

Halfon, N., Larson, K., & Russ, S. (2010). Why Social Determinants? *Healthcare Quarterly, 14*(Special edition), 8–20.

Hamer, R. (1999). Goals 2000: For MDs: Managerial competency. For HMOs: Administrative retooling. *Managed Care, 8*(11), 38.

Heller, B. R., Oros, M. T., & Durney-Crowley, J. (2000). The future of nursing education: Ten trends to watch. *Nursing and Health Care Perspectives, 21*(1), 9–13.

Hurley, J. (2004). Regionalization and the allocation of healthcare resources to meet population health needs. *Healthcare Papers, 5*(1), 34–39.

Joint Commission on Accreditation of Healthcare Organizations (2001). Healthcare at the crossroads: Strategies for addressing the evolving nursing crisis. Retrieved from www.jointcommission.org/assets/1/18/health_care_at_the_crossroads.pdf

Kelly, L. Y., & Joel, L. A. (1999). *Dimensions of professional nursing* (8th ed.). New York: McGraw-Hill.

Kodner, D. (2009). All Together Now: A Conceptual Exploration of Integrated Care. *Healthcare Quarterly, 13*(Special issue), 6–15.

Lancaster, J. (1999). *Nursing issues in leading and managing change.* St. Louis, MO: Mosby.

Lang, N. M. (1999). Discipline approaches to evidence-based practice: A view from nursing. *Joint Commission Journal on Quality Improvement, 25*(10), 539–544.

Lea, D. H., & Lawson, M. T. (2000). A practice-based genetics curriculum for nurse educators: An innovative approach to integrating human genetics into nursing curricula. *Journal of Nursing, 39*(9), 418–421.

Levine, D. (2005). A healthcare revolution: Quebec's new model of healthcare. *Healthcare Quarterly, 8*(4), 38–46.

Lindeman, C. A. (2000). The future of nursing education. *Journal of Nursing Education, 39*(1), 5–12.

Lohr, K. N., & Carey, T. S. (1999). Assessing "best evidence": Issues in grading the quality of studies for systematic reviews. *Joint Commission Journal on Quality Improvement, 25*(9), 470–479.

Lovern, E. (2001a, January 1). JCAHO's new tell-all: Standards require that patients know about below-par care. *Modern Healthcare, 31*(1), 2, 15.

Lovern, E. (2001b, May 7). Another makeover: JCAHO moves to rewrite many rules to lessen hospitals' regulatory burden. *Modern Healthcare, 31*(19), 5, 16.

Lovern, E. (2001c, May 28). Oh no, not that type of review: JCAHO singling out more hospitals for noncompliance with standards. *Modern Healthcare, 31*(22), 4–5.

McLaughlin, C. P., & Kaluzny, A. D. (1999). *Continuous quality improvement in health care* (2nd ed.). Gaithersburg, MD: Aspen.

Milstead, J. A. (Ed.). (1999). *Health policy and politics: A nurse's guide* (3rd ed.). Gaithersburg, MD: Aspen.

Nicklin, W., & Graves, E. (2005). Nursing and patient outcomes: It's time for healthcare leadership to respond. *Healthcare Management Forum, 18*(1), 9–13.

Nicklin, W., & McVeety, J. E. (2002). Canadian nurses' perceptions of patient safety in hospitals. *Canadian Journal of Nursing Leadership, 15*(3), 27–29.

Norton, D., & Kaplan, R. (2001). *The strategy-focused organization: How balanced scorecard companies thrive in the new business environment.* Boston: Harvard Business School Press.

O'Grady, E. (2000). Access to health care: An issue central to nursing. *Nursing Economics, 18*(2), 88–90.

Pesut, D. J., & Rezmerski, C. J. (2000). Future think. *Nursing Outlook, 48*(1), 9.

Phipps, S. (2003). *The impact of poverty on health: A scan of research literature.* Ottawa: Canadian Institute for Health Information. Retrieved from http://secure.cihi.ca/cihiweb/dispPage.jsp?cw_page=GR_323_E

Poochikian-Sarkissian, S., Hunter, J., Tully, S., Lazar, N.M., Sabo, K., & Cursio, C. (2008). Developing an innovative care delivery model: Interprofessional practice teams. *Healthcare Management Forum, 21*(1), 6–18.

Postl, B., Cook, C., & Moffatt, M. (2010). Aboriginal child health and the social determinants – Why are these children so disadvantaged? *Healthcare Quarterly, 14*(Special edition), 42–51.

Sackett, D. L., Rosenberg, W. M. C., Gray, J. A. M., Haynes, R. B., & Richardson, W. S. (1996). Evidence-based medicine: What it is and what it isn't. *British Medical Journal, 312*(7023), 71–72.

Scobie, K. B., & Russell, G. (2003). Vision 2020, part 1: Profile of the future nurse leader. *Journal of Nursing Administration, 33*(6), 324–330.

Sinclair, D. G. (2002). Speaking with Michael Kirby. *Hospital Quarterly, 5*(4), 32–39.

Sinclair, D. G. (2004). The big thing we haven't done yet. *Healthcare Papers, 4*(4), 69–73.

Spitzer, W. O. (1998). Quality of life. In D. Burley & W. H. W. Inman (Eds.), *Therapeutic risk: Perception, measurement, and management.* New York: Wiley.

Storch, J. L. (2005). Patient safety: Is it just another bandwagon? *Canadian Journal of Nursing Leadership, 18*(2), 39–55.

Strasen, L. (1999). The silent health care revolution: The rising demand for complementary medicine. *Nursing Economics, 17*(5), 246–256.

Sullivan, E. J. (1999). *Creating nursing's future: Issues, opportunities, and challenges.* St. Louis, MO: Mosby.

Suter, E., Arndt, J., Lait, J., Jackson, K., Kipp, J., Taylor, E., & Arthur, N. (2007). How can frontline managers demonstrate leadership in enabling professional practice? *Healthcare Management Forum, 20*(4), 38–43.

Sutherland, R., & Fulton, J. (1994). *Spending smarter and spending less: Policies and partnerships for health care in Canada*. Ottawa: The Health Group.

Taylor, D. W. (2003). 2020. Healthcare management in Canada: A new model home next door. *Healthcare Management Forum,* 16(1), 6–10.

Tepfers, A., Hruska, C., Stone, J., & Moser J. (2009). New accreditation program: University health network's experience with Qmentum. *Healthcare Quarterly,* 12(3), 90–97.

Thompson, L. J., & Martin, M. T. (2004). Integration of cancer services of Ontario: The story of getting it done. *Healthcare Quarterly,* 7(3), 42–48.

Tieman, J. (2001). Coming of age: Disease management making a case for itself clinically and financially. *Modern Healthcare,* 31(28), 26–27, 38.

Tieman, J., & Bellandi, D. (2001). HIPAA will be no holiday: Experts say exhaustive rules may require significant cultural and administrative changes. *Modern Healthcare,* 31(1), 3, 15.

Trofino, J. (1997). The courage to change: Reshaping health care delivery. *Nursing Management,* 28(11), 50–53.

Villeneuve, M., & MacDonald, J. (2006). *Toward 2020: Visions for nursing*. Ottawa: Canadian Nurses Association.

Walt, G. (1994). Health policy: *An introduction to process and power.* London and New Jersey: Zed Books.

Weatherill, S. (2004). Public/private pragmatism. *Healthcare Papers,* 4(4), 74–78.

Weeks, W. B., Hamby, L., Stein, A., & Batalden, P. B. (2000). Using the Baldridge Management System framework in health care: The Veterans Health Administration experience. *Joint Commission Journal on Quality Improvement,* 26(7), 379–387.

Wilkins, R., Berthelot, J.-M., & Ng, E. (2002). Trends in mortality by neighbourhood income in urban Canada from 1971 to 1996. *Health Reports (StatsCan),* 13(Supplement), 1–28.

Wilson, L. M. (1999). Healthy people: A new millennium. *Journal of Nursing Administration's Healthcare Law, Ethics, and Regulation,* 1(2), 29–32.

CHAPTER ENDNOTES

1. Health Canada, "Aboriginal Diabetes Initiative." Retrieved from http://www.hc-sc.gc.ca/fniah-spnia/diseases-maladies/diabete/index-eng.php

2. Health Canada, "Canada Health Act Overview." Retrieved from http://www.hc-sc.gc.ca/ahc-asc/media/nr-cp/2002/2002_care-soinsbk4_e.html

3. Health Canada, "Health Care System Federal Transfers to Provinces/Territories." Retrieved from http://www.hc-sc.gc.ca/hcs-sss/delivery-prestation/fedrole/index-eng.php

4. Health Canada, "Federal Transfers to Provinces/Territories." Retrieved from http://www.hc-sc.gc.ca/hcs-sss/delivery-prestation/fedrole/pttransfer/index_e.html

5. Health Canada, Department of Finance, "A History of the Health and Social Tax Transfers." Retrieved from http://www.fin.gc.ca/fedprov/his-eng.asp

6. Canadian Institute for Health Information, "Regulated Nurses: Canadian Trends, 2005 to 2009." Retrieved from http://secure.cihi.ca/cihiweb/products/nursing_report_2005-2009_en.pdf

7. CIHI. (2010). National Health Expenditure Trends, 1975 to 2010. p. xii.

8. Ibid.

9. Ibid., pp. 17–20.

10. Ibid., p. 57.

11. CIHI, "About the Canadian Population Health Initiative." Retrieved from http://www.cihi.ca/CIHI-ext-portal/internet/en/document/factors+influencing+health/environmental/cphi

12. Public Health Agency of Canada, "The Federal Strategy: What are the responsibilities of a public health system." Retrieved from http://www.phac-aspc.gc.ca/about_apropos/federal_strategy-eng.php

13. Public Health Agency of Canada, "Why was the Agency created?" Retrieved from http://www.phac-aspc.gc.ca/about_apropos/faq-eng.php

14. Pan Canadian Public Health Network, Partners in Health, "About the Network: The Pan-Canadian Public Health Network: An Overview." Retrieved from http://www.phn-rsp.ca/About_e.html

15. Canadian Public Health Association, "About CPHA: Mission Statement." Retrieved from http://www.cpha.ca/en/about.aspx

16. Centre for Aging, "Chronic Disease Self-Management Program History." Retrieved from http://www.coag.uvic.ca/cdsmp/cdsmp_history.htm

17. Ibid.

18. Accreditation Canada, "Accreditation Programs, Qmentum." Retrieved from http://www.accreditation.ca/accrediation-programs/qmentum

19. Accreditation Canada, "Organ and Tissue Donation and Transplant." Retrieved from http://www.accreditation.ca/accreditation-programs/new-initiatives/organ-and-tissue-donation-and-transplant/

20. Accreditation Canada, "ISQua Accredited." Retrieved from http://www.accreditation.ca/accreditation-programs/international/

21. Institute for Clinical Evaluative Sciences, "Our Research." Retrieved from http://www.ices.on.ca/webpage.cfm?site_id=1&org_id=26

22. Canadian Health Services Research Foundation, "What We Do. Strategic Priorities." Retrieved from http://www.chsrf.ca/AboutUs/Accountability/annual2009.aspx

23. Canadian Health Services Research Foundation, "About EXTRA, History." Retrieved from http://www.chsrf.ca/Programs/EXTRA/history.aspx

24. Ibid.

25. Canadian Health Services Research Foundation, "2009 EXTRA Competition Results." Retrieved from http://www.chsrf.ca/Programs/EXTRA/intervention_projects/Cohorts/2009EXTRACompetitionResults.aspx

26. Canadian Health Services Research Foundation, "Primary Healthcare." Retrieved from http://www.chsrf.ca/Programs/PrimaryHealthcare.aspx

27. Accreditation Canada, "Knowledge Exchange, Patient Safety, Surgical Checklist." Retrieved from http://www.accreditation.ca/knowledge-exchange/patient-safety/surgical-checklist/

28. Canadian Health Services Research Foundation, 2006. Ottawa: Canadian Health Services Research Foundation. "What's Ailing Our Nurses? A Discussion of the Major Issues Affecting Nursing Human Resources in Canada." Retrieved from http://www.chsrf.ca/SearchResults.aspx?search=ailing%20our%20nurses

29. McGillis Hall, L., Irvine Doran, D., Baker, G. R., Pink, G. H., Sidani, S., O'Brien-Pallas, L., et al. *A study of the impact of nursing staff mix models and organizational change strategies on patient, system and nurse outcomes.* Retrieved from http://www.chsrf.ca/SearchResults.aspx?search=impact%20nursing%20staff%20mix%20models

30. Office of the Privacy Commissioner of Canada, "Fact Sheet, Privacy Legislation in Canada." Retrieved from http://www.privcom.gc.ca/fs-fi/02_05_d_15_e.asp

31. Canadian College of Health Leaders, "Professional Development." Retrieved from http://www.cchl-ccls.ca/default_conferences.asp?active_page_id=6492

CHAPTER 2

Basic Clinical Health Care Economics

Laura J. Nosek, PhD, RN
Ida M. Androwich, PhD, RNC, FAAN
Adapted by Heather Crawford, BScN, MEd, CHE

The Institute of Health Economics is based in Edmonton, Alberta. Its mission, as an independent, not-for-profit organization, is to make useful contributions to health policy and practice by performing research in health economics and to synthesize evidence in health technology assessment.[1]

OBJECTIVES

The purpose of this chapter is to enable the reader to

- identify three functions of a health care system;
- identify the health reforms related to financing, funding, and delivery;
- identify four main models of alternative physician remuneration;
- describe costing systems in health care; and
- describe the issues surrounding the public/private health care debate.

Terry Chan/Shutterstock

You have been struggling with progressive pain and disability in your knees. You have finally been able to access a physician, and he has agreed to be your family doctor. He has suggested numerous remedies to you, but you have already tried most of them. He will set up an appointment with a specialist to determine whether you need a knee replacement. You are becoming progressively discouraged because you will have to wait an estimated seven or eight months before getting any relief. In the meantime, you are starting to lose your ability to walk independently. However, a private clinic will afford you the ability to get treatment sooner.

What do you think is the problem?

Do you perceive the problem to be the same as the problem perceived by politicians? The economists? The physicians?

When cost is removed from the equation, what drives the decision to provide or not provide health care?

Is that driver a universal value or is it culturally dependent?

Regardless of how expert, creative, collaborative, and altruistic a health care system may be, it cannot function without money. Over the ages, that money has flowed from varying sources, including philanthropy, volunteerism, fee-for-service, insurance, and government subsidies. Securing the bottom line is basic to achieving the mission of providing health care and is now viewed as the shared responsibility of people around the world.

We once thought that nurses needed only to be educated in the art and the science of providing clinical care to clients. Today, we recognize that nurses must be much more broadly educated. In addition to clinical care expertise, nurses must demonstrate at least minimal competence in the humanities, management science, and computer science, as well as be skilled in evaluating and applying new knowledge suggested by scientific research.

Canada spends significant dollars on health care on an annual basis, yet morbidity and mortality statistics, in terms of improved health outcomes, lead us to question the value that we receive for our dollars. Researchers commonly focus on life expectancy as an indicator of overall health of a population because it is a relatively reliable measure, especially when making international comparisons. For example, the United States spends considerably more on health care than Canada, but Canadians tend to live longer. In 2005 Canadians' life expectancy at birth was 80.4 years compared to the Americans' life expectancy of 77.9 years. Japan spends less than both countries, but has a higher life expectancy: 82 years.[2]

Florence Nightingale's early search for the "good" versus "mischievous" outcomes of the money spent on health care may have initiated an unspoken commitment to financial stewardship among nurses. It seems fitting, then, that all nurses are required to participate knowledgeably in designing care systems that provide the best possible care at the lowest cost (Chang, Price, & Pfoutz, 2001). Consequently, every nurse today needs to have a basic understanding of clinical health care **economics**—the study of how scarce resources are allocated among possible uses—in order to make appropriate choices among the increasingly scarce resources of the future.

The study of economics is based on three general premises: (1) scarcity—resources exist in finite quantities and consumption demand is typically greater than resource supply; (2) choice—decisions are made about which resources to produce and consume among many options; and (3) preference—individual and societal values and preferences influence the decisions that are made. In a traditional market economy, the sellers sell to the buyers who buy, with each trying to maximize their gains from the transactions. Health care does not fit well in this model. For example, consider the concept of price elasticity, which is related to the price that an individual is willing to pay for a given item. Normally, as the price goes up, the demand goes down. When the purchase is health care, however, the price may be viewed as irrelevant to the decision to purchase. Think of a wristwatch that you might always purchase for $5, but you would likely not buy at $50, and would never consider at $500. Now, imagine that instead of a wristwatch, the item in question is a medication or therapy needed to save your sick child. The consideration of price in the decision-making process is likely quite different. Thus, health care is much less "elastic" with reference to price than many other consumer goods.

Another aspect of health care's difference from the traditional economic model relates to the knowledge of options and payment mechanisms available to the consumer. In a typical market, the buyer is also the payer. In health care, the health care provider (buyer) ordering a hospitalization or treatment is a doctor or nurse. The provider is not the payer, nor is the client (buyer) using the hospital or treatment the payer. The actual **payer** is the third-party reimburser (i.e., the insurance company or government). Consequently, the financial impact of the decision on the provider (buyer) and the client user (buyer) is skewed. Neither of these buyers is the payer.

This chapter presents basic concepts of clinical health care economics that are important to the novice nurse entering clinical practice. The following topics are included: perspectives on the role that cost has played—and will play—in directing health care delivery, methods for determining the cost of delivering nursing care, and the effect of health care policy on the delivery of nursing care. Recognized nurse experts provide projections for the future impact of economics on clinical nursing.

Traditional Perspective on the Cost of Health Care: Health Care as Altruism

The long-standing tradition of health care is to help people achieve their optimal level of health so that they can enjoy their maximum quality of life. **Altruism** refers to the unselfish concern for the welfare of others, and **ethics** refers to the doctrine that the general welfare of society is the proper goal of an individual's actions. These are opposed to **egoism**, which is the tendency to be self-centred or to consider only oneself and one's own interests (Agnes, 2000). Altruism and ethics traditionally drove the way health care was viewed and provided. Several early nursing leaders, including Florence Nightingale, Isabel Adams Hampton Robb, and Adelaide Nutting were members of socially prominent families instilled with the value that altruistic service was the expected role of the privileged. Such feelings of dedication to the less fortunate stemmed from medieval infirmaries established by convents and monasteries to care for the aged, orphaned, poor, and disabled. The first hospitals to care for the sick and injured were also charitable institutions established around the 14th century to provide illness care to those who did not have a home or who could not afford home care (Ross-Kerr & Wood, 2003). The people cared for in hospitals were called patients—from the Latin *patiens*, meaning "to suffer" (vos Savant, 2001). The term *client* is used throughout the text to include all individuals who access the health care system as customers.

Need for Health Care Determined by Provider

Health care was traditionally delivered from a paternalistic model of governance and control. Health professionals, led by physicians, controlled a vast body of scientific knowledge

and skill, and this was rendered awesome and mystical by complex scientific language. A command of that scientific knowledge and skill required extensive and expensive education and was not shared with so-called outsiders. The physician determined the type of health care that was needed, independent of the client and even independent of professional colleagues. The physician also decided how much to charge for that care. Decision making about all aspects of health care was the exclusive domain of the professionals.

Less than 40 years ago, no significant difference between Canada and the United States existed in the provision of health care. However, since 1971 the countries have proceeded in dramatically different directions. To prevent Canadians from having to incur the costs associated with health care, and to prevent them from being financially disadvantaged, a series of steps took place, which ultimately ended with what we now know as medicare. On the other hand, the United States still has a system of private and public health care, with more than 40 million Americans uninsured.

Esmail and Walker (2008) suggest that, based on comparative evidence, the Canadian health care model is not as good as models in place in other countries of the Organisation for Economic Co-operation and Development (OECD) (see Table 2-1). They also state that Canada has the following health care problems: inferior age-adjusted access to physicians and technology, longer wait times, less success in preventing deaths that are preventable, and higher costs than almost all other health systems with comparable objectives. Models that produce better results, and cost less than Canada's, charge user fees; offer alternative, comprehensive private insurance; and include private hospitals that compete for clients. According to Esmail and Walker (2008), comparatively speaking, Canada underperforms and needs to consider the more successful models in other countries that offer their citizens universal access to health care (see Figure 2-1).

The Right to Health Care at Any Cost

At the beginning of the 1990s the cost of providing health care spiralled. Health care expenditures continue to increase annually. Spending on health care is substantial in Canada, but it is not uniform across the provinces and territories. At a pan-Canadian level, per capita spending in 2010 was $5,614 per person, ranging from a low of $5,096 in Québec to a high of $6,266 in Alberta. In the territories, total per capita spending ranged from $7,977 in Yukon to $12,356 in Nunavut in 2010.[3] The higher spending in the territories may be related to the costs associated with travel to receive certain types of care. Factors that may have contributed to the spending differences among provinces and territories include differences in populations and their health status, patterns of health service delivery

TABLE 2-1   PERFORMANCE OF HEALTH SYSTEMS IN OECD COUNTRIES

ExSum Table 1: Performance of Health Systems in OECD Countries

	Mortality Based on Population Statistics			Mortality Closely Related to the Effectiveness of Health Care ("Disease-level Indicators")				
	Healthy Life Expectancy/ Life Expectancy Rank 2003	Infant Mortality Rank 2005	Perinatal Mortality Rank 2005	Mortality Amenable to Health Care Rank 2002/03	Potential Years of Life Lost Rank 2004	Breast Cancer Mortality Rank 2002	Colon/ Rectum Cancer Combined Mortality Rank 2002[1]	Cumulative Rank
Australia	7	20	3	3	6	5	2	1
Japan	2	4	1	2	3	11	4	2
Sweden	6	2	6	9	2	1	9	3
Iceland	20	1	1	12[2]	1	4	7	4
Switzerland	10	16	25	12[2]	4	9	1	5
France	8	10	27	1	9	6	11	6
Canada	17	24	17	6	10	10	2	7
Italy	5	13	11	5	8	11	5	8
Luxembourg	1	3	10	12[2]	7	6	6	9
Norway	12	6	9	7	5	8	14	10
Finland	13	5	4	13	11	2	14	11
Korea	27	23	8	12[2]	19	3	7	12
Germany	3	13	13	12	14	14	12	13
New Zealand	21	20	19	14	18	13	10	14
Spain	3	10	11	4	13	21	18	15
Netherlands	15	19	20	8	12	23	16	16
Austria	17	16	15	11	16	16	17	17
Greece	19	10	14	10	15	17	19	18
United Kingdom	10	22	25	16	20	15	13	19
Belgium	8	9	15	12[2]	20[2]	18	20	20
Poland	26	26	20	12[2]	24	20	22	21
Ireland	23	15	23	17	17	24	21	22
Denmark	13	18	22	15	21	21	25	23
Portugal	25	8	7	18	22	19	23	23
Czech Republic	15	7	5	12[2]	23	25	24	25
Turkey	28	28	28	12[2]	20[2]	28	28	26
Slovak Republic	23	27	18	12[2]	25	27	26	27
Hungary	22	25	23	12[2]	26	26	27	28

Note 1: Combined mortality is the average of male and female mortality percentages.
Note 2: Not all information was available for all nations. Where data was unavailable, the rank of average values has been inserted.

Source: Esmail, M., & Walker, M. (2005). How Good is Canadian Health Care? *2005 Report: An International Comparison of Health Care Systems.* The Fraser Institute, p. 8. Reprinted with Permission.

and coverage, geography and population density, and the costs of providing care.[4] Approximately 12 percent of the gross domestic product (GDP) was dedicated to health care spending in 2010 (CIHI, 2010c, p. 92).

There remains no consensus on the right amount of money to spend or the right distribution of resources within the system. The complex question of fiscal sustainability also arises frequently. In 2002 Roy Romanow stated, "Medicare

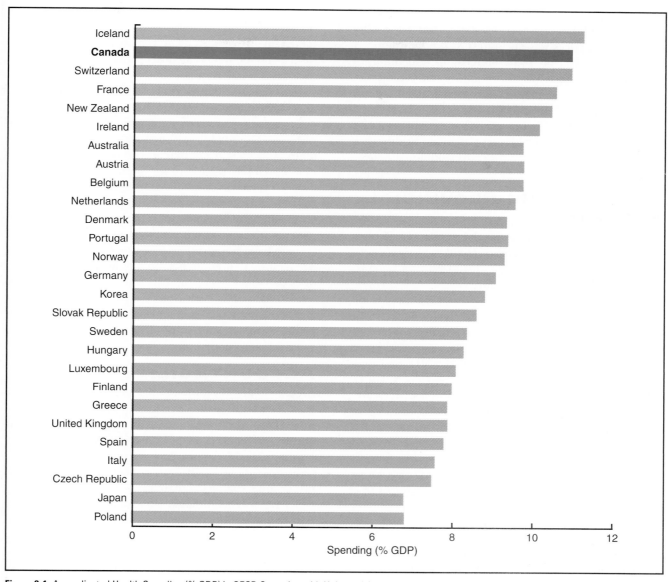

Figure 2-1 Age-adjusted Health Spending (% GDP) in OECD Countries with Universal Access to Health Care, 2005
Source: Esmail, M., & Walker, M. (2005). How Good is Canadian Health Care? *2005 Report: An International Comparison of Health Care Systems.* The Fraser Institute, p. 4. Reprinted with Permission.

is as sustainable as Canadians want it to be."[5] It is a system funded by tax dollars; as long as Canadians are willing to pay, the system will be there. With an annual increase of anywhere from 1 percent to 18 percent over the past 35 years, Canada's health care spending reached an estimated $191.6 billion in 2010. Although health spending in 2010 continued to increase, the estimated increase in health care spending from 2009 to 2010 was the smallest observed since 1997. The proportion of the provincial and territorial budgets spent on health care has remained stable since 2004.[6]

Internationally, Canada's per capita spending is among the highest when compared with other OECD countries. In 2008 Canada ranked fourth out of 24 OECD countries with comparable data. Canada also ranked 9th

out of 33 OECD countries for life expectancy. Health care spending and life expectancy are often linked together, but the variation in the two measures does not appear to be highly correlated. Jurisdictions that have higher per capita health care spending do not appear to have similarly higher life expectancy. The reverse is also true. For example, British Columbia and Québec spend the least per person compared to the other provinces ($5,355 in B.C. and $5,096 in Québec), yet they both fall in the top three for average life expectancy (81.2 years in B.C. and 80.7 in Québec) in Canada.[7]

The Canadian media took note of the cutbacks and began to report on clients being untreated, long waiting lists, and anecdotal reports of catastrophe. Canadians began to lose confidence in their health care system. They were told that costs were escalating, but that quality of care and services was declining. At the same time, a number of provincial royal commissions and inquiries concluded that there was still room for additional rationalization and cost containment within hospital systems (Barer, Morgan, & Evans, 2003).

It didn't take long before questions were being asked about the sustainability of the Canadian health care system. In response to these concerns, additional reports were commissioned.

FEDERAL AND PROVINCIAL REPORTS

The two federal reports were the Romanow Report, *Building on Values, the Future of Health Care in Canada* (Commission on the Future of Health Care in Canada, 2002), and the Kirby Report, *Reforming Health Protection and Promotion in Canada: Time to Act* (Standing Committee on Social Affairs, Science, and Technology, 2002). A number of provincial reports included, from Alberta, *A Framework for Reform*, known as the Mazankowski Report (Premier's Advisory Council on Health, 2001); Saskatchewan's *Caring for Medicare: Sustaining a Quality System*, known as the Fyke Report (Commission on Medicare, 2001); and from Québec, *Emerging Solutions*, known as the Clair Report (Commission d'étude sur les services de santé et les services sociaux, 2000). These reports all varied in their recommendations, but together they set the stage for Canada's future. The two federal reports are referenced most frequently. Whereas Senator Kirby is considered to be an advocate of privatization, Romanow is a proponent of the public system.

In the early days, medicare was equated with doctors and hospitals. Although considerable change has occurred over the past 40 years, medicare is still largely organized around hospitals and doctors. Home care, however, is rapidly becoming a critical element of our health system. Not long ago, what are currently day procedures were performed in hospital and required an in-hospital stay of weeks, including convalescence. Today, medication costs are increasing, and they now represent some of the highest costs in the system. Drugs associated with some therapies are not covered by the public system, outside of hospitals, and these costs can be financially devastating for some families. This situation is incompatible with the medicare philosophy (Commission on the Future of Health Care in Canada, 2002).

Canadians want and need a more accountable health care system. Canadians do not accept that things will get better—they want to *know* that things will get better. How? According to Romanow (Commission on the Future of Health Care in Canada, 2002, p. xix), Canadians want to know what is happening with their money: with health care budgets, hospital beds, nurses, doctors,

access, wait lists, community care, diagnostic testing, and whether outcomes are improving. Aboriginal people and some Canadians in rural and remote parts of the country cannot always access medical services where and when they need them (Commission on the Future of Health Care in Canada 2002, p. 220). Also, some medical procedures have unacceptable wait times. These are only a few of the reasons why accountability needs to be addressed. Although Canada is a top spender, ranking sixth, tenth, tenth, and second in comparisons of types of mortality that are closely related to the performance of a health system, Canada's cumulative rank is seventh, behind Australia, Japan, Sweden, Iceland, Switzerland, and France.[8] Canadian patients experience longer wait times than patients in other comparable countries and, generally, seem to have more trouble accessing health care services. Six nations deliver higher quality health services than does Canada. Each of these nations have private alternatives to the public health care system, some form of user fees at the point of access, and all but one (Iceland) allow private hospitals and surgical clinics to deliver at least some publicly funded care.[9]

ACCOUNTABILITY

Accountability was a theme of *Looking Back, Looking Forward*, (Ontario Health Services Restructuring Commission, 2000), the Romanow Report (Commission on the Future of Health Care in Canada, 2002), and the First Ministers Health Accord.[10] Shortt and Macdonald (2002) state that public discussions concerning accountability often imply that accountability is synonymous with the collection of quantifiable indicators. However, operationalizing accountability is far more complex than that and needs to be tailored to individual relationships. According to Brown, Porcellato, and Barnsley (2006), accountability is the catchall word for Canadian health care today. Policymakers, managers, researchers, and providers all refer to accountability in a different way—from the quality of our relationships, to transparency in business dealings, to balanced budgets.

The stakeholders in Canadian health care accountability include the federal government, the provincial governments, the territorial governments, regional health authorities or their equivalents, hospitals, individual providers, physicians, and the public (Shortt & Macdonald, 2002).

Accountability instruments and processes include citizen involvement, through their involvement on boards of health care institutions or regions, or through consultation. Citizens also hold the government accountable through the electoral process. Government ministers are accountable to their legislatures for the operation of their departments. Information that increases the transparency of the government assists in making the government accountable to the people who receive the information.

Some governments review the accreditation process as a form of accountability, because an external source confirms the quality of the organization's services. Licensing of professionals, by virtue of their registration, is evidence that they have met the entry-to-practice standards of their profession. Complaints committees of professional bodies will hold the professionals accountable if that is not done by the profession (Shortt & Macdonald, 2002).

In an accountability framework, stakeholder identity predominantly determines the type of relationship. See Table 2-2 for a complete list of accountability instruments associated with accountability processes.

TABLE 2-2	ACCOUNTABILITY INSTRUMENTS ASSOCIATED WITH ACCOUNTABILITY PROCESSES
Process	**Instruments**
Citizen involvement	consultations
	board service
Political activity	elections
	legislature transparency
Constitutional practice	ministerial responsibility
	public accounts committee
Provision of information	business and strategic plans
	annual reports
	access to information
Delegated activity	independent review boards
	self-governing professions
Review functions	Auditor General and provincial auditors
	Comptroller General
Managerial functions	program evaluation
	guideline development
	report cards
	performance indicators
	quality assessment and assurance
Legal contracts	personal service contracts
	purchase service agreements
	performance agreements
	partnerships
Accreditation and credentialing	regional and facility accreditation
	professional licensing
Complaints procedures	ombudsperson
	client representatives
	professional disciplinary committees
	litigation
Ethical judgments	implicit social standards
	individual conscience
	laws

Source: Shortt, S.E.D. & Macdonald, J.K. (2002). Toward an Accountability Framework for Canadian Healthcare. *Healthcare Management Forum,* 15(2): 30. Reprinted with Permission.

The province of Ontario introduced Bill 8, the Commitment to the Future of Medicare Act, in November 2003. This bill was designed to create clear accountability and governance mechanisms between the Ministry of Health and Long-Term Care and health care providers. The hospital boards were made accountable through accountability agreements, and the hospital CEOs were made accountable for the effective and efficient management of the hospitals (Chester, Quigley, & Scott, 2004). Hospitals and the Ministry of Health and Long-Term Care differed in their opinions of Sections 26 and 27 of the bill. Those sections proposed that CEO compensation could be rolled back under certain undefined conditions, a power that was to be used only under exceptional circumstances. The accountability agreements complemented the powers of the minister of health and long-term care that then existed in the Public Hospitals Act. The bill reinforced corporate governance and structures to promote accountability by putting reliance on the accountability chain rather than bypassing it through Sections 26 and 27 (Chester et al., 2004) (see Figure 2-2).

On June 3, 2010, Ontario passed health care accountability legislation: Bill 46, the Excellent Care for All Act, 2010. The Act makes health care providers and executives accountable for improving client care and enhancing the client experience. Although aimed at the hospital sector specifically, the Ontario government indicated these requirements may be extended to other health sectors as well. The Ministry of Health in British Columbia has signed performance agreements with the six health authorities that hold them accountable for the delivery of client care, health outcomes, and how health dollars are spent. Newfoundland and Labrador's health minister, Jerome Kennedy, in a CBC News clip on March 11, 2010 warned health care managers that they could be fired if they failed to live up to new accountability standards. The province of Saskatchewan has an accountability document that sets out the ministry's expectations of regions for the funding that is provided – both high level governance and directional expectations and program specific expectations for the regions. Manitoba's document, Achieving Health System Accountability 2009: Getting There Together, defined accountability, the accountability process (establish expectations; measure, monitor, and report; and evaluation and feedback), and the relationships in their health system.

Accountability is still a work in progress that is evolving rapidly, and there is growing acceptance of accountability by individuals who have authority. It is important that not only health care but also all jurisdictions demonstrate accountability. For an illustration of accountability in the Canadian health care system, see Figure 2-3. See Figure 2-4 for the Accountability Model for the Health System in Manitoba, and Figure 2-5 for the Accountability Framework for the Health System of Manitoba.

FUNCTIONS OF THE HEALTH CARE SYSTEM

Three functions of the health care system were mentioned briefly in Chapter 1: financing, funding, and delivery.

The **financing** of the system refers to how health care is paid for. Because the Canadian health care system is government financed, most money is raised in the form of taxes, including income taxes and federal and provincial sales taxes. The federal government transfers funds to the provincial and territorial governments to assist them to fund health care in the provinces and territories. In addition, equalization payments (i.e., cash transfers) are made to the provinces from the federal government so that the less wealthy Canadian provinces have the ability to deliver government services. These payments are unconditional, which means that the receiving provinces are able to spend the funds on public services according to their own priorities (Hibberd & Smith, 2006, p. 32)

Some Canadians and their employers pay insurance premiums to a private insurer, such as Blue Cross. Canadians can also pay directly out-of-pocket to the health care provider. Figure 2-6 shows the financial flows of the Canadian health care system.

The **funding** function of the health care system refers to the way provincial and territorial health plans pay the provider of care. The main form of funding for physicians has been **fee-for-service** (FFS). Physicians are paid separately for each service they provide. Hospitals have been funded on the basis of a global budget, which

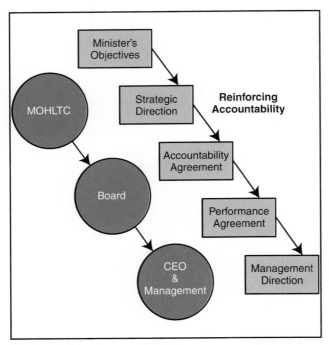

Figure 2-2 Reinforcement of Proper Relationships by Accountability Structures (Bill 8)
Source: Chester, S., Quigley, M., & Scott, G. (2004). Bill 8: Accountability and Control. *Healthcare Quarterly*, 7(3): 67. Reprinted with Permission.

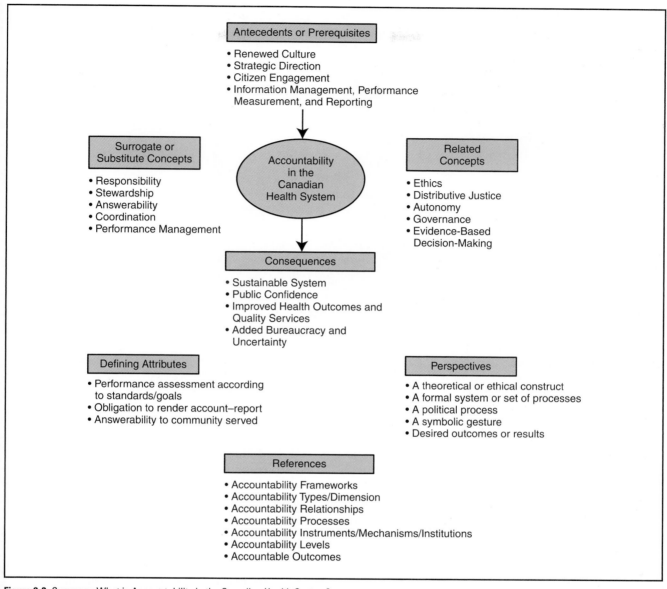

Figure 2-3 Summary: What is Accountability in the Canadian Health System?
Source: Penney, C. (2004). Understanding Accountability in the Canadian Health System. *Healthcare Management Forum*, 17(2): 10. Reprinted with Permission.

is a lump-sum payment given to the hospital, based on the number and types of cases they treat (i.e., case mix groups) or their number of client days. Public health is funded by a budget, but home care and nursing home care are funded on a fee-for-service basis or by fees per day (Hibberd & Smith, 2006, p. 33). Since global budgets are largely based on prior budgets, there is a risk of perpetuating historical inequities or inefficiencies and cultural spending norms within hospitals (Canadian Health Services Research Foundation, 2010).

The **delivery** function refers to the method used to provide health care to the public. Each delivery method has operated more or less separately. For example, most

health facilities have their own boards of directors, and physicians function independently, often as private entities similar to businesses. Although hospitals are mostly not-for-profit, some long-term care facilities operate for profit. Client prescriptions are ordered by physicians, but are funded by private insurance or by out-of-pocket expenses.

HEALTH CARE FINANCE REFORM

Neither Kirby nor Romanow suggests changing the basic funding structure that pays for medically necessary hospital and doctor services. User fees and co-payments were still against the principles of the 1984 Canada Health Act.

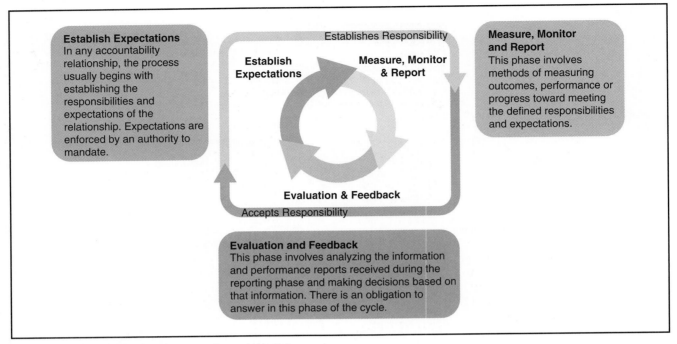

Establish Expectations
In any accountability relationship, the process usually begins with establishing the responsibilities and expectations of the relationship. Expectations are enforced by an authority to mandate.

Measure, Monitor and Report
This phase involves methods of measuring outcomes, performance or progress toward meeting the defined responsibilities and expectations.

Evaluation and Feedback
This phase involves analyzing the information and performance reports received during the reporting phase and making decisions based on that information. There is an obligation to answer in this phase of the cycle.

Figure 2-4 Accountability Model for the Health System in Manitoba
Source: Manitoba Health and Healthy Living Accountability Support Branch. (2009). *Achieving Health System Accountability 2009: Getting There Together. Manitoba:* Winnipeg. Retrieved from http://www.gov.mb.ca/health/rha/docs/ahsa2009.pdf, March 20, 2011. Permission to reproduce this figure is provided by the Queen's Printer for Manitoba. The Queen's Printer does not warrant the accuracy or currency of the reproduction of this information.

However, finance reform is currently being considered in a number of ways. Some procedures previously covered by health insurance are no longer covered; for example, some provinces no longer cover the cost of circumcision or routine eye exams for a percentage of the population. These de-insured services are no longer considered necessary. Variations also exist in the services that are insured from province to province.

FUNDING HEALTH REFORM

Physician remuneration is the second largest component of public sector health expenditures in Canada. Hospital services are the largest. According to the 2007 National Physician Survey, about half of the family physicians would like to change the way they are compensated. The majority of physicians receive their income from fee-for-service payments. However, the past 10 years has seen a shift towards alternative payment schemes (Devlin, Sarma, & Hogg, 2006). Data from the Canadian Institute for Health Information (CIHI) show that in 2004–05 roughly 80 percent of payments to family physicians were fee for service, whereas 20 percent were alternative payments (Wranik & Durier-Copp, 2009). Determining how physicians should be remunerated is not easy. For example, how many minutes should be allocated by a physician to assess a client's condition? How much time does the client think the physician should spend in conversation? Is the social nature of the client's situation important? Does it have an impact on the physical state the client presents? Both the physician and the client have different perspectives and different pieces of information that may affect the treatment being considered. What is the right balance, and how much money should be paid? The client and the government are unable to determine the appropriate quantity and quality of care for a particular condition, and must rely on the physician's advice (Devlin et al., 2006). Physician payment schemes provide a powerful tool to align the preferences of physicians, clients, and insurers (i.e., the government) to produce the best possible health outcomes (Devlin et al., 2006). Figure 2-7 depicts how government choices affect decisions made by physicians, which in turn, influence clients' (patients') choices.

Physician remuneration in Canada has four main models: fee-for-service, **capitation**, salary, and blended payments. In the fee-for-service (FFS) model, physicians are paid for each unit of service provided to clients. Physicians are able to deliver more services if they reduce the length of time for their consultations. Fee-for-service payments lead to higher use of primary care services than do other forms of physician payment. Devlin et al. (2006) state that health care utilization, defined as per-capita consultations, is higher with FFS than with either capitation or a **blended payment scheme**.

Most provinces fund regions through a global budget. Annually, each region submits a plan that articulates how it will meet the health needs of its residents.

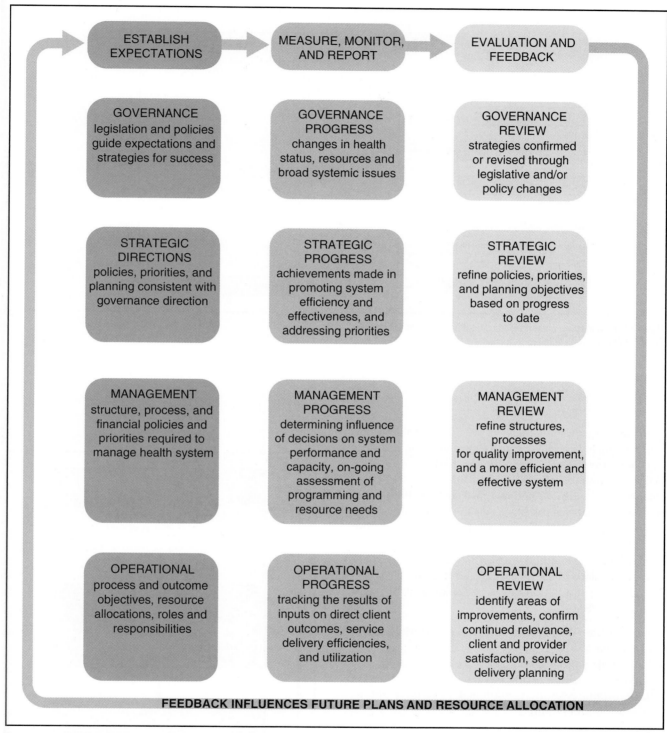

ESTABLISH EXPECTATIONS → **MEASURE, MONITOR, AND REPORT** → **EVALUATION AND FEEDBACK**

GOVERNANCE
legislation and policies guide expectations and strategies for success

GOVERNANCE PROGRESS
changes in health status, resources and broad systemic issues

GOVERNANCE REVIEW
strategies confirmed or revised through legislative and/or policy changes

STRATEGIC DIRECTIONS
policies, priorities, and planning consistent with governance direction

STRATEGIC PROGRESS
achievements made in promoting system efficiency and effectiveness, and addressing priorities

STRATEGIC REVIEW
refine policies, priorities, and planning objectives based on progress to date

MANAGEMENT
structure, process, and financial policies and priorities required to manage health system

MANAGEMENT PROGRESS
determining influence of decisions on system performance and capacity, on-going assessment of programming and resource needs

MANAGEMENT REVIEW
refine structures, processes for quality improvement, and a more efficient and effective system

OPERATIONAL
process and outcome objectives, resource allocations, roles and responsibilities

OPERATIONAL PROGRESS
tracking the results of inputs on direct client outcomes, service delivery efficiencies, and utilization

OPERATIONAL REVIEW
identify areas of improvements, confirm continued relevance, client and provider satisfaction, service delivery planning

FEEDBACK INFLUENCES FUTURE PLANS AND RESOURCE ALLOCATION

Figure 2-5 Accountability Framework for the Health System of Manitoba
Source: Manitoba Health and Healthy Living Accountability Support Branch. (2009). *Achieving Health System Accountability 2009: Getting There Together.* Manitoba: Winnipeg. Retrieved from http://www.gov.mb.ca/health/rha/docs/ahsa2009.pdf, March 20, 2011. The Queen's Printer does not warrant the accuracy or currency of the reproduction of this information.

The resource requirements and performance evaluation measures are also included. Minor revisions are usually made from year to year. According to Hurley (2004), almost all provinces had declared their intent to develop a needs-based funding formula for allocating the budget to regional health authorities. Ontario, Alberta, Saskatchewan, and British Columbia have all adopted such a formula for home care and community support services.

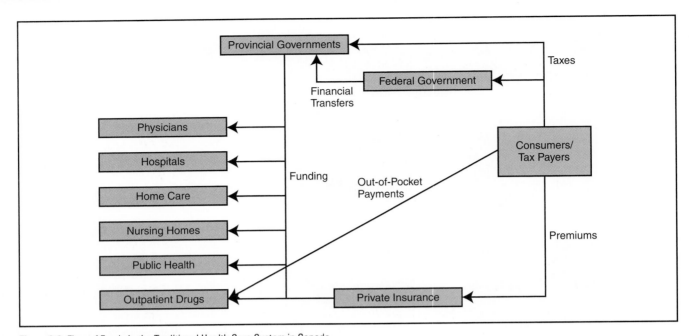

Figure 2-6 Flow of Funds in the Traditional Health Care System in Canada
Source: From Judith M. Hibberd & Donna Lynn Smith, *Nursing Leadership and Management in Canada, 3rd edition* (Figure 2.2 from p. 32). Copyright ©
Elesevier Canada, a division of Reed Elsevier Canada, Ltd. All rights reserved. Reprinted by permission of Elsevier Canada, 2011.

Many organizational leaders are aware of the importance of including physicians as managers, or if not as managers, then at least as contributors to their governance activities. However, Harrison and Mitton (2004) believe that **program budgeting and marginal analysis** (PBMA) is a mechanism that can link physicians to organizational decision-making processes. Physicians' knowledge and expertise in client care make their input into organizational processes imperative. These authors highlighted the Alberta experience, particularly in the Calgary Health Region.

Harrison and Mitton (2004, p. 22) identify the stages involved in PBMA:

1. Determine the aim and scope of the priority setting exercise.
2. Compile a program budget.
3. Form a stakeholder advisory panel.
4. Determine relevant decision-making criteria and consultation required.
5. Advisory panel identifies options for service growth, resource release for producing the same outcome with fewer resources, or resource release through scaling back or stopping some services.
6. Advisory panel recommends funding growth areas with new resources, decisions to move resources from one area to another, or to trade-off decisions to move resources to another service if proof is demonstrated.
7. Use evidence from a variety of sources to make final decisions to inform budget planning process.

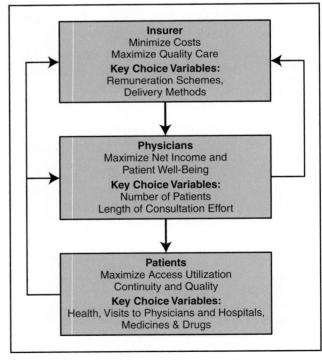

Figure 2-7 Interactions among the Key Players in the Canadian Health Care System
Source: Devlin, R.A., Sarma, S. & Hogg, W. (2006). Remunerating Primary Care Physicians: Emerging Directions and Policy Options for Canada. *Healthcare Quarterly,* 9(3): 36. Reprinted with Permission.

REAL WORLD INTERVIEW

I accompanied my mother to her doctor's appointment. She asked me to advocate on her behalf because her physician had told her that she could only ask him about one issue at each visit. On this particular day, she had two issues and was worried that she would have to visit the doctor again in the near future. When I arrived at the physician's office, a sign in the waiting room confirmed my mother's concern. The sign stated that only one issue could be discussed with the doctor per visit. I accompanied my mother into the doctor's office, and he told us that she would need to decide which issue was the priority. I was mortified!

Helen Salter, RN

CRITICAL THINKING

Is the physician practice appropriate? Should it be different for the young and for the elderly?

Given the circumstances in this example, what would you have done?

LITERATURE APPLICATION

Citation: Sarre-McGregor, D., & Knoefel, F. D. (2005). Lessons learned: The implementation of an alternative funding plan at SCO Health Service in Ottawa. *Healthcare Management Forum, 18*(4), 46–49.

Discussion: The authors describe the Alternative Funding Plan agreement that the physicians of SCO Health Service, in Ottawa, entered into with the Ministry of Health and Long-Term Care. The negotiation and process for establishing the plan are described. Lessons learned are also outlined.

Implications: Physicians have supported the concept and will probably renew the contract when it expires in 2006. Others may wish to take advantage of a similar scheme or adapt the process used in this example.

LITERATURE APPLICATION

Citation: Wranik, D. W., & Durier-Copp, M. (2009). Physician Remuneration Methods for Family Physicians in Canada: Expected Outcomes and Lessons Learned. *Health Care Annal*, retrieved from http://www.bing.com/search?q=physician+remuneration+methods+for+family+physicians+in+canada++expected+outcomes+and+lesson+learned&src=IE-SearchBox, April 11, 2011.

Discussion: A series of qualitative interviews were held with 27 stakeholders in the Canadian health care system to assess the reasons and expectations behind the implementation of payment methods for family physicians.

Implications: Blended payments have had some positive effects on preventive care delivery, collaboration, and care continuity. Salaries have provided a stable, predictable, and high source of income for physicians, thereby improving recruitment and retention. The implementation of salaries has led to concerns about declining physician productivity and brought to light the need for improved measurement and monitoring systems.

The PMBA approach was successful in six of the seven examples cited in the study. The case studies included urban, regional, and rural centres with pediatric, medical surgical, and acute and chronic care populations. Physician involvement in this budgeting process highlighted the importance of including both medical and managerial representatives in the process. The participants thought they would not have been as successful if the physicians had not been involved. Also noted was the improvement in communication among the medical groups with managers. This PBMA approach to budgeting can be used even if the relationship between the region and the physicians is not aligned. The studies reinforced the idea that if managers ask physicians for their opinion, the managers must be prepared to listen. In addition, the physicians learned more about resource allocation and the impact of shifts in resources on the client population being served. With this type of budgeting, physicians can contribute to their health care organizations in ways that use their clinical expertise but don't require them to give up their clinical practice.

LITERATURE APPLICATION

Citation: O'Neill, M. L., & Downer, P. (2004). Change readiness for SAP in the Canadian healthcare system. *Healthcare Management Forum,* 17(1), 18–25.

Discussion: The study described in this article contributes to the literature that assesses whether the Canadian health care system is ready to embrace the idea of e-business cost management systems. One hundred fifty-four Canadian chief executive officers were surveyed to determine change readiness. A deductive design methodology was used. Although the majority of the CEOs had no e-business cost management system experience, the majority were interested in the concept. Change readiness was found to affect system implementation significantly.

Implications: More information is required as the Canadian health care system considers e-business cost management implementation. The authors of this study recommend that consideration be given to the development of national performance indicators in this area.

In this era of increased efficiency, it is important for Canada's health care organizations to understand the costs associated with client care. Many Canadian hospitals are meeting their need for client-specific financial information by using costs based on resource intensity weights (RIWs), which are calculated by the Canadian Institute of Health Information (CIHI), instead of using an in-house case-costing system.

Activity-based costing (ABC) has been recommended as a way to achieve better management accounting information in health care. **Case-costing** systems provide a way to operationalize the ABC concepts. However, because of the expense involved, many hospitals have opted to use the RIW costs. Activity-based costing was developed to improve the way indirect costs were assigned to hospital departments (e.g., how does one assign the costs of the human resources department to the emergency department?). The traditional client-accounting system allocated the costs of the human resources department equally to all direct care departments. In activity-based costing, however, the costs of human resources are shared by the direct care departments, based on either the department's square footage or its number of employees. The ABC approach, therefore, required increased definition and specificity, such as types and cost of supplies per procedure. The Guidelines for Management Information Systems in Canadian Health Service Organizations (MIS Guidelines) specify the use of simultaneous equations for hospital costing systems. This is because that method meets the theoretical requirement of accounting for the services that indirect departments provide to each other (Borsa & Anis, 2005, p. 21).

Borsa and Anis (2005) compared resource intensity weight costs at St. Paul's Hospital in British Columbia with case costs for selected client groups. They found that average case costs for surgical clients were 23.9 percent higher than their resource intensity weight costs, but the case costs for non-surgical clients were 14.8 percent lower. Average case costs for clients receiving surgical implants were 32.8 percent higher than the resource intensity weight costs. For clients receiving internal defibrillators, average case costs were three times higher.

Borsa and Anis (2005) conclude that the national RIW assignment process in Canada has the potential to provide valuable information for resource benchmarking and provincial funding, but the results of their analysis suggest that further work is needed in order to align the measures with actual resource consumption.

The **Health-Based Allocation Model** (HBAM) is a new, made-in-Ontario, funding methodology that is based on direct measures of health status, and takes into account both population and provider-based factors. The HBAM, which estimates the shares in the available funding in the system that go to the LHIN and the health service provider, has two components: the utilization model and the cost model. The utilization model estimates the annual health requirements of each Ontario resident, taking into account social, clinical (disease and health status), and demographic conditions. The unit cost model considers the unit costs for each health service provider, taking into account recognized provider characteristics, such as teaching activity, that justifiably lead to higher unit costs.

The population-based funding model for Regional Health Authorities was implemented in Alberta for the 1997–98 fiscal year, and was fully implemented by 1999–2000. It remains in place today. At the time of writing this chapter, it was unknown what impact the restructuring of Alberta Health Services with one Board would have on the population-based funding model.

DELIVERY HEALTH REFORM

The main type of reform referred to here is privatization. Much debate and confusion surrounds public–private partnerships in Canada. Romanow didn't recommend any changes to the tax-based funding source for Canada Health Act services. Kirby put forward some ideas concerning user fees and private insurance, but his final report rejected anything other than tax-based methods to fund Canada Health Act services. Marchildon (2004) suggested that the question is really whether private for-profit delivery should replace private not-for-profit or public arm's-length delivery in three situations. The first situation he described relates to the contracting out of ancillary services, such as food and laundry services, to existing private, for-profit services. The second context concerns the role of public–private partnerships (P3s) in the building of new health facilities; in the United Kingdom these partnerships are known as private finance initiatives (PFIs).

The possibility of private delivery of advanced diagnostic services by First Nations on urban reserves or reserves near large urban centres has raised a third private-delivery issue. Because provincial laws and regulations have no jurisdiction on reserves, the potential to have a parallel private-for-profit alternative to the public system exists. In addition, the legal status of the Canada Health Act on First Nations' territories is also questioned (Marchildon, 2004, p. 67).

Alberta has led the way with privately owned clinics and hospitals, but other provinces have also launched similar services. The April 13, 2006 newsweekly, *Health Edition*, reported that Québec has decided to implement public–private partnerships (P3s) to build two new multibillion-dollar hospitals in Montréal, but that the province is scaling down private sector involvement in order to maximize public control. In October 2007 the McGill University Health Centre and Québec government qualified two bidding consortia to participate in a PPP competition to build the entire Glen Campus, including the new adult facilities (Royal Victoria Hospital), Montréal Children's Hospital and research facilities. The tender did not include medical equipment or "soft" maintenance, such as hotel services. The Mountain Campus proceeded conventionally.[11] Ontario is also

using private capital as part of its $5 billion overhaul of health care infrastructure. Some 29 separate projects have been announced so far using "alternative financing and procurement" arrangements (Health Edition, 2006). Negotiations for P3 contracts can take up to two years to complete.

FUTURE PERSPECTIVE ON THE COST OF HEALTH CARE

Futurists are in demand to guide health care in organizing for success. Health care providers have been thrashing in chaos for nearly 20 years, reinventing their structures and processes, right-sizing their enterprises, outsourcing to better focus on their core business, and merging to share scarce or expensive resources. Despite some short-term cost savings and a slowdown in the rise in health care spending, several evolving trends keep the overall cost growing.

The need for highly complex and expensive technology, including microsurgery, continues to develop. New diseases that require expensive or long-term treatment, such as AIDS and Ebola, continue to emerge. With the eradication or successful management of selected

REAL WORLD INTERVIEW

An early focus for interest in public/private partnerships is the "P3" approach to facility construction and operation, and in this area we have had particular success. In the long-term sector, all our new facilities are being built and operated on an award-winning tendering and partnership model. We've opened nearly 300 beds in the past year and are planning another 1,000 beds by 2010. Projects are tendered on equal terms to public, voluntary, and for-profit operators. Operators are full partners in planning and designing their own facilities, instead of taking over buildings designed by the regions or government. They share in the capital costs and then receive standard formula-based operating funding from the region.

The result is that we've built twice as many beds as we could have on the old model. That has enabled us to cut the waiting list for long-term care to less than two months' average turnover, and cut the number of acute care beds blocked by patients awaiting placement by half in the past year. Just as important, we've seen a remarkable leap forward in the design of our facilities and the quality of life for residents. All our new facilities are designed on the aging-in-place model, coordinated with commercial housing, enabling a continuum of service levels and living environments according to need.

With our experience in long-term care, we're looking at the potential for P3s to deliver the same kinds of benefits in other areas.

Sheila Weatherill
former President and CEO Capital Health, Edmonton, Alberta

Source: Weatherill, S. (2004). Public/Private Pragmatism. *Healthcare Papers,* 4(4): 74–78. Reprinted with Permission.

REAL WORLD INTERVIEW

The age of "volume" as a measure of anything is long past. In health care, for so many years, the notion of unparalleled growth and expansion and anything for anyone was common. Subsequent introduction of broader concepts reflecting an understanding of value and sustainability now drive rational thinking about availability and delivery of health services. The issue of "value" now drives all elements of health service from access to delivery and, ultimately, to making a difference. Now we can more clearly enumerate the relationship between inputs and outcomes, process and product. Health services now must be able to establish the connection between what is done and what is achieved. Professions' addictions to what they do now give way to tightening the connection between what is done and what difference it makes. The noise for both nurses and physicians is a closer look by everyone at the "value" of action in the light of the promise it holds. The issue: either deliver, or rethink why you're doing what you're doing. This critical examination and expectation will radically alter the economics and values of health care for the next two decades.

Tim Porter-O'Grady, EdD, PhD, RN, FAAN
Prolific Nurse Author and Speaker on New-Edge Health Care

Source: Tim Porter-O'Grady, EdD, PHD, RN, FAAN; Prolific Nurse Author and Speaker on *New Edge Health Care.*

diseases, such as tuberculosis, populations are surviving longer. With lengthening survival rates come debilitating diseases of aging.

We look to futurists to help us make decisions about the business we ought to be prepared to provide. Will the Veterans Affairs hospitals go out of business when all the veterans with illness or injuries related to their military service and all the indigent veterans die? Will a few strategically located hospitals provide an intensive level of care only, while acute care is managed on an ambulatory basis without invasive procedures? Will preventive, primary, and restorative care be the purview of advanced nurse practitioners practising in community sites? Will the call for duty no longer be the basis for caring careers (Reverby, 2001)? Will nurses be ordered to care in a society that no longer values caring (Reverby, 1987)?

KEY CONCEPTS

- Health care economics is grounded in past values and culture. Nearly 150 years ago, Florence Nightingale recognized that the resources being used to care for sick people ought to be tracked and analyzed to improve clinical and business outcomes.

- In Canada the health care system has three main functions: financing, funding, and delivery. Reform is taking place in each of these areas.

- Most physicians wish to be remunerated in a way other than fee-for-service.

- All jurisdictions, including health care, need to demonstrate accountability.

- There is much debate about public–private partnerships.

KEY TERMS

accountability
altruism
blended payment schemes
capitation
case-costing
delivery
economics
egoism
ethics

fee-for-service
financing
funding
health-based allocation model (HBAM)
payer
program budgeting and marginal analysis (PBMA)

REVIEW QUESTIONS

1. Economics is the study of which of the following?
   A. the cost: quality interface
   B. cost accounting
   C. the cost of doing business
   D. how to manage scarce resources

2. Which of the following nurse leaders was not mentioned in this chapter as having a perspective on economics?
   A. Abdellah
   B. Chang
   C. Barton
   D. Henderson

REVIEW ACTIVITIES

1. Interview the chief financial officer of a health care organization to gain an understanding of how various costs are managed. Use the following questions to guide the interview:

   What method is used to measure nursing costs?

What level of confidence does financial services have in its accuracy, and why?

2. Consult a seasoned member of the medical staff of a health care organization. Ask for a personal perspective on any adjustments in practice that person made relating to cost and quality issues as his or her career unfolded. Compare and contrast what you discover to the experiences of a second medical staff person who has been in practice for only the past 10 years. What level of passion about the discussion was demonstrated by each interviewee? What did they view as their greatest challenge?

3. Explore with a chief nursing officer the most current challenging clinical economic issue for nursing in the organization and how it is being addressed.

EXPLORING THE WEB

What sites could you recommend to a colleague interested in tracking health care cost trends over time?

Go to the sites for the Institute of Health Economics and The Centre for Health and Policy Studies (CHAPS). How does the information differ on each site?

■ *http://www.ihe.ca*

■ *http://www.chaps.ucalgary.ca*

Go to the site for the Canadian Institute for Health Information (CIHI). What statistics does the site offer?

■ *http://www.cihi.ca.*

Go to a site designed for nurses, such as the Canadian Nurses Association. What type of information is available on the site? Is it relevant to cost or quality issues?

■ *http://www.cna-nurses.ca*

Search the following websites for information of interest to nurses:

■ *http://www.nurseone.ca/*

■ http://www.cna-aiic.ca/CNA/documents/pdf/publications/BG8_Social_Determinants_e.pdf

■ *http://www.rnao.org/Page.asp?PageID=861&SiteNodeID=133*

■ *http://www.cadth.ca/*

■ *http://www.gaiam.com/*

■ *http://www.coachorg.com/*

REFERENCES

Agnes, M. (2000). (Ed.). *Webster's new world collegiate dictionary* (4th ed.). Foster City, CA: IDG Books Worldwide.

Barer, M. L., Morgan, S. G., & Evans, R. G. (2003). Strangulation or rationalization: Costs and access in Canadian hospitals. *Long-woods Review,* 1(4), 10–19.

Borsa, J., & Anis, A. (2005). The cost of hospital care in Canada: A comparison of two alternatives. *Healthcare Management Forum,* 18(1), 19–27.

(British Columbia Government). (2008). British Columbia Health Authorities Performance Agreements. Retrieved from http://www.health.gov.bc.ca/socsec/performance.html

Brown, A. D., Porcellato, C., & Barnsley, J. (2006). Accountability: Unpacking the suitcase. *Healthcare Quarterly,* 9(3), 72–75.

Canadian Health Services Research Foundation. (2010). *Evidence-informed options for hospital funding. Are hospital funding mechanisms in Canada designed to provide efficient care?* Retrieved from http://www.chsrf.ca/Libraries/Hospital_Funding_docs/PolicyBrief_Hospital_Funding_ENG_Final.sflb.ashx

Canadian Institute for Health Information. (2010a). *A primer on activity-based funding. Discussion Paper: Activity-based funding unit.* Retrieved from http://www.ihe.ca/documents/A%20Primer%20on%20Activity-Based%20Funding%20_web.pdf

Canadian Institute for Health Information. (2010b). Choice of a case mix system for use in acute care activity-based funding—options and considerations. Discussion Paper: Activity-based funding unit. Retrieved from http://www.cihi.ca/CIHI-ext-portal/pdf/internet/case_mix_system_for_use_en

Canadian Institute for Health Information. (2010c). *Health Care in Canada 2010.* Ottawa: Author.

CBC News. (2010). Health Minister puts managers on notice—Newfoundland and Labrador. Retrieved from http://www.cbc.ca/news/canada/newfoundland-labrador/story/2010/03/11/kennedy-health-warning-311.html

Chang, C., Price, S., & Pfoutz, S. (2001). *Economics and nursing: Critical professional issues.* Philadelphia: F. A. Davis.

Chester, S., Quigley, M., & Scott, G. (2004). Bill 8: Accountability and control. *Healthcare Quarterly,* 7(3), 66–68.

Commission d'étude sur les services de santé et les services sociaux. (2000). *Emerging solutions: Report and recommendations.* Québec: Author. Chair: Michel Clair.

Commission on the Future of Health Care in Canada. 2002. *Building on values: The future of health care in Canada.* Saskatoon: Author. Commissioner: Roy J. Romanow.

Devlin, R. A., & Sarma, S. (2008). Do physician remuneration schemes matter? The case of Canadian family physicians. *Journal of Health Economics,* 17(5), 1168–1181.

Devlin, R. A., Sarma, S., & Hogg, W. (2006). Remunerating primary care physicians: Emerging directions and policy options for Canada. *Healthcare Quarterly,* 9(3), 34–42.

Esmail, N., & Walker, M. (2008). *How good is Canadian health care? 2008 report: An international comparison of health care systems.* Vancouver: The Fraser Institute.

Government of Ontario. (2010). *Ontario's health-based allocation model (HBAM) overview.* Retrieved from http://www.waterloowellingtonlhin.on.ca/uploadedFiles/HBAMOverview.pdf

Government of Saskatchewan. (2011). Regional Health Governance. Accountability. Regina: Author. Retrieved from http://www.health.gove.sk.ca/accountability

Harrison, A., & Mitton, C. (2004). Physician involvement in setting priorities for health regions. *Healthcare Management Forum, 17*(4), 21–27.

Health Edition. (2006, March 31.) Quebec embracing P3s for new hospital projects. *Health Edition, 10*(13).

Hibberd, J. M., & Smith, D. L. (2006). *Nursing leadership and management in Canada* (3rd ed.). Toronto: Elsevier Mosby.

Hurley, J. (2004). Regionalization and the allocation of healthcare resources to meet population health needs. *Healthcare Papers, 5*(1), 34–39.

Manitoba Health and Healthy Living. (2009). *Achieving health system accountability 2009. Getting there together.* Manitoba: Author. Retrieved from *www.gov.mb.ca/health/rha/docs/ahsa2009.pdf*

Marchildon, G. P. (2004). The public/private debate in the funding, administration and delivery of healthcare in Canada. *Healthcare Papers, 4*(4), 61–68.

O'Neill, M. L., & Downer, P. (2004). Change readiness for SAP in the Canadian healthcare system. *Healthcare Management Forum, 17*(1), 18–25.

Ontario Health Services Restructuring Commission. (2000). *Looking back, looking forward: A legacy report.* Toronto: Author.

Penney, C. (2004). Understanding accountability in the Canadian health system. *Healthcare Management Forum, 17*(2), 9–15.

Premier's Advisory Council on Health. (2001). *A framework for reform: Report of the premier's advisory council on health.* Edmonton: Author. Chair: Donald Mazankowski.

Reverby, S. (1987). *Ordered to care: The dilemma of American nursing, 1850–1945.* New York: Cambridge.

Reverby, S. (2001). A caring dilemma: Womanhood and nursing in historical perspective. In E. Hein (Ed.), *Nursing issues in the 21st century: Perspectives from the literature.* Philadelphia: Lippincott.

Ross-Kerr, J., & Wood, M. J. (2003). *Canadian nursing issues and perspectives* (4th ed.). Toronto, Philadelphia, London, New York, St. Louis, Sydney: Mosby.

Saskatchewan Standing Committee on Health Care. (2001). *Caring for Medicare: Sustaining a quality system: Final report of the Commission on Medicare.* Regina: Author. Chair: Ken Fyke.

Shortt, S. E. D., & Macdonald, J. K. (2002). Toward an accountability framework for Canadian healthcare. *Healthcare Management Forum, 15*(2), 24–32.

Smith, N., & Church, J. (2008). Shifting the lens: The introduction of population-based funding in Alberta. *Healthcare Management Forum, Summer,* 36–42.

Standing Committee on Social Affairs, Science and Technology. (2002). *Reforming health protection and promotion in Canada: Time to act.* Ottawa: Author. Chair: Michael Kirby.

Weatherill, S. (2004). Public/private pragmatism. *Healthcare Papers, 4*(4), 74–78.

Wranik, D. W., & Durier-Copp, M. (2009). Physician remuneration methods for family physicians in Canada: Expected outcomes and lessons learned. *Health Care Analysis.* doi: 10.1007/s10729-008-0105-9. Retrieved from http://toolkit.cfpc.ca/en/files/wranik.pdf

SUGGESTED READINGS

Bégin, M. (2004). Public/private boundaries in Canadian healthcare: Some clarification. *Healthcare Papers, 4*(4), 35–40.

Chodos, H., & MacLeod, J. J. (2004). Romanow and Kirby on the public/private divide in healthcare: Demystifying the debate. *Healthcare Papers, 4*(4), 10–25.

Christensen, C., Bohmer, R., & Kenagy, J. (2000, September/October). Will disruptive innovations cure health care? *Harvard Business Review,* 102–112, 199.

Christman, L. (2001). The future of the nursing profession. In E. Hein (Ed.), *Nursing issues in the 21st century: Perspectives from the literature.* Philadelphia: Lippincott.

Copeland, T. (2001, September/October). Cutting costs without drawing blood. *Harvard Business Review,* 155–156, 159–160, 162, 164.

Deber, R., Lam, K. C. K., Roos, N., Walld, R., Finlayson, G. S., & Roos, L. (2008). Canadian healthcare: Need and utilization in an almost-universal system. *Harvard Health Policy Review, 9*(1), 46–55.

Feldstein, P. (1993). *Health care economics* (5th ed.). Clifton Park, NY: Delmar Learning.

Finkler, S. (2001). *Budgeting concepts for nurse managers* (3rd ed.). Philadelphia: Saunders.

Finkler, S., & Kovner, C. (2000). *Financial management for nurse managers and executives* (2nd ed.). Philadelphia: Saunders.

Friedman, E. (2001). Managed care devils, angels, and the truth in between. In E. Hein (Ed.), *Nursing issues in the 21st century: Perspectives from the literature.* Philadelphia: Lippincott.

Fuller, R. L., McCullough, E. C., Bao, M. Z., & Averill, R. F. (2009). Estimating the costs of potentially preventable hospital acquired complications. *Health Care Financing Review, 30*(4), 17–32.

Gillani, A., Jarvi, K., & De Angelis, A. (2005). Fostering a culture of accountability through a performance appraisal system. *Healthcare Management Forum, 18*(1), 35–38.

Hackbarth, G., Reischauer, R., & Mutti, A. (2008). Collective accountability for medical care – toward bundled payments. *New England Journal of Medicine, 359*(1), 3–5.

Hein, E. (2001). *Nursing issues in the 21st century: Perspectives from the literature.* Philadelphia: Lippincott.

Hoppszallern, S. (2001, January). 2001 benchmarking guide. *Hospitals and Health Networks,* 43–50.

Kantarevic, J., Kralj, B., & Weinkauf, D. (2011). Enhanced fee-for-service model and enhanced physician productivity: Evidence from family health groups in Ontario. *Journal of Health Economics, 30*(1), 99–111.

Kenny, N. (2004). Value(s) for money? Assessing Romanow and Kirby. *Healthcare Papers, 4*(4), 28–34.

McAllister, J. (2010). A better way of funding hospitals. *Canadian Healthcare Manager. January–February,* 17–21.

McCullough, C. (2001). *Creating responsive solutions to healthcare change.* Indianapolis, IN: Sigma Theta Tau International.

McGowan, T. (2004). Does the private sector have a role in Canadian healthcare? *Healthcare Papers,* 4(4), 45–50.

McLean, R. (1997). *Financial management in health care.* Clifton Park, NY: Delmar Learning.

Mor, V., Intrator, O., Feng, Z., & Grabowski, D. C. (2010). The revolving door of rehospitalisation from skilled nursing facilities. *Health Affairs* 29(1): 57–64.

Philpott, T. G. (2007). Public-private partnerships: A Canadian hospital's perspective. *Healthcare Management Forum. Winter,* 33–36.

Pink, G. H., Brown, A. D., Daniel, I., Hamlette, M. L., Markel, F., McGillis Hall, L., et al. (2006). Financial benchmarks for Ontario hospitals. *Healthcare Quarterly,* 9(1), 40–45.

Rachlis, M. M. (2005). Medicare: Innovation is the key to sustainability? *Healthcare Management Forum,* 18(1), 28–31.

Rachlis, M. M. (2008). Health equity and Ontario's health-based allocation model. Wellesley Institute. Retrieved from http://wellesleyinstitute.com/files/healthequity/healthequityhbam.pdf

Rowland, H., & Rowland, B. (1997). *Nursing administration handbook* (4th ed.). Gaithersburg, MD: Aspen.

Sarre-McGregor, D., & Knoefel, F. D. (2005). Lessons learned: The implementation of an alternative funding plan at SCO Health Service in Ottawa. *Healthcare Management Forum,* 18(4), 46–49.

Savage, G., Hoelscher, M., & Walker, E. (1999). International health care: A comparison of the United States, Canada, and Western Europe. In L. Wolper (Ed.), *Health care administration: Planning, implementing, and managing organized delivery systems* (3rd ed.). Gaithersburg, MD: Aspen.

Senge, P. M. (2006). *The fifth discipline: The art & practice of the learning organization.* Toronto: Doubleday.

Shamian, J., & Lightstone, E. (1997). Hospital restructuring initiatives in Canada. *Medical Care,* 35(10), OS62–OS69.

Statistics Canada. (2010). *Canada year book 2010.* Ottawa: Author.

Taylor, W. (2003). 2020 healthcare management in Canada: A new model home next door. *Healthcare Management Forum,* 16(1), 6–10.

Vertesi, L. (2004). Romanow versus Kirby: Resolving the differences. *Healthcare Papers,* 4(4), 41–44.

vos Savant, M. (2001, May 6). Ask Marilyn. *Parade,* 26.

Werle, J., Dobbelsteyn, L., Feasel, A. L., Hancock, B., Job, B., Makar, L., et al. (2010). A study of the effectiveness of performance-focused methodology for improved outcomes in Alberta public healthcare. *Healthcare Management Forum, Winter,* 169–174.

CHAPTER ENDNOTES

1. Institute of Health Economics, "Mission Statement." Retrieved from http://www.ihe.ca

2. Human Resources and Skills Development Canada, "Health-Life Expectancy at Birth, Summary." Retrieved from http://www4.hrsdc.gc.ca/.3ndic.1t.4r@-eng.jsp?iid=3

3. Canadian Institute for Health Information (CIHI). (2010c). Health Care in Canada 2010. Ottawa: Author. p. 93.

4. Ibid.

5. Commission on the Future of Health Care in Canada. (2002). *Building on values: The future of health care in Canada.* Saskatoon: Author. Commissioner: Roy J. Romanow.

6. CIHI, 2010c, p. 92.

7. Ibid., p. 94.

8. Esmail, N., & Walker, M. (2008). *How good is Canadian health care? 2008 report: an international comparison of health care systems,* p. 85. Vancouver: Fraser Institute.

9. Ibid.

10. Health Canada. "2003 First Ministers Health Accord." Retrieved from http://www.hc-sc.gc.ca/hcs-sss/delivery-prestation/fptcollab/2003accord/fs-if_1-eng.php

11. Philpott, T. G. (2007). Public-private partnerships: A Canadian hospital's perspective. *Healthcare Management Forum, Winter,* 33–36.

UNIT II
A New Health Care Model

CHAPTER
3

Evidence-Based Practice

Rinda Alexander, PhD, RN, CS
Adapted by Victoria E. Pennick, RN, MHSc

Evidence-based practice is the integration of best research evidence with clinical expertise and patient values to facilitate clinical decision making.[1]

OBJECTIVES

The purpose of this chapter is to enable the reader to

- understand the history of evidence-based practice in nursing;
- discuss the importance of evidence-based practice;
- identify terminology used in research and evidence-based practice;
- understand the issues that stimulated the development of an evidence-based practice model for health care delivery;
- understand the steps used in evidence-based practice processes; and
- understand the roles of Canadian organizations in the funding, creation, and dissemination of research to inform evidence-based decision making at the individual, organizational, and policy levels.

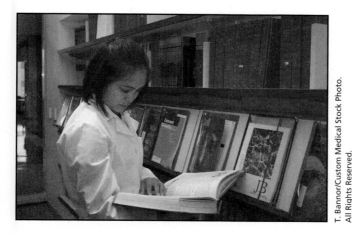

You are at the Nurses' Week luncheon at your institution. Your unit manager and the nursing director to whom she reports stop to chat with you. They tell you that they have recently attended the Nursing Leadership conference at which some of them discussed Janet Squire's (Squires, 2011) recently updated systematic review on determinants of RN utilization of research. They also wonder how the nurses in our facility measure up. During your last performance review, you indicated that you were interested in learning more about research and how it may impact your practice. So they are wondering if you are interested in representing your unit on the newly formed nursing journal club.

Nursing journal clubs are becoming more common in health care institutions as managers of care explore new ways to engage nurses in evidence-based practice and improve the quality of care.

What do you know about evidence-based practice?

As the staff nurse, how will you prepare yourself for this task?

As the manager, how will you facilitate the success of the journal club?

Nurses represent the largest group of health care personnel, and it is widely accepted that they are the coordinators of care. However, as health care continues to evolve, nurses must consider innovative ways to deliver more effective and efficient interventions. In fact, there is not a greater challenge for nursing than to ensure that nurses have the competencies needed for health care delivery in the 21st century. Nursing leaders at all levels are particularly well positioned to ensure that health care organizations have resources and processes in place that enable professional nurses to meet new challenges in the clinical delivery of care. Evidence-based decision making is an important element of quality care in all domains of nursing practice. It is essential to optimize outcomes for clients, improve clinical practice, achieve cost-effective nursing care, and ensure accountability and transparency in decision making (Canadian Nurses Association, 2002). The purpose of this chapter is to discuss the importance of evidence-based practice

to both clients and nursing and to define what constitutes evidence for clinical practice. Evidence-based decision making is here to stay—at least for the foreseeable future. The future of health care demands the use of sophisticated evidence-based tools to deliver care and to measure outcomes of care. Nurses must be proficient in balancing a scientific process driven by evidence-based standards and practice guidelines with continuing quality improvement initiatives. Are they different concepts or different expressions of providing quality care along the same continuum?

HISTORY OF EVIDENCE-BASED PRACTICE

The evidence-based movement began with medicine. The term **evidence-based medicine** was coined during the 1980s at McMaster University's Michael G. DeGroote School of Medicine, in Hamilton, Ontario. It referred to a clinical learning strategy that had been in use at McMaster University since the 1970s (Evidence-Based Medicine Working Group, 1992). David Sackett, well known in the evidence-based medicine movement, and his Oxford colleagues encouraged the practice of evidence-based medicine to integrate individual clinical medical experience with external clinical evidence using systematic research. Sackett and his colleagues defined evidence-based medicine as the "conscientious, explicit, and judicious use of current best evidence in making decisions about the care of individual patients" (Sackett, Rosenberg, Gray, Haynes, & Richardson, 1996, p. 71). Evidence-based medicine integrates the clinical expertise of individual clinicians with the best available external clinical evidence from systematic research into the accuracy and precision of diagnostic tests; the clinical examination; and other elements of the therapeutic, rehabilitative, and preventive regimens prescribed for clients.

But health care decision making extends beyond medicine. Before long, the more encompassing and neutral term **evidence-based practice** was coined. This form of practice incorporated evidence-based medicine with **evidence-based care**. The result was a blend of the beliefs, values, and attitudes of clients, families, and practitioners with the most current knowledge of the incidence and prevalence of the particular health care problem at hand and an understanding of the organization and delivery of health care (Silagy & Haines, 1998). Evidence-based clinical decision making should incorporate consideration of the client's clinical state, the clinical setting, and the clinical circumstances (DiCenso, Guyatt, & Ciliska, 2004). In Canada there are different health care systems in each provincial and territorial jurisdiction, each representing

Q. Can you give me an example of a clinical situation where you used evidence to inform your practice?

A. Drug use is an example. Is sublingual Fentanyl really superior to Dilaudid for prior-to-care comfort or is there value in the longer lasting effect of Dilaudid? Wound care is more straight-forward. There is good research with objective outcomes that are measurable.

Q. Where do you go to find evidence?

A. Almost every week, someone has read, or heard of, a procedure or new way of using a drug (off label). Most of our decisions regarding client care are informed by College standards, RNAO Nursing Best Practice Guidelines, organizational policy and procedures, and a constant stream of research articles — quantitative and qualitative primarily, but often expert opinion (popular content experts) and anecdotal.

Margaret Lynn Furman, RN
Staff Nurse, Palliative Care

Source: Margaret Lynn Furman

vast areas with scant populations, large urban areas, and the most heterogeneous population in the world. Client expectations and available resources vary widely from setting to setting. Guidelines and care plans, which are based on the best current evidence and developed with local values and resources in mind, help nurses to incorporate evidence into their practice.

IMPORTANCE OF EVIDENCE-BASED PRACTICE

Nothing is more important to clients and professional nurses than evidence-based clinical interventions that can be linked to clinical outcomes and used as a basis for care within the organization. However, it wasn't until the 1970s that outcome data were systematically collected, and the 1990s before nursing minimum data sets (NMDS) were agreed and collected (Doran, 2011). The development of the Canadian Institute for Health Information (CIHI) in 1994 afforded the opportunity for the systematic collection and analysis of Canadian data to identify Canadian trends.

As a result, the "new" approach of evidence-based practice and the evolving methodology of systematic reviews of scientific literature and the development of guidelines, standards, and processes began to be based on evidence.

Over the past two decades, nursing, medicine, health care institutions, and health policymakers have come to understand that evidence-based clinical decision making refers to decisions based on state-of-the-art science reports. This involves a process approach to collecting, reviewing, interpreting, critiquing, and evaluating research and other relevant literature for direct application to client care. In nursing, **best research evidence** refers to methodologically sound, clinically relevant research on the effectiveness and safety of nursing interventions, the accuracy and precision of nursing assessment measures, the power of prognostic markers, the strength of causal relationships, the cost-effectiveness of nursing interventions, and the meaning of illness or client experiences. Clinical expertise refers to nurses' abilities to (1) use clinical skills and past experience to identify the health state of clients or populations, their risks, their preferences and actions, and the potential benefits of interventions; (2) to communicate information to clients and their families; and (3) to provide them with an environment they find comforting and supportive (DiCenso et al., 2004).

Applying the best available evidence does not guarantee good decisions, but it is one of the keys to improving outcomes that affect health. When critical thinking and sound clinical judgment support it, evidence-based practice should be viewed as the highest standard of care. Nurses and doctors will always need to search for the best available evidence to support their clinical decisions. Despite the attention paid to evidence-based practice, much clinical practice is not supported by research, and debate continues about how long it takes for new knowledge—created by research— to find its way into daily clinical practice (Squires, 2011).

Demonstrating that outcomes of nursing care are appropriate, effective, efficient, and safe is a major responsibility for nursing. By recognizing the importance of not only evidence-based practice but also stimulating an organizational environment in which evidence-based models of care can flourish, nurses will see improved outcomes of clinical care. Organizations that create a supportive environment for evidence-based practice are likely to do the following: compensate managers and frontline nurses for their participation in academic activities, provide easy access to library resources and computers, include clinical nurse specialists in the staffing mix, use evidence in their management decision making, and adopt evidence-based corporate goals (Udod & Care, 2004).

Until the 1990s nursing practice and its impact were not generally captured in the major administrative databases that informed many funding and human resource decisions. Some nursing-related outcomes were collected through the Canadian Standards for Management Information Systems (MIS), which were developed in the 1980s and rolled into the data that was routinely collected when CIHI was formed in 1994. In the early 1990s the Canadian Nurses Association convened the first Nursing Minimum Data Set Conference to start the conversation on developing, collecting, and using nursing outcomes. In 1998 the Ontario Ministry of Health and Long-Term Care created the Ontario Nursing Task Force with mandates to examine the impact of health care reform on both the delivery of nursing services and the nursing profession in Ontario, and to recommend strategies to ensure and enhance quality of care through effective use of nursing human resources (Joint Provincial Nursing Committee, 2001). As a result, the Ontario government funded the Nursing and Health Outcomes Project (now called the Health Outcomes for Better Information and Care (HOBIC), to reflect the expanded scope of the project. The goals were to identify nursing-sensitive client outcomes, determine appropriate ways of measuring these outcomes, and identify databases where these outcomes could be stored. Similar projects were started in Saskatchewan and Manitoba (Canada—HOBIC) and in a variety of other health care settings internationally (Doran, 2011).

As these projects evolve, there is growing acknowledgement and recognition that their results will be important sources of evidence that can inform nursing policy and practice. The development of evidence-based guidelines, care plans, and other decision-aid tools will help to transfer the research-based knowledge in ways that facilitate its use by busy clinicians. Input from the end-users will improve the likelihood that these tools will be used.

Evidence-based nursing practice has deep roots. During the Crimean War, Florence Nightingale used her records of nursing interventions (i.e., sanitation, basic hygiene, good nutrition, rest, and a healing environment) and outcomes (i.e., reduced mortality of the wounded soldiers under care from 50 percent to 2 percent) to prove that more nursing services and supplies were needed (Rafael, 2000). In the 1960s the Royal College of Nurses in the United Kingdom assessed the clinical effectiveness of their members and discovered that practice lagged behind the scientific evidence (Estabrooks, Scott-Findlay, & Winther, 2004). The 1990s marked the beginning of several evidence-based nursing programs and initiatives. In 1990 Linda O'Brien-Pallas, at the University of Toronto, and Andrea Baumann, at McMaster University, received provincial funding for the forerunner of the Nursing Health Services Research Unit. In 1996 the Joanna Briggs Institute for Evidence-based Nursing and Midwifery was opened in Australia, and the Centre for Evidence-based Nursing was established at University of York in the United

Kingdom, followed in 1998 by the Sarah Cole Hirsch Institute for Best Nursing Practice Based on Evidence in the United States. More recently, the School of Nursing at Queen's University in Kingston, Ontario, has become a collaborating centre of the Joanna Briggs Institute. Over the past 20 years significant work has been accomplished worldwide to implement evidence-based practice within health care organizations. Evidence-based nursing centres have also been established in Hong Kong, New Zealand, Thailand, Russia, and Finland. The World Health Organization (WHO) in Europe has formed partnerships with organizations such as the International Council of Nurses (ICN) and the European Federation of Nurses Associations (EFN). Their goal is to help nurses and midwives cope with advancing technology and deliver high-quality, evidence-based care.[2]

In the United States, the Agency for Healthcare Research and Quality (AHRQ) has stimulated the evidence-based practice movement by recognizing a need for evidence to guide practice throughout the health care system. In 1997 the AHRQ launched an initiative that established 12 evidence-based practice centres (EPCs). The initiative was renewed in 2002 with 13 EPCs, three of which are located in Canada: McMaster University, University of Ottawa, and University of Alberta. The EPCs develop evidence reports and technology assessments on a variety of relevant topics: clinical, social, and behavioural sciences; economics; and health care organization and delivery issues. The initiative facilitates the translation of evidence-based research findings into clinical practice by including the input of stakeholders at key decision points along the process.[3]

The Canadian Agency for Drugs and Technologies in Health (CADTH) is a national body that provides Canada's federal, provincial, and territorial health care decision makers with credible, impartial advice and evidence-based information about the effectiveness and efficiency of drugs and other health technologies. Several provincial governments fund similar health technology assessment initiatives. To ensure the information is relevant and useful to decision makers, CADTH has established liaison officers, who work with local health care stakeholders to develop strategies that will enable more consistent uptake to practice.[4]

In 1999, with funding from the Ministry of Health and Long-Term Care, the Registered Nurses' Association of Ontario (RNAO) began the Nursing Best Practice Guidelines (NBPG) project, an initiative to facilitate clinical decisions that were based on the best available evidence. In 2004 Health Canada provided further funding to enable the initiative to disseminate its guidelines and related products across Canada, including translation into French. There are currently 42 completed guidelines in English, a number of which are in the process of being updated to incorporate new evidence; 16 are available in French. They are also available in Chinese, Italian, Japanese, and Spanish, and as a BPG mobile application.[5] In 2006, with funding from the Ontario Ministry of Health and Long-Term Care, the RNAO partnered with the University of Ottawa to form the Nursing Best Practice Research Unit (NBPRU) with a focus on nursing best practice research.[6]

ATTRIBUTES OF EVIDENCE-BASED PRACTICE

Davies and colleagues identified organizational factors that facilitate the implementation of best practice guidelines (BPGs) in a variety of settings: ongoing and supportive leadership, continuing education, an organizational culture supportive of evidence-informed practice, and the integration of guideline recommendations into organizational policies and procedures (Davies et al., 2002). To encourage the "new" behaviour to continue, organizations needed many factors to be in place: ongoing leadership by champions, management support, ongoing staff education, the integration of the guidelines into policies and procedures, staff buy-in and ownership, synergy with partners, and multidisciplinary involvement. The barriers to successful integration and ongoing use of the best practice guidelines were in fact the opposite to the positive conditions as outlined above. These were often seen to coincide with changes in staffing and organizational structure, departure of champions, heavy workload, and limited time for staff to participate in ongoing staff education. In turn, this led to staff resistance and a decline in follow-up and feedback, management commitment, and support (Davies, 2006). Tregunno and colleagues evaluated pilot sites for the implementation of Health Outcomes for Better Information and Care (HOBIC) and found similar challenges. Learning how to use the assessment protocols and technology were the easy parts, but changing the system to enable nurses the time to keep up their skills and integrate the tools into their daily practice were the biggest barrier to their ongoing use (Tregunno Gordon, & Gardiner-Harding, 2010). These findings are also in line with earlier work by Stetler and colleagues (Stetler, 1998), a recent systematic review by Thompson and colleagues (Thompson, 2007) and organizational change literature (Knox, 2001; Reddy, 2001).

In 1996 Carole Estabrooks conducted a survey of nurses in Alberta to identify the frequency with which they used various sources of information to inform their practice. The respondents most frequently said they used experiential information sources (e.g., client data and personal experience), followed by basic nursing

education programs, in-service programs and conferences, policy and procedure manuals, physician sources, intuition, and "what has worked for years." Articles published in nursing research journals were ranked 15th out of 16 possible sources. The nurses' reliance on nonscientific knowledge and on basic nursing education—despite having graduated from their nursing education programs an average of 18 years earlier—was considered a troubling trend (Estabrooks, 1998). In 2011 an updated systematic review of the literature looked at factors that impacted nurses' decisions to use research to inform their practice. The review included 45 reports of 41 studies. The review authors concluded that the following most important personal factors impacted nurses' use of research: having a positive attitude towards research, attending conferences or in-services; having a graduate degree (compared to a bachelor's degree or diploma); their current role (i.e., leadership or advanced practice compared to staff nurse); clinical specialty (working in critical care areas compared to general hospital units); and job satisfaction (Squires, 2011).

REAL WORLD INTERVIEW

I f I am looking for a systematic review for a specific clinical situation, I usually needed it pretty quickly; so I will search online. Should it be a matter that I can take some time to look up, I will use the online library through the hospital and use a search engine such as MEDLINE.

One of the challenges I face when trying to use systematic reviews is the lack of them in my specific area of work, pediatric palliative care. Since there is still so much research to be done in this field, often there is not enough completed research for a clinically informative systematic review. So then we have to see if the adult-based research and systematic reviews are applicable for that given situation.

We are fortunate that at our hospital the nursing policies and procedures are all evidence-based. So, often we can refer to the references cited in the policy when looking for the research to support why we do what we do.

Gurjit Sangha, RN, BSc, MN
Clinical Nurse Specialist, Palliative & Bereavement Care Service

Source: Gurjit Sangha.

Sonia Udod and W. Dean Care at the University of Manitoba conducted a survey to determine which managerial competencies were important in creating an environment where evidence-based practice could flourish. Nursing leaders were expected to be role models for evidence-based practice—that is, searching for and appraising the evidence and using it when making their decisions. They were expected to create opportunities for staff to develop networks to facilitate the development of important skills needed in an evidence-based environment, such as computer skills for searching the literature, or critical appraisal skills to assess the quality of what they read. Finally, sharing leadership and decision making among the team and providing psycho-social support to help sustain new behaviours were identified as other important attributes (Udod & Care, 2004).

MISCONCEPTIONS ABOUT EVIDENCE-BASED PRACTICE

Despite the importance and many attributes of evidence-based medicine, physicians have taken almost 20 years to accept that it was not meant to devalue the "art" of clinical medicine, and that clinical expertise, individual preference, and local availability continued to be important components and must be balanced with the current best evidence (Tracy, 2003). Nurses and other health care professionals voice similar concerns. Nurses are particularly concerned that evidence-based practice ignores client preferences and values, is atheoretical, uses only quantitative research, and overemphasizes randomized controlled trials and systematic reviews. In an effort to overcome these beliefs, it is incumbent on nursing managers to provide a practice environment that encourages nurses to incorporate the best evidence with their clinical skills, client preferences, and clinical circumstance (DiCenso, 2003).

Since not all clinical questions are best answered with a randomized trial, other study designs may offer the best available evidence to answer a particular question. Our nursing knowledge base is built on different theoretical frameworks and sources of information. We have developed theories that identify, analyze, and clarify our moral obligations and values, our interpersonal relationships, and our understanding of client behaviour. Systematic reviews are only a tool for systematically searching, appraising, and synthesizing the literature in an attempt to answer a clinical question. Although the methods used to synthesize results from randomized trials are more advanced, both the Cochrane Collaboration[7] and the Campbell Collaboration[8] are working on systematic

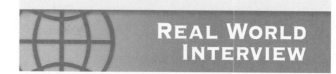

review methods to synthesize data from different study designs, including studies of prognosis, non-randomized clinical trials, and qualitative research (DiCenso et al., 2004; Thomas et al., 2004).

EVIDENCE: SOURCES, TYPES, AND EVALUATION

Depending on the question, sources of evidence can vary widely. The efficacy of a treatment is best tested with a randomized controlled trial, where the potential for bias is limited by the study design. In contrast, qualitative research is better suited to answering questions that increase our understanding of attitudes, beliefs, and experiences of groups or individuals. Both approaches to scientific inquiry have developed methodological criteria to minimize bias. On the other hand, nursing administrators must make decisions based on evidence that comes from outside the scientific realm. They use **organization evidence** that gives them information about the organization's capacity to execute tasks. This information may be in the form of financial reports, program evaluations, utilization data, and report cards. **Political evidence,** on the other hand, gives a sense of how the various stakeholders may respond to policies: for example, the barriers or facilitators that may have to be managed. This information may be found by conducting environmental scans, holding focus groups, or convening expert panels. In all circumstances, decisions and implementation strategies must be evaluated to determine their effectiveness (Canadian Health Services Research Foundation, 2004).

Scientific literature is published in a growing number of nursing-oriented journals: Online Journal of Knowledge Synthesis for Nursing, Evidence-Based Nursing, Canadian Journal of Nursing Leadership, Clinical Effectiveness in Nursing, Internet Journal of Advanced Nursing Practice, Canadian Journal of Nursing Research, Clinical Nursing Research, and Worldwide Nursing, to name just a few. Access to the nursing literature is slowly starting to increase with the advent of Open

Access internet journals, for example, BMC Nursing. Canadian nursing leaders continue to be leaders and active participants in many of these journals. In an attempt to assist the busy practitioner in keeping abreast of the literature, Evidence-Based Nursing and BioMed Central's Nursing and Health Care Gateway select articles from the health-related literature that warrant immediate attention by nurses, appraises them, summarizes them, and adds comments from clinical experts. A growing number of web-based sources are also available. A selection is listed at the end of the chapter. See also Table 3-1 for a list of the funded Canadian nursing research chairs. Research from these programs continues to be a very important source of evidence for health care decision makers.

The publication of systematic reviews helps busy clinicians find relevant information. Since the early work of the McMaster group, methods for the review and synthesis of evidence have undergone dramatic advances. Archie Cochrane, a British epidemiologist, was a pioneer in the movement and the impetus behind the development of the Cochrane Collaboration. This is an international organization that aims to help people make well-informed decisions about health care by preparing, maintaining, and promoting the accessibility of

TABLE 3-1	CANADIAN NURSING RESEARCH CHAIRS, JUNE 2011	
University	**Name**	**Funding Agency/ Area of Research**
University of British Columbia, Okanagan campus	Dr. Barbara Pesut	Canada Research Chair (CRC) in Health, Ethics and Diversity
University of Alberta	Dr. Wendy Austin	CRC in Relational Ethics in Health Care
	Dr. Carole Estabrooks	CRC in Knowledge Translation (Tier 2)
	Dr. Kathy Hegadoren	CRC in Stress-Related Disorders in Women
	Dr. Gina Higginbottom	CRC in Ethnicity and Health
	Dr. Wendy Duggleby	Endowed Nursing Research Chair in Aging and Quality of Life
	Dr. Gwen Rempel	Alberta Heritage Foundation for Medical Research. (AHFMR) Population Health Investigator—Building Capacity in Parents with Complex Congenital Heart Disease
	Dr. Shannon Scott	AHFMR Population Health Investigator— Understanding Implementation Processes of Clinical Pathways and Clinical Practice Guidelines in Paediatric Contexts

(Continued)

TABLE 3-1	CANADIAN NURSING RESEARCH CHAIRS, JUNE 2011 (CONTINUED)

	Dr. Miriam Stewart	AHFMR Health Senior Investigator Promoting Health Equity for Vulnerable Children Affected by Chronic Lung Conditions
	Dr. Greta Cummings	AHFMR Population Health Investigator— Connecting Leadership, Education and Research (CLEAR) Outcomes Research Program
University of Manitoba	Dr. Maureen Heaman	Canadian Institutes of Health Research (CIHR) Research chair in New Perspectives in Gender, Sex and Health
Lawrence S. Bloomberg Faculty of Nursing, University of Toronto	Dr. Ellen Hodnett	Heather M. Reisman Chair in Perinatal Nursing Research
	Dr. Bonnie Stevens	The Signy Hildur Eaton Chair in Paediatric Nursing Research
	Dr. Doris Howell	The RBC Chair in Oncology Nursing Research
	Dr. Cindy-Lee Dennis	Canada Research Chair in Perinatal Community Health (Tier 2)
	Dr. Arlene Bierman	Ontario Women's Health Council Chair in Women's Health
	Dr. Patricia McKeever	Bloorview Kids Foundation Chair in Childhood Disability Studies
	Dr. Sean Clarke	The RBC Financial Group UHN Chair in Cardiovascular Nursing Research
	Dr. Cindy-Lee Dennis	Shirley Brown Chair in Women's Mental Health Research
York University	Dr. Pat Armstrong	CHSRF/CIHR Applied Health Services and Nursing Research.
University of Western Ontario	Dr. Heather Laschinger	The Arthur Labatt Family Nursing Research Chair in Human Resource Optimization (causes and impacts of the nursing shortage)
McMaster University	Dr. Alba DiCenso	CHSRF/CIHR Chair in Advanced Practice Nursing Roles and Interventions
Children's Hospital of Eastern Ontario (CHEO) and University of Ottawa	Dr. Denise Harrison	CHEO Research Chair in Nursing Care of Children, Youth and Their Families.
Université de Montréal	Dr. Francine Ducharme	Desjardins Chair in Nursing Care for Older Persons and Families
	Dr. Louise Potvin	CHSRF/CIHR Chair in Approches communautaires et inégalités de santé [Community Approaches to Inequities in Health Care]

(Continued)

TABLE 3-1	CANADIAN NURSING RESEARCH CHAIRS, JUNE 2011 (CONTINUED)		
	open	Newton Foundation Research Chair in Nursing Care Development and Evaluation is reserved for McGill University and Université de Montréal
McGill University School of Nursing	open	Susan E. French Chair in Nursing Research and Innovative Practice
Dalhousie University, Nova Scot	Dr. Ingrid Sketris	CHSRF/CIHR Chair Developing and Applying Drug Use Management Strategies and Policies for Nova Scotia's Provincial Drug Programs: A Partnership of Researchers, Healthcare Professionals, Consumers and Government.

Note: This list is not meant to be exhaustive, but to show the range of Canadian Nursing Research Chairs that are currently funded. Many of them were funded by CHSRF and CIHR to support capacity-building for health services and policy research in Canada. Many teaching hospitals also have endowed chairs to support nursing research. The Internet search (June 13, 2011) started with a Google search for "Canadian Nursing Research Chairs" and then snowballed from the Faculties of Nursing listed with the Chair Holders.

systematic reviews of the effects of health care interventions. The U.K. Cochrane Centre started in 1992 and was followed shortly by the Canadian Cochrane Centre, hosted by McMaster University in 1993.[9] Used initially as a resource to inform medical practice, it wasn't long before nurses became involved in the Cochrane Collaboration as authors, review group co-ordinators, trial search coordinators, and editors. The Nursing Care Field was established in 2009, with the explicit goals of improving care by increasing the use of the Cochrane Library by nurses, engaging nurses in research activities, and providing an evidence-base for nursing care.[10] Systematic reviews in the Cochrane Library cover a range of nursing interventions, methods in nursing research, and economic analyses of a variety of nursing policies and practices.[11]

Some basic methodological differences distinguish the more traditional narrative review from a systematic review. A systematic review attempts to "collate all empirical evidence that fits pre-specified eligibility criteria in order to answer a specific research question. It uses explicit, systematic methods that are selected with a view to minimizing bias, thus providing more reliable findings from which conclusions can be drawn and decisions made" (Higgins & Green, 2011). Systematic reviews typically start with a focused question, develop and execute a comprehensive search strategy, select studies based on explicitly stated inclusion criteria, appraise the risk of bias of the relevant studies, extract and synthesize the data using either a statistical (i.e., a meta-analytical) or qualitative approach, and come to conclusions that are based on the evidence. A narrative review may follow some of the same steps, but it is likely to be answering a broader question, is usually less comprehensive about the literature included, and its results and recommendations may extend beyond the data.[12]

The evidence-based practice process comprises a number of steps: (1) define the clinical question, (2) search the literature, (3) select and critically appraise the most relevant reports, (4) decide whether and how to use the information, and (5) evaluate the effects of your decision. The question and available resources will dictate the extent of the literature search. The decision on how to use the information will be influenced by client preferences and circumstances, by the provider's skill and preference, and by local resources, policies, and practices. Not all inquiries will result in a full systematic review; however, it is always important to evaluate the effects of your decisions and actions. See Table 3-2 for details on the five steps. Table 3-3 gives an overview of research terminology that is useful in developing skills in evidence-based practice (EBP).

TABLE 3-2	**FIVE STEPS IN EVIDENCE-BASED PRACTICE**
1. Define the clinical question	The clinical question may be defined from the perspective of different parties: the client, the clinician, the policymaker, the organization's administrator, or the pharmaceutical industry, to name a few. Each perspective will produce a different question, such as What are the effects of the introduction of clinical practice guidelines in nursing (including health visiting), midwifery, and other professions allied to medicine? Are nursing-led inpatient units effective in preparing clients for discharge from hospital, compared to usual inpatient care?
2. Search the literature	If you have the time, skills, and resources, you can search the literature yourself. In most cases, it makes more sense to ask a trained health sciences librarian for assistance. This solution may be problematic for clinicians who are not affiliated with an academic institution or a health care facility with a good library. PubMed (http://www.ncbi.nlm.nih.gov/sites/entrez?db=pubmed), sponsored by the National Library of Medicine and the National Institutes of Health in the United States, is a large, freely accessible database of medical, nursing, and allied health journals, but not all journals are indexed in PubMed. Unfortunately, CINAHL, the specialized database for nursing and allied health, is only available by subscription (see http://www.cinahl.com/). The recent increase in Free Access journals, such as those published by PubMed Central, has resulted in increased access for health care workers who are not able to freely access a health sciences library.
3. Critically appraise the literature	Before you can have confidence in the results of the literature, you first need to determine the quality of the data. Therefore, when accessing an intervention trial, it is important to determine the following risks of bias:

3. Critically appraise the literature (continued)

- random sequence generation (selection bias)
- allocation concealment (selection bias)
- blinding of participants and providers (performance bias and detection bias)
- blinding of outcome assessors (performance bias and detection bias)
- incomplete outcome data (attrition bias)
- selective reporting (reporting bias)
- other biases not addressed elsewhere (Higgins & Green, 2011)

For qualitative studies you need to ask the following questions:

- Is the research question clear and adequately substantiated?
- Is the design appropriate for the research question?
- Was the sampling appropriate for the research design and question?
- Were data collected and managed systematically?
- Were data analyzed appropriately?
- Is the description of the results thorough? (DiCenso et al., 2004)

If you have found a systematic review, determine the following:

- What study designs were synthesized?
- Was the literature search described?
- How was the validity of the studies assessed?
- Were the results consistent across studies?
- Were individual or aggregate data used in the analysis? (Oxman & Guyatt, 1991)

(Continued)

TABLE 3-2	FIVE STEPS IN EVIDENCE-BASED PRACTICE
	For clinical practice guidelines, assessing the following six domains will help you determine the methodological rigour and transparency of the development of the guideline: ■ scope and purpose ■ stakeholder involvement ■ rigour of development ■ clarity of presentation ■ applicability ■ editorial independence (AGREE Collaboration, 2010, http://www.agreetrust.org/about-agree/introduction0/)
4. **Decide whether and how to use the information**	To decide whether the information you found is likely to help you with the question at hand, determine the size and precision of the treatment results; that is, ask whether the effects of the treatment were both statistically and clinically important. Decide whether your clients are similar to the clients in the study, whether the treatment is feasible in your setting, and whether all clinically important outcomes (e.g., harms and benefits) were considered. Finally, based on local practice, administrative constraints, and client preferences, ask whether the anticipated benefits are worth the harms and costs. If you are looking at qualitative research, decide what meaning and relevance the results have for your client care, whether the results will help you understand the context of your client care, and whether the study will enhance your knowledge about your client care (DiCenso et al., 2004).
5. **Evaluate the effects of your decision**	Deciding how you will evaluate the effects of your decision should be as carefully thought out as the other steps. Can you determine what would have happened if you had taken another route? Are the parameters by which you are evaluating your decision appropriate for the clinical question you asked in Step 1? (DiCenso et al., 2004)

TABLE 3-3	RESEARCH TERMINOLOGY IN EVIDENCE-BASED PRACTICE
Absolute Risk Reduction (ARR)	The absolute arithmetic difference (i.e., the risk difference) in rates of harmful outcomes between experimental and control groups. Use of this term is restricted to a beneficial exposure or intervention.
Allocation concealment	Randomization is concealed when the person making the decision about enrolling a client is unaware of whether the next client enrolled will be entered in the intervention group or the control group (e.g., by using techniques such as central randomization or sequentially numbered opaque, sealed envelopes). When randomization is not concealed, clients with better prognoses may tend to be preferentially enrolled in the active treatment arm resulting in exaggeration of the apparent benefit of the intervention (or even falsely concluding that the intervention is efficacious).

(*Continued*)

TABLE 3-3	**RESEARCH TERMINOLOGY IN EVIDENCE-BASED PRACTICE**
Bias	A systematic error in the design, conduct, or interpretation of a study that may cause a systematic deviation from the underlying truth.
Case control study	A study designed to determine the association between an exposure and an outcome in which clients are sampled by outcome. Those with the outcome (i.e., the cases) are compared to those without the outcome (i.e., the controls) with respect to exposure to the suspected harmful agent.
Case reports	Descriptions of individual clients.
Case series	A study reporting on a consecutive collection of clients treated in a similar manner, without a control group. For example, a clinician might describe the characteristics of an outcome for 25 consecutive clients with diabetes who received education for prevention of foot ulcers.
Clinical practice guidelines	Systematically developed statements or recommendations to assist practitioner and client decisions about appropriate health care for specific clinical circumstances. Clinical practice guidelines present indications for performing a test, procedure, or intervention, or the proper management for specific clinical problems.
Cohort study	A study that identifies two groups (i.e., cohorts) of clients: one group received the exposure of interest and one group did not receive the exposure. The cohort study follows the two groups forward for the outcome of interest (also called a longitudinal study).
Co-intervention	An intervention other than the intervention under study that may be differentially applied to the intervention groups and the control groups and, thus, potentially introduces bias in the results of a study.
Comparative research	A research design that either compares two or more groups, compares a single group at two or more points in time, or compares a single group under different circumstances or experiences.
Confidence interval	A range between two values within which it is probable that the true value lies for the population of clients from which the study clients were selected.
Confounder	A factor that distorts the true relationship of the study variable of interest by virtue of also being related to the outcome of interest. Confounders are often unequally distributed among the groups being compared. Randomized studies are less likely to have their results distorted by confounders than are observational studies.
Control group	Subjects in an experiment who do not receive the experimental treatment and whose performance provides a baseline against which the effects of the treatment can be measured.
Dependent variable	The outcome variable of interest; the variable that is hypothesized or thought to depend on or be caused by another variable, called the independent variable (also called the outcome).
Descriptive research	Research studies that have as their main objective the accurate portrayal of the characteristics of people, situations, or groups, and the frequency with which certain phenomena occur.
Dichotomous data	Data that can take one of two possible values, such as dead/alive, smoker/non-smoker, present/not present. (Also called binary data.) Sometimes continuous data or ordinal data are simplified into dichotomous data (e.g. age in years could become <75 years or ≥75 years).

(Continued)

TABLE 3-3	RESEARCH TERMINOLOGY IN EVIDENCE-BASED PRACTICE (CONTINUED)
Dose-response gradient	The risk of an outcome increasing as the quantity or the duration of exposure to the putative harmful agent increases.
Effect size	The difference in outcomes between the intervention and control groups divided by some measure of variability, typically the standard deviation.
Generalizability	The degree to which the results of a study can be generalized to settings or samples other than those being studied (external validity).
Incidence	The number of new cases of a disease occurring during a specified period of time; expressed as a percentage of the number of people at risk during that time.
Independent variable	The variable that is believed to cause or influence the dependent variable; in experimental research, the independent variable is the variable that is manipulated.
Intention-to-treat analysis	The analyzing of study participant outcomes based on the group to which the participants were randomized, even if they dropped out of the study or for other reasons did not actually receive the planned intervention. This analysis preserves the power of randomization, thus maintaining the likelihood that important unknown factors that influence outcome are equally distributed across comparison groups.
Internal validity	The ability of a study to provide valid results, dependent on whether it was designed and conducted well enough that the study findings accurately represent the direction and magnitude of the underlying true effect (risk of bias).
Interrupted-time series	A study design in which data are collected at several times both before and after the intervention. Data collected before the intervention allow the underlying trend and cyclical (e.g., seasonal) effects to be estimated, whereas data collected after the intervention allow the intervention effect to be estimated, while accounting for underlying secular trends. The time series–design monitors the occurrence of outcomes or end points over a number of cycles and determines whether the pattern changes coincident with the intervention.
Matched case-controlled study	A research technique that uses select sample characteristics to match experimental subjects with a control group (matched sample).
Meta-analysis	A statistical technique for quantitatively gathering the results of multiple studies that measure the same outcome and combining those results into a single pooled estimate or a summary estimate.
Non-randomised study	Any quantitative study estimating the effectiveness of an intervention (harm or benefit) that does not use randomisation to allocate units to comparison groups (including studies where 'allocation' occurs in the course of usual treatment decisions or peoples' choices, i.e. studies usually called 'observational'). To avoid ambiguity, the term should be substantiated using a description of the type of question being addressed. For example, a 'non-randomised intervention study' is typically a comparative study of an experimental intervention against some control intervention (or no intervention) that is not a randomised controlled trial. There are many possible types of non-randomised intervention study, including cohort studies, case control studies, controlled before-and-after studies, interrupted-time-series studies and controlled trials that do not use appropriate randomisation strategies (sometimes called quasi-randomised studies).
Number-Needed-to-Treat (NNT)	The number of clients who need to be treated over a specific period of time to achieve one additional good outcome. When discussing NNT, the intervention, its duration, and the good outcome should be specified. NNT is the inverse of the absolute risk reduction.
Observational studies	Studies in which a participant or clinician preference determines whether a participant is assigned to the intervention group or the control group.

(*Continued*)

TABLE 3-3	RESEARCH TERMINOLOGY IN EVIDENCE-BASED PRACTICE (CONTINUED)
Odds ratio	A ratio of the odds of an event in an exposed group to the odds of the same event in a group that is not exposed.
Outcome evaluation	An assessment of the impact of an intervention, which examines the changes that occurred as a result of the intervention and whether the intervention is having the intended effect. It answers the question, What is the impact of this intervention? It may also answer the question, Are the benefits of the intervention worth the costs?
Phenomenology	An approach to inquiry that emphasizes the complexity of human experience and the need to understand the experience holistically, as it is actually lived.
Power	The ability of a study to reject a null hypothesis when it is false (and should be rejected). Power is linked to the adequacy of the sample size: if a sample size is too small, the study will have insufficient power to detect differences between groups, if differences exist.
Prevalence	The proportion of persons in a population who are affected with a particular disease at a specified time. Prevalence rates obtained from high-quality studies can inform pretest probabilities.
Probability	The quantitative estimate of the likelihood of either a condition existing (e.g., in a diagnosis) or of subsequent events occurring (e.g., in an intervention study).
Prognostic study	A study that enrols clients at a particular point in time and follows them forward to determine the frequency and timing of subsequent events.
Program evaluation	Research that investigates how well a program, practice, or policy is working.
Qualitative research	The investigation of phenomena in a non-quantitative, in-depth, and holistic fashion, through the collection of rich narrative materials. Examples of data collection include observation, interviews, and document analysis.
Quality improvement project	The selection of a particular diagnostic group, unit, or other measurement that needs scientific investigation to identify needed improvement.
Quantitative research	The investigation of phenomena that lend themselves to test well-specified hypotheses through precise measurement and the quantification of predetermined variables that yields numbers suitable for statistical analysis.
Quasi-experiment	A study in which subjects are systematically, rather than randomly, assigned to treatment conditions, although the researcher manipulates the independent variable and exercises certain controls to enhance the internal validity of the results.
Random allocation	A method that uses the play of chance to assign participants to comparison groups in a trial, e.g. by using a random numbers table or a computer-generated random sequence. Random allocation implies that each individual or unit being entered into a trial has the same chance of receiving each of the possible interventions. It also implies that the probability that an individual will receive a particular intervention is independent of the probability that any other individual will receive the same intervention. See also quasi-random allocation, randomisation.
Randomized controlled trials	Experiments in which individuals are randomly allocated to receive or not receive an experimental preventive, therapeutic, or diagnostic procedure and then followed to determine the effect of the intervention.
Research utilization	The use of some aspect of a research or scientific investigation in an application unrelated to the original research.
Relative Risk Reduction (RRR)	The proportional reduction in rates of harmful outcomes between experimental and control participants. Used with a beneficial exposure or intervention.

(Continued)

TABLE 3-3	**RESEARCH TERMINOLOGY IN EVIDENCE-BASED PRACTICE (CONTINUED)**
Statistical significance	A description of results obtained in an analysis of study data that are unlikely to have occurred by chance, and the null hypothesis is rejected. When statistically significant, the probability of the observed results, given the null hypothesis, falls below a specified level of probability (most often $P < 0.05$).
Systematic review	A review of a clearly formulated question that uses systematic and explicit methods to identify, select, and critically appraise relevant research, and to collect and analyze data from the studies included in the review. Statistical methods (i.e., meta-analyses) may or may not be used to analyze and summarize the results of the included studies.
Time series design	A quasi-experimental design that involves the collection of information over an extended period of time, with multiple data collection points both before and after the introduction of a treatment.
Variable	A characteristic or attribute of a person or object that varies (i.e., takes on different values) within the population under study (e.g., body temperature, heart rate).

Source: The Cochrane Collaboration. Glossary of Terms in *The Cochrane Collaboration Version 4.2.5* (Updated May 2005). Available from: http://www.cochrane.org/training/cochrane-handbook

LEVELS OF EVIDENCE

As you may have noticed, not all science is equally well designed and executed, nor are all the published reports equally well written. It is impossible for busy clinicians to keep abreast of advances in the field by reading all the original research. Fortunately, groups of clinicians and researchers synthesize the information into systematic reviews, and develop clinical guidelines and quality assessment tools to help us to decide which studies are well conducted. Subjective decisions are inherent during the synthesis of the data. Review authors should be transparent in the reporting of their decisions and clinicians should learn to read and understand a little of the theory behind the science.

Following is a list of national organizations and programs concerned with nursing research in Canada. (See the website for the Office of Nursing Policy for details: http://www.hc-sc.gc.ca/hcs-sss/pubs/nurs-infirm/onp-bpsi-fs-if/2006-res-eng.php)

1. The Canadian Health Services Research Foundation (CHSRF)
2. The Canadian Institutes of Health Information (CIHR)
3. Partnership Programs by CHSRF and CIHR
4. The Canadian Association for Nursing Research (CANR)
5. The Canadian Nurses Foundation (CNF)
6. The Consortium for Nursing Research and Innovation (CNRI)

When the results of the original studies are unequivocal and all of the data can be statistically pooled (e.g., in a meta-analysis), the conclusions in systematic reviews and recommendations for practice in clinical guidelines are likely to be straightforward. The challenge arises when results from a systematic review may not be statistically or clinically significant, and yet are the best available evidence for use in developing evidence-based clinical guidelines. Since guidelines are in part dependent on the norms and available resources of a jurisdiction, it is not unusual to find different recommendations in guidelines from different practice environments, which are based on the same evidence.

A related challenge for health care decision makers is to understand the quality of the evidence upon which guideline recommendations are made. Some guideline development groups use alphabetic assignments, others use numeric assignments. Some consider the highest level of evidence to be a well-conducted systematic review; others assign the highest level to a well-conducted randomized controlled trial. This situation is very confusing for those who must use these sources of evidence to inform their practice. Understanding the differences is important (Glasziou, Vandenbroucke, &

LITERATURE APPLICATION

Citation #1: Akbari, A., Mayhew, A., Al-Alawi, M.A., Grimshaw, J., Winkens, R., Glidewell, E., Pritchard, C., Thomas, R., & Fraser, C. (2008). Interventions to improve outpatient referrals from primary care to secondary care. *Cochrane Database of Systematic Reviews*, Issue 4. Art. No.: CD005471. DOI: 10.1002/14651858.CD005471.pub2 Copyright Cochrane Collaboration, reproduced with permission.

Discussion: The objective of this review was to estimate the effectiveness and efficiency of interventions to change outpatient referral rates or improve outpatient referral appropriateness. This article includes 17 studies involving 23 separate comparisons. Nine studies (14 comparisons) evaluate professional educational interventions. Ineffective strategies include (1) passive dissemination of local referral guidelines (two studies), (2) feedback of referral rates (one study), and (3) discussion with an independent medical adviser (one study). Generally effective strategies include dissemination of guidelines with structured referral sheets (four out of five studies) and involvement of consultants in educational activities (two out of three studies). Four studies evaluate organizational interventions: patient management by family physicians compared to general internists, attachment of a physiotherapist to general practices, a new slot system for referrals, and the requirement of a second "in-house" opinion prior to referral—all of these interventions were effective. Four studies (five comparisons) evaluate financial interventions. One study that evaluates the change from a capitation-based system to mixed capitation and FFS system and from a FFS system to a capitation-based system (with an element of risk-sharing for secondary care services) and shows a reduction in referral rates. Modest reductions in referral rates of uncertain significance were observed following the introduction of the general practice fundholding scheme in the United Kingdom. One study evaluating the effect of providing access to private specialists demonstrates an increase in the proportion of patients referred to specialist services but no overall effect on referral rates.

Implications for practice: There are a limited number of rigorous evaluations on which to base policy. Based on current evidence, active, local, educational interventions involving secondary care specialists and structured referral sheets are the only interventions that have an impact on referral rates. The effects of in-house second opinion and other intermediate primary-care-based alternatives to outpatient referral appear promising.

Citation #2: Foxcroft, D. R., & Cole, N. (2000). Organisational infrastructures to promote evidence based nursing practice. *Cochrane Database of Systematic Reviews*, Issue 3. Art. No.: CD002212. DOI: 10.1002/14651858.CD002212.

Discussion: The objective of this review is to identify and summarize organizational infrastructure developments that are aimed at promoting evidence-based nursing practice. No studies were sufficiently rigorous to be included in this systematic review. Seven case studies were identified but excluded from the review because of poor research design and lack of controls. The review describes several conceptual models on organizational processes to promote evidence-based practice and a number of organizational infrastructural interventions were described, but none of these were evaluated properly.

Implications for practice: There are no clear implications for practice. The next step in this field should be to conduct well-planned evaluations of well-planned interventions.

Chalmers, 2004; Schünemann, Best, Vist, & Oxman, 2003; Upshur, 2003).

An international group of epidemiologists and clinicians, (the Grading of Recommendations Assessment, Development and Evaluation [GRADE] Working Group), developed a "common sense approach" to grading the evidence and strength of recommendations. The methodology is now widely used to grade the quality of evidence in a systematic review (e.g., Cochrane Reviews), prioritize important client-centred outcomes, and inform recommendations in clinical practice guidelines.

GRADE combines information on the study design, risk of bias, consistency, and robustness of the results, and the applicability to the target population for each outcome, across all studies that measured the outcome. The quality of the evidence decreases by one level for poor performance against each of the criteria.[13] Readers wishing more information on the process are directed to the GRADE website, http://www.gradeworkinggroup.org/.

KNOWLEDGE TRANSFER AND EVIDENCE-BASED DECISIONS IN POLICY

During the 1990s a number of federally funded organizations were created in Canada to enable evidence-based decision making and policy development. In 1997 the National Forum on Health, a committee established to advise the federal government on innovative ways to improve our health care system and the health of Canadians, recommended that long-term plans for restructuring Canada's health care system be informed by the values of Canadians and current research findings. Today, Health Canada uses scientific expertise to inform its decisions on health standards, health policy, regulations, and health programs, and to provide evidence-based information to help Canadians make well-informed health care decisions.[14] Cochrane Canada has been instrumental in providing a ready source of systematic reviews in one easy-to-access database. Health and policy decision makers can access *Health Systems Evidence* at www.healthsystemsevidence.org for over 1000 evidence summaries

of governance, finance, and delivery systems within health care systems.

Clinical researchers have traditionally disseminated their findings among themselves, in peer-reviewed journals and at scientific conferences. Clinicians who have read the journals and attended the conferences, were apprised of the new information, which sometimes informed practice. However, as the evidence-based practice paradigm spread during the 1990s, funding organizations began to expect that researchers would make their results more widely known, in formats that could be readily used by decision makers at all levels. This approach to dissemination is now commonly known as Knowledge Transfer and Exchange (KTE). The KTE process is built on the concept that decision makers are more likely to incorporate research results into their decisions if they have a vested interest in the process (i.e., if they have input into the important questions and other steps of the research). In 1997 the Canadian Health Services Research Foundation (CHSRF) was created to "support the evidence-informed management of Canada's healthcare system by facilitating knowledge transfer and exchange—bridging the gap between research and healthcare management and policy."[15] In 1999 the Canadian Population Health Initiative (CPHI) was created to promote the development of evidence-based healthy public policy with a population health focus. CPHI's 2001 report, *An Environmental Scan of Research Transfer Strategies*, which surveyed 17 organizations across Canada, is an excellent resource for anyone who wishes to gain an understanding of the KTE process.[16] The Canadian Institutes of Health Research (CIHR), the federal health research funding agency established in 2000, incorporated both the creation and translation of new research into its mandate.[17] The CIHR and the Canadian Agency for Drugs and Technologies in Health (CADTH) are primary funders of the Canadian Cochrane Centre and the Cochrane review groups, methods groups, and fields located in Canada.[18] The CHSRF and CIHR co-fund a number of nursing research chairs that have set up research programs to examine nursing practice, nursing resources, and effective strategies to transfer the knowledge into policy and practice. The Institute for Work & Health, in Toronto, has been a leader in developing KTE and have developed five key principles for evidence-based KTE.

1. What? Key messages must be clear, compelling "ideas" backed by a body of rigorous research.
2. To whom? The interaction should be specific to the audience.
3. By whom? The messenger must be considered credible by the audience.
4. How? Interactive engagement between the messenger and the audience is ideal.

CRITICAL THINKING

You have just started work in a new palliative care hospital. You have been working in the community for many years and have enjoyed an environment where you were a respected member of the health care team, received encouragement and assistance to attend conferences, and had the opportunity to lead a couple of Nursing Best Practice Guideline initiatives in your agency. As you begin to take account of your new surroundings, you notice some aspects of care that you thought were revised years ago! You are conscious of being "the new kid on the block," but you finally summon the courage to ask your preceptor how evidence-based nursing is practised and supported on the floor. She looks at you suspiciously and says, "We've been giving excellent care around here for many years. Our clients are kept comfortable and their families appreciate what we do for them. We can't see any good reason to change."

What do you do now?

CRITICAL THINKING

You are a community health nurse visiting Mrs. McTavish to change the dressings on her stasis ulcers. She is upset when you get there and hasn't prepared things as she usually does for your visit. You have barely taken off your coat when she starts talking.

"My daughter went to her doctor recently because she was having really heavy periods again. I suffered from the same problems when I was her age. They weren't sure I could have any children. In those days, they kept trying to find out if I had any glandular problems and when I would have a really bad bleed, they would bring me into hospital for a D&C. She has been on contraceptives forever. I really worry about her. Don't they say that if you are on hormones for too long you increase your risks of cancer, heart disease, bone fractures, and things like that? Her doctor also said he might consider a hysterectomy. She's only 35. She's too young to go through menopause."

Where do you turn for your information?

What do you tell her?

What evidence informs your care of her stasis ulcers?

5. With what effect? Performance measures must be audience-specific and appropriate to the context.[19]*

An important player in this field is the Nursing Health Services Research Unit (NHSRU), developed jointly by Dr. Linda-Lee O'Brien-Pallas at the University of Toronto and Dr. Andrea Bauman at McMaster University. Its goals are to (1) conduct research and other academic inquiry; (2) provide the information necessary for evidence-based policy and management decisions about the effectiveness, quality, equity, utilization, and efficiency of health care and health services in Ontario, with a particular focus on nursing services; and (3) develop a joint mechanism for knowledge transfer between the Ontario Ministry of Health and Long-Term Care (MOHLTC) and the NHSRU ensure that recent and accurate evidence is used to guide evidence-based policy and management decision making.

The NHSRU has proven to be a valuable source of evidence for policy decisions on understanding and planning for health human resources, quality work environments for nurses, performance standards and practice, and the impact of organizational restructuring and downsizing, to name a few.[20, 21] In spring 2010 Dr. O'Brien-Pallas

stepped down from her co-directorship of the Nursing Health Services Research Unit and ended her term as the inaugural CHSRF/CIHR National Chair, Nursing Health Human Resources. Nursing colleagues summarized some of the research that had been influenced by and conducted at the NHSRU over the past 10 years in a *Festschrift* in honour of Dr. O'Brien-Pallas; *Mapping the field: Nursing scholarship in health human resources* is a valuable overview of how nursing research has flourished.

According to the Canadian Institute for Health Information, in 2010 government spending on health care was projected to reach $135.1 billion, while private-sector spending, which includes both private insurance and out-of-pocket expenses, was projected at $56.6 billion, which is an estimated 11.7 percent of the gross domestic product (GDP).[22]

Given our fragile economy, an aging population, and the anticipated impact these demographics will have on Canada's ability to provide publically funded, high quality health care, it is incumbent on all health care decision makers to use the best available evidence to inform sound healthcare decisions. Policymakers, clinicians, nursing leaders, nursing managers, and clients must promote the use of evidence-based practice to develop best practices at all levels of care. Many health care organizations support research programs, the results of which are used locally and internationally. Not all organizations have the resources to conduct large research projects, but, at the very least, they should be engaged in evaluating current practices and programs to ensure they are meeting the best standards of care. Changes in practice can only be facilitated through the collaboration of all disciplines working in an atmosphere that fosters evidence-based health care delivered to obtain quality outcomes.

KEY CONCEPTS

- The focus on evidence-based practice is expected to remain a driving force in the health care arena in the foreseeable future.

- Nursing can make significant contributions to the advancement of evidence-based care.

- Nursing leaders and managers can promote a culture receptive to the practice of evidence-based care, and all nurses can support this culture.

- Ultimately, evidence-based care is the gold standard in clinical care.

- By accepting the challenge to provide evidence-based care, nursing can pursue its future, confident of its ability to contribute to an increasingly complex health care system.

*Institute for Health and Work.

KEY TERMS

best research evidence
evidence-based medicine
evidence-based care
evidence-based nursing
    practice

evidence-based practice
organization evidence
political evidence

REVIEW QUESTIONS

1. What is the major purpose of evidence-based practice?
    A. to increase variability of care
    B. to create a missing link in clinical care
    C. to determine which medical models can be applied by nursing
    D. to provide evidence-based care that is incorporated with clinical competency, client preferences, and local resources

2. Concerning evidence-based practice, which of the following is an accurate statement?
    A. Evidence-based practice takes the place of continuous quality improvement.
    B. Because we can already demonstrate effective and efficient care, evidence-based practice is redundant.
    C. Leaders and managers in nursing are not clinicians, generally speaking, and so do not have a role in evidence-based practice processes.
    D. Generally speaking, evidence-based practice is recognized by nursing, medicine, and health policymakers as state-of-the-art clinical practice.

3. Which of the following organizations develops clinical practice guidelines?
    A. National Guideline Clearinghouse
    B. Public Health Agency of Canada
    C. Registered Nurses' Association of Ontario
    D. Guidelines Advisory Committee
    E. Canadian Medical Association

4. Which of the following is a research design that always involves testing of a clinical treatment with assignments of research subjects to either experimental or control conditions?
    A. longitudinal study
    B. randomized controlled trial
    C. meta-analysis
    D. time-series design

REVIEW ACTIVITIES

1. Review Table 3-2, on pages 71 and 72. Are the steps for evidence-based practice clear to you? Consider a client that you recently cared for. What clinical questions do you have about that client's care? How would you try to answer them? Are any clinical pathways or standards in use to help you care for this client?

2. To understand some of the studies used in evidence-based care, it is necessary to understand some of the research terminology. Review the research terminology in Table 3-3, on pages pages 72–76. Think of a clinical question related to a client you cared for. What kind of research study would best answer your question? Check the library and see whether you can answer your question.

3. Go to the RNAO Best Nursing Practice Guidelines website. Consider a client you cared for during your clinical experience. Which level of evidence supports the care delivery approaches to this client? How can you incorporate this guideline into your daily practice?

EXPLORING THE WEB

- Agency for Healthcare Research and Quality: *http://www.ahcpr.gov/*

- Appraisal Tools: *http://www.phru.nhs.uk/casp/casp.htm*

- Canadian Health Services Research Foundation: *http://www.chsrf.ca/home_e.php*

- Canadian Institute for Health Information: *www.cihi.ca*

- Canadian Institutes of Health Research: *http://www.cihr-irsc.gc.ca/*

- Canadian Medical Association infobase of clinical practice guidelines: *http://mdm.ca/cpgsnew/cpgs/index.asp*

- Canadian Population Health Initiative: *http://www.cihi.ca/CIHI-ext-portal/internet/ en/document/factors+influencing+health/ environmental/cphi*

- Centre for Evidence-based Nursing: *http://www. library.yorku.ca/ccm/Steacie/nursing/ systematic-reviews---resources.en*

- Centre for Reviews and Dissemination: *http://www.york.ac.uk/inst/crd/*

- Cochrane Collaboration: *http://www.cochrane.org/index.htm*

- CONSORT Statements: *http://www.consort-statement.org/*

- GRADE Working Group: *http://www.gradeworkinggroup.org/intro.htm*

- Guidelines Advisory Committee: *http://www.gacguidelines.ca/*

- Health Canada: *http://www.hc-sc.gc.ca/sr-sr/index_e.html*

- Institute for Work & Health: *http://www.iwh.on.ca*

- National Guideline Clearinghouse:
  http://www.guideline.gov/

- Newcastle-Ottawa Scale (Observational Studies):
  http:// www.ohri.ca/programs/clinical_epidemiology/oxford.htm

- Nursing Best Practice Guidelines:
  http://www.rnao.org/bestpractices/index.asp

- Nursing Health Services Research Unit:
  http://www.nhsru.com/

- Nursing Ideas.ca: a website designed to share ideas of research, innovation and leadership with nurses. *http://nursingideas.ca/*

- OHA Hospital Reports: *http://www.oha.com/oha/reprt5.nsf*

- Quality in Qualitative Evaluation: A Framework for Assessing: *http://www.pm.gov.uk/files/pdf/Quality_framework.pdf*

- Health Outcomes for Better Information and Care: *http://www.rnao.org/ehealth/mar07/mar07_hobic.htm*

REFERENCES

AGREE Collaboration. (2010). Retrieved from http://www.agreet-rust.org/about-agree/introduction0/

Canadian Health Services Research Foundation (CHSRF). (2004, March 11). *What counts? Interpreting evidence-based decision-making for management and policy: Report of the 6th CHSRF Annual Invitational Workshop*, pp. 1–14. Retrieved from http://www.chsrf.ca/SearchResults.aspx?search=What%20counts?%20Interpreting%20evidence-based%20decision-making%20for%20management%20and%20policy:%20Report%20of%20the%206th%20CHSRF%20Annual%20Invitational%20Workshop

Canadian Nurses Association. (2002). *Position statement on evidence-based decision-making and nursing practice*. Retrieved from http://www.cna-nurses.ca/cna/, June 13, 2011.

Davies, B., Edwards, N., Ploeg, J., Virani, T., Skelly, J., & Dobbins, M. (2006). Determinants of the sustained use of research evidence in nursing: Final report. Canadian Health Services Research Foundation & Canadian Institutes for Health Research. Ottawa, Ontario, Canada.

DiCenso, A. (2003). Evidence-based nursing practice: How to get there from here. *Nursing Leadership*. 16(4): 20–26.

DiCenso, A., Guyatt, G., & Ciliska, D. (2004). *Evidence-based nursing: A guide to clinical practice*. Philadelphia: Elsevier Publishing & AMA Press.

DiCenso, A., Virani, T., Bajnok, I., Borycki, E., Davies, B., Graham, I., Harrison, M., Logan, J., McCleary, L., Power, M., & Scott, J. (2002). A toolkit to facilitate the implementation of clinical practice guidelines in healthcare settings. *Healthcare Quarterly*, 5(3), 55–60.

Doran, D., Mildon, B., & Clarke, S. (2011). Toward a national report card in nursing: A knowledge synthesis. Prepared for the planning committee for the thinktank entitled Toward a National Report Card for Nursing.

Estabrooks, C. A. (1998). Will evidence-based nursing practice make practice perfect? *Canadian Journal of Nursing Research*, 30(1), 15–36.

Estabrooks, C. A., Scott-Findlay, S., & Winther, C. (2004). A nursing and allied health sciences perspective on knowledge utilization. In L. Lemieux-Charles & F. Champagne (Eds.), *Using knowledge and evidence in health care* (pp. 242–280). Toronto: University of Toronto Press.

Evidence-based Medicine Working Group. (1992). Evidence-based medicine: A new approach to teaching the practice of medicine. *JAMA*, 268(17), 2420–2425.

Glasziou, P., Vandenbroucke, J., & Chalmers, I. (2004). Assessing the quality of research. *British Medical Journal*, 328(7430), 39–41.

Higgins, J. P. T., & Green, S. (Eds.). *Cochrane Handbook for Systematic Reviews of Interventions*. Version 5.1.0 [updated March 2011]. The Cochrane Collaboration, 2011. Available from www.cochrane-handbook.org and *Glossary of Terms in the Cochrane Collaboration*. Version 4.2.5 [updated May 2005].

Higgings, J.P.T., & Green, S. (Eds). This reference may change related to the number of emails I have seen between the publisher and the chapter author. Please check directly with publisher for the correct citation.

Joint Provincial Nursing Committee. (2001). Progress report on the nursing task force strategy in Ontario: Good nursing, good health: A good investment. Toronto: Author.

Knox, A. B., Underbaake, G., McBride, P. E., & Mejicano, G. C. (2001). Organization development strategies for continuing medical education. *The Journal of Continuing Education in the Health Professions*. 21(1),15–23.

Lavis, J. N., Davies, H. T. O., Gruen, R. L., Walshe, K., & Farquhar, C. (2006). Working within and beyond the Cochrane collaboration to make systematic reviews more useful to healthcare managers and policy makers. *Healthcare Policy*, 1(2), 21–33.

Nelson, S., & Doran, D. (Eds.). (2011). *Mapping the field: Nursing scholarship in health human resources. Festschrift* in honour of Dr. Linda O'Brien-Pallas. Lawrence S. Bloomberg Faculty of Nursing, University of Toronto.

Ontario Ministry of Health and Long-Term Care. (2002). *Health outcomes for better information and care project*. Retrieved from http://www.health.gov.on.ca/english/providers/project/nursing/overview/overview.html

Oxman, A. D., & Guyatt, G. H. (1991). Validation of an index of the quality of review articles. *Journal of Clinical Epidemiology, 44*, 1271–1278.

Rafael, A. R. F. (2000). Evidence-based practice: The good, the bad, the ugly. *Registered Nurse, September/October*, 7–9.

Reddy, J. C., Katz, P. P., Goldman, L., & Wachter, R. M. (2001). A pneumonia practice guideline and a hospitalist-based reorganization lead to equivalent efficiency gains. *American Journal of Managed Care*, 7(12), 1142–1148.

Sackett, D. L., Rosenberg, W. M. C., Gray, J. A. M., Haynes, R. B., & Richardson, W. S. (1996). Evidence-based medicine: What it is and what it isn't. *British Medical Journal (BMJ)*, 312 (7023), 71.

Sackett, D. L., Straus, S. E., Richardson, W. S., Rosenberg, W. M. C., & Haynes, R. B. (2000). *Evidence-based medicine: How to practice and teach EBM.* London: Churchill Livingstone.

Schünemann, H. J., Best, D., Vist, G., & Oxman, A. D. (2003). Letters, numbers, symbols and words: How to communicate grades of evidence and recommendations. *CMAJ,* 169(7), 677–680.

Silagy, C., & Haines, A. (Eds.). (1998). *Evidence-based practice in primary care.* London: BMJ Books.

Squires, S. E., Estabrooks, C. A., Gustavsson, P., & Wallin, L. (2011). Individual determinants of research utilization by nurses: A systematic review update. *Implementation Science, 6*,1. Retrieved from http://www.implementationscience.com/content/6/1/1

Stetler, C. B., Brunell, M., Giuliano, K., Morsi, D., Prince, L., & Newell-Stokes, V. (1998). Evidence-based practice and the role of nursing leadership. *Journal of Nursing Administration,* 28(7/8), 45–53.

Thomas, J., Harden, A., Oakley, A., Oliver, S., Sutcliffe, K., Rees, R., et al. (2004). Integrating qualitative research with trials in systematic reviews. *British Medical Journal,* 328(7446): 1010–1012.

Thompson, D. S., Estabrooks, A., Scott-Findlay, S., Moore, K., & Wallin, L. (2007). Interventions aimed at increasing research use in nursing: A systematic review. *Implementation Science,* 11(2), 15.

Tracy, C. S., Dantas, G. C., & Upshur, R. E. G. (2003). Evidence-based medicine in primary care: Qualitative study of family physicians. *BMC Family Practice,* 4, 6. doi: 10.1186/1471-2296-4-6.

Tregunno, D., Gordon, S., & Gardiner-Harding, P. (2010). Implementing health outcomes for better information and care (HOBIC): Lessons from an early adopter site. *Nursing Leadership,* 23(3), 56–68.

Udod, S. A., & Care W. D. (2004). Setting the climate for evidence-based nursing practice: What is the leader's role? *Canadian Journal of Nursing Leadership,* 17(4), 64–75.

Upshur, R. E. (2003). Are all evidence-based practices alike? Problems in the ranking of evidence. *CMAJ,* 169(7), 672–673.

SUGGESTED READINGS

Angel, B. F., Duffey, M., & Belyea, M. (2000). An evidence-based project for evaluating strategies to improve knowledge acquisition and critical-thinking performance in nursing students. *Journal of Nursing Education,* 39, 219–228.

Bakken, S., & McArthur, J. (2001). Evidence-based nursing practice: A call to action for nursing informatics. *Journal of the American Medical Informatics Association,* 8, 289–290.

Beason, C. (2000). Creating an innovative organization. *Nursing Clinics of North America,* 35, 443–452.

Bradham, D., Mangan, M., Warrick, A., Geiger-Brown, J., Reiner, J. I., & Saunders, H. J. (2000). Linking innovative nursing practice to health services research. *Nursing Clinics of North America,* 35, 557–568.

Ciliska, D. (2006a). Educating for evidence-based practice. *Journal of Professional Nursing,* 21(6), 345–350.

Ciliska, D. (2006b). Evidence-based nursing: How far have we come? What's next? *Evidence-Based Nursing,* 9, 38–40.

Coyte, P. C., Wise, L. M., & Motivala, S. (2008). *An evaluation of the Nursing Research Fund: Lessons to date and recommended next steps.* Report prepared for the Canadian Health Services Research Foundation (includes CHSRF comments and response to the recommendations).

Cullum, N. (2000). Users' guides to the nursing literature: An introduction. *Evidence-based Nursing, 3,* 71–72.

Dobbins, M., Davies, B., Danseco, E., Edwards, N., & Virani, T. (2005). Changing nursing practice: Evaluating the usefulness of a best practice guideline implementation toolkit. *The Canadian Journal on Nursing Leadership,* 18(1), 34–45.

Dobbins, M., & DeCorby, K. (2004). A knowledge transfer strategy for public health decision makers. *Worldviews on Evidence-Based Nursing,* 2, 100–108.

Goldman, J., Meuser, J., Lawrie, L., Rogers, J., & Reeves, S. (2010). Interprofessional primary care protocols: A strategy to promote an evidence-based approach to teamwork and the delivery of care. *Journal of Interprofessional Care,* 24(6), 653–665.

Goode, C. J. (2000). What constitutes the "evidence" in evidence-based practice? *Applied Nursing Research, 13,* 222–225.

GRADE Working Group. (2004). Grading quality of evidence and strength of recommendations. *BMJ,* 328, 1490–1497. Retrieved from http://bmj.bmjjournals.com/

Greer, N., Mosser, G., Logan, G., & Halaas, G. W. (2000). A practical approach to evidence grading. *Joint Commission Journal on Quality Improvement,* 26, 700–712.

Grimshaw, J. (2004). So what has the Cochrane Collaboration ever done for us? A report card on the first 10 years. *CMAJ,* 171(7), 747–701.

Haynes, E. (2000). Research as a key to promoting and sustaining innovative practice. *Nursing Clinics of North America,* 35, 453–463.

Hollander, M. J., Corbett, C., & Pallan, P. (2010). Time for a paradigm shift: Managing smarter by moving from data and information to knowledge and wisdom in healthcare decision-making. *Healthcare Quarterly,* 13(2), 49–54.

Jansen, M. W., van Oers, H. A., Kok, G., & de Vries N. K. (2010). Public health: Disconnections between policy, practice and research. *Health Research. Policy and Systems, 8,* 37. Retrieved from http://www.health-policy-systems.com/content/8/1/37

Khan, K. S., Kunz, R., Kleijnen, J., & Antes, G. (2003). *Systematic reviews to support evidence-based medicine: How to review and apply findings of healthcare research.* London: Royal Society of Medicine Press.

Kitson, A. (2000). Towards evidence-based quality improvement: Perspectives from nursing practice. *International Journal for Quality in Health Care,* 12, 459–464.

Kizer, K. (2000). Promoting innovative nursing practice during radical health system change. *Nursing Clinics of North America, 35,* 430–449.

Lankshear, S., Huckstep, S., Lefebre, N., Leiterman, J., & Simon, D. (2010). The ALIVE program: Developing a web-based professional development program for nursing leaders in the home healthcare sector. *Nursing Leadership, 23*(Special issue), 61–74.

Lemieux-Charles, L., & Champagne, F. (Eds.). (2004). *Using knowledge and evidence in health care.* Toronto: University of Toronto Press.

McIntosh, H. M., Woolacott, N. F., & Bagnall, A. M. (2004). Assessing harmful effects in systematic reviews. *BMC Medical Research Methodology, 4,* 19.

Munro, B. H. (2005). *Statistical methods for health care research* (5th ed.). Philadelphia: Lippincott Williams & Wilkins.

Rosenfeld, P., Duthie, E., Bier, J., Bowar-Ferres, S., Fulmer, T., Iervolino, L., et al. (2000). Engaging staff nurses in evidence-based research to identify nursing practice problems and solutions. *Applied Nursing Research, 13*(4), 197–203.

Shaw, B. L., Taylor, W., & Roach, C. (2006). Focus on clinical best practices, patient safety and operational efficiency. *Healthcare Quarterly, 10*(Special issue), 50–57.

Shorten, A., Wallace, M. C., & Crookes, P. A. (2001). Developing information literacy: A key to evidence-based nursing. *International Nursing Review, 48,* 86–92.

"STROBE statement: STrengthening the Reporting of OBservational studies in Epidemiology." Retrieved from http://www.strobe-statement.org/

Urbshott, G. B., Kennedy, G., & Rutherford, G. (2001). The Cochrane HIV/AIDS review group and evidence-based practice in nursing. *Journal of the Association of Nurses in AIDS Care, 12*(6), 94–101.

van Tulder, M., Furlan, A., Bombarier, C., Bouter, L., & the Editorial Board of the Cochrane Collaboration Back Review Group. (2003). Updated methods guidelines for systematic reviews in the Cochrane Collaboration Back Review Group. *Spine, 28*(12), 1290–1299.

CHAPTER ENDNOTES

1. Sackett, D. L., Straus, S. E., Richardson, W. S., Rosenberg, W. M. C., & Haynes, R. B. (2000). *Evidence-based medicine: How to practice and teach EBM.* London: Churchill Livingstone.

2. World Health Organization, "Nursing and midwifery." Retrieved from http://www.euro.who.int/en/what-we-do/health-topics/Health-systems/nursing-and-midwifery

3. Agency for Healthcare Research and Quality, "Evidence-based Practice Centres, Overview, Centres." Retrieved from http://www.ahrq.gov/clinic/epc/

4. Canadian Agency for Drugs and Technologies in Health, "About CADTH." Retrieved from http://www.cadth.ca/index.php/en/cadth

5. Registered Nurses Association of Ontario, "Nursing Best Practice Guidelines." Retrieved from http://www.rnao.org/Page.asp?PageID=861&SiteNodeID=133

6. Registered Nurses Association of Ontario, "Nursing Best Practice Research Unit." Retrieved from http://www.rnao.org/researchunit

7. Cochrane Collaboration, "What Is the Cochrane Collaboration?" Retrieved from http://www.cochrane.org/

8. Campbell Collaboration, "About the Campbell Collaboration." Retrieved from http://www.cochrane.org/about-us/campbell-collaboration

9. Cochrane Collaboration, "What Is the Cochrane Collaboration?" Retrieved from http://www.cochrane.org/docs/descrip.htm

10. Cochrane Nursing Care Field, "The Joanna Briggs Institute – a field of the Cochrane Collaboration." Retrieved from http://cncf.cochrane.org/home

11. Cochrane Library, "About Cochrane." Retrieved from http://www.thecochranelibrary.com/view/0/index.html

12. Ibid.

13. GRADE Working Group, "Grading the Quality of Evidence and the Strength of Recommendations." Retrieved from http://www.gradeworkinggroup.org/intro.htm

14. Health Canada, Canada's Health Infostructure, "National Forum on Health." Retrieved from http://www.hc-sc.gc.ca/hcs-sss/ehealth-esante/infostructure/nfoh_nfss-eng.php

15. Canadian Health Services Research Foundation, "About CHSRF." Retrieved from http://www.chsrf.ca/home_e.php

16. Canadian Population Health Initiative, "About CPHI." Retrieved from http://www.cihi.ca/CIHI-ext-portal/internet/en/document/factors+influencing+health/environmental/cphi

17. Canadian Institutes of Health Research, "An Overview of CIHR, Mandate." Retrieved from http://www.cihr-irsc.gc.ca/e/30240.html#slide1_e

18. Canadian Cochrane Centre, "Funding and Support." Retrieved from http://www.cochrane.org/about-us/funding-support

19. Institute for Work and Health, "KTE: what works best in measuring its impact?" Retrieved from http://www.iwh.on.ca/knowledge-transfer-exchange

20. Nursing Health Services Research Unit, "Welcome to the Nursing Health Services Research Unit." Retrieved from http://www.nhsru.com/

21. Canadian Health Services Research Foundation, Retrieved from http://www.chsrf.ca/home_e.php

22. CIHI Annual Report: National Health Expenditure Trends, 1975 to 2010. Retrieved from http://www.cihi.ca/CIHI-ext-portal/internet/en/Document/spending+and+health+workforce/spending/RELEASE_28OCT10)

CHAPTER 4

Nursing and Health Care Informatics

Leslie H. Nicoll, PhD, MBA, RN
Adapted by Heather Crawford, BScN, MEd, CHE

From then on, when anything went wrong with a computer, we said it had bugs in it. (Admiral Grace Murray Hopper, on the removal of a two-inch-long moth from an experimental computer at Harvard University, September 9, 1945)

OBJECTIVES

The purpose of this chapter is to enable the reader to

- list the components that define a nursing specialty and discuss how nursing informatics meets these requirements;
- discuss educational opportunities for nurses interested in pursuing a career in nursing informatics;
- describe highlights in the history of modern computing;
- discuss how ubiquitous computing and virtual reality have the potential to influence nursing education and practice; and
- use established criteria to evaluate the content of health-related sites found on the Internet.

Nathan Gleave/iStockphoto

What is the most important card in your wallet? Your driver's licence? Your nursing registration? Your library card? In a few years, it might be your electronic health record. This record, a collection of all of your interactions with the health care system, would be available electronically to health care professionals anywhere in Canada. A swipe of the card in a barcode reader, and your complete health history would be available, no matter where you are or the nature of your complaint. At each encounter, the card would be updated, ensuring that every health care provider you come in contact with has the most complete and current health information available for your care.

Does this scenario sound like science fiction, or do you think it will be a reality within the coming years?

Like it or not, computers are here to stay. Technology has changed the way we communicate, obtain information, work, and, most recently, shop. As evidence, during 2010 a total of 26,224,900 Canadians, or 77.7 percent of the Canadian population, used the Internet. This was 9.9 percent of the North American population (Internet World Stats, 2011).

Consumers are also going online for health information. Seventy per cent of the online activity for home Internet users in 2009 was for seeking medical or health-related content (Statistics Canada, 2010). There has been a shift in the role of the client from passive recipient to active consumer of health information. Health professionals are responding to the more "Internet-informed" client (McMullan, 2006).

Computers and the Internet are also changing health care delivery. For example, myPatientAccess.ca was launched in September 2010. This was Canada's first interactive client portal to be fully integrated with an electronic medical record (EMR) system. It allowed clients to gain full, real-time access to their health records, and schedule appointments, review lab results after their physicians had reviewed them, request prescription refills, receive clinical alerts and reminders, and review care plans and educational materials provided by their doctor. In another example, in 2003 David Kaufman, a professor

in the Faculty of Education at Simon Fraser University, British Columbia, received funding for a project called Assessment of Technology in Context to study how game and simulation technology can be used to educate people in the field of health. One of the researchers developed a computer game for 9- to 12-year-olds to teach them about contagious diseases, such as HIV/AIDS and West Nile virus.

In another study, in the fall of 2005, Sunnybrook and Women's College Hospital was the first hospital in Ontario to evaluate a new software program, called New Age, which claims to improve client safety by instantly alerting clinicians of abnormal lab results. New Age is handheld software that displays Sunnybrook and Women's College Hospital's electronic client record data, including lab results, radiology reports, admission and discharge information, and client-specific transcription—all in an integrated fashion. The software allows physicians to monitor a client's condition in real-time and creates instant alerts (Bristow, 2005). *Giiwednong* Healthlink is a health and information management project between Manitoulin and North Shore First Nation health organizations. The project focuses on developing an integrated knowledge base to improve decision making, gain efficiencies, and integrate into larger systems. The aim is to electronically collect, manage, and store health data. In 2011 Share-Point became part of the project.

Nurses are not immune to the changes that computers bring to both everyday life and nursing practice. Computer technology can help nurses to achieve the goals of quality client care and positive client outcomes. Whether you are a student learning a clinical procedure using a computer-based instruction program or an administrator using a spreadsheet and database to plan a budget, computer technology is an essential part of professional nursing practice, at the individual, group and organizational level.

Although nearly everyone today is involved with computers to a certain degree, some have specialized within the field of computer science, information, and technology. Within nursing, this specialty is known as nursing informatics. Nurses in informatics have taken on a wide variety of roles and are involved in a myriad of activities, ranging from the design and implementation of clinical information systems to research on the use of technology to improve client outcomes. Although this specialty is fairly new within the profession, informatics nurses are already having a major impact on the way care is planned and delivered in the current health care environment.

This chapter will introduce you to two dimensions of computing in professional nursing: the world of nursing informatics and the world of computing "for the rest of us." Although it may not be your career choice to become an informaticist, professional registered nurses of the 21st century will not be effective in their roles without a solid knowledge base related to computers and technology and their impact on nursing practice, client care, and client outcomes.

WHAT IS NURSING INFORMATICS?

The term *informatics* was derived from the French word *informatique*. Gorn (1983) first defined the term as computer science plus information science. Informatics involves more than just computers—it includes all aspects of technology and science, from the theoretical to the applied. Another important part of the field of informatics concerns learning how to use new tools and maximizing the capabilities provided by computers and related information technologies (Ball, Hannah, & Douglas, 2000).

Nursing informatics refers to that component of informatics designed for and relevant to nurses. The first definition of nursing informatics was developed by Ball and Hannah in 1984 (Ball & Hannah, 1984). Various authors modified and embellished the definition during the ensuing decade (see Table 4-1). The definition proposed by the 1999 National Nursing Informatics Project (NNIP) discussion paper has been generally accepted in Canada.

The sponsors for this project included the Canadian Association of Schools of Nursing (CASN), the Canadian Nurses Association (CNA), the Registered Nurses Association of British Columbia (RNABC), the Academy of Canadian Executive Nurses (ACEN), and the Nursing Informatics Special Interest Group of the Canadian Organization for Advancement of Computers in Health (COACH). Note that this definition includes many components of nursing informatics: information management, knowledge from sciences other than nursing, and the importance of informatics within all areas of nursing practice.

THE SPECIALTY OF NURSING INFORMATICS

Specialties in nursing cover a range of interests and clinical domains, such as critical care nursing, community health nursing, and nursing administration. Key attributes of a specialty were identified by Styles[*] (1989) as follows:

- differentiated practice
- research program
- representation of the specialty by at least one organized body
- mechanism for credentialing nurses in the specialty
- educational programs for preparing nurses to practise in the specialty

TABLE 4-1	EVOLUTION OF A DEFINITION: NURSING INFORMATICS

The discipline of applying computer science to nursing process
(Ball & Hannah, 1984)

A focus that uses information technology to perform functions with nursing
(Hannah, 1985)

The application of the principles of information science and theory to the study, scientific analysis, and management of nursing information for the purposes of establishing a body of nursing knowledge
(Grobe, 1988)

The combination of nursing science, information science, and computer science to manage and process nursing data, information, and knowledge to facilitate the delivery of health care
(Graves & Corcoran, 1989)

Nursing Informatics (NI) is the application of computer science and information science to nursing. NI promotes the generation, management, and processing of relevant data in order to use information and develop knowledge that supports nursing in all practice domains.
(National Nursing Informatics Project (NNIP) discussion paper, 1999)

Nursing Informatics science and practice integrates nursing, its information and knowledge, and their management with information and communication technologies to promote the health of people, families, and communities worldwide.
(Redefinition by International Medical Informatics Association—Nursing Informatics. In 2009 the Canadian Nursing Informatics). Association adopted the definition.

[*] M.M. Styles (1989), *On Specializing in Nursing: Toward a New Empowerment*, Kansas City, MO, American Nurses Foundation.

In 1992 the American Nurses Association (ANA) acknowledged that nursing informatics possessed these attributes and designated nursing informatics as an area of specialty practice.

In 2001 the Canadian Nursing Informatics Association (CNIA) was formed. The mission of the CNIA is to be the voice for health informatics in Canada. The Canadian Nurses Association granted Associate Group status to the CNIA, which is also affiliated with the Canadian Organization for Advancement of Computers in Health (COACH). Through this strategic alliance, the CNIA is the Canadian nursing nominee to the International Medical Informatics Association–Special Interest Group in Nursing Informatics. In 2002–03 the CNIA conducted a study, Educating Tomorrow's Nurses: Where's Nursing Informatics?[1] This project built on the 1999 National Nursing Informatics Project. It was influenced by the Canadian Nurses Association national Health Information: Nursing Components (HI-NC) policy initiative and Health Canada's Office of Health and the Information Highway (OHIH) work in conjunction with the Canadian Nurses Association, 2006 (Toward 2020 - Visions for Nursing) and with the University of Victoria Summit on health informatics competencies (Canadian Nursing Informatics Association, 2003). The Canadian Nurses Association (CNA) developed an E-Nursing Strategy for Canada in 2006. At that time CNA launched the Canadian Nurses Portal Project, shortened to NurseONE, to address the vision of the e-nursing strategy. The purpose of the strategy was to guide the development of informatics, communication, and technology (ICT) initiatives in nursing to improve nursing practice and client outcomes (Canadian Nurses Association, 2006).

The Canadian Nursing Informatics Association exists to help nurses across Canada to learn, share, research, and create informatics-related projects and experiences that can help to boost the competencies, theory, and practice of informatics on a national level.[2] As part of this commitment, the Canadian Journal of Nursing Informatics (CJNI) was initiated—an online publication that is available to everyone.

EDUCATION IN INFORMATICS

Both formal and informal opportunities exist for education in health informatics. The first formal programs to offer specific degrees in nursing informatics were established within the past 15 years, and the number of programs has increased steadily. However, because educational options were originally limited, many nurses practising in informatics prepared for their role through on-the-job training or by receiving education outside of nursing. For example, a nurse may have a bachelor's degree of science in nursing (BSN) plus a second degree in computer science or information technology. However, nurses are now able to pursue a double degree in both Nursing and Science in Health Informatics at the University of Victoria in British Columbia.

FORMAL PROGRAMS There are many formal programs in nursing informatics available in Canada. Kwantlen Polytechnic University in British Columbia offers the Bachelor of Science in Nursing program, which integrates both the theory and practice of nursing informatics across the program. The British Columbia Institute of Technology (BCIT) offers the Advanced Specialty Certificate in Health Informatics Technology Management. Centennial College in Toronto offers a diploma in health informatics technology. Conestoga College Institute of Technology and Advanced Learning has a bachelor's degree program in health informatics management. It also offers coop programs leading to the Graduate Certificate in Applied Health Informatics and the Graduate Certificate in Information Management for Health Care. Dalhousie University in Halifax, has master's and PhD programs in health informatics (HI), and a bachelor's degree in informatics (major in HI). George Brown College in Toronto, Ontario, has a post-graduate certificate in health informatics. McGill University offers master's, PhD, and diploma programs in epidemiology, biostatistics, and occupational health. McMaster University offers both a master's degree and PhD in clinical epidemiology and biostatistics and eHealth. Memorial University in Newfoundland has a master's program in health services research. Université de Montréal had a master's program in évaluation des technologies de la santé. The University of Sherbrooke in Québec has a master's and a PhD program in clinical sciences, and it offers the Diploma in Microprogramme in Health Informatics. A master's degree in health informatics is offered at the University of Ontario Institute of Technology (UOIT). The University of Toronto offers a master's degree in health informatics. The University of Victoria has a bachelor's degree in health information science and both a master's and PhD program in health informatics. The University of Waterloo has bachelor, master's, and PhD programs in health informatics options. York University has a bachelor's degree and the Certificate of Attendance in Health Informatics and HI & Information Technology.[3]

The Canadian Nursing Informatics Association's education bursary is directed at advancing the informatics education of a selected nurse recipient. The registered nurse or registered practical nurse must be a member in good standing in the Canadian Nurses Informatics Association, and be enrolled or accepted in an informatics certificate, diploma, or degree program.[4] The Health Informatics Training System (HITS) is the world's leading online resource for learning and understanding about health informatics and its contribution to administrative and clinical best practice. Frontline Informatics Training is the North American provider of HITS.

HITS was originally created in Ireland but has undergone significant review and modification for Canada.[5]

INFORMAL EDUCATION Many opportunities are available for nurses in Canada to be involved in informal education. In Ontario, the government has announced that the 14 Local Data Management Partnerships will link information technology and health care professionals from the 14 Local Health Integration Networks. Many hospitals now have formal positions in clinical informatics. Organizations have also implemented eHealth Councils. All of these initiatives present opportunities for nurses to learn through an informal route.

For many nurses, graduate education is not an option or personal choice, but they still desire to become more knowledgeable about informatics. For these nurses, many informal opportunities exist, including networking through professional organizations, keeping abreast of the literature by reading journals, and attending professional conferences.

Organizations vary in the scope of services and educational opportunities offered to their members and the types of educational programs offered. Nelson and Joos (1992) describe five types of organizations*:

1. *Special interest groups*, such as the Nova Scotia Nursing Informatics Group, the Ontario Nursing Informatics Group, the Saskatchewan Nursing Informatics Association, the Manitoba Nursing Informatics Provincial Group, the Association québécoise des infirmières et infirmiers en systèmes et technologies de l'information (AQIISTI), and the New Brunswick Nursing Informatics Group Non-nursing organizations also have special interest groups that may offer benefit to nurses, including the Ontario Hospital Association, the Canadian Medical Association, the Canadian Society of Telehealth, and the Canadian Organization for the Advancement of Computers in Health.[6]
2. *Information science and computer organizations*, such as the Canadian Information Processing Society (CIPS)
3. *Health computing organizations*, such as the Canadian Institute for Health Information (CIHI) and Smart Systems for Health Agency
4. *User groups*, which consist of individuals working with a specific language, software, or vendor. One such group of interest to nurses is the Microsoft Healthcare Users Group (MS-HUG), which focuses on applications of Microsoft products in health care environments.
5. *Local groups*, such as the nursing informatics special interest groups

Nurses interested in learning more about informatics should become active in at least one related organization. As a member, a nurse has access to the meetings, publications, and educational offerings that the organization provides. Being on mailing lists and visiting organizations' websites also allows a nurse to keep abreast of different opportunities available through each organization.

Reading journals and newsletters is another way to become more knowledgeable about informatics. Offerings include trade magazines that are not related to health but are important sources of information, such as *PC Magazine* or the online magazine *Byte,* and specialized nursing journals, such as *CIN: Computers, Informatics, Nursing,* which offers continuing education contact hours in every issue. The American Medical Informatics Association (AMIA) publishes the *Journal of the American Medical Informatics Association,* a publication source for much of the research that has been conducted related to informatics. Healthcare Information Management & Communications Canada, published quarterly, is the official journal of COACH, Canada's Health Informatics Association. The Canadian Journal of Nursing Informatics (CJNI) is an online publication available to anyone. A nurse interested in informatics should become familiar with the journals that are available, subscribe to those that are most interesting, and read others in the library. Unfortunately, more information is published every month than anyone could possibly hope to keep abreast of—and that is where networking comes in! Colleagues can alert others to articles of interest that are in journals they might not regularly read.

Finally, conferences are excellent sources of education. At a conference, nurses are able to hear the latest information directly from experts in the field. Larger conferences usually have vendor exhibits that provide hands-on demonstrations for a variety of commercial products. Conferences vary in size, focus, location, and cost. For those interested in nursing informatics, nursing conferences are especially helpful. COACH: Canada's Health Informatics Association and the Canadian Institute for Health Information have an annual conference related to e-Health. Traditional themes have related to electronic health records, privacy, and telehealth. However, in 2011, new areas of focus included models of care, using evidence to affect change, and Health 2.0 (Technologies for a New Decade, and Building Readiness – education/capacity/pathways/change management).[7] The 11th International Congress on Nursing Informatics, sponsored by IMIA-NI, is being held in Montréal in June, 2012.

CERTIFICATION

Whether a nurse has pursued a formal or informal educational path in nursing informatics, many practising in the specialty choose to become certified. Certification in a

---

* R. Nelson & I. Joos. (1992). *Strategies and resources for self-education in nursing informatics. Computer applications in nursing education and practice.* Reprinted with permission of National League for Nursing, New York, NY.

specialty is a formal, systematic mechanism whereby nurses can voluntarily seek a credential that recognizes their quality and excellence in professional practice and continuing education (American Nurses Credentialing Center, 1993). For many nurses, becoming certified is both a professional milestone and a validation of their qualifications, knowledge, and skills in a defined area of nursing practice. The American Nurses Credentialing Center (ANCC) and the Canadian Nurses Association (CNA) offer certification examinations for a variety of specialties in nursing. The ANCC offers certification examinations in informatics. To be eligible for the nursing informatics examination, which was first offered in 1995, a nurse must meet the following requirements:

- Possess an active registered nursing licence in the United States or its territories
- Have a baccalaureate or higher nursing degree
- Have at least two years of active practice as a registered nurse
- Have at least 2,000 hours of practice in the field of nursing informatics within the past five years or completed at least 12 semester hours of academic credits in informatics in a graduate nursing program and a minimum of 1,000 hours in informatics within the past five years
- Have 20 contact hours of continuing education credit applicable to the specialty area within the past two years (American Nurses Credentialing Center, 2001b)

The nurse who successfully passes the examination is certified as a generalist in informatics nursing. The ANCC is planning to offer an examination for a specialist in informatics nursing in the future. Once certified, the nurse must be recertified every five years. In the first year the examination was offered, 83 nurses in the United States became certified in informatics (Newbold, 1996). Currently, there are more than 400 nurses who are certified in the specialty (American Nurses Credentialing Center, 2001a). The Canadian Nurses Association does not offer a certification in informatics.

CAREER OPPORTUNITIES

Career opportunities in the fields of computer science and information technology are growing at an exponential rate, and nursing is no exception. Nurses working in informatics can look forward to multiple job opportunities, with new roles continuously being developed as technology changes and matures. Changes in health care delivery have caused shifts in computer systems to case management, clinical systems, clinical data repositories, care mapping, and outcomes measures (Hersher, 2000).

Career opportunities for nurses in informatics exist in a number of different types of industries. Health care institutions, such as hospitals, are an obvious choice, but nurses also work for vendors of clinical information systems, insurance companies, and consulting firms.

CLINICAL INFORMATION

Clinical information systems are changing the way health care is delivered, whether in the hospital, the clinic, the provider's office, or the client's home. With capabilities ranging from advanced instrumentation to high-level decision support, a **clinical information system (CIS)** offers nurses and other clinicians information when, where, and how they need it. Increasingly, CIS applications function as the mechanisms for delivering client-centred care and for supporting the move toward the electronic health record.

What exactly is a CIS? Definitions vary, often from organization to organization. Semancik (1997) describes a CIS as a collection of software programs and associated hardware that supports the entry, retrieval, update, and analysis of client care information and associated clinical information related to client care. The CIS is primarily a computer system used to provide clinical information for the care of a client.

CLINICAL INFORMATION SYSTEMS

A CIS can be client focused or departmental. In client-focused systems, automation supports client care processes. Typical applications found in a **client-focused clinical information system** include client demographics, order entry, results reporting, clinical documentation, care planning, and clinical pathways. As data are entered into the system, data repositories are established that can be accessed to identify trends in client care. The **departmental clinical information system** evolved to meet the operational needs of a particular unit, such as the laboratory, radiology, pharmacy, health records, or the finance or accounting department. Early systems often were stand-alone systems designed for an individual department. A major challenge facing CIS developers is to integrate these stand-alone systems to work with each other and with the newer client-focused systems.

ELECTRONIC HEALTH RECORD

A CIS is not the same as an **electronic health record (EHR).** Ideally, the EHR will include all information about an individual's lifetime health status and health care. The EHR is a replacement for the paper health record as the primary source of information for health care, meeting all clinical, legal, and administrative requirements. However, the EHR is more than today's health record. Information technology permits much more data to be captured, processed, and integrated, which results in information that is broader than that found in a linear paper record.

REAL WORLD INTERVIEW

Mount Sinai Hospital uses technology to provide its staff with the best possible environment to care for its clients. Sinai e-learning enables busy clinical staff to combine the best of computer-based learning with the best of instructor-based training. Through Sinai e-learning, it is simple for clinicians to get up to speed with new and upgraded applications, and test their knowledge in scenarios that accurately reflect real-world clinical situations—accelerating training, ensuring competency, and guaranteeing clinical staff can spend the maximum time caring for clients.

Dr. Lynn Nagle
Former Senior Vice-President, Technology and Knowledge Management, Mount Sinai Hospital

Source: Nagle, L. (2005). Dr. L. Nagle and The Case for Nursing Informatics, *Canadian Journal of Nursing Leadership,* 18(1): 16-18. Reprinted with Permission.

The EHR is not a record in the traditional sense of the term. *Record* connotes a repository with limitations of size, content, and location. The term traditionally has suggested that the sole purpose for maintaining health data is to document events. Although documentation is an important purpose, the EHR permits health information to be used to support the generation and communication of knowledge.

The health care delivery system is dramatically changing, with a strong emphasis on improving outcomes of care and maintaining health. The EHR needs to be considered in a broader context and is not applicable to clients only, that is, individuals with the presence of an illness or disease. Rather, in the EHR, the focus is on the individuals' health, encompassing both wellness and illness.

As a result of this focus on the individual, the EHR is a virtual compilation of non-redundant health data across a person's lifetime, including facts, observations, interpretations, plans, actions, and outcomes. Health data include information on allergies, history of illness and injury, functional status, diagnostic studies, assess-

ments, orders, consultation reports, and treatment records. Health data also include wellness information, such as immunization history, behavioural data, environmental information, demographics, health insurance, administrative data for care delivery processes, and legal data (e.g., consents). The who, what, when, and where of data capture also are identified. The structure of the data includes text, numbers, sounds, images, and full-motion video. These structures are thoroughly integrated so that any given view of health data may incorporate one or more structural elements.

Within an EHR, an individual's health data are maintained and distributed over different systems in different locations, such as a hospital, clinic, physician's office, and pharmacy. Intelligent software agents with appropriate security measures are necessary to access data across these distributed systems. The nurse or other user who is retrieving these data must be able to assemble the data in such a way as to provide a chronology of health information about the individual.

The EHR is maintained in a system that captures, processes, communicates, secures, and presents the data about the client. This system may include the CIS. Other components of the EHR system include clinical rules, literature for client education, and expert opinions. When these elements work together in an integrated fashion, the EHR becomes much more than a client record—it becomes a knowledge tool. The system is able to integrate information from multiple sources and provides decision support; thus, the EHR serves as the primary source of information for client care.

A fully functional EHR is a complex system. Consider a single data element (i.e., a datum), such as a person's weight. The system must be able to record the weight; store it; process it; communicate it to others; and present it in a different format, such as a bar graph or chart. It may also be necessary to convert a weight from kilograms to pounds or vice versa. All of this processing must be done in a secure environment that protects the client's confidentiality and privacy. The complexity of these issues and the development of the necessary systems help to explain why few fully functional EHR systems are in place today.

DATA CAPTURE

Data capture refers to the collection and entry of data into a computer system. The origin of the data may be local or remote, with the data coming from client-monitoring devices; from telemedicine applications; directly from the individual recipient of health care; and even from others who have information about the recipient's health or environment, such as relatives, friends, and public health agencies. Data may be captured by multiple means, including key entry, pattern recognition (e.g., voice, handwriting, or biological characteristics), and medical device transmission.

All data entered into a computer are not necessarily structured for subsequent processing. Document-imaging systems, for example, provide for creation of electronically stored text but have limitations on the ability to process that text. Data capture includes the use of controlled vocabularies and code systems to ensure common meaning for terminology and the ability to process units of information. As noted earlier, great strides have been made in the development of standardized nursing languages. These languages provide structured data entry and text processing that result in common meaning and processing.

Data capture also encompasses authentication to identify the author of an entry and to ensure that the author has been granted permission to access the system and change the EHR.

STORAGE

Storage refers to the physical location of data. In EHR systems, health data are distributed across multiple systems at different sites. For this reason, there need to be common access protocols, retention schedules, and universal identification.

Access protocols permit only authorized users to obtain data for legitimate uses. The systems must have backup and recovery mechanisms in the event of failure. Retention schedules address the maintenance of the data in active and inactive forms and the permanence of the storage medium.

A person's identity can be determined by many types of data, in addition to common identifiers such as name and number. Universal identifiers or other methods are required for integrating health data of an individual distributed across multiple systems at different sites.

INFORMATION PROCESSING

Computer processing functions provide for effective retrieval and processing of data into useful information. These functions include decision-support tools, such as alerts and alarms for drug interactions, allergies, and abnormal laboratory results. Reminders can be provided for appointments, critical path actions, medication administration, and other activities. The systems also may provide access to consensus- and evidence-driven diagnostic and treatment guidelines and protocols. The nurse could integrate a standard guideline, protocol, or critical path into a specific individual's EHR, modify it to meet unique circumstances, and use it as a basis for managing and documenting care. Outcome data communicated from various caregivers and health care recipients themselves also may be analyzed and used for continuous improvement of the guidelines and protocols.

INFORMATION COMMUNICATION

Information communication refers to the interoperability of systems and linkages for exchange of data across disparate systems. To integrate health data across multiple systems at different sites, identifier systems (e.g., unique numbers or other methodology) are essential for health care recipients, caregivers, providers, and sites. Local, regional, and national health information infrastructures that tie all participants together using standard data communication protocols are key to the linkage function. Hundreds of types of transactions or messages must be defined and agreed to by the participating stakeholders. Vocabulary and code systems must permit the exchange and processing of data into meaningful information. EHR systems must provide access to point-of-care information databases and knowledge sources, such as pharmaceutical formularies, referral databases, and reference literature.

SECURITY

Computer-based health record systems provide better protection of confidential health information than paper-based systems because of their support controls that ensure that only authorized users with legitimate uses have access to health information. Security functions address the confidentiality of private health information and the integrity of the data. The design of security functions must ensure compliance with applicable legislation, regulations, and standards. Security systems must ensure that access to data is provided only to those who are authorized and have a legitimate purpose for using the data. Security functions also must provide a means to audit for inappropriate access.

Three important terms are used when discussing security: privacy, confidentiality, and security. It is important to understand the differences between these concepts.

- Privacy refers to the right of individuals to keep information about themselves from being disclosed to anyone. If a client had an abortion and chose not to tell a health care provider this fact, the client would be keeping that information private.
- Confidentiality refers to the act of limiting disclosure of private matters. After a client has disclosed private information to a health care provider, that provider has a responsibility to maintain the confidentiality of that information.
- Security refers to the means of controlling access and protecting information from accidental or intentional disclosure to unauthorized people and from alteration, destruction, or loss. When private information is placed in a confidential EHR, the system must have controls in place to maintain the security of the system and not allow unauthorized people access to the data (CPRI Work Group on Confidentiality, Privacy & Security, 1995).

CRITICAL THINKING

In your clinical practice, you have likely interacted with a clinical information system to both enter and access data for the client you were caring for.

What security systems were in place to maintain the confidentiality of client data, for example, passwords, identification cards, and other features? Do you believe the security system was effective? Was it updated on a regular basis? Did the security system present any barriers to your obtaining necessary information for providing quality client care—for example, were the results of certain tests or past history restricted in any way?

REAL WORLD INTERVIEW

Elizabeth Borycki, an RN and assistant professor at the University of Victoria's School of Health Information Science, has studied the impact of technology on client care and says EHRs can allow nurses to make well-informed, timely decisions about client care. Technology also makes it easier to access nursing research relevant to their clients. But Borycki cautions that some research suggests technology can lead to medical errors if it isn't designed in a clinician-friendly way. That's why she says it's essential for nurses to provide their expertise when new client documentation methods are being developed and introduced. "Nurses can identify aspects of technology that don't allow for its easy introduction to the clinical practice setting," she says. "They can identify functions, features, and components of technology that don't meet nursing's needs, and suggest elements that should be changed."

Source: Shaw, J. (2006). From Paper to Programming. *Registered Nurse Journal*, 18(2). Reprinted with Permission.

INFORMATION PRESENTATION

The wealth of information available through EHR systems must be managed to ensure that authorized caregivers (e.g., nurses) and others with legitimate uses have the information they need in their preferred presentation form.

For example, a nurse may prefer to see data organized by source, caregiver, encounter, problem, or date. Data can be presented in detail or summary form. Tables, graphs, narrative, and other forms of information presentation must be accommodated. Some users may need to know only of the presence or absence of certain data, not the nature of the data itself. For example, blood donation centres test blood for HIV, hepatitis, and other conditions. If a donor has a positive test result, the centre may not be given the specific information regarding the test but just general information that a test result was abnormal and that the client should be referred to an appropriate health care provider.

CANADA HEALTH INFOWAY

Canada Health Infoway, established in 2001, is an independent not-for-profit corporation created by Canada's First Ministers to foster and accelerate the development and adoption of electronic health record systems with compatible standards and communications technologies. It is funded by the federal government to work with the ten provinces and three territories to implement private, secure EHR systems, enabling best practices and successful projects in one region to be shared or replicated in other regions of the country.[8] Infoway developed Vision 2015 which was an information and communications technology roadmap for health care in Canada. This initiative is made up of the following five key priorities:

1. Complete work underway in Electronic Health Records, Telehealth, and Public Health Surveillance
2. Implement Electronic Medical Record (EMR) systems in physician offices and Provider Order Entry systems in hospitals
3. Deploy Wait Time Management Systems
4. Implement Consumer Health Solutions to support self-care
5. Integrate Chronic Disease Management systems, starting with Diabetes[9]

The February 11, 2011 *Health Edition* reported that almost 50 percent of Canada (by population) has an electronic health record accessible to their health providers.[10]

INTERFACE BETWEEN THE INFORMATICS NURSE AND THE CLINICAL INFORMATION SYSTEM

Information demands in health care systems are pushing the development of CISs and EHRs. The ongoing development of computer technology—smaller, faster machines with extensive storage capabilities and the ability for cross-platform communication—is making the goal of an integrated electronic system a realistic option, not just a long-term dream. As these systems evolve, informatics nurses will play an important role in their development, implementation, and evaluation.

Informatics nurses, because of their expertise, are in an ideal position to assist with the development, implementation, and evaluation of CISs. Their knowledge of policies, procedures, and clinical care is essential as workflow systems are redesigned within a CIS. It is not unusual for nurses within an institution to have more hands-on interaction with and knowledge of different departments than any other group of employees in an institution.

TRENDS IN COMPUTING

As noted earlier, computers have moved from the realm of a "nice to have" luxury item to a "NEED to have" essential resource for professional practice. Nurses are knowledge workers who require accurate and up-to-date information for their professional work. The explosion in information—some estimate that all information is replaced every 9 to 12 months—requires nurses to be on the cutting edge of knowledge to practise ethically and safely. Trends in computing will also affect the work of professional nurses and not just through the development of CISs and EHRs. Research advances, new devices, monitoring equipment, sensors, and "smart body parts" will all change the way that health care is conceptualized, practised, and delivered.

Within this context, not every nurse will need to be an informatics specialist, but every nurse must be computer literate. **Computer literacy** is defined as the knowledge and understanding of computers combined with the ability to use them effectively (Joos, Whitman, Smith, & Nelson, 1996). Computer literacy may be interpreted as different levels of expertise for different people in various roles. At the most basic level, computer literacy involves knowing how to turn on a computer, start and stop simple application programs, and save and print information. For health care professionals, computer literacy requires an understanding of systems used in clinical practice, education, and research settings. In clinical practice, for example, electronic health records and clinical information systems are widely used. The computer-literate nurse is able to use these systems effectively and can address issues discussed earlier, such as confidentiality, security, and privacy. At the same time, the nurse must be able to effectively use applications typically found on personal computers (PCs), such as word-processing software, spreadsheets, presentation graphics,

and statistical programs used for research. Finally, the computer-literate nurse must know how to access information from a variety of electronic sources and how to evaluate the appropriateness of the information at both the professional and client level. The remainder of this chapter is designed to help you gain a broader understanding of computer literacy and the computing environment of PCs and the online world, and includes a discussion of future trends.

DEVELOPMENT OF MODERN COMPUTING

Weiser and Brown (1996) have characterized the history and future of computing as having three phases. The first phase, known as the "mainframe era," is characterized by many people sharing one computer. Computers were found behind closed doors and run by experts with specialized knowledge and skills. Although we have mostly moved beyond the mainframe era, it still exists in CISs (hence, some of the problems discussed previously) and other situations with large mainframe systems, such as banking, weather forecasting, and academic institutions.

The archetypal computer of the mainframe era must be the ENIAC, developed at the University of Pennsylvania in 1945. The Electronic Numerical Integrator and Computer (ENIAC) was conceived by John Mauchly, an American physicist, and built at the Moore School of Engineering by Mauchly and J. Presper Eckert, an engineer. The ENIAC is regarded as the first successful digital computer. It weighed more than 60,000 pounds and contained more than 18,000 vacuum tubes. About 2,000 of the computer's vacuum tubes were replaced each month by a team of six technicians. Despite one vacuum tube blowing approximately every 15 minutes, the functioning of the ENIAC was still considered to be reliable! Many of the ENIAC's first tasks were for military purposes, such as calculating ballistic-firing tables and designing atomic weapons. Because the ENIAC was initially not a stored-program machine, it had to be reprogrammed for each task.

Phase II in modern computing is the "PC era," which is characterized by one person to one computer. In this era, the personal computing relationship is personal and intimate. Similar to a car, the computer is seen as a special, relatively expensive item, which requires attention but provides a valuable service in one's life.

The first harbinger of the PC era was in 1948, with the development of the transistor at Bell Telephone Laboratories. The transistor, which could act as an electric switch, replaced the costly, energy-inefficient, and unreliable vacuum tubes in computers and other devices, including televisions. By the late 1960s, integrated circuits, tiny transistors, and other electrical components arranged on a single chip of silicon replaced individual transistors in computers. Integrated circuits became miniaturized, enabling more components to be designed into a single computer circuit. In the 1970s refinements in integrated circuit technology led to the development of the modern microprocessor, integrated circuits that contained thousands of transistors. Weiser and Brown (1996) date the true start of the second phase as 1984, when the number of people using personal computers surpassed the number of people using shared computers.

Manufacturers used integrated circuit technology to build smaller and cheaper computers. The first PCs were sold by Instrumentation Telemetry Systems. The Altair 8800 appeared in 1975. Graphical user interfaces were first designed by the Xerox Corporation in a prototype computer, the Alto, developed in 1974. This prototype computer incorporated many of the features found on computers today, including a mouse, a graphical user interface, and a user-friendly operating system. However, the Xerox Corporation made a corporate decision to not pursue commercial development of the PC, the rationale being that the core business strategy of Xerox was copiers, not computers. One only has to look at how PCs have proliferated throughout the world to realize that this choice may not have been the smartest business decision ever made. In fact, this whole episode has become a bit of a computer history legend (Hiltzik, 2000; Smith & Alexander, 1988). Continuing development of sophisticated operating systems and miniaturization of components (modern microprocessors contain as many as 10 million transistors) have enabled computers to be developed that can run programs and manipulate data in ways that were unimaginable in the era of the ENIAC.

UBIQUITOUS COMPUTING

Phase III has been dubbed the era of **ubiquitous computing (UC),** characterized by many computers to each person. In 1996 Weiser and Brown (1996) estimated that the crossover with the PC era would occur between 2005 and 2020. Their prediction was not far off; many of their forecasts have already become reality. According to Weiser and Brown, in the ubiquitous computing phase, computers would be everywhere—in walls, chairs, clothing, light switches, cars, appliances, and so on. In the UC era, computers are so fundamental to our human experience that they will "disappear" and we will cease to be aware of them. The result will be "calm technology," in which computers do not cause stress and anxiety for the user but, rather, recede into the background of life.

For those who are skeptical that this era has either already come or will come to pass, consider two other ubiquitous technologies: writing and electricity (Weiser, 1991). In Egyptian times, writing was a secret art, known and performed only by specially trained scribes who lived on a level close to royalty. Clay tablets and, later, papyrus were precious commodities. Many people died without ever having seen a piece of paper in their lives! Now, paper and writing are everywhere. Within the course of an average day, most people use and discard hundreds of pieces of paper, never giving them a second thought. Electricity has a similar history. When electricity was first invented in the 19th century, entire factories were designed to accommodate the presence of light bulbs and bulky motors. The placement of workers, machines, and parts was designed around the need for electricity and motors. Today, electricity is everywhere. It is hidden in the walls and stored in tiny batteries. The average car has more than 22 motors and 25 solenoids.

We only have to look around a typical house to see how UC is becoming part of our lives. Microprocessors exist in every room: appliances in the kitchen, remote controls for the TV and stereo in the den, and clock radios and cordless phones in the bedroom. And the bathroom? Matsushita of Japan has developed a prototype toilet (dubbed the "smart toilet") that includes an online, real-time health-monitoring system. It measures the user's weight, fat content, and urine sugar level; plots the recorded data on a graph; and sends the data instantaneously to a health care provider for monitoring (Watts, 1999).

Another dimension of UC is the Internet. Each time you connect to the Internet, you are connecting with millions of information resources and hundreds of information delivery systems. A person truly does become one person to hundreds of computers. It is ironic that the interface to the UC world of the Internet is still through a PC. But this is changing. Wireless, infrared connections eliminate wires; handheld devices eliminate the bulky PC. We have become wireless and mobile—UC is a reality.

Ubiquitous computing integrates computation into the environment, instead of having computers which are distinct objects. Ubiquitous health care is the delivery of health related services and information via ubiquitous computing technologies (Figure 4-1). Examples could be two physicians discussing a case over the telephone, or a physician at one hospital performing surgery at another facility miles away, using videoconferencing equipment and robotic technology. Ubiquitous health care is an expansion of the functionality around Telemedicine and encompasses preventive, promotive, and curative aspects.[11]

VIRTUAL REALITY

According to Weiser (1991), virtual reality (VR) is roughly the opposite of ubiquitous computing. Virtual reality puts people inside a computer-generated world, whereas UC puts the computer out in the world with people. Virtual reality, although still limited in its development, has enormous potential in health care applications.

Virtual reality, despite its recent popularization, is not new. Similar to the Internet, it had its beginnings within the U.S. Department of Defense with innovations developed during the 1960s. During the time of

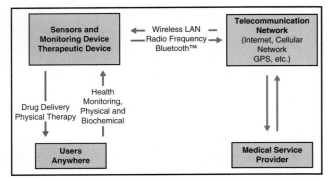

Figure 4-1 Concept of Ubiquitous Healthcare

Source: MELab. *Ubiquitous Healthcare in MELab.* Retrieved from http://melab.snu.ac.kr/dokuwiki/doku.php?id=research:melab:uhealthcare, April 12, 2011. Reprinted with permission.

the Cold War, great fear focused on the possibility of a nuclear attack. Military leaders sought to develop systems that would remain intact in the face of great destruction. The Internet, a worldwide network of computers, was developed so that the electronic communication infrastructure could not be destroyed. Electronic mail (email) was created to ensure rapid and secure communication in the event the wire-based telephone system was destroyed. Virtual reality simulations were developed so that jet pilots' training would mimic a world turned upside down: flying through fire, mushroom clouds, and poisonous gases in planes that might lack air-to-ground control systems.

Current virtual reality systems have developed from these early applications. With VR, a person can see, move through, and react to computer-simulated items or environments. Using certain tools, such as a head-mounted computer display and a handheld input device, the user

CRITICAL THINKING

Think of the freedom of going wireless. Wireless phones allow us to walk around the house, fold laundry, make the bed, straighten up a room, and yes, even go to the bathroom, all while talking on the phone. Remember being tethered by a phone cord?

Many businesses still do not provide their workers with wireless technology. Think of possible reasons why. Would wireless applications in health care settings improve the efficiency of care delivery systems? Why or why not?

feels immersed in and can interact with this world. The virtual world can represent the current world or a world that is difficult or impossible to experience first-hand—for example, the world of molecules, the interior of the human body, or the surface of Pluto. By putting the sensors on the person (e.g., a head-mounted computer display or sensors in gloves, shoes, and glasses), the person can move and experience the world in a typical way—by walking, moving, and using the senses of touch, sight, smell, and hearing.

To date, VR applications have been more developed in medicine and other fields, but interest is growing for its applications in nursing. Within medicine, VR has allowed physicians to develop minimally invasive surgical techniques. Traditionally, surgery is performed by making incisions and directly interacting with the organs and tissues. Recent innovations in video technology allow direct viewing of internal body cavities through natural orifices or small incisions. The surgeon is able to perform laparoscopic cholecystectomy and laparoscopic bowel surgeries, enabling clients to have shorter lengths of stay in hospital and faster recoveries.

Applications in medical education also exist. Virtual reality allows information visualization through the display of enormous amounts of information contained in large databases. Through 3-D visualization, students can understand important physiological principles or basic anatomy. Students can go inside a human body to visualize structures and see how they work. Changes in physiologic functioning can also be observed. For example, students can use clinical simulation equipment to hear heart and lung sounds, bowel sounds, and even see the consequence of administering the wrong medication to the mannequin.

IDT is a company that specializes in simulation consultancy and engineering. They act as project integrators of the Challenging Environment Assessment Lab (CEAL) simulator and the falls laboratory simulator at the Toronto Rehabilitation Institute in Ontario.[12] Toronto Rehab is home to one of the world's most advanced rehabilitation research facilities known as iDAPT (Intelligent Design for Adaptation, Participation and Technology). iDAPT brings together the brightest research minds and state-of-the-art technology, with CEAL as its centrepiece. CEAL features the world's first hydraulic motion simulator that mimics everyday environmental challenges faced by older people and those with disabling illness and injury. The simulator has different chambers that can be lifted on and off the base to generate snow and ice, different motions, slopes, and terrain. Scientists will use this lab to safely and accurately measure the difficulties encountered in the real world and to evaluate the impact of new treatments, devices, and technologies.[13]

Applications in nursing are similar. For students learning clinical procedures, VR provides the opportunity to practise invasive and less commonly occurring procedures in the lab so they will have both the skill and confidence necessary when encountering a client requiring the procedure. Likewise, VR will enhance client education materials. Diabetic clients needing to understand the physiologic processes of the pancreas could visualize the organ to more fully understand their disease and treatment. Clients requiring painful or unusual procedures could experience a VR simulation as a means of preparation. By providing an alternate environment, VR also has the potential to mitigate or minimize the side effects of certain procedures, such as chemotherapy in clients with cancer.

THE INTERNET

The Internet will continue to change the way we communicate and obtain information. Many mistakenly believe that the Internet is a recent development. But, like VR, it has been around for almost four decades. The modern Internet started out in 1969, as a U.S. Defense Department network called ARPAnet. Scientists built ARPAnet with the intention of creating a network that would still be able to function efficiently if part of the network were damaged. Since then, the Internet has grown, changed, matured, and mutated, but the essential structure of interconnected domains randomly distributed throughout the world has remained the same. ARPAnet no longer exists, but many of the standards established for that first network still govern the communication and structure of the modern Internet.

In 1989 English computer scientist Timothy Berners-Lee introduced the World Wide Web (WWW). Berners-Lee initially designed the WWW to aid communication between physicists who were working in different parts of the world for the European Laboratory for Particle Physics, known in French as Conseil Européen pour la Recherche Nucléaire (CERN). As it grew, however, the WWW revolutionized the use of the Internet. During the early 1990s increasingly large numbers of users who were not part of the scientific or academic communities began to use the Internet, in large part because of the ability of the WWW to easily handle multimedia documents. Other changes have also influenced the growth of the Internet, such as the U.S. government's High-Performance Computing Act of 1991, the decision to allow computers other than those used for research and military purposes to connect to the network, and the development of user-friendly software and tools that allowed less experienced computer users to obtain information quickly and easily.

USING THE INTERNET FOR CLINICAL PRACTICE

A major use of the Internet is to obtain information. In clinical practice, this dimension of the Internet is becoming essential to ensure that you have accurate and up-to-date information for your nursing work. To use information that exists on the Internet, skills must be developed for searching quickly and efficiently. A variety of strategies can be used for searching, including quick and dirty searching, links, and brute force. Keep in mind that you must be persistent: no single search strategy will work all the time, nor is any one search engine more effective than any other. Search engines are good starting points, but you can augment their effectiveness by adding a few other strategies to your Internet exploration tool kit.

THE P-F-A ASSESSMENT

One strategy to develop your search is to conduct a purpose-focus-approach (P-F-A) assessment. To determine your purpose, ask yourself why you are doing the search and why you need the information. Consider questions such as the following:

- Is it for personal interest?
- Do you want to obtain information to share with co-workers or a client?
- Are you verifying information given to you by someone else?
- Are you preparing a report or writing a paper for a class or project?

Based on your purpose, your focus may be as follows:

- broad and general (e.g., basic information for yourself)
- lay-oriented (e.g., to give information to a client) or professionally oriented (e.g., to locate information for colleagues)
- narrow and technical, with a research orientation

Purpose combined with focus determines your approach. For example, information that is broad and general can be found using brute force methods or quick and dirty searching. Lay information can be quickly accessed at a few key sites, including MEDLINE*plus* and consumer health organizations. Similarly, professional associations and societies are a good starting point for professionally oriented information. Scientific and research information usually requires literature resources that can be found in databases such as MEDLINE or CINAHL (Cumulative Index to Nursing and Allied Health Literature).

QUICK AND DIRTY SEARCHING

Quick and dirty searching is a very simple but surprisingly effective search strategy. First, start with a search engine, such as Google (www.google.ca). Next, type in the term of interest. At this point, do not worry about being overly broad or general. You will retrieve an enormous number of found references (called hits), but you are interested only in the first 10 to 20. Look at the uniform resource locators (URLs), that is, the addresses of the sites that are returned by your search, and try to decipher what they mean. Pay attention to the domains: .com is commercial; .org refers to an organization; and .ca identifies a Canadian website. Quickly visit a few sites. Look for the information you need and useful links. If a site is not relevant, use the back button on your browser to return to your search results and go to the next site. When you find a site that appears to be useful, begin to explore the site. Many sites will connect you to other sites, using links, or hot buttons. If you click on a link, it will take you to a related site. Most sites have links you can follow to connect to other relevant sites. This process—quick search, quick review, clicking, and linking—can provide a starting point for finding useful information in a relatively short period of time.

BRUTE FORCE

Brute force searching is another alternative: type in an address in the URL box (the address box at the top of the browser window) and see what happens. The worst outcome is an annoying error message, but you may land on a site that is exactly what you want. To be effective, think of how URLs work: they usually start with www (for World Wide Web), then a word or phrase in the middle is followed by a domain. Perhaps you are trying to find a school of nursing at a certain university. What is the common name for the university? The very logical URL for the University of Victoria is www.uvic.ca. Organizations are also quite logical in their URLs: www.caccn. ca is the Canadian Association of Critical Care Nurses (CACCN); www.srna.org is the Saskatchewan Registered Nurses Association (SRNA).

LINKS AND BOOKMARKS

As noted earlier, just about every website has links to other websites of related interest. Take advantage of these links, because the site developer has already done some work finding other useful resources. Combine quick and dirty searching or brute force with links to find the information you need. Each site you visit will have more links, and in this way, the resources keep building. Visiting a variety of sites will open up the vistas of information that are available. When you find a site of interest, bookmark it or add it to your list of favourites. A bookmark list, or list of favourites, is like a personal address book. Each time you find a site that is particularly useful, add it to your list of favourites, using the appropriate feature in your browser. Eventually, you will have a comprehensive list of sites that are relevant to your work and interests. Use this list to quickly return to websites in the future.

RESOURCES FOR PROFESSIONALS AND CONSUMERS

The preceding discussion has focused on strategies to use when you are faced with a "needle in a haystack" searching situation—just dive in and see what you find. The advantage of this method is that it is fast and easy. The disadvantages include sites of dubious quality that may be accessed, and the process, though fast, is not terribly efficient.

Another approach is to develop a short list of well-known, well-researched sites that can be used as starting points for further exploration. Such a list is useful to share with others so that they can begin their own exploration. These should be sites that you have determined are trustworthy and reliable, for example, organizations and associations with which we are all familiar, such as the Canadian Cancer Society (CCS). The CCS has client education and consumer information materials that can be obtained through www.cancer.ca. In addition to the traditional types of resources available from the CCS website, you can also email the society to request more information, sign up for regular updates and news, read news items, and obtain updated statistical information. The website is truly a value-added version of the CCS. Practically any health organization you can think of has created a virtual storefront on the Internet. Professional associations, in nursing, medicine, and other disciplines, are also becoming comprehensive resource websites. Canadianrn.com (www.canadianrn.com) has a handy list of Canadian associations in nursing and related disciplines. Other resources include Canadian government agencies, such as the Canadian Institutes for Health Research (CIHR) (www.cihr-irsc.gc.ca) and Canada Health Infoway (www.infoway-inforoute.ca). Once again, all these agencies have been busy creating virtual institutes. A useful resource is Canadian Health Services Research Foundation (www.chsrf.ca/links/gov_e.php), which can point you to news, information, tools, and databases.

Although these resources are the web versions of known and useful organizations, some virtual resources exist only on the Internet. One such site that is particularly impressive is MEDLINE*plus* (http://www.nlm.nih.gov/medlineplus/), developed by the National Library of Medicine. A similar resource, specific to oncology, is OncoLink at the University of Pennsylvania (www.oncolink.org). OncoLink, created in 1994, was the first multimedia oncology information resource on the Internet. It continues to adhere to the following objectives: dissemination of information relevant to the field of oncology, education of health care personnel, education of patients, families and others, and rapid collection of information pertinent to oncology (Oncolink, 2011).

LITERATURE RESOURCES

Thinking back to P-F-A, if you are searching for scientific, technical, or research-oriented information then you must search literature databases. The first place to turn to is the National Library of Medicine, which is the home of the **MEDLARS (Medical Literature Analysis and Retrieval System),** a computerized system of databases and databanks offered by the National Library of Medicine (NLM). A person may search the computer files either to produce a list of publications (bibliographic citations) or to retrieve factual information on a specific question. The most well-known of all the databases in the MEDLARS system is MEDLINE, NLM's premier bibliographic database covering the fields of medicine, nursing, dentistry, veterinary medicine, and the preclinical sciences. Journal articles are indexed for MEDLINE, and their citations are searchable using NLM's controlled vocabulary, called MeSH (Medical Subject Headings). MEDLINE contains all citations published in *Index Medicus* and corresponds in part to the International Nursing Index and the Index to Dental Literature. Citations include the English abstract when it is published with the article (approximately 76 percent of the current file). MEDLINE contains more than 11 million records from 7,300 health science journals. The file is updated weekly. An individual can search MEDLINE for free, using PubMed, a specially designed search engine (http://www.ncbi.nlm.nih.gov/sites/entrez). With this search engine, there are no fees to the user to access the MEDLINE database.

Two other literature resources to investigate are the U.S. National Guideline Clearinghouse (NGC) (http://www.ngc.gov/) and the Canadian Agency for Drugs and Technologies in Health (CADTH) (http://www.cadth.ca/), which until April 2006 was known as the Canadian Coordinating Office for Health Technology Assessment (CCOHTA). Whereas MEDLINE includes citations to articles in professional journals, the NGC is a comprehensive database of evidence-based clinical practice guidelines and related documents produced by the Agency for Healthcare Research and Quality (AHRQ) in partnership with the American Medical Association (AMA) and the American Association of Health Plans (AAHP). The NGC mission is to provide an accessible mechanism for obtaining objective, detailed information on clinical practice guidelines and to further their dissemination, implementation, and use. The NGC database is important for physicians, nurses, and other health professionals and health care providers; it is also useful for health plans, integrated delivery systems, and purchasers.

CADTH is a primary resource for unbiased health information on drugs, devices, health care systems, and best practices. It is funded by the Canadian federal, provincial, and territorial governments.

A variety of other literature resources are available on the Internet, some of which have fees attached. However, do not automatically assume that you must pay the fee. Your workplace or school may have licensing agreements in place with different vendors, and as an employee or student you may have access to the literature resources. Check with your library or information services department to see whether any of these arrangements apply.

The final element of searching for literature online is locating full-text articles. The databases discussed (e.g., MEDLINE and others) do not contain full-text articles: they provide literature citations only. However, most academic journals now have full-text articles online, available to university students through their library access. You can also visit the publisher's website to see whether access to the journal is available, or research the old-fashioned way, that is, by taking a trip to the library and photocopying articles. A final option is to access a service such as Ingenta (http://www.ingentaconnect.com/) to gain access to its collection of scholarly research materials. This resource allows you to conduct a search. It identifies which articles can be sent to you and what the fees will be (including article fees, service charges, and copyright fees).

EVALUATION OF INFORMATION FOUND ON THE INTERNET

When using Internet resources, one must always use critical thinking skills to evaluate the information that is found. The wide-open nature of the Internet means that just about anyone with a computer and online access can create a home page and post it for the world to see. Although there are many excellent health- and nursing-related sites, others do not measure up in terms of accuracy, content, or currency.

In recent years, criteria for website evaluation have proliferated. They range from the simple and cursory to the elaborate and expansive. I have found a simple mnemonic, "Are you PLEASED with the site?" to be very helpful (see Table 4-2).

The mnemonic makes the seven criteria very easy to remember, and I have found these criteria, in hundreds of hours of surfing and evaluating, to be extremely comprehensive (Nicoll, 2000, 2001). To determine whether you are PLEASED, consider the following:

- *P—Purpose.* What is the author's purpose in developing the site? Are the author's objectives clear? Many people will develop a website as a hobby or a way of sharing information they have gathered. The true purpose of the site should be immediately evident. At the same time, consider your purpose; that is, think back to your P-F-A assessment. Congruence

TABLE 4-2	WEBSITE EVALUATION: ASK YOURSELF, "AM I PLEASED WITH THE SITE?"
P	Purpose
L	Links
E	Editorial (site content)
A	Author
S	Site navigation
E	Ethical disclosure
D	Date site last updated

should exist between the author's purpose and yours.

- **L—Links.** Evaluate the links at the site. Are they working? Links that do not take you anywhere are called dead links. Do they link to reliable sites? Critically evaluate the links at sites hosted by organizations, businesses, or institutions because these entities are usually presenting themselves as authorities on the subject at hand. Some pages, such as those created by individuals, are really nothing more than a collection of links. These can be useful as a starting point for a search, but it is still important to evaluate the links that are provided at the site.

- **E—Editorial (site content).** Is the information contained in the site accurate, comprehensive, and current? Is there a particular bias, or is the information presented in an objective way? Who is the consumer of the site: is it designed for health professionals, clients, consumers, or other audiences? Is the information presented in an appropriate format for the intended audience? Look at details, too. Are there misspellings and grammatical errors? "Under construction" banners that have been there forever? These types of errors can be very telling about the overall quality of the site.

- **A—Author.** Who is the author of the site? Does that person or group of people have the appropriate credentials? Is the author clearly identified by name and is contact information provided? One suggestion is to double-check an author's credentials by doing a literature search in MEDLINE. When people advertise themselves as "the leading worldwide authority" on a topic, they should have a few publications to their credit to establish their reputations. It is surprising how many times this search brings up nothing.

Be wary of how a person's credentials are presented. Consider a site where Dr. X is touted as an expert. Upon further exploration, you may find that, in fact, Dr. X does have a PhD (or an MD or an EdD), but the discipline in which this degree was obtained has nothing to do with the subject matter of the site. Remember that there is no universal process of peer review on the Internet and people can present themselves in any way that they want. Be suspicious.

Keep in mind that the webmaster and the author may be two (or more) different people. The webmaster is the person who designed the site and is responsible for its upkeep. The author is the person responsible for the content and the expert in the subject matter provided. In your evaluation, make sure you determine the qualifications of these people.

- **S—Site.** Is the site easy to navigate? Is it attractive? Does it download quickly or have too many graphics and other features that make it inefficient? A site that is pleasing to the eye will invite you to return. Sites that cause your computer to crash should be viewed with a skeptical eye.

- **E—Ethical.** Is contact information available for the site developer and the author? Is full disclosure available on the author and the purpose of the site? Is this information easy to find or is it buried deep in the website? Many commercial services, particularly pharmaceutical companies, have excellent websites with very useful information. Some of them, however, exist only to sell their product, although this purpose may not be immediately evident.

- **D—Date.** When was the site last updated? Is it current? Does the information need to be updated regularly? Generally, with health and nursing information, information needs to be updated both frequently and regularly. You should be concerned with sites that have not been updated within 12 to 18 months. The date the site was last updated should be prominently displayed. Keep in mind that different pages within the site may be updated at different times. Be sure to check the date on each of the pages that you visit.

CRITICAL THINKING

PubMed has made the vast resources of the NLM available, for free, to anyone with a computer and Internet access. Some argue that scientific publications, such as the *New England Journal of Medicine,* are too technical and sophisticated for laypeople. Others contend that the resources of the NLM are maintained with taxpayer dollars and, therefore, should be available to all taxpayers.

Which point of view do you support? Why? As a health care professional, what resources for understanding and clarification would you suggest to your clients who are accessing abstracts and article citations from the professional health care literature?

As you become more proficient at evaluating websites, you may have additional criteria to add to this list or criteria that are important to you for a specific purpose, but, in general, this simple group of seven criteria is surprisingly comprehensive. Test them for yourself.

LITERATURE APPLICATION

Citation: McMullan, M. (2006). Patients using the Internet to obtain health information: how this affects the patient-health professional relationship. *Patient Education and Counseling,* October 63(1-2): 24-28. Copyright © 2006 Elsevier. Reprinted with permission from Elsevier.

Discussion: A review of the literature was carried out to determine the use of the Internet for health information by the client and how this could affect the client-health professional relationship. The review showed that the majority of health related Internet searches by clients are for specific medical conditions. There has been a shift in the role of the client from passive recipient to active consumer of health information.

Implications for Practice: It is important that health professionals acknowledge clients' search for knowledge and that they discuss the information offered by clients and guide them to reliable and accurate health websites.

Do a quick search on a topic of interest, visit a number of sites, and determine just how PLEASED you are with what you find.

CASE STUDY 4-1

You are working in a women's health clinic with a number of nurse practitioners and family physicians. The clinic receives at least two to three telephone calls a day from women with a urinary tract infection (UTI). The question is asked, "Do all these women need to be seen by a practitioner, or can some of the cases be managed by telephone?" You are asked to be on a committee to explore this issue and possibly come up with a protocol. Where do you begin? Is a protocol for telephone management of UTI realistic?

KEY CONCEPTS

- Computers are no longer a novelty but a fact of life, with exponential growth on a worldwide basis.

- Within nursing, the combination of computer science and information science with clinical expertise allows us to develop systems that have the ultimate goal of improving client outcomes.

- Nursing informatics is the application of computer science and information science to nursing. It promotes the generation, management, and processing of relevant data in order to use information and develop knowledge that supports nursing in all practice domains.

- Nurses can pursue formal education in nursing informatics at both the graduate and undergraduate levels. Informal education in informatics can be pursued through self-study, attendance at conferences, and reading the informatics literature.

- Certification in nursing informatics is voluntary and recognizes superior achievement and excellence in the specialty.

- The history of modern computing is described in three phases: phase I, the era of the mainframe computer; phase II, the era of the personal computer; and phase III, ubiquitous computing. The phase of ubiquitous computing, characterized by many computers to one person, was predicted to occur between 2005 and 2020. It has already begun.

- Virtual reality simulations have been used in education and client care. Minimally invasive surgery has been developed in large part through the technology of virtual reality.

- Effective searching for information on the Internet requires that you target your search. One technique is to conduct a P-F-A: a purpose-focus-approach assessment to determine what you are looking for and the best way to find it.

- PubMed is a search engine developed by the National Library of Medicine that allows you to search the databases of the MEDLARS system, including MEDLINE. It is free to anyone with Internet access.

- Information found on the Internet should be critically evaluated. Ask yourself, "Am I PLEASED with the site?"

  P—Purpose
  L—Links
  E—Editorial (site content)
  A—Author
  S—Site navigation
  E—Ethical disclosure
  D—Date site last updated

KEY TERMS

client-focused clinical
   information system
clinical information system (CIS)
computer literacy
data capture
departmental clinical
   information system
electronic health record
   (EHR)

information
   communications
MEDLARS (Medical
   Literature Analysis and
   Retrieval System)
storage
ubiquitous computing
   (UC)

REVIEW QUESTIONS

1. E-health includes which of the following activities?
   A. obtaining health information online
   B. shopping for health products online
   C. online case management
   D. all of the above

2. Which of the following describes certification in nursing informatics?
   A. It is mandatory in certain states or for certain jobs.
   B. It is voluntary and recognizes superior achievement in the specialty.
   C. It is a component of Category II education in informatics.
   D. It is automatic after practising in the field for five years.

3. A person is HIV-positive and chooses not to reveal this information to a nurse during an admission assessment. Which of the following describes what the person is doing with this information?
   A. keeping it anonymous
   B. keeping it secure
   C. keeping it confidential
   D. keeping it private

4. If a client came to you asking for a website to learn more about diabetes, which of the following would be appropriate for you to suggest?
   A. MEDLINE at the National Library of Medicine
   B. OncoLink
   C. MEDLINE*plus*
   D. all of the above

5. Decipher the following URL: www.uvic.ca. This is the URL for which of the following websites?
   A. University of Victoria
   B. Victoria Visitors and Convention Bureau
   C. Victoria State Government
   D. Victoria Nurses Association

6. You are interested in learning more about amyotrophic lateral sclerosis (ALS). You find a website where the author states that he is a worldwide leading researcher into causes for this disease. Which of the following describes what you do as part of your evaluation of the author's credentials?
   A. take him at his word
   B. email him and ask for a list of references
   C. ask several colleagues whether they are familiar with his research
   D. conduct an author search on MEDLINE

REVIEW ACTIVITIES

1. An immediate priority of Canada Health Infoway is the development and implementation of effective electronic health record solutions in Canada. Is there a fully functional electronic health record system in place in your community today? If not, what are the barriers to implementation? Check the Canada Health Infoway website at http://www.infoway-inforoute.ca/en/home/home.aspx.

2. A popular area of research in nursing informatics has been the attitudes of nurses toward computers and technology. Another topic that has been studied widely is ergonomics, that is, the relationship of a person's body to the computer equipment and the negative health outcomes that may occur (e.g., repetitive motion injury is a

common problem associated with computer use). As we move into the era of ubiquitous computing, do you think these research areas will continue to receive priority? Why or why not?

EXPLORING THE WEB

- Pick a specialty area in nursing that interests you. Visit the Canadian Nurses Association (http://www. cna-nurses.ca) to determine whether the CNA certifies nurses in this specialty. If yes, what are the requirements? If no, is there another organization that credentials nurses in this specialty? Do a search to find another organization and its requirements for certification.

- Find a current health news item, either in the newspaper or in a report on the television or radio. Search the Internet to find the original source of the news item. Was the way it was reported (e.g., newspaper, television, or radio) accurate? What information was included? What was omitted?

REFERENCES

American Nurses Credentialing Center. (1993). *Statement of philosophy.* Washington, DC: American Nurses Publishing.

Ball, M. J., & Hannah, K. J. (1984). *Using computers in nursing.* Reston, VA: Reston Publishers.

Ball, M. J., Hannah, K. J., & Douglas, J. (2000). Nursing and informatics. In M. Ball, K. Hannah, S. Newbold, & J. Douglas (Eds.), *Nursing informatics: Where caring and technology meet* (3rd ed., pp. 6–14). New York: Springer-Verlag.

Bard, M. R. (2000). The future of e-health. *Cybercitizen Health,* 1(1), 1–13.

Bristow, L. (2005, November/December). Sunnybrook tests new patient-safety alert system. *Canadian Healthcare Technology.* Retrieved from http:// www.canhealth.com/current%20issue.html

Canadian Nurses Association. (2006). *Toward 2020 – Visions for Nursing.* Ottawa: Author.

Canadian Nurses Association. (2006). *E-nursing strategy for Canada.* Ottawa: Author.

Canadian Nursing Informatics Association. (2003). *Educating tomorrow's nurses: Where's Nursing Informatics?* Project G3-6B-DP1-0054, p. 8. Retrieved from http://www.cnia.ca/OHIHfinaltoc.htm

COACH: Canada's Health Informatics Association. *Health informatics education in Canada.* Retrieved from http://coachorg.com/health_informatics/health_informatics_education/hi_education_in_Canada.htm

CPRI Work Group on Confidentiality, Privacy & Security. (1995). *Guidelines for establishing information security policies at organizations using computer-based patient records.* Schaumburg, IL: Computer-based Patient Record Institute.

DeLoitte. (2010). Did you know? *Healthcare Information Management & Communications Canada,* 24(3), 60.

Giiwednong Health Link (2011). Retrieved from http://www.giiwednonghealth.ca/

Graves, J. R., & Corcoran, S. (1989). The study of nursing informatics. *Image: The Journal of Nursing Scholarship,* 21, 227–231.

Grobe, S. J. (1988). Introduction. In H. E. Petersen & U. G. Jelger (Eds.), *Preparing nurses for using information systems: Recommended informatics competencies* (p. 4). New York: National League for Nursing.

Hannah, K. J. (1985). Current trends in nursing informatics: Implications for curriculum planning. In K. J. Hannah, E. J. Guillemin, & D. N. Conklin (Eds.), *Nursing uses of computer and information science* (pp. 181–187). Amsterdam: Elsevier.

Health Edition. (2011). Almost half the country has an electronic health record. *Health Edition,* February 11 2011.

Hersher, B. (2000). New roles for nurses in health care information systems. In M. J. Ball, K. J. Hannah, S. Newbold, & J. Douglas (Eds.), *Nursing informatics: Where caring and technology meet* (3rd ed., pp. 80–87). New York: Springer-Verlag.

Hiltzik, M. (2000). *Dealers of lightning: Xerox PARC and the dawn of the computer age.* New York: Harper Business.

Hodges, L., Rothbaum, B., Kooper, R., Opdyke, D., Meyer, T., North, M., et al. (1995). Virtual environments for treating the fear of heights. *IEEE Computer,* 28(7), 27–34.

Internet World Stats. (2011). Internet Usage and Population Statistics. Retrieved from http://www.internetworldstats.com/stats14.htm

Jenkins, S. (2000). Nurses' responsibilities in the implementation of information systems. In M. J. Ball, K. J. Hannah, S. Newbold, & J. Douglas (Eds.), *Nursing informatics: Where caring and technology meet* (pp. 207–223). New York: Springer-Verlag.

Joos, I., Whitman, N., Smith, M., & Nelson, R. (1996). *Computers in small bytes: The computer workbook* (2nd ed.). New York: National League for Nursing.

Lau, F. (2006). A collaborative approach to building capacity in health informatics. *Electronic Healthcare,* 4(4), 88–92.

McMullen, M. (2006). Patients using the Internet to obtain health information: How this affects the patient-health professional relationship. *Patient Education and Counseling,* 63(1–2), 24–28.

Nagle, L. (2005). Dr. Lynn Nagle and the case for nursing informatics. *Canadian Journal of Nursing Leadership,* 18(1), 16–18.

National Nursing Informatics Project (NNIP) discussion paper. (1999). Project sponsored by CAUSN, CNA, Registered Nurses Association of British Columbia, Academy of Canadian Executive Nurses, and the Nursing Informatics Special Interest Group of COACH.

Nelson, R., & Joos, I. (1992). Strategies and resources for self-education in nursing informatics. In J. M. Arnold & G. A. Pearson (Eds.), *Computer applications in nursing education and practice* (pp. 9–19). New York: National League for Nursing.

Newbold, S. K. (1996). The informatics nurse and the certification process. *Computers in Nursing,* 14(2), 84–85, 88.

Nicoll, L. H. (2000). *Nurses' guide to the Internet* (3rd ed.). Philadelphia: Lippincott, Williams & Wilkins.

Nicoll, L. H. (2001). Quick and effective website evaluation. *Lippincott's Case Management,* 6(4), 220–221.

OncoLink. (2011). About Oncolink. Abramson Cancer Center of the University of Pennsylvania. Retrieved from http://www.oncolink.org/about/article.cfm?id=11

Pilarski, T. (2011). Where is nursing informatics in undergraduate nursing education? *CJNI: Canadian Journal of Nursing Informaticsm, 5*(4), Article Two. Retrieved from http://cjni.net/journal/?p=1041

Sanli, M. (2005). Mount Sinai Hospital develops "Sinai e-Learning": Making it simpler for busy clinical staff to master healthcare applications. *Healthcare Quarterly, 8*(2), 82–84.

Semancik, M. (1997). *The history of clinical information systems: Legacy systems, computer-based patient record and point of care.* Seattle, WA: SpaceLabs Medical.

Shaw, J. (2006). From paper to programming. *Registered Nurse Journal, 18*(2), 14–17.

Sieburg, R., Mattheus, & Christensen, J. P. (Eds.). *Interactive technology and the new paradigm for healthcare* (pp. 334–339). Washington, DC: IOS Press.

Smith, D., & Alexander, R. (1988). *Fumbling the future: How Xerox invented, then ignored, the first personal computer.* New York: Morrow.

Statistics Canada. (2009). Canadian Internet Use Survey. *The Daily,* May 10, 2010. Retrieved from http://www.statcan.gc.ca/daily-quotidien/100510/dq100510a-eng.htm

Styles, M. M. (1989). *On specialization in nursing: Toward a new empowerment.* Kansas City, MO: American Nurses Foundation.

Ward, B. O. (1999). "Internet-positive patients" driving you crazy? Find out how to get online and cope. *Internet Medicine: A Critical Guide, 4*(7), 1, 6.

Watts, J. (1999). The healthy home of the future comes to Japan. *Lancet, 353*(9164), 1597–1600.

Weiser, M. (1991). The computer for the 21st century. *Scientific American, 265*(3), 94–102.

Weiser, M., & Brown, J. (1996, October 5). *The coming age of calm technology.* Retrieved from http://www.ubiq.com/hypertext/weiser/acmfuture2endnote.htm

SUGGESTED READINGS

Bassendowski, S. (2011). How are you using Social Networking Tools? *Canadian Journal of Nursing Informatics, 6*(1). Technology in Education Column. Retrieved from http://cjni.net/journal/?p=1199

Biem, H. J., Klimaszewski, A., & Chen, F. (2004). Computer telephony in healthcare. *Electronic Healthcare, 3*(2), 80–86.

Canadian Nurses Association. (2001) What is nursing informatics and why is it so important? *Nursing Now: Issues and Trends in Canadian Nursing,* 11, 1–4.

Canadian Nurses Association. (2002). Demystifying the electronic health record. *Nursing Now: Issues and Trends in Canadian Nursing,* 13, 1–4.

Canadian Nurses Association. (2003). Measuring nurses' workload. *Nursing Now: Issues and Trends in Canadian Nursing,* 15, 1–4.

Carter-Langford, A. (2010). Is privacy dead? *Canadian Healthcare Manager,* 17(4), 54.

Ellis, J., Langford, S., Mathews, J., Bourbonnais, F. F., Alain, D., & Cragg, B. (2011). Clinical evaluation online: Implementation of a clinical evaluation tool into a web-based format for baccalaureate nursing students. *CJNI: Canadian Journal of Nursing Informatics, 6*(1), Article One. Retrieved from http://cjni.net/journal/?p=1166

Health Canada. (2006). eHealth Resources: Initiatives. Retrieved from http://www.hc-sc.gc.ca/ohih-bsi/res/init_e.html

Lau, F. (2006). A collaborative approach to building capacity in health informatics. *Electronic Healthcare, 4*(4), 88–92.

Lau, F., Protti, D., & Coward, P. (2005). A review of information management practices for health ministries. *Healthcare Management Forum, 18*(2), 14–21.

Office of Health and the Information Highway (OHIH), Health Canada. (2006). *eHealth.* Retrieved from http://www.hc-sc.gc.ca/hcs-sss/ ehealth-esante/index_e.html

Pastore, M. (2002). *Internet Part of the Family in Canada.* Retrieved from http://www.clickz.com/stats/big_picture/geographics/article/php/964381

Pederson, L., & Leonard, K. (2005). Measuring information technology investment among Canadian academic health sciences centres. *Electronic Healthcare, 3*(3), 94–101.

Protti, D. (2003). Issues, musings and trends IT & EHR Governance: Who should the leaders be? *Healthcare Management Forum, 16*(1), 40–42.

Protti, D. (2004). England's revolutionary change in approach to the electronic health record. *Healthcare Management Forum, 17*(1), 32–35.

Sandhu, J. S., Anderson, K., Keen, D., & Yassi, A. (2005). Implementing information technology to improve workplace health: A web-based information needs assessment of managers in Fraser Health, British Columbia. *Healthcare Management Forum, 18*(4), 6–10.

Shaw, C. (2004). Who needs health information management professionals?—Every Healthcare Entity Does! *Healthcare Quarterly, 7*(3), 107–108.

Shop.org. (2002). "Statistics: Holiday 2002, Transactions and Spending." Retrieved from http://www.shop.org/learn/stats_intshop_canada.asp

Staggers, N., & Gassert, C. (2002). Results of a Delphi study to determine informatics competencies for nurses at four levels of practice. *Nursing Research,* 51(6), 383–390.

Strating, D., MacGregor, J., & Campbell, N. (2006). Bridging Information "islands": Designing an electronic health record that meets clinical needs. *Electronic Healthcare, 4*(4), 94–98.

Underhill, C., & McKeown, L. Getting a second opinion: Health information and the Internet. *Health Reports,* 19(1), 1–5.

Zytkowski, M. (2003). Nursing informatics: The key to unlocking contemporary nursing practice. *AACN Clinical Issues Advanced Practice in Acute Critical Care,* 14(3), 271–281.

CHAPTER ENDNOTES

1. Canadian Nursing Informatics Association. (2003). *Educating tomorrow's nurses: Where's nursing informatics?* Canadian Nursing Informatics Association, p. 8. Retrieved from http://www.cnia.ca/ OHIHfinaltoc.htm

2. Canadian Journal of Nursing Informatics, "About CJNI." Retrieved from http://cjni.net/journal/?page_id=2

3. Canada's Health Informatics Association (COACH), "Health Informatics Education in Canada." Retrieved from http://www.coachorg.com/health_informatics/health_informatics_education/hi_education_in_canada.htm

4. Canadian Nursing Informatics Association, "CNIA Nursing Informatics Education Bursary." Retrieved from http://cnia.ca/education.htm

5. Canadian Nursing Informatics Association, "Informatics Education – HITS Health Informatics Training System." Retrieved from http://www.cnia.ca/education.htm

6. Canadian Nursing Informatics Association, "Collaborating Associations." Retrieved from http://www.coachorg.com/COACH/health_informatics/health_informatics_associations.htm

7. e-Health 2011: Enabling Healthy Outcomes Conference (2011). Topics for Submission. Retrieved from http://www.e-healthconference.com/present-learn/topics-for-submission/

8. Canada Health Infoway. "Who we are." Retrieved from https://www.infoway-inforoute.ca/lang-en/about-infoway

9. Canada Health Infoway, "2011–2012 Summary Corporate Plan." Retrieved from http://www2.infoway-inforoute.ca/Documents/Infoway_Sum.Corp.Plan.2011-2012_EN.pdf

10. Health Edition. (2011). Almost half the country has an electronic health record. *Health Edition*, February 11 2011.

11. MELab website. Ubiquitous healthcare in MELab. Retrieved from http://melab.snu.ac.kr/dokuwiki/doku.php?id=research:melab:uhealthcare

12. IDT International Development of Technology website. "Company Background." Retrieved from http://www.idt-engineering.com/Company.html

13. Toronto Rehabilitation Institute website. "Facilities (iDAPT)." Retrieved from http://www.torontorehab.com/Research/Facilities.aspx

CHAPTER 5

Population-Based Health Care Practice

Patricia M. Lentsch Schoon, MPH, RN
Adapted by Victoria E. Pennick, RN, MHSc

The selection of groups for care should be based on the questions: What difference might nursing care be expected to make in this situation? Is it more or less than would be expected in other groups?
(Ruth B. Freeman, 1957)

OBJECTIVES

The purpose of this chapter is to enable the reader to

- discuss the social mandate to provide population-based health care at the global, national, provincial, and local levels;

- describe how population-based nursing is practised within the community and the health care system;

- identify vulnerable and high-risk population groups for whom specific health promotion and disease prevention services are indicated; and

- outline a multidisciplinary population-based planning and evaluation process that includes partnerships with the community and health care consumers.

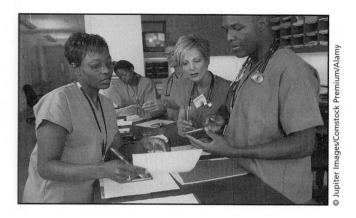

© Jupiter Images/Comstock Premium/Alamy

You are completing a clinical experience with the public health nurse in an elementary school located in a large metropolitan area. This school has 1,600 students from kindergarten to Grade 6. Forty percent of the families in the surrounding neighbourhood are in the low-income bracket; 46 percent immigrated to Canada within the past five years; 92 percent rent, rather than own their homes; virtually all of them live in high-rise apartments. Sixty-eight percent are Canadian citizens. Of those considered to be visible minorities 42 percent are South Asian, 11 percent are Filipino, 4 percent are Black, 4 percent are Asian, and 3 percent are Middle Eastern. Twenty-two percent of the total population in the area is under the age of 14; 93 percent of the students speak English as a second language. The school nurse encourages you to think about some of the social problems these children might encounter that will affect their health and the nursing actions you might take to help them overcome those problems.

> *What health problems might you expect to identify in this group of schoolchildren?*

> *What social and environmental factors might contribute to these health problems?*

> *What nursing actions directed at groups of children, rather than individuals, could you take to help these children?*

Nurses have acted to improve the health of populations and communities since the time of Florence Nightingale. Nightingale's actions to improve the health care of soldiers on the battlefields of the Crimean War and of the poor and infirm in London were directed at vulnerable population groups. Nightingale's actions were based on the recognition that vulnerable population groups were not able to advocate effectively for themselves. She became their advocate. Nightingale was able to intervene to improve the health status of disenfranchised groups of people by influencing the health policies of the English government and changing the health care delivery systems in London and on the battlefield. That same spirit of advocacy and call-to-action is alive today among nurses throughout the world.

The primary thrust of this advocacy is on behalf of vulnerable groups in our society—those who, because of biological, social, and environmental factors, are not able to attain a level of health generally enjoyed by many people. Nurses are united in partnership with other health care disciplines, the community, and health care consumers to achieve population-based global, national, provincial, and local health care goals. This chapter provides readers with an understanding of the theory and practice of population-based health care.

Population-based care requires active partnership of both providers and recipients of care. The phrase *health care consumer* includes recipients of care and those who make health care–related decisions at the individual or group level.

POPULATION HEALTH

Through the Alma-Ata Declaration, proclaimed in 1978, the international community, led by the World Health Organization (WHO), made a commitment to the principles of primary health care and global strategies that would see "health for all people of the world" (World Health Organization, 1978). In 1986 the WHO's First International Conference on Health Promotion was held in Ottawa. The Ottawa Charter, based on the principles of primary health care, was a blueprint for health promotion that stood the test of time (World Health Organization, 1986). Building on previous meetings, participants at the Fourth International Conference on Health Promotion, held in 1997, in Jakarta, Indonesia, examined what was known about health promotion, re-examined the determinants of health, and invited the private sector to contribute resources needed to promote health in the 21st century (World Health Organization, 1997). In September 2005 the Declaration of Montevideo, co-sponsored by the Pan American Health Organization (PAHO) and the WHO, stated that the principles outlined in the Declaration of Alma-Ata must be integrated into the community health systems rather than implemented as a separate program or objective (Pan American Health Organization, 2005). To facilitate this, the 2010 WHO world health report set out strategies that countries can follow to enable the development of universal health coverage, still considered to be the pillar of health for all.[1] In 2012 the World Health Report will discuss the impact of health research and highlight the significance of conducting and translating health research to help promote healthy behaviours and reduce individual risk factors that can be modified.[2]

Population health is the concept that a population—or a community—as a whole, has a particular state of health. This concept goes beyond the health of individuals and looks at the health of the entire population. The health of a population is strongly affected by social and environmental factors that are now widely known as **determinants of health.** Within Canadian society, groups of vulnerable individuals have an increased risk of experiencing health disparities because of their lack of stable income, lack of education, reduced access to secure jobs, and inadequate housing.

In the Declaration of Alma-Ata, primary health care (PHC) was defined as "essential health care based on practical, scientifically sound and socially acceptable methods and technology, made universally accessible to individuals and families in the community through their full participation and at a cost that the community and country can afford to maintain at every stage of their development in the spirit of self-reliance and self-determination" (World Health Organization, 1978). The Ottawa Charter defined **health promotion** as "the process of enabling people to increase control over and to improve their health."[3]

Individual **health risk factors** are variables that increase or decrease the probability of illness, disability or death. Risk factors may be either modifiable (i.e., they can be changed) or non-modifiable (i.e., they cannot be changed). Modifiable risk factors include smoking, lack of exercise, unsafe sexual practices, alcohol and drug use, and lack of health screening. Non-modifiable risk factors include age, sex, race, or other inherent physical characteristics. On the other hand, determinants of health are variables that include biological, psychosocial, environmental (physical and social), lifestyle, behavioural, and health system factors that may cause changes in the health status of individuals, families, and communities or populations. In the Jakarta Declaration, determinants or prerequisites for health were specifically identified as peace, shelter, education, social security, social relations, food, income, the empowerment of women, a stable ecosystem, sustainable resource use, social justice, respect for human rights, and equity. Poverty was identified as the greatest threat to health.[4]

The Ottawa Charter* set out five strategies for health promotion:

1. Build healthy public policy.
2. Create supportive environments.
3. Strengthen community action.
4. Develop personal skills.
5. Reorient health services.[5]

The Jakarta Declaration† built upon the strategies from the Ottawa Charter and set the following five priorities:

1. Promote social responsibility for health.
2. Increase investments for health development.
3. Consolidate and expand partnerships for health.

4. Increase community capacity and empower the individual.
5. Secure an infrastructure for health promotion.[6]

Health status is the level of health of an individual, family, community, or population. It is a combination of individual and societal factors, and one's perception of how they all fit together. **Quality of life** is the level of satisfaction one has with the actual conditions of one's life. This includes satisfaction with socioeconomic status, education, occupation, home, family life, recreation, and the ability to enjoy life, freedom, and independence. The following factors are reviewed during a quality of life assessment: a person's perceived and actual ability to be autonomous and independent in making life choices; one's sense of happiness, satisfaction, and security; and the ongoing ability to strive to reach one's potential. **Health-related quality of life** refers to one's level of satisfaction with those aspects of life that are influenced either positively or negatively by one's health status and risk factors.

Functional health status is the ability to care for oneself and meet one's human needs. Functional abilities are the combined abilities to be independent both in the activities of daily life and in the instrumental activities of daily living. **Activities of daily living** are activities related to toileting, bathing, grooming, dressing, feeding, mobility, and verbal and written personal communication. **Instrumental activities of daily living (IADLs)** are activities related to food preparation and shopping; cleaning; laundry; home maintenance; verbal, written, and electronic communications; financial management; and transportation, along with activities to meet social and support needs, manage health care needs, access community services and resources, and meet spiritual needs. Functional health status affects health-related quality of life.

The WHO's International Classification of Functioning, Disability and Health (ICIDH-2), adopted in 2001, recognizes the importance of defining health domains and health-related domains and their interrelationship to further our understanding of health status. Using the ICIDH-2 framework, health status is the result of the interaction between personal characteristics and environmental factors: the three main domains are impairment (i.e., body function and structure), activities (i.e., person-level functioning), and participation (i.e., societal functioning).[7]

Health and illness are on a continuum, with total health at one end and severe illness on the other. All of the aforementioned factors interact to determine an individual's position on the health–illness continuum.

Nurses working with our most vulnerable populations must develop strategies to target finite health care

*Ottawa Charter for Health Promotion, "Health Promotion Action Means." Retrieved from http://www.who.int/hpr/NPH/docs/ottawa_charter_hp.pdf, June 16, 2011. Reprinted by permission of WHO.
† Jakarta Declaration on Leading Health Promotion into the 21st Century, "Priorities for Health Promotion in the 21st century." Retrieved from http://www. who.int/hpr/NPH/docs/jakarta_declaration_en.pdf, June 16, 2011. Reprinted by permission of WHO.

resources effectively. Despite the fact that we have universal health insurance in Canada, **vulnerable population groups** are often underserved. They often have a diminished health status and are at increased risk for morbidity and mortality because of multiple and complex medical and social problems. These people are vulnerable because of their poverty, lack of education, lack of opportunity, and their history of mental health and drug and alcohol abuse. Vulnerable population groups include Aboriginal people, elderly people, poor children, and people with disabilities (Shah, chap. 6). These groups often exist at the margins of mainstream society and have a reduced ability to participate in, or influence, decisions that affect their health care status.

Population-based health care initiatives to help and work with these groups exist at the global, national, provincial, and local level. Table 5-1 gives examples of population-based health care initiatives.

CRITICAL THINKING

Laura is a 40-year-old woman with MS, who is desperate to keep living in her own home. Laura is an artist and loves classical music. She is now bed-bound, has a g-tube, a Foley catheter, and pneumonia. The home care system expects her 78-year-old father to do much of the needed care. Even though she was receiving the maximum in-home hours, her care was still very exhausting. Assessing, implementing, and evaluating the plan of care involved continuously balancing nursing, assessing health status, problem solving and preventing skin breakdown against the need for caregiver relief —with the backdrop of Homecare cutbacks.

Margaret Lynn Furman, RN
Staff Nurse, Community Health Organization

What determinants of health would you identify in this situation and what is their impact on Laura's health? If you had no resource constraints, what would you do to improve Laura's health?

Source: Margaret Lynn Furman

CRITICAL THINKING AND REAL WORLD INTERVIEW

Program Planning In my practice as a health care administrator and professional practice leader, I locate and use different levels of evidence depending on the question at hand. For example, in a past role, my health care organization identified the advancement of development and use of clinical practice guidelines as a strategic priority. A literature search was conducted of online databases (e.g., MEDLINE and CINAHL). The resulting evidence included observational studies and systematic reviews of studies regarding various aspects of clinical practice guidelines. Experiential or anecdotal evidence was gathered from key informants who had implemented clinical practice guidelines in their settings or from case studies.

My current role involves making recommendations or decisions about many aspects of health care services. These include care-delivery models with a staff mix, budget allocation, and the content, credibility or effectiveness of clinical policies. On a daily basis I access and review evidence to inform these decisions. My sources of evidence include the following:

- the weekly "E-Watch Newsletter" produced by the Québec Population Health Research Network (*http://www.santepop. qc.ca/en/index.html*)
- the weekly Longwood's E-Letter (*http://www.longwoods.com/newsletters*)
- hard-copy journals such as the Journal of Nursing Scholarship, the Canadian Journal for Nursing Leadership, and the Forum (Canadian College of Health Leaders

(Continued)

CRITICAL THINKING AND REAL WORLD INTERVIEW (CONTINUED)

- reports produced by the Canadian Institute for Health Information (*http://www.cihi.ca*) and the Canadian Health Council (*http://www.healthcouncilcanada.ca/en/*)
- the website for the Canadian Health Services Research Foundation (*http://www.chsrf.ca/Home.aspx*).

Barbara Mildon, RN, PhD, CHE
Vice President, Professional Practice & Research
and Chief Nurse Executive, Ontario Shores
Centre for Mental Health Sciences

Think of an example of another vulnerable population you may encounter as a nursing manager.

What information would you gather to determine the needs of the population?

What steps would you undertake to plan programs to meet these needs?

What are some of the barriers and facilitators you may encounter on the way?

Source: Barbara Mildon

TABLE 5-1	POPULATION-BASED HEALTH CARE INITIATIVES
Global Groups	**Initiatives**
World Health Organization and the Pan American Health Organization (PAHO) (http://new.paho.org/hq/index.php?option=com_frontpage&Itemid=1)	To help achieve the United Nations' Millennium Development Goals, members of PAHO and other WHO affiliate organizations agreed to advocate for the integration of primary health care (PHC) as an integral part of their health and social structure. Their strategies would be based on the following elements: 1. commitment to facilitate social inclusion and equity in health 2. recognition of the critical roles of both the individual and the community in the development of PHC-based systems 3. orientation toward health promotion and comprehensive and integrated care 4. development of intersectoral work 5. orientation toward quality of care and client safety. 6. strengthening of human resources in health 7. establishment of structural conditions that allow PHC renewal 8. guarantee of financial sustainability 9. research and development and appropriate technology 10. network strengthening and partnerships of international cooperation in support of PHC

Source: Draft "DECLARATION OF THE AMERICAS ON RENEWAL OF PRIMARY HEALTH CARE." <www.paho.org/english/ad/ths/os/phc-regionaldeclaration.pdf> Retrieved March 20, 2011. Reprinted by permission of World Health Organization.

(Continued)

TABLE 5-1	POPULATION-BASED HEALTH CARE INITIATIVES (CONTINUED)
United Nations: Millennium Development Goals (http://www.un.org/millenniumgoals/)	The eight Millennium Development Goals (MDGs),agreed to by all the world's countries and all of the world's leading development institutions, formed a blueprint for goals to be met by 2015. 1. Eradicate extreme poverty and hunger. 2. Achieve universal primary education. 3. Promote gender equality and empower women. 4. Reduce child mortality. 5. Improve maternal health. 6. Combat HIV/AIDS, Malaria and other diseases. 7. Ensure environmental sustainability. 8. Develop a global partnership for development.
National Groups	**Initiatives**
Public Health Agency of Canada (www.publichealth.gc.ca)	The Public Health Agency of Canada (PHAC) was created in September 2004. Its mission is to promote and protect the health of Canadians through leadership, partnership, innovation and action in public health. For example, in partnership with CIHI, the Canadian Network of Multiple Sclerosis (MS) Clinics and the MS Society of Canada, PHAC has initiated a new MS monitoring system.
Northern Ireland Public Health Agency (http://www.publichealth.hscni.net/)	The Public Health Agency was established in April 2009 as part of the reforms to Health and Social Care (HSC) in Northern Ireland to address the causes and associated inequalities of preventable ill-health and lack of wellbeing. For example, the Agency initiated the use of National Breastfeeding Awareness Week (NBAW) to emphasize the message that breastfeeding is the healthiest option for both mother and baby.
Great Britain Health Protection Agency (http://www.hpa.org.uk/)	The Health Protection Agency's role is to provide an integrated approach to protecting UK public health. Examples of initiatives for vulnerable populations include their services for IV drug users.
U.S. Department of Health and Human Services (HHS) (http://www.hhs.gov/)	The U.S. Department of HHS works with state and other government departments to protect the health of Americans. Their range of current includes promoting self-efficacy in view of the new health-reform law; supporting a person's exploration of insurance coverage options, raising awareness of signs of bullying, and providing information on how to protect oneself from the flu.
Provincial and Territorial Groups	**Initiatives**
Northwest Territories Health and Social Services (http://www.hlthss.gov.nt.ca/default.htm)	Aboriginal Head Start (AHS) is an early intervention program for First Nations, Inuit, and Métis children and their families. It is primarily a preschool program that prepares young Aboriginal children for school by meeting their spiritual, emotional, intellectual, and physical needs. This program is funded by Health Canada. Other programs aim to prevent and treat fetal alcohol syndrome, family violence, mental health and addictions, to name a few.

Source: Reproduced with permission of the United Nations.

(Continued)

TABLE 5-1	POPULATION-BASED HEALTH CARE INITIATIVES (CONTINUED)
Yukon Health and Social Services Department (http://www.hss.gov.yk.ca/communityhealthprograms.php)	The Yukon Health and Social Services Department provides a variety of community and public health services throughout the territory: for example, mental health and addictions, blood-borne infections, children's dental health, and peer counselling.
Nunavut Department of Health and Social Services (http://www.hss.gov.nu.ca/en/Home.aspx)	The Department of Health and Social Services is responsible for the health and well-being of citizens of Nunavut. Its mission is to promote, protect, and enhance the health and well-being of all Nunavummiut, incorporating Inuit *Qaujimajatuqangit* at all levels of service delivery and design. They support a number of programs for mental health and addictions, and family violence.
British Columbia Centre for Disease Control (http://www.bccdc.ca/default.htm)	Chee Mamuk is a program developed to provide culturally appropriate onsite community-based education and training on HIV/AIDS and sexually transmitted diseases to Aboriginal communities, organizations, and professionals within British Columbia.
Alberta Health and Wellness (http://www.health.alberta.ca/)	Raising Children is an initiative across a number of ministries to provide services to ensure children reach their potential.
Saskatchewan Health (http://www.health.gov.sk.ca/)	The goals of Saskatchewan Health are to increase the health and well-being of individuals and families. Initiatives include programs for breastfeeding, mental health and substance use, nutritional health, and parenting. Everyone living in Saskatchewan has free access to The Cochrane Library (www.thecochranelibrary.com) to help inform their decisions.
Manitoba Health–Public Health (http://www.gov.mb.ca/health/publichealth/index.html)	Public health initiatives include, for example, communicable disease control, environmental health, emergency preparedness.
Public Health Ontario (PHO) (http://www.oahpp.ca/index.html)	An arm's-length government agency, PHO aims to protect and promote the health of all Ontarians and reduce inequities in health. It provides information, knowledge and support to health care decision makers at all levels.
Québec Ministère de la Santé et des Services Sociaux (http://www.msss.gouv.qc.ca/en/)	The Ministère provides programs and services to address public health issues and social determinants of health, particularly for seniors, adults, youth and individuals with disabilities. One initiative is The SexEducator, a magazine for educators and individuals providing sex-education activities to adolescents.
New Brunswick Department of Health (http://www.gnb.ca/0051/index-e.asp)	The health department supports all aspects of health and well-being for New Brunswick citizenry—in French and English. Everyone living in New Brunswick has free access to The Cochrane Library (www.thecochranelibrary.com) to help inform their decisions.

(Continued)

TABLE 5-1	POPULATION-BASED HEALTH CARE INITIATIVES (CONTINUED)
Nova Scotia Department of Health and Wellness (http://www.gov.ns.ca/health/)	Recent initiatives include (1) in September 2010 adopting the Declaration on Prevention and Promotion —along with other federal, provincial, and territorial health departments—a public statement to "make the promotion of health and the prevention of disease, disability, and injury a priority for action"; and (2) the working together of provincial and Mi'kmaq leaders of Unama'ki (Cape Breton) to improve health care for First Nations people on the island.
Prince Edward Island (PEI) (http://gpei.ca/infopei/index.php3?number=43156&lang=E)	Eighty-three percent of the population of PEI have at least one of the major risk factors for stroke, and 45 percent have at least two. In 2009 the provincial government committed to an Organized Stroke Care Model for PEI. The model includes a comprehensive 3-Phase implementation plan.
Newfoundland and Labrador Health and Community Services (http://www.health.gov.nl.ca/health/)	This department provides leadership in health and social services programs and policy. In partnership with the federal, provincial and territorial governments, the Aboriginal Health Transition Fund is intended to improve the health and well-being of Aboriginal people. Some of the initiatives in Newfoundland include culturally aware foster care, mental health and addictions, and e-health.

POPULATION-BASED NURSING PRACTICE

Population-based nursing practice has been an integral part of nursing since the profession began. Florence Nightingale's use of aggregated statistics as population-based indices and outcome measures demonstrates her population-focused practice. Canadian community health nurses have a long and important history. Over the years, they have understood the importance of social, economic, environmental, and political determinants of health. They considered social activism and collaboration with community organizations and governments to be fundamental aspects of public health nursing practice (Falk Rafael, Fox, Mildon, & O'Donnell, 1998). In 1905 Ottawa's Anti-Tuberculosis League hired Canada's first tuberculosis (TB) nurse—a public health role—to visit the homes of TB clients, and in 1907 the Toronto Health Department became the first municipal health department in Canada to hire a TB nurse, Christina Mitchell. In 1909, Ontario extended public health nursing by starting medical inspection programs under the department of education, to counteract high levels of school absenteeism due to widespread childhood disease. Working outside the strict structure of hospitals, public health nurses were the most independent nurses of this period. In 1920 the Ontario Red Cross Society funded a one-year university program for public health nurses at the University of Toronto, a program that would continue to be recognized as the preferred postgraduate training for Ontario public health nurses until the 1960s.[8]

Today, community health nurses work in a broad spectrum of situations. Their populations include school children, homeless and at-risk youth, individuals with mental health problems, individuals with alcohol and drug abuse problems, individuals in the sex trade, Aboriginal people, and new Canadians. According to statistics from the Canadian Institute for Health Information (CIHI), 30,544 (13.2 percent) of a total 230,957 registered nurses were working in the community in 2003. In January 2004 community health nursing became one of the 17 nursing specialties certified by the Canadian Nurses Association.[9]

NURSING IN NONTRADITIONAL SETTINGS

Community Health Centres (CHCs) are nonprofit organizations that provide primary health and health promotion programs for individuals, families, and communities. A health centre is established by the community and governed by a community-elected board of directors; the health centre receives its base funding from the Local Health Integrated Networks in Ontario and may obtain program-specific funds from other sources. CHCs work with others in the community on health promotion initiatives within schools, in housing developments, and in the workplace. Depending on the needs of the community, staff will include a mix of nurses, physicians, health

REAL WORLD EXAMPLE

In 1986 a group of homeless people in Toronto met to discuss health care issues they were facing. They felt discriminated against within the health care system, and given their circumstances, they were often unable to follow prescribed treatments. The group identified nurses as the people they would feel most comfortable approaching for health care.

Upon learning of the initial discussions, a group of volunteer nurses opened the first Street Health nursing station in September 1986, at a church in downtown Toronto. Other nursing clinics followed, located where homeless people congregated. The purpose was to provide hands-on health care and assistance in accessing and navigating the health care system.

Street nurses provide services on the street, in alleys, along the lakeshore, in parks and ravines, and in homeless shelters and drop-in centres. Their clients' lives are characterized by extreme poverty, chronic unemployment, insecurity in housing, poor nutrition, high stress, and loneliness. They have more frequent and serious illnesses and die younger, on average, than the general population. The nurses provide outreach nursing, mental health support and case management, and HIV/AIDS prevention. They support those with Hepatitis C, provide prevention strategies for individual who are at risk for the disease, and strongly advocate for supportive public policy to make a more lasting difference for the population as a whole.[10]

Source: Streat Health, "About Us," Retrieved from http://www.streathealth.ca/home.htm, June 16, 2011

REAL WORLD EXAMPLE

Cathy Crowe was granted the prestigious Atkinson Economic Justice award in January 2004. The award, which provides $100,000 per year for up to three years, was renewed twice (2004–09). Upon receipt of the award, Cathy said, *"I want to inspire and engage Canadians from all walks of life, to empathize and respond to the injustice of homelessness in their community and motivate them to become involved in calling for the solution —a national housing program"* (http://cathycrowe.ca/).

Cathy has worked as a street nurse since 1988 and has been involved in numerous coalitions and public education work regarding the homeless. In 1998 she co-founded the Toronto Disaster Relief Committee, an organization that has dramatically increased the public's understanding of homelessness.[12] She currently holds a part-time position with the Faculty of Nursing at McMaster University.

These two real-world examples demonstrate what nurses can do when they choose to advocate on behalf of their vulnerable clients. Policymakers can facilitate these initiatives by recognizing the true cost to society of non-action. Government departments are expected to manage their own budgets. There is little incentive to work across departments to assess how action in one area can affect outcomes in another. Nursing managers may find themselves in similar situations within their organizations. In the current atmosphere of accountability and the ultimate importance of the bottom line, all stakeholders—including the client, the service provider, and the payer—must come together to develop creative strategies. Regionalization of health and social services across Canada (the most recent example being the Local Integrated Health Networks in Ontario) has been cited by governments as initiatives to coordinate services to improve access and care. However, since in most cases the emphasis is on organizations that provide health care, organizations and initiatives that address determinants of health that fall outside the traditional health care system will, with rare exception, be excluded.[13]

promoters, social workers, nutritionists, and vocational counsellors; all staff are on salary. Traditionally, CHCs were developed to help vulnerable groups overcome issues of access to service. As a result, CHCs focus on providing primary care, linking with other community partners, advocating for determinants of health for their community, and empowering their clients to advocate on their own behalf.[11]

LITERATURE APPLICATION

Citation: Smith, D., & Davies, B. (2006) Participatory model: Creating a new dynamic in Aboriginal health. *Canadian Nurse*, 102(4): 36–39. © Canadian Nurses Association. Reprinted with permission. Further reproduction prohibited.

Discussion: This report outlines the challenges of using current research to inform nursing practice in Aboriginal communities, and it highlights the value of using a participatory model of research transfer to help overcome these challenges. An evidence-based prenatal workshop for community health nurses working in First Nations' communities in British Columbia was used as a venue to test the acceptability of the model and to increase the uptake of research to improve care.

Implications for Practice: The nurses identified that "without participation, nothing would change" in the Aboriginal communities. They said that understanding the beliefs, lifestyle, and expectations of the individuals with whom they worked was "critical to success and capacity building."

CRITICAL THINKING

Consider the previous literature application. Can this approach be used successfully when planning services for other vulnerable populations? Think of a vulnerable population with whom you work. What steps would you take to address one of their social determinants of health? As the nursing manager, what actions would you take to support your staff in this initiative?

CRITICAL THINKING

The local food bank was scheduled to close in six months. The agency that had hosted it for the past decade was reassessing its mandate and resources, and felt it could no longer provide this service. The community was devastated! With 40 percent of the local population identified as living in a low-income bracket, this closure was not good news. Sally, the local school nurse, and Carol, the outreach worker at the local Community Health Centre, hastily called a meeting of other community partners and clients. Over the next six months, the community was able to articulate their specific needs, identify why the food bank was important to them, and successfully convey their message to local politicians and the media. They successfully negotiated with another agency to host the service temporarily, until more permanent plans could be made—a commitment to which the community agencies and politicians agreed.

Do you think this was an effective effort? Why, or why not?

Aboriginal Health Centres are similar to CHCs but offer culturally appropriate primary care to Aboriginal families, individuals, and communities. Programs may include family medicine and nurse practitioner services, nutrition counselling, health education, disease prevention, mental health counselling, and traditional healing and others approaches, depending on the need of the community.[14]

CRITICAL THINKING

Betty is a parish nurse who works in a low-income neighbourhood that is home to many new Canadians. Ten percent of the population is between the ages of 15 and 24. Most of the parents, although university-educated, have been able to find only menial jobs that pay poorly, necessitating long hours and often a second job. Many families are headed by a single parent. City-sponsored activities are available, but the registration process is frustrating even for long-time city dwellers who are fluent in English and understand the system. New Canadians who have poor command of English, little time, and no understanding of the system find the system virtually inaccessible. The teens have limited access to age-appropriate health care and spend long hours left to their own devices—but are observed by the neighbourhood to make sure they act in culturally appropriate ways. Collaborative efforts between the parish nurse, public health, and the neighbouring community health centre resulted in the development of a youth health care clinic in one of the local secondary schools. Also in collaboration with other community agencies, Betty started "Saturday Night at the Movies" at a local community centre, giving the youth an opportunity to go to a chaperoned outing and still interact with their peers. When the local community health centre offered a number of small grants for community programs, the youth were successful recipients of a grant, when they applied for money to expand their recreational program.

What needs would you identify for this population?

What strategies from the Ottawa Charter have been employed in this example? What other strategies do you think should be considered?

CRITICAL THINKING

While working at a health centre for homeless youth, the nurses identified the lack of parenting skills displayed by many of the teen parents. They knew from the literature and from their own experience that without good parenting, these children of children would never "spin out," and the cycle would be perpetuated. Through reviewing journals and conferring with colleagues who worked with the same population, they discovered a new teaching tool—a computer-programmed doll that cried and could not be consoled until the root cause was discovered and alleviated. The doll would only calm down if she was fed, her wet diapers changed, her tender loving care (TLC) needs were met, etc. The doll, used primarily in "family studies" classes in the secondary schools, as a tool to teach parenting skills to non-pregnant teens, cost $800. One of the other agencies had a doll donated, so the nurses were able to see her and glean information from the other agency's experience. The other agency staff raved about its usefulness. The nurses determined that they had to have one—but it was a little expensive for their small budget, and they couldn't justify buying the doll for a few of their clients, instead of medication and medical supplies that would benefit so many more. So, they decided to ask someone to donate it. They were sure the youth would be fascinated by it and would learn basic skills to deal with some of the challenges they would face in the months to come.

What health needs can you identify for this population?

What strategies, besides those outlined above, would you initiate to help meet these needs?

As the manager, what strategies and activities would you develop and implement to facilitate these initiatives?

PROGRAM PLANNING AND EVALUATION

The nursing process, which is integral to our care at the individual-client level, is also used in population-based nursing practice to assess, diagnose, plan, implement, and evaluate programs developed to meet the needs of a community. Several models of program planning and evaluation are outlined in the literature, although all have similar components.

One model to consider when planning and evaluating programs to meet the needs of the community is the Precede-Proceed Model, developed by Lawrence Green and colleagues at the University of British Columbia. They outline nine steps to establish, evaluate, and maintain community programs. Steps one through five assess the health, social, and environmental issues; step six covers the implementation; and steps seven to nine address the evaluation (Green, 1999; Johnson, 2006).

ASSESSMENT

Population assessment follows a structured model for data collection. Table 5.2 is a template for collecting population-level data on the determinants of community health as outlined in the Jakarta Declaration. To complete the full assessment, the following steps are important: identify the issue, determine its importance to the community, back it up with epidemiological evidence if available, determine the educational and organizational needs of the community if a program were to be implemented, and define the administrative and policy components of program implementation (Green & Kreuter, 1999).

PLANNING AND IMPLEMENTATION

During the planning and implementation stages, collaboration with all partners is imperative—including collaboration with clients, care providers, and other community and government agencies. When you establish buy-in, determine logistical factors, and develop strategies to deal with

TABLE 5-2	POPULATION-BASED NEEDS ASSESSMENT

Determinants of Health	Is There Information to Assess These Determinants of Health?	Assessment of Situation
Information from observation and discussions with members of the community (i.e., primary data)	Information from health data sources (i.e., secondary data, such as census data and mortality data)	Review the data from the two sources of information. Do they agree or disagree? If they disagree, why?
Physical Environment ■ Shelter ■ Stable Ecosystem ■ Peace ■ Sustainable Resource		
Social Environment ■ Income ■ Education ■ Social Security ■ Social Relations		
Biological and Behavioural Determinants of Health Equity ■ Social Justice ■ Respect for Human Rights		
Genetic Endowment Access to Health Care Services		

Source: Johnson, I. (Ed.). (2006). *Determinants of Community Health, Year 1, Semester 2: Course Manual & Readings 2006–2007.* Toronto: University of Toronto.

them, you help to guarantee the success of your program. Defining measurable outcomes and a means of evaluation at this stage will facilitate the evaluation process.

EVALUATION

The programs should be measured in three ways: (infra) structure (e.g., manuals and finances); implementation processes (e.g., are people participating in the program?); and outcomes (e.g., did the program actually make a difference for the community?) (Green & Kreuter, 1999). Outcomes of population-based nursing practice focus on health status, functional abilities, and the quality of life of at-risk population groups. Justification of both resources and budget is necessary. A cost-benefit analysis is appropriate. This involves comparing improvements in health status, functional abilities, and quality of life of the targeted at-risk population with expenditures of human and material resources. Ethical guidelines, as well as guidelines for culturally competent care, should be used to evaluate the effectiveness of interactions between the health provider and the vulnerable or marginalized population group.

During the evaluation stage, data are collected that reflect the aggregated response of the total group for each specified outcome. Descriptive statistics, such as mean, range, and percentages may be used in the analysis of group data. These data may be collected at the program level, or may be forwarded to a provincial or national data-collection program to allow between-program comparisons. Case studies illustrating how services provided to clients "made a difference" are also very effective.

Questions such as the following will help guide your data collection:

- Did we find the high-risk, underserved, vulnerable population groups in the community or service area and provide timely and accessible services?
- Did we offer service regardless of age, gender, race, ethnicity, health care status, or location?
- Did our services meet the greatest unmet health needs of the community or the at-risk, vulnerable, underserved population groups?
- Did their health status improve?
- Were their health risks reduced?
- Were they satisfied with the services they received?
- Did we manage to stay within our budget?
- Did we use our resources in the most effective way?
- Did we use our resources in a way that met the priority health needs of all of our high-risk client groups?
- Did we target our services and use our resources to improve the health status of those who were the most underserved?
- Did we have enough resources left over to meet the essential health needs of lower-risk population groups?

LITERATURE APPLICATION

Citation: Kristjansson, B., Petticrew, M., MacDonald, B., Krasevec, J., Janzen, L., Greenhalgh, T., Wells, G.A., MacGowan, J., Farmer, A.P., Shea, B., Mayhew, A., Tugwell, P., & Welch, V. School feeding for improving the physical and psychosocial health of disadvantaged students. *Cochrane Database of Systematic Reviews* 2007, Issue 1. Art. No.: CD004676. DOI: 10.1002/14651858. CD004676.pub2

Discussion: The main objective was to determine the effectiveness of school feeding programs in improving physical and psychosocial health for disadvantaged school pupils. Lack of food security affects many aspects of child health and development. School feeding programs are designed to provide food to hungry children and to improve their physical, mental and psycho-social health. This systematic review includes 18 studies. In the trials from Lower Income Countries, experimental group children gained an average of 0.39 kilograms (95 percent C.I: 0.11 to 0.67) over an average of 19 months and 0.71 kilograms (95 percent C.I.: 0.48 to 0.95) over 11.3 months respectively. Results were mixed in higher income countries. Results were mixed for height; gains were greater for younger children. School attendance in lower income countries was higher in experimental groups than in controls; results showed an average increase of four to six days a year. Math gains were consistently higher for experimental groups in lower income countries. In short-term studies, small improvements in some cognitive tasks were found.

Implications for Practice: Imagine you are the school health nurse in a poor neighbourhood and have been consulted by the principal about the possibility of starting a breakfast program. Based on this systematic review, what advice would you give her? For what other sources of information would you search in trying to advise her?

CRITICAL THINKING AND REAL WORLD INTERVIEW

As we look at Canada's aging population, the demand for acute care services is increasing, particularly emergency department care for older adults and those with chronic conditions— especially for the frail elderly. Using population health projections, that is, historical service demand by disease type and age, we recognized the need to develop and strengthen ambulatory clinics for chronic disease management to help keep people well and living in the community. Using the information collected, several chronic disease management clinics were developed or enhanced. For example, we implemented the New Diabetic Day Hospital and significantly expanded the CHF and COPD clinics by implementing self-management programs. A number of outreach initiatives are currently under development, including programs for electronic monitor (remote), telehealth, and interprofessional outreach.

We used local population and service data and, of course, found a lot of information in the scientific literature. We also drew from provincial and national secondary data through organizations such as the Canadian Institute for Health Information (CIHI) and the Institute for Clinical Evaluative Sciences (ICES).

The most common sources of evidence are those that reflect current uses of resources and services. When looking to new ways to solve problems, we use literature to determine what worked well in other jurisdictions, recognizing that the "context matters" and one may need to adapt to one's own local environment.

David McNeil
Vice President Clinical Program and Chief Nursing Executive,
Sudbury Regional Hospital

Using the Precede-Proceed Model, describe the program-planning process that was undertaken in this situation.

How did the program address the issues at the levels of the community, the targeted population, and the system?

What outcomes were identified to evaluate the success of the program? How were they measured?

Source: David McNeil

The evaluation process involves the multidisciplinary team, clients, and community partnerships. A regular evaluation of the program allows adjustments to be made, unmet needs of the at-risk groups to be identified, and further interventions developed if necessary. Community planning is an iterative process. Ongoing assessment of the structure, process, and outcomes is used to improve existing programs and develop new programs as the need arises.

CRITICAL THINKING

In many developing countries, high rates of maternal and child morbidity and mortality are everyday realities. Access to health care may be many hours' walk away. Supplies are often limited, and the health care providers may have been poorly trained. Nurses from the School of Nursing, University of Ottawa, recently embarked on a collaborative program with the Yunnan Provincial Public Health Bureau in southern China in attempt to improve the health of vulnerable members of that society. Working collaboratively with their project partners in Yunnan, the Canadian team discovered that (1) isolation and mountainous terrain were major barriers to transportation and communication; (2) health care personnel were poorly trained and poorly equipped to handle emergencies; and (3) fees for health care providers were not adequate to reimburse them when they have to leave their farms to deliver health care, and the fees for visits to either the midwife or the local hospital were prohibitive for the women

(Continued)

CRITICAL THINKING (CONTINUED)

themselves. Through their sharing of experiences in other poor settings, the Canadians were able to stimulate their Yunnan partners to think of ways to overcome some of these barriers. Their ideas were taken to the government, who agreed to pilot the strategies in a number of isolated communities. When the health of pregnant women and their children improved and mortality rates decreased, the government agreed to provide the programs throughout the province (Edwards & Roelofs, 2005).

Can you give other examples of international initiatives in which you or your colleagues have participated?

What are some of the access-to-care challenges faced by pregnant new Canadian women in your community?

What initiatives in your community help these women to overcome these challenges? Were they successful? How was success measured?

CRITICAL THINKING

Pregnant women in northern Aboriginal communities must be flown to southern centres (a 6- to 10-hour flight) to have their babies. This displacement takes them out of their familiar surroundings— away from their families and support systems— and places them in a foreign environment, surrounded by strangers who often speak in a language they don't understand. In the late 1980s these women started to explore alternatives. Working with local nurses, midwives, doctors, local health centres, and the federal government, they were instrumental in establishing a local, collaborative, maternity program that ensured quality care for themselves and their babies, but kept them close to home.

An evaluation of the program showed that the women were receiving comprehensive perinatal care in their communities. Perinatal and maternal mortality and morbidity rates became comparable to the rest of the province of Québec. Rates of premature births declined, and the numbers and costs of transfers to southern hospitals decreased. The program was considered successful because it had been developed collaboratively with the at-risk group it was meant to serve (Peterson & Mannion, 2005).

What access-to-care issues were identified by the community?

What strategies were initiated to meet these needs?

What other questions might you want to ask to determine whether this program was successful?

The goal for the World Health Organization (WHO) is the attainment by all peoples of the highest possible level of health. WHO defines health as a state of complete physical, mental, and social well-being, not merely the absence of disease or infirmity.[15] We know that personal, social, and political factors, commonly known as determinants of health, extend beyond the boundaries of traditional health care. As health care costs continue to rise, and governments around the world attempt to meet growing needs with finite budgets, society must recognize that, in order to ensure good health, these factors are no less critical than high-quality health care. We must identify vulnerable populations who are at highest risk for ill health. As well, we need to advocate for programs that will enable these people to obtain food and income security, safe and sound housing, and strong support systems. We must enable them to find their own voice so they learn to advocate for themselves. We must not let valuable human capital go untapped.

CRITICAL THINKING

In March 2011 Sheilah Fraser, auditor general, released her report on the success of the Nunavut Government to deliver health and social services to support children, youth, and families. Despite the fact that the Nunavut Government has stated that the health and welfare of their children is a priority, the auditor general's report found it was "not adequately meeting its key responsibilities for the protection and well-being of children, youth, and their families." A new and rapidly growing jurisdiction, Nunavut finds itself unable to collect sufficient information about children in care; the health and social services department cannot accurately track their status, understand their needs, and adjust its activities to provide appropriate support.[16] In her June 2011 report to the federal government, Ms. Fraser reports not only on the overall health and well-being of First Nations in Canada, but also that the social determinants of health are negatively impacting them at every step of the way.[17] The lack of adequate housing, potable drinking water, appropriate education, health and social services continue to be the norm rather than the exception.

Pick one social determinant of health.

Using the Precede-Proceed Model, determine how you would define the problem, plan a program to mitigate it, and assess the success of your program.

Who are the key stakeholders you would call to the planning table?

How did the program address the issues at the levels of the community, the targeted population, and the system?

What outcomes were identified to evaluate the success of the program? How were they measured?

KEY CONCEPTS

■ The focus of population-based health care is to reduce health disparities that exist among diverse population groups.

■ The goal of population-based health care is for all members of a community to have equitable access to the resources they need to acquire and maintain the highest health status possible.

■ Health promotion is the process of enabling people both to increase control over their health and to improve their health.

■ Population-based nursing practice focuses on at-risk, vulnerable, and underserved population groups.

■ Determinants, or prerequisites, for health include peace, shelter, education, social security, social relations, food, income, the empowerment of women, a stable ecosystem, sustainable resource use, social justice, respect for human rights, and equity.

■ Population-based nursing practice starts with either a community health needs assessment that identifies health priorities and at-risk vulnerable population groups or the identification of needs by the vulnerable population groups themselves.

■ Population-based health care involves multidisciplinary partnerships with the health care consumer and the community.

■ To improve the health of the population as a whole, population-based intervention strategies need to be focused at the general population and integrated into the community health and social systems.

■ Outcomes of population-based health care are measured at the population level. Three domains of population outcomes are health status, functional abilities, and quality of life.

■ Nurses play key roles in the successful development and implementation of population-based health care services.

KEY TERMS

activities of daily living
Community Health
  Centres (CHCs)
determinants of health
functional health status

health promotion
health-related quality of life
health risk factors
health status
population health

instrumental activities of
  daily living (IADLs)
population-based
  nursing practice

quality of life
vulnerable population
  groups

REVIEW QUESTIONS

1. Which of the following is the goal of population health?
   A. access, cost, empowerment, equity
   B. access, cost, equity, resilience
   C. access, cost, equity, quality

2. have equitable access to resources for all members of a population

3. Population-based nursing interventions are directed at which of the following?
   A. all individuals who need health services
   B. people without health care insurance
   C. the health needs of the total community
   D. vulnerable groups within the community

4. Major causes of health disparities include which of the following?
   A. gender, race, ethnicity, and poverty
   B. lack of sustainable health care systems
   C. poverty, public policy, and national economic conditions
   D. TB, diarrhea, malaria, and AIDS

5. Which of the following are included in the priorities of population-based nursing interventions for at-risk families who have limited access to health care and many unmet health needs?
   A. advocacy, community organizing, social marketing, coalition building
   B. disease and health event investigation, screening, referral, consultation
   C. outreach, screening, referral and follow-up, health teaching, and counselling
   D. screening, referral and follow-up, case management, surveillance

REVIEW ACTIVITIES

1. Compare and contrast individual-focused nursing practice with population-based nursing practice. Compared to individual-focused nursing, what specific nursing knowledge and skills do you need to practice population-based nursing care?

2. If you were developing a framework for the empowerment of new-Canadian women, what features would you include? How could you become a nursing advocate for the empowerment of these women at local, national, and international levels?

3. Survey your classmates using the health determinants assessment framework. Analyze your data and identify common health-risk factors within the group.

EXPLORING THE WEB

- Canada Public Health Agency of Canada: *http://www.phac-aspc.gc.ca/about_apropos/index.html*

- Canadian Public Health Association: *http://www.cpha.ca/*

- Canadian Nurses Association: *http://www.cna-nurses.ca/cna/*

- Community Health Nurses' Initiatives Group: *http://www.chnig.org/*

- Community Health Nurses Association of Canada: *http://www.chnc.ca/*

- Health Canada: *http://www.hc-sc.gc.ca/*

- Local Health Integrated Networks: *http://www.health.gov.on.ca/transformation/lhin/lhin_mn.html*

- Office of the Auditor General of Canada: *http://www.oag-bvg.gc.ca/internet/index.htm*

- United Nations: *http://www.un.org*

- World Bank: *http://www.worldbank.org/*

- World Health Organization: *http://www.who.int/en/*

REFERENCES

British Columbia Centre for Disease Control. (2002). "*Chee Mamuk.*" Retrieved from http://www.bccdc.org/content.php?item=96

Edwards, N., & Roelofs, S. (2005). Participatory approaches in the co-design of a comprehensive referral system. *Canadian Nurse, 101*(8), 21–24.

Falk Rafael, A. R., Fox, J., Mildon, B., & O'Donnell, R. (1998). *Public health nursing: Position statement.* Toronto: The Community Health Nurses' Interest Group of the Registered Nurses Association of Ontario.

Freeman, R. B. (1957). *Public health nursing practice* (2nd ed.). Philadelphia: Saunders.

Green, L. W., & Kreuter, M. W. (1999). *Health promotion planning: An educational and ecological approach.* New York: McGraw-Hill.

Johnson, I. (Ed.). (2006). *Determinants of Community Health, Year 1, Semester 2: Course Manual & Readings 2006–2007.* Toronto: University of Toronto.

Kristjansson, B., Petticrew, M., MacDonald, B., Krasevec, J., Janzen, L., Greenhalgh, T., et al. (2007). School feeding for improving the physical and psychosocial health of disadvantaged students. *Cochrane Database of Systematic Reviews,* Issue 1. Art. No.: CD004676. doi: 10.1002/14651858.CD004676.pub2.

Mitchell, P. (1999). UK government aims to prevent 300,000 deaths over ten years. *Lancet, 354,* 139.

Office of the Auditor General. (2001). Report of the Auditor General of Canada to the Legislative Assembly of Nunavut. Children, Youth and Family Programs and Services in Nunavut. Ottawa, 8 March 2011. Retrieved from http://www.oag-bvg.gc.ca/internet/English/nun_201103_e_35006.html

Office of the Auditor General. (2011). Canada Status Report of the Auditor General of Canada to the House of Commons: Chapter 4, Programs for First Nations on Reserves. Ottawa, 3 May 2011. Retrieved from http://www.oag-bvg.gc.ca/internet/English/parl_oag_201106_00_e_35368.html

Peterson, W. E., & Mannion, C. (2005). Multidisciplinary collaborative primary maternity care project: A national initiative to address the availability and quality of maternity services. *Canadian Nurse, 101*(9), 24–28.

Shah, C. P. (2003). *Public health and preventive medicine in Canada* (5th ed.). Toronto: Elsevier.

Smith, D., & Davies, B. (2006). Participatory model: Creating a new dynamic in Aboriginal health. *Canadian Nurse, 102*(4), 36–39.

World Health Organization. (1978). *Declaration of Alma-Ata: Report of the International Conference on Primary Health Care.* Alma-Ata, USSR, September 1978. Geneva: WHO. Retrieved from http://www.who.int/hpr/NPH/docs/declaration_almaata.pdf

World Health Organization. (1986). *Ottawa charter for health promotion.* Retrieved from http://www.who.int/healthpromotion/conferences/previous/ottawa/en/

World Health Organization. (1997). *The Jakarta declaration on leading health promotion into the 21st century.* Jakarta, Indonesia. Retrieved from http://www.who.int/hpr/NPH/docs/jakarta_declaration_en.pdf

SUGGESTED READINGS

Bronskill, S. E., Stevenson, J. E., Hirdes, J. P., Henry, D. A., & the Chartbook Advisory Group. (2011). Aging in Ontario: Using population-based data in the evaluation of trends in health system use. *Healthcare Quarterly, 14*(2), 21–25.

Diem. E. (2004). *Community health nursing projects: Making a difference.* Philadelphia: Lippincott Williams & Wilkins.

Lapeyre, J., & Nelson, S. (2010). The "old internationals": Canadian nurses in an international nursing community. *Nursing Leadership, 23*(4), 33–44.

Haddad, M. J. (Editor-in-Chief). (2010). Issue 1: Social Determinants: Child health in Canada. *Healthcare Quarterly, 14* (Special issue), 1–3.

Heymann, J., Hertzman, C., Barer, M. L., & Evans, R. G. (Eds.). (2006). *Healthier societies: From analysis to action.* New York: Oxford University Press.

Hilfinger, D. K. (2001). Globalization, nursing, and health for all. *Journal of Nursing Scholarship, 33*(1), 9–11.

Kothari, A., & Armstrong, R. (2011). Community-based knowledge translation: Unexplored opportunities. *Implementation Science, 6* (1), 59. doi: 10.1186/1748-5908-6-59.

Kurland, J. (2000). Public health in the new millennium II: Social exclusion. *Public Health Reports, 115*(4), 298.

Leeseberg Stamler, L. (2004). *Community health nursing: A Canadian perspective.* Toronto: Pearson Education Canada.

Lindeman, C. A. (2000). The future of nursing education. Journal of *Nursing Education, 39*(1), 5–12.

National Collaborating Centre for Determinants of Health. (2011). *Integrating Social Determinants of Health and Health Equity into Canadian Public Health Practice: Environmental Scan 2010.* Retrieved from http://www.nccdh.ca/

Orchard, C. A., Smillie, C., & Meagher-Stewart, D. (2005). Community development and health in Canada. *Journal of Nursing Scholarship, 32*(2), 205–207.

Registered Nurses Association of British Columbia. (1992). *Determinants of health: Empowering strategies for nursing practice.* Vancouver: Registered Nurses Association of British Columbia.

Robinson Vollman, A. (2003). *Canadian community as partner.* Philadelphia: Lippincott Williams & Wilkins.

Uys, L. R. (2001). Universal access to health care: If not now, when? *Reflections on Nursing Leadership, 27*(2), 21–23.

Young, L. E., & Hayes, V. E. (2002). *Transforming health promotion practice: Concepts, issues, and applications.* Philadelphia: F. A. Davis Company.

CHAPTER ENDNOTES

1. World Health Organization, "The World Health Report, Health Systems Financing, the path to universal coverage." Retrieved from http://www.who.int/whr/2010/en/index.html

2. World Health Organization, "World Health Report 2012, No health without research." Retrieved from http://www.who.int/rpc/whr2012/en/index.html

3. Ottawa Charter for Health Promotion. Retrieved from http://www.who.int/hpr/NPH/docs/ottawa_charter_hp.pdf

4. Jakarta Declaration on Leading Health Promotion into the 21st Century (1997). Retrieved from http://www.who.int/hpr/NPH/docs/jakarta_declaration_en.pdf

5. Ottawa Charter for Health Promotion, "Health Promotion Action Means." Retrieved from http://www.who.int/hpr/NPH/docs/ottawa_charter_hp.pdf

6. Jakarta Declaration on Leading Health Promotion into the 21st Century (1997). Retrieved from http://www.who.int/hpr/NPH/docs/jakarta_declaration_en.pdf

7. Tate, D. G., & Nieuwenhujsen, E. "The ICIDH–2: A New Classification of Disablement." Retrieved from http://www.psychosocial.com/policy/icidh.html

8. Ontario. Ministry of Health and Long-Term Care, "Public Health Nurses: Bringing Health Home." Retrieved from http://www.archives.gov.on.ca/english/on-line-exhibits/health-promotion/health-home.aspx

9. Canadian Nurses Association, "Obtaining CNA Certification." Retrieved from http://cna-aiic.ca/cna/nursing/certification/specialties/initials/default_e.aspx

10. Street Health, "About Us," Retrieved from http://www.streethealth.ca/home.htm

11. Ministry of Health and Long-Term Care, "Community Health Centres." Retrieved from http://www.health.gov.on.ca/english/public/contact/chc/chc_mn.html

12. Cathy Crowe's website. Retrieved from http://cathycrowe.ca/

13. Ministry of Health and Long-Term Care, "Local Health Integration Networks." Retrieved from http://www.health.gov.on.ca/transformation/lhin/lhin_mn.html

14. Aboriginal Health Access Centres, "Programs and Services." Retrieved from http://www.ahwsontario.ca/programs/prog_top.html

15. World Health Organization, "About WHO." Retrieved from http://www.who.int/about/en/index.html

16. Office of the Auditor General of Canada, 2011 March Report of the Auditor General of Canada, "Children, Youth and Family Programs and Services in Nunavut." Retrieved from http://www.oag-bvg.gc.ca/internet/English/nun_201103_e_35006.html#hd3a

17. Office of the Auditor General of Canada, 2011 March Report of the Auditor General of Canada, "Chapter 4 – Programs for First Nations on Reserves." Retrieved from http://www.oag-bvg.gc.ca/internet/English/parl_oag_201106_04_e_35372.html

CHAPTER 6

Personal and Interprofessional Communication

Jacklyn L. Ruthman, PhD, RN

Adapted by John P. Angkaw, RN, BScN, MEd, MBA(c) and Heather Crawford, BScN, MEd, CHE

Communication among healthcare providers is a prerequisite for safe client management, and it accounts for the major part of the information flow in healthcare. (J. Tija, K. Mazor, T. Field, V. Meterko, A. Spenard, & J. Gurwitz, 2009)

OBJECTIVES

The purpose of this chapter is to enable the reader to

- detail current trends in society that affect communication;
- describe the communication process;
- identify the characteristics of verbal and nonverbal communication;
- increase effectiveness of communication by using basic communication skills;
- identify barriers to communication; and
- describe typical nursing communication activities in the workplace.

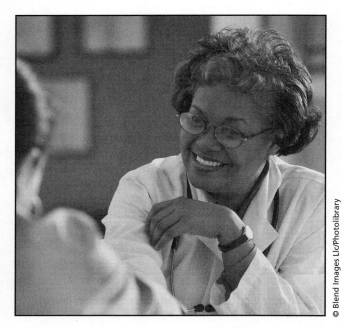

© Blend Images Llc/Photolibrary

As a new graduate nurse working on a medical unit in your community hospital, you begin your shift by making rounds of your clients to perform initial assessments and obtain their vital signs. You enter the room of Mr. Davis, who has a long history of asthma and chronic obstructive pulmonary disease. He was admitted yesterday with aspiration pneumonia. While conducting a respiratory assessment, he tells you, "I don't think I'm going to survive this one. My body has gone through enough." His wife, who is at his bedside, replies, "What's wrong with you? Don't talk like that."

What are your thoughts about this situation?

What nonverbal cues might be used to help you interpret this message?

What communication skills will you use to respond appropriately?

Today's nurses use basic principles of communication to facilitate interactions with clients and their family members, peers, and practitioners in other disciplines. These principles allow nurses to adapt to trends that affect the profession of nursing and its practice. The dictionary defines *communication* as a process by which information is exchanged. Nurses follow a widely used process of communication, rather than one that is unique to nursing. In an increasingly diverse society, they must rely on good communication skills to effectively promote client care and professionalism in a variety of settings. These skills enable nurses to engage in a complex, interactive process of communication that uses both verbal and nonverbal modes. Nurses are aware of the context in which communication occurs. They must be aware of potential barriers to communication and be able to overcome those barriers. Awareness of the principles and skills of communication empowers nurses to manage a variety of communication demands in the workplace.

TRENDS IN SOCIETY THAT AFFECT COMMUNICATION

Increasingly, good communication is important because of cultural trend in Canadian society. Among the trends affecting nursing practice is the increasing social diversity. Canada has been called the melting pot, and that is evident in the presence and influence of many different ethnic, racial, cultural, and socioeconomic backgrounds (Peach, 2005). With increased diversity, the once-dominant values and beliefs tend to be replaced or diluted with new values and beliefs. Differences can become a source of misunderstanding, but these can be bridged by effective communication.

Another trend is Canada's aging population. Approximately 23 percent to 25 percent of the population will be 65 years of age or older by 2036. The rate of growth of this age group will rise to 24 percent to 28 percent by 2061, compared to a 14 percent growth rate in 2009 (Statistics Canada, 2010). By 2036 the number of seniors will likely double the number in 2009—between 9.9 million and 10.9 million people. In 2061 the number would increase to between 11.9 million and 15.0 million people (Statistics Canada, 2010). An aging society will challenge nurses to maintain effective communication, particularly to compensate for the diminished sensory abilities that typically accompany aging. Because multiple sensory deficits can occur simultaneously, clients may experience combined sensory losses that include hearing, seeing, smelling, tasting, and touching. As a result, the older person's potentially diminished input will challenge both the nurse and the client to creatively compensate for these deficits.

At the same time as the population is aging, there is a cultural shift to electronic modes of communication: computer technology plays an increasing role. Consequently, it will be important for nurses to be able to communicate effectively in writing. A reliance on written, electronic communication will mean a shift away from the traditional sources of input through visual, auditory, and kinesthetic modes. In future, nurses will require keen writing skills. These trends have influenced recommendations for current nursing competencies. Communication is so central to nursing that most of competencies required of nurse managers contain a communication component (Jeans & Rowat, 2005).

The intensity and pervasiveness of social media and the cyber world cannot be ignored. With four generations of nursing staff—from the youngest staff members, the millennials, who've rarely been without instant connectivity to information and communication, to the baby boomers—social media can and must be used successfully by nurse managers or they risk becoming the dreaded "dinosaur" and possibly even inadequate leaders (Raso, 2010).

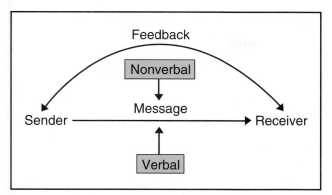

Figure 6-1 Basic Communication Model

ELEMENTS OF THE COMMUNICATION PROCESS

Communication is the exchange of information or opinions. Communication is most often an interactive process that is a means to an end and is influenced by the context in which it occurs. Communication typically involves a sender, a message, a receiver, and feedback. Face-to-face communication allows the process to proceed almost immediately, that is, to be synchronous. Electronic media can be either synchronous or asynchronous. Figure 6-1 illustrates the communication process.

SENDER

A message originates with the **sender**. Laswell's classic model of communication (1948) describes the sender as the "who" in communication. When nurses initiate communication, they are the senders.

MESSAGE

The **message** originates with the sender and consists of verbal and nonverbal stimuli that are taken in by the receiver. The message is the "what" in communication.

RECEIVER

The **receiver** takes in the message and analyzes it. When nurses listen to client-initiated conversations, they are the receivers. When the receiver reacts by returning a new message, the receiver and sender reverse roles.

FEEDBACK

The new message that is generated by the receiver in response to the original message from the sender is the **feedback.** Grohar-Murray and DiCroce (2003) state that feedback informs the sender that the receiver had understood the message transmitted. Feedback is effective when the two communicators are sensitive to each other's messages and they change behaviours based on

the message exchanges. Feedback can be either direct or indirect. Direct feedback is the receiver's explicit response to the sender's message. On the other hand, indirect feedback is more subtle and implicit.

CHANNELS OF COMMUNICATION

In almost every nursing interaction, there is **visual** (seeing), **auditory** (hearing), and **kinesthetic** (touching) input. According to Potter and Perry (2001), these sensory stimuli may be processed at different levels, with the simplest level reporting what is actually seen, heard, or touched. The next level of sensory processing orders and structures information from the usual auditory or kinesthetic input and integrates the stimulus so that one reports observing, listening, or feeling. The highest level of processing interprets and integrates information from all the inputs leading to perception and interpretation.

The processing occurs in each person who is involved in the communication, and may occur at different levels, depending on each person's cognitive abilities. For example, a toddler who is just beginning to communicate effectively using words delights in sharing labels such as "snow." This is the simplest level of communication. Upon touching the snow, the toddler might demonstrate an ability to integrate the experience with touching snow by exclaiming, "Snow cold." The mother delights in the child's sophistication and interprets the first encounter at the higher level of processing by responding to the child at the highest level and telling the child that's right and offering that snow is cold and white and beautiful and fun to play in.

THE VISUAL CHANNEL

All visually capable people take in information from the surrounding environments through sight. The amount of detail available is limited primarily by how much one is able to see. For nurses, visual data offer a wealth of information that can lead to rapid interpretation. For example, a nurse who is caring for a fresh postoperative client looks at the dressing to validate that it is dry, intact, and free of discharge. The nurse interprets these negative findings as a stable situation.

THE AUDITORY CHANNEL

Hearing is another sensory channel that is focused on words that are spoken, but also takes into account the volume, pitch, tone, rhythm, and speed with which they are delivered. Hearing involves identifying not only the words spoken but also how a message is delivered. Babies are typically born with the ability to hear, but they must learn to listen. Listening involves making sense out of what was said.

To listen effectively, the nurse must put together accurately what is said and how it is said. The nurse who is assessing the fresh postoperative client asks, "How would you rate your pain on a scale of 0 to 10, with 0 being no pain and 10 being the worst pain you can imagine?" The client replies, "Oh, I don't know, maybe a four." The nurse begins the feedback by inquiring of the client whether a pain rating of four is acceptable. The words the nurse speaks are also filled with cues based on the volume, rhythm, tone, pitch, and speed. The client tells the nurse that the pain is acceptable, but a nurse who is truly listening must also process cues based on the client's volume, rhythm, tone, pitch, and speed.

THE KINESTHETIC CHANNEL

All aspects of communication that relate to feelings are considered kinesthetic. At the most basic level, these feelings involve touch and physiological responses. Kinesthetic stimuli have cognitive and emotional components that are integrated to become feelings, or the quality of things as imparted through touch. For example, as the nurse repositions the client, the nurse may touch the client's skin and note that it is warm and dry. The nurse interprets these stimuli favourably. However, the nurse also notices that the client grimaces when moved. A client's body actions or body language communicate additional kinesthetic information. Body language is important because it may accompany, substitute, or modify input from other channels. Integrating information from all channels, the nurse perceives that the client may be in pain that is unacceptable. The nurse offers verbal feedback that matches that perception, thereby continuing the communication process using all channels until the exchange is complete.

MODES OF COMMUNICATION

The two traditional modes of communication, verbal and nonverbal, are exemplified in the nurse–client scenario in the Real World Interview. Because face-to-face encounters usually allow for verbal and nonverbal exchange, they have been regarded as the most effective modes of communication and hence have been preferred. When face-to-face encounters are not possible or practical, other approaches are used. Historically, the next most effective approach is the telephone, followed by voice messages, email messages, and written documents. These electronic methods comprise the third mode of communication, which will grow in importance as nurses increasingly rely on technology, particularly computers, to communicate interpersonally. As was previously mentioned, using email requires that nurses have keen writing skills.

VERBAL COMMUNICATION

Verbal communication relies on speaking words to convey a message. It also involves the use of the auditory channel previously discussed. The accuracy of the message is dependent on the sender's vocabulary and the receiver's ability to make sense of the words used to send the message. In addition, the verbal message is influenced by the sender's tone. According to Yogo, Hashi, Tsutsui, and Yamada (2000), when conveying a message, the tone is more influential than the content. Other factors that influence verbal communication are the pacing, timing, and context of the message.

The Institute for Healthcare Communication Canada is a nationally accredited not-for-profit organization that has partnered with hundreds of health care organizations since 1987 to train more than 150,000 physicians and other health care professionals throughout North America in effective communication skills.[1] The Institute stresses the concept that effective communication between clinician and client is a necessity, and it will work with health care organizations to provide educational opportunities to make it possible for clinicians to develop the communication skills they need to be effective.[2]

NONVERBAL COMMUNICATION

Nonverbal communication consists of aspects of communication that are outside what is spoken. The communicator's appearance, facial expressions, posture, gait, body movements, position, gestures, and touch all influence how the message is processed. Futhermore, although tone is more important than the words spoken, it has long been suggested that facial expression is even more important than either tone or the words used. Nonverbal communication tends to be unconscious and more difficult to control.

ELECTRONIC COMMUNICATION

As previously mentioned, communication is shifting to an electronic mode, with computer technology playing an increasingly dominant role. Clients are being monitored long distance and connecting to their health care providers through a variety of technologies, including telephone, voice mail, and email. These methods—which may be asynchronous because caregiver and care receiver must interact using technology rather than the traditional face-to-face or voice-to-voice encounter— require careful communication. For example, email allows almost instantaneous communication around the world, but it also accommodates individual preferences with respect to the timing of the response. For example, a client can provide an update on a condition early in the day, and the caregivers can respond as their schedules permit. Using email may save a client and caregiver from travel or loss of work; however, nurses acting in such a caregiver role need to have keen writing skills.

All the considerations that are important to effective writing are beyond the scope of this text; however, a few tips can be given here. The speed with which exchanges can now be made using computers has reduced the acceptable response time. Therefore, the first tip when communicating using computers is to respond in a timely manner. Next, keep in mind that accurate spelling, correct grammar, and organization of thought are very important, especially when the verbal and nonverbal cues provided by face-to-face encounters are absent. Finally, always proofread your correspondences prior to sending them. Imagine yourself the recipient of the document. Look for complete sentences; a logical development of thought and reasoning; accuracy; and an appropriate use of grammar, such as punctuation and capitalization.

SOCIAL MEDIA

Email is relatively simple compared to the interactive and multidimensional networking of current web technology. Sites such as Facebook, Twitter, LinkedIn, and YouTube allow people to create a wide social network. Responses to questions or articles on a website are immediately posted for the world to see. What is different in the world of social media is the interactive nature of information sharing. Blogging and online discussion boards allow for direct disclosure of feelings, facts, and thoughts with immediate unfiltered feedback. The unpredictable and spontaneous nature of social networks and blogs may add authentic content, but it also adds risk. Remember that the Internet is considered public domain. That means that anything you publish online, whether in a chat room, on a Facebook page, or in a Tweet, is legally considered public material. As such, everyone is personally responsible for their publications.

Organizational policy is paramount. Multiple departments, such as legal, human resources, and compliance, will have input into organizational policy pertaining to social media. The sharing of policy and the boundaries to be followed should occur during staff orientation, as well as with incumbent staff (Raso, 2010). Critical points to address include avoidance of violation of client confidentiality, slander, and anything that destroys public confidence in the organization. Privacy and confidentiality are just as important with

REAL WORLD INTERVIEW

When working on a cardiac and vascular surgery unit, it is fairly infrequent that the nurses must care for tracheostomy clients. When we do, these clients often are unable to speak or are deconditioned to the point where it is impossible for them to even write with a pen or pencil. When they are unable to communicate or voice their concerns, nursing care for these clients becomes very task oriented, and the client may not be involved in any decision making. Unfortunately, the nurses on the unit also voice feeling frustrated and helpless because they are unable to effectively communicate with their client. The results are feelings of distress, and inadequacy as they believe they are not providing optimal care.

One client we cared for recently had a tracheostomy and tried to verbalize what he wanted but was unable to speak through his trach. Almost every nurse that was assigned to him could not understand him. Feelings of frustration mounted for the client in such a way that his behaviours were misconstrued and labelled as agitation or confusion. One day a nurse created a letter board for the client. He was then able to point to different letters and spell words. Both the nurse and the client were ecstatic that this seemingly simple method worked. Of course, not all tracheostomy clients are cognitively able to communicate in this same manner. Similarly, as nurses we encounter clients that are difficult to communicate with for different reasons. What is important to remember is that nurses need to cater to individual clients according to their communication needs.

Communication can sometimes take a back seat when managing clients and various nursing tasks. The nurse in this scenario demonstrated client-centred care and made communication a priority. Such a simple task ended up being a significant turning point for the client, as it meant involving the client in his own care. Furthermore, this established trust and ensured that the needs of the client were not being ignored. Communication facilitated the therapeutic nurse–client relationship as they worked together toward positive client outcomes.

Larissa Clemente, RN, BScN, MN(c), CCN(c)
Staff Nurse, Cardiac and Vascular Surgery

Source: Larissa Clemente.

social media as within the workplace. Do not reveal your own personal information, or any confidential information related to your job or your organization itself. Also, respect the privacy of others, and do not post or discuss inappropriate or personal information about others on your own sites. Think before you post. Ask yourself, "Would I put this up on a bulletin board or in a common area at work?" Above all, do not post any materials or comments that could be read as offensive, hurtful, insulting, or demeaning to your co-workers, staff, community partners, or the organization itself. If you are unsure about any content, discuss it with your manager. Another area to address is permission to use an organization email address—employees should use their personal email to post anything on social media sites, not the organization's email.

LEVEL OF COMMUNICATION

The level of communication depends on the audience for the message. Consequently, communication can be thought of as having three levels: public, intrapersonal, and interpersonal.

PUBLIC COMMUNICATION

Public communication directs the message to an audience or group of people with a common interest. For example, the nurse educator presenting a workshop on signs and symptoms of menopause to a room full of middle-aged women engages in public communication. Her audience is a group of people with a common interest. As the presenter, she acts primarily as a sender of information. By design, feedback is typically limited in public speaking, though it does occur. Strategies abound to enhance public speaking skills, but it is beyond the scope of this text to discuss them.

INTRAPERSONAL COMMUNICATION

Intrapersonal communication can be thought of as self-talk. As the name suggests, this level of communication refers to how individuals communicate within themselves, which can present as doubts or affirmations. New nurses may engage in intrapersonal communication while, simultaneously, doubting and affirming their ability to complete a procedure. For example, the first time newly registered RNs have to catheterize a client, they may simultaneously doubt their ability to insert a Foley catheter, with one message to themselves—"I haven't done this for months"—and affirm their ability to insert a Foley catheter with another—"I can do this." They are engaging in intrapersonal communication. The so-called competing voices within them act as sender and receiver

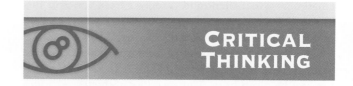
in this intrapersonal conversation, whose outcome will be influenced by the feedback that follows.

Simms, Price, and Ervin (2000) present communication with self, or intrapersonal communication, as the first important element in developing a sphere of communication. From self-awareness and understanding of oneself, a nurse can progress confidently to one-on-one interactions with others, and then into interactions with smaller and larger groups. See Figure 6-2 for some spheres of communication and their related skills.

INTERPERSONAL COMMUNICATION

Interpersonal communication involves communication between individuals, either person-to-person or in small

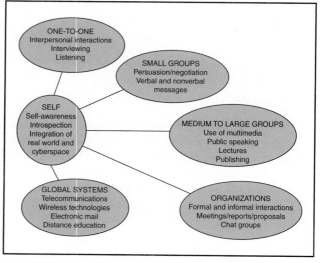

Figure 6-2 Spheres of Communication and Related Skills

CRITICAL THINKING

A diabetic client who lives in the rural North is excited to have recently become connected to the World Wide Web with the acquisition of a computer and Internet services. His wife, who accompanies him to the office visit, wonders whether some of the monitoring that currently occurs during office visits might not be accomplished using email. Winters are hard and travel is difficult, the client's circulation is poor, he fatigues easily, and using email could save them the six-hour round trip to the primary care clinic. By using email, they can maintain contact as needed without these drawbacks.

Do you agree with their idea? What are the advantages of this suggestion for the client? For the caregiver? What are the drawbacks of this suggestion for the client? For the caregiver? What safeguards can you think of to facilitate communicating using email and to ensure quality care?

groups. Not surprisingly, nurses engage in this level of communication regularly. Interpersonal communication allows for a very effective level of communication as it incorporates all of the elements, channels, and modes previously discussed. The nurse, who observes a client grimace when he moves, interprets the nonverbal cue as indicating that the client is experiencing pain. Using verbal communication, she clarifies her perception by asking the client to describe and rate his pain. He describes it as tolerable and states he is expecting a visitor and he does not want to be drowsy. The communication goes back and forth until, ideally, both parties' understanding of the message match, achieving the goal of communication.

ORGANIZATIONAL COMMUNICATION

Avenues of communication are often defined by an organization's formal structure, which establishes who is in charge and identifies how different levels of personnel and various departments relate within the organization. The chief executive officer of an organization announces that the company will adopt a new policy that all employees will follow; such an announcement is a downward communication. The message starts at the top and is usually disseminated by levels through the chain of communication.

Upward communication is the opposite of downward communication. The idea originates at some level below the top of the structure and moves upward. For example, upward communication has occurred when a nurse recommends a more efficient approach to organizing care to his nurse manager, who takes the recommendation to her superior, who uses the recommendation to develop a new policy. Lateral communication occurs among people with similar status. Two nurses who are discussing how best to change a client's dressing are engaged in lateral communication. Diagonal communication occurs when members of the team, who may be on different levels of the organizational chart, discuss a client care concern, such as discharge planning.

The organizational structure within nursing also determines who is responsible for representing nursing concerns in this type of interaction. For example, if the department practises within a primary nursing model, the primary nurse is responsible for representing nursing concerns. In team nursing, the team leader rather than the nurse delivering the care is responsible.

A final avenue that organizes communication is the grapevine. The **grapevine** is an informal avenue in which rumours circulate. It ignores the formal chain of command. The major benefit of the grapevine is the speed with which information is spread, but its major drawback is that it often lacks accuracy. For example, nurses who inform an oncoming shift about a rumour that layoffs or mandatory overtime is imminent, in the absence of any information from the hospital's administration, are participating in grapevine communication.

COMMUNICATION SKILLS

Because nurses are often placed in positions of leadership and are responsible for representing nursing's concerns to others, including the client, they must have the requisite skills to be effective communicators. No single correct method ensures effective communication. Rather, effective communication requires that both the parties engaged in communicating use skills that enhance that particular interaction. Baker, Beglinger, King, Salyards, and Thompson (2000) believe that the most important considerations for facilitating communication are openness and willingness to give and receive feedback. Some of the most important skills that nurses rely on to facilitate communication are attending, responding, clarifying, and confronting skills. Additional skills are listed in Table 6-1.

| TABLE 6-1 | ADDITIONAL COMMUNICATION SKILLS |

Skill	Description
Supporting	Siding with another person or backing up another person: "I can see that you would feel that way."
Focusing	Centres on the main point: "So your main concern is …"
Asking open-ended questions	Allows for client-directed responses: "How did that make you feel?"
Providing information	Supplies knowledge that an individual did not previously have: "It's common for people with pneumonia to be tired."
Using silence	Allows for intrapersonal communication
Reassuring	Restores confidence or removes fear: "I can assure you that tomorrow …"
Expressing appreciation	Shows gratitude: "Thank you" or "You are so thoughtful."
Using humour	Provides relief and gains perspective, but may also cause harm; so use humour carefully
Conveying acceptance	Makes known that one is capable or worthy: "It's okay to cry."
Asking related questions	Expands the listener's understanding: "How painful was it?"

ATTENDING

Attending involves active listening, the most important skill used by nurses to gain an understanding of the client's message. Active listening requires that the nurse pays close attention to what the client is saying. In addition, the nurse uses the sensory and visual channels, looking for congruence between what is said and how it is said. Attending involves the nurse's nonverbal cues. Facing the client and maintaining eye contact are two skills that facilitate attending. Sitting down and leaning forward sends a message that the nurse is willing to listen. Distracting behaviours, such as tapping, send a message that the nurse is not interested in the message; therefore, such behaviours should be avoided.

RESPONDING

Responding entails verbal and nonverbal acknowledgment of the sender's message. When a nurse nods affirmatively while listening, this nonverbal response says that the message has worth. A response can be as simple as an acknowledgment that the message was received, for example, "I hear you." Sometimes, however, responding involves more. Two verbal skills that elevate the level of responding are questioning and rephrasing. Questioning allows the nurse to clarify the message by asking related questions. Rephrasing involves restating what the nurse believes to be the important points. These techniques refine perceptions and enhance understanding.

CLARIFYING

Clarifying helps the message become clear by using such skills as restating, questioning, and rephrasing. As with most communication, clarifying can be accomplished using a variety of approaches. For example, if the nurse does not follow a client's account of his presenting complaint, the nurse can respond with "I lost you there." Perhaps the nurse tries to process information that is confusing or conflicting. The nurse can then restate what was heard, in an effort to clarify the information. Clarifying involves communicating as specifically as possible. Questioning and rephrasing, which were described previously, are used not only to respond but also to clarify.

CONFRONTING

Confronting describes working jointly with others to resolve a problem or conflict. Given that definition, confronting is an effective means of resolving conflict.

It involves, first of all, identifying the conflict, which can arise from either perceived or real differences. A nurse might identify a conflict with a simple "we have a problem here." Next, the problem is clearly delineated so that those involved understand what it is and what it is not. Then, using knowledge and reason, attempts are made to resolve the problem. The goal is to achieve a win-win solution in which both parties' needs are met, which sounds easier than it sometimes is because emotions can get in the way and cloud reason. Cooling-off periods are sometimes needed between problem identification and conflict resolution. Acceptable motives for confronting are to resolve conflict, further growth, and improve relationships.

BARRIERS TO COMMUNICATION

Barriers are obstacles to effective communication. The nurse who can identify potential barriers to communication will be better equipped to avoid them or to compensate for them. Some of the most common barriers are gender, culture, anger, incongruent responses, and conflict. Environmental barriers such as managerial philosophy, organizational structure, and power and status relationships between the sender and the receiver can also impact communication (Longest, Rakich, & Darr, 2006).

GENDER

Gender interferes with communication when men and women lack the understanding that they sometimes process information differently. Gender differences and patterns do not preclude working together. Rather, both sides must realize the other's preference and make accommodations so that effective communication results.

Gender differences have been attributed, in part, to gender socialization in which males are provided with more opportunities to develop confidence and assertiveness than females. Fortunately, the feminist movement and increased sexual equality in Western society, in general, have lessened traditional sociological patterns of competitiveness and decisiveness in men and passivity and nurturing in women. However, remnants of the traditional model persist, particularly in health care settings. Nurses who lack assertiveness and confidence are encouraged to acquire the requisite skills to be assertive and confident, be an effective client advocate, and also communicate in a confident manner.

CULTURE

As stated previously, Canadian culture is becoming increasingly diverse. This diversity reduces the likelihood that clients and nurses will share a common cultural background. In turn, the number of safe assumptions about beliefs and practices decreases and the probability for misunderstanding increases. For example, shortly after delivering a baby, women are often hungry and thirsty. Some cultures believe that women should eat hot foods and beverages to appropriately restore their energies, whereas other cultures believe cold foods and beverages are appropriate. A well-intentioned nurse who does not consult with the client about her preferences may arrange culturally inappropriate nourishment.

Broadly defined, *culture* encompasses the beliefs and practices of different groups, including different perspectives on gender, race, age, economic status, health, and disability. Poole, Davidhizar, and Giger (1995) suggest six cultural phenomena that a person needs to consider when delegating to a culturally diverse staff: communication, space, social organization, time, environmental control, and biological variations. They emphasize that culture and communication are intrinsically intertwined (see Literature Application).

Nurses are responsible for bridging gaps between themselves and their clients, first of all through accepting of differences. They can also overcome cultural differences by learning about other cultures. Finally, nurses can bridge cultural differences by being vigilant in applying the skills previously described to facilitate communication.

ANGER

Anger is a universal, strong feeling of displeasure that is often precipitated by a situation that either frustrates someone or prevents them from attaining a goal or getting what they want from life. Anger is often a response to conflict and is influenced by one's beliefs. Ellis (1997) describes anger as an irrational response that arises from one of four irrational ideas: (1) sensing that the treatment one received was awful (awfulizing); (2) feeling that one can't stand having been treated so irresponsibly and unfairly (can't-stand-it-itis); (3) believing that one should not and must not behave as he did (shoulding and musting); and (4) thinking that one is a terrible person because one acted in a terrible manner (undeservingness and damnation). Ellis maintains that beliefs remain rational as long as the evaluation of the action does not involve an evaluation of the person. Rational and appropriate responses are feelings of disappointment. Anger, on the other hand, can be unmanageable and self-defeating. According to Ellis, we all have the ability to choose our response to anger. Potter and Perry (2001) state that anger has the following implications for nursing: (1) the nurse must not take the anger personally; (2) the nurse must meet the need that caused the angry response; and (3) when necessary, the nurse must encourage the client and the family to further express their feelings.

Anger can be dealt with in one of several ways. Three methods that may work from time to time, but that may have serious and potentially destructive drawbacks, are denying and repressing anger. These responses may lead to resentment; expressing anger, which may lead to defensiveness on the part of the respondent; and turning the other cheek, which may lead to continued mistreatment and lack of trust. Because anger stems from carrying things further and viewing the situation as awful, terrible, or horrible, Ellis (1997) advocates disputing irrational beliefs. Anger can stem from deep-seated feelings of unassertiveness. Assertion involves taking a stand, whereas aggression involves putting another person down. If unassertiveness is the source of anger, then one solution is to learn to act assertively.

INCONGRUENT RESPONSES

When words and actions in a communication do not match the inner experience of self or are inappropriate to the context, the response is incongruent. Some common incongruent responses are blaming, placating, being super reasonable, and using irrelevant information

to make decisions. Blaming is finding fault or error and occurs when a response lacks respect for others' feelings. For example, a nurse who attributes a medication error to her overloaded assignment might blame the nurse who made the assignment, saying, "It's all her fault." This reaction can be avoided by standing up for one's rights while respecting the rights of others.

Placating is soothing by concession, which occurs when one lacks self-respect. For example, a nurse who consents to a client assignment that she believes is unfair or unsafe just to keep the peace is placating. Placating

LITERATURE APPLICATION

Citation: Hall. P. (2005). Interprofessional teamwork: Professional cultures as barriers. *Journal of Interprofessional Care.* 19: 188–196.

Discussion: Careful consideration must be given by nurses to the professional cultures of their colleagues, as barriers may arise that may inhibit professional interaction and communication. Health disciplines and professions have evolved under their own or societal forces, but so too have their identities, values, and scopes of practice. With the shift toward interprofessional practice in today's health care environment, nurses must be aware of the specific professional roles and scopes of practice that each health team member contributes. They also must be able to collaborate with other team members to identify issues, and jointly develop a plan of action to address the issues and accomplish goals. In order to do this, they must be able to communicate effectively.

Implications for Practice: Nurses must become aware of the cultural barriers associated with their colleagues, and develop skills to address them.

LITERATURE APPLICATION

Citation: Lingard, L., Espin, S., Rubin, B., Whyte, S., Colmenares, M., Baker, G. R., Doran, D., Grober, E., Orser, B., Bohnen, J., & Reznick, R. (2005). Getting teams to talk: development and pilot implementation of a checklist to promote interprofessional communication in the OR. *Quality and Safety in Health Care,* 14: 340–346. Copyright © 2005 BMJ Publishing Group Ltd.. Reproduced with permission from BMJ Publishing Group Ltd.

Discussion: When medical errors occur, they are regularly traced back to breakdowns in communication among members of the health care team. Communication research has often found that critical information is often transferred in a reactive, ad hoc manner and communicative tension is frequent. As a result, a pilot implementation of a preoperative team communication checklist was conducted. The objectives of the study were as follows: to assess the feasibility of the checklist

(that is, team members' willingness and ability to incorporate it into their work processes); to describe how the checklist tool was used by operating room teams; and to describe perceived functions of the checklist discussions.

Implications for Practice: The preoperative team checklist shows promise as a feasible and efficient tool that promotes information exchange and team cohesion. Further research is needed to determine the sustainability and generalizability of the checklist intervention, to fully integrate the checklist routine into workflow patterns, and to measure its impact on client safety.

Author's note: See Safer Healthcare Now! website, http://www.saferhealthcarenow.ca/EN/Pages/default.aspx, and look at "Safe Surgery Checklist."

can be overcome by paying attention to one's own needs and by negotiating what one believes to be a fair and safe assignment.

Being super reasonable means going beyond reason and lacking respect for others' and one's own feelings. The nurse described previously, who, when approached by the house supervisor, agrees to whatever solution is offered, has become super reasonable when she says, "You're always right; I'll do whatever you need." This ineffective approach can be sidestepped by considering each other's feelings when arriving at a solution.

Finally, using irrelevant information for decision-making shows lack of respect for others' and one's own feelings. A nurse who challenges a colleague's abilities based solely on the colleague's out-of-work activities or political preference is using irrelevant information. Likewise, arguing against a colleague's ability to function as a charge nurse because of an incident that occurred a year prior during the nurse's orientation is often irrelevant. Respecting feelings and context can avert irrelevance.

CONFLICT

Conflict arises when ideas or beliefs are opposed. Not surprisingly, it occurs at different levels: interpersonal and organizational. As previously stated, conflict resolution is one way to resolve conflict. To resolve conflict, the nature of the differences and the reasons for the differences must be considered. These differences arise for an array of reasons. Some of these reasons include variations in facts, goals, and methods to achieve goals, values, or standards (Grohar-Murray & DiCroce, 2003). Conflict resolution can typically occur by using one of five distinct approaches: avoiding, accommodating, competing, compromising,

and collaborating. Two conflict management strategies, avoiding and compromising, were used predominantly by all categories of nurses in this research study (Valentine, 2001).

Avoiding or retreating disregards the needs of self and others but sometimes offers the benefit of allowing tempers to cool. An example of avoidance is the nurse who walks away from a heated discussion with a peer, after a change-of-shift report.

Accommodating satisfies the needs of others at the expense of self. The nurse who forfeits after-work plans to staff the unit by working overtime is accommodating. Accommodating can lead to disappointment or anger.

Competing can lead to personal victory at the expense of others, which can lead to ill will. For example, two nurses who want the same weekend off may plead their cases to the nurse manager, each in hopes of getting her own way.

Compromising leads to a middle-ground solution in which each party makes a concession. The charge nurse who gives each of the nurses above a day off on the weekend they requested has resolved the conflict by compromising.

Collaborating resolves conflict so that both parties are satisfied. It involves seeking creative, integrative solutions, while also working through emotions. Collaborating is the best strategy for successful conflict resolution, but it is more difficult than it may appear. The charge nurse who clarifies the above nurses' requests for the same weekend off discovers one nurse wants the weekend off to attend her sister's wedding, whereas the other nurse wants to plan a getaway that can be moved to another weekend. Each nurse can be satisfied through collaboration.

Additional barriers to communication are described in Table 6-2.

TABLE 6-2	ADDITIONAL BARRIERS TO COMMUNICATION
Barrier	**Description**
Offering false reassurance	Promising something that cannot be delivered
Being defensive	Acting as though one has been attacked
Stereotyping	Unfairly categorizing others based on their traits
Interrupting	Speaking before others have completed their message
Inattention	Not paying attention
Stress	A state of tension that gets in the way of reasoning
Unclear expectations	Ill-defined tasks or duties that make successful completion unlikely

WORKPLACE COMMUNICATION

How individuals communicate depends, in part, on where communication occurs and the relationship between the sender and the receiver. Patterns of communication in the workplace are sensitive to organizational factors that define relationships. Nurses have diverse roles and relationships in the workplace that call for different communication patterns with superiors, co-workers, subordinates, physicians, and other health care professionals, clients, families, and mentors.

SUPERIORS

Communicating with a superior can be intimidating, especially for a new nurse. Observing professional courtesies is an important first step. For instance, when a problem arises, begin by requesting an appointment to discuss the issue. This approach demonstrates respect and allows for the conversation to occur at an appropriate time and place. Dress professionally. Arrive for the appointment on time, and be prepared to state the concern clearly and accurately. Provide supporting evidence, and anticipate resistance to any requests. Separate your needs from your desires. State a willingness to cooperate in finding a solution and then match your behaviours to words. Persist in the pursuit of a solution.

CO-WORKERS

Nurses depend on their co-workers to collectively provide quality client care. Nowhere is this relationship more important than in the acute care setting, where nursing services are non-stop around the clock. Transfer of client care from nurse to nurse is one of the most important and frequent communications between co-workers. It depends on fluid communication in end-of-shift reports to achieve quality nursing care. However, time constraints demand that the change-of-shift report be accurate, informative, and succinct. How the nursing care is organized influences the person who receives the report. For example, nurses who practise using a team model will require that, at a minimum, the charge nurse or team leader receives the report.

The method of delivery of the report also varies from setting to setting and may include walking rounds, written communication, or tape recording. Regardless of the method used, information that is typically exchanged during a change-of-shift report, either in writing or orally, includes the client's age, gender, admitting problem, needs, other health care concerns, activity, diet, intake and output, IV therapy, treatments, tests, and family concerns. Significant physical findings and client responses to any of the items just listed are often elaborated. The organization of the information varies and may, for example, follow a head-to-toe model if assessment forms also use this organizing approach. The most important consideration for nurses as they organize their reports is to paint an accurate picture of the client's condition and needs.

SUBORDINATES

An excellent guide for directing communication with subordinates is the golden rule: Do unto others as you would have them do unto you. As a nurse who will be responsible for overseeing others' work, a valuable perspective to maintain is that all members of the team are important to successfully realize quality client care. Communication between nurses and subordinates will most likely involve delegating, which is covered in Chapter 13, and you are encouraged to review this material as it relates to subordinates. In addition to delegating, a few other communications skills are worth mentioning. Offering positive feedback, such as, "I appreciate the way you interacted with Mr. T. to get him to ambulate twice this shift," goes a long way toward team building, and it improves subordinates' sense of worth.

Nurses also have an opportunity to act as teachers to subordinates. Often in a hospital setting, nurses teach by example. Demonstrating the desired behaviour allows the subordinate to copy the behaviour. Allow time for return demonstrations to evaluate whether the subordinate has learned the intended skill. For example, as the nurse, you may demonstrate how to position a client with special needs, encouraging the subordinate to assist and ask questions. The next time repositioning is indicated, accompany the subordinate and observe that person's ability to successfully complete the task. Offer constructive feedback. Be patient. Remember your own learning curves when mastering new skills and behaviours, and allow those you supervise the opportunity to grow. Be open to the possibility that subordinates, particularly those with experience, may have a few pearls of wisdom to share with you as well. For example, this author is forever indebted to a nurse aide who shared how to really position clients comfortably. Likewise, a veteran registered practical nurse (RPN) who knew the politics of the institution mentored a batch of new graduates as they learned to be charge nurses on the evening shift.

PHYSICIANS AND OTHER HEALTH CARE PROFESSIONALS

One of the most intimidating experiences for new nurses is communicating with physicians. Despite gender and role challenges, such communications need not be stressful events. The nurse's goal is to strive for collaboration, keeping the client goal central to the discussion. As previously discussed, collaboration allows both parties to be satisfied. It involves seeking creative, integrative solutions while also working through emotions.

To communicate effectively with the physician, the nurse presents information in a straightforward manner, clearly delineating the problem, supported by pertinent evidence. This approach is especially important when reporting changes in client conditions. Nurses are responsible for knowing the classic symptoms of conditions, orally informing the physician of changes, and recording all observations in the chart (Potter & Perry, 2001). Dr. Josh McDonald offers a recent real-life example from an occupational health care setting in the Real World Interview feature. It is important that the nurse remain calm and objective even if the physician does not cooperate.

Potter and Perry (2001) offer suggestions for handling telephone miscommunications. For example, if a physician sounds hurried over the phone, use clarification questions to avoid a misunderstanding. If a physician hangs up, document that the call was terminated and fill out an incident report. If the physician gives an inappropriate answer or gives no orders, for example, for a client complaint of pain, document the call, the information relayed, and the fact that no orders were given. In addition, document any other steps that were taken to resolve the problem, for example, notifying the charge nurse or nursing supervisor. If a physician cannot be reached, first follow the institution's procedure for treating the client and then document the actions taken.

REAL WORLD INTERVIEW

A night shift RN working in a busy emergency room was presented with a client who was hypertensive and complaining of a headache. When she did her initial triage assessment, including the client's vital signs, she found no abnormalities other than the slightly elevated blood pressure. The nurse was aware that in her place of work it was important to distinguish the truly urgent cases from those that could be sent to the waiting room. She further assessed the client's headache. She discovered that the client was not having any visual disturbances, such as photophobia, and his pupils were equal and reactive. She knew what to assess and look for and how to relate these findings to the physician in order to provide her client with the necessary care. By performing these assessments the nurse was prepared to discuss the basics, such as the client's chief complaint, his vital signs, his medications, and any changes from baseline. Know why you are worried about observed changes and communicate this to the physician.

Josh McDonald, MD

CLIENTS AND THEIR FAMILIES

Communication with clients and their families is optimized by the many skills previously described in this chapter. A few additional skills have not yet been mentioned. The first is touch. Nurses routinely use touch as a way to communicate caring and concern. Occasionally, language barriers will limit communication to the nonverbal mode. For instance, a stroke client who cannot process words can still interpret a gentle hand on his shoulder.

Communication requires an openness and honesty with concurrent respect for clients and their families. In addition, clients' privacy needs to be honoured and protected by the nurse's actions and words. Information that clients share with nurses and other health care providers is to be held in confidence. Verbal exchanges regarding client conditions are private matters that should not occur in the hallway or just outside a client's room where they could be overheard by others. Nurses

LITERATURE APPLICATION

Citation: Narasimhan, M., Eisen, L., Mahoney, C., Aceerra, F., & Rosen, M. (2006). Improving nurse-physician communication and satisfaction in the intensive care unit with a daily goals worksheet. *American Journal of Critical Care*, 15(2): 217–222.

Discussion: The development of effective communication between nurses and physicians is an essential element that has the potential to impact both staff satisfaction and client outcomes. Enhanced interaction and coordination among nurses and physicians have been shown to decrease mortality rates and increase achievement of client goals. Nurses can take a proactive role in initiating the process to enhance the communication, coordination, and interaction among nurses and physicians within a unit or organization. Furthermore, consider several quality initiatives that would seek to improve communication pathways and tools, not only enhancing the sharing of information among the health care team, but also be in alignment with your organization's strategic mission, vision, and direction.

Implications for Practice: Learn to be proactive, and initiate processes that would result in the development or improvement of a communication pathway or tool within your unit or organization. Build the rationale and case for urgency, and engage the key stakeholders, including physicians and administrators.

are obligated to not discuss client conditions with others, even family members, without the client's permission.

MENTOR AND PRODIGY

The final pattern of communication in the workplace that will be discussed is between mentor and prodigy. Mentoring is typically an informal process that occurs between an expert nurse and a novice nurse, but it may also be an assigned role. This one-on-one relationship focuses on professional aspects and is mutually beneficial. The optimal novice is hardworking, willing to learn, and anxious to succeed (Shaffer, Tallarica, & Walsh, 2000). Communication entails using the skills previously described in this chapter to help the novice develop expert status and career direction by gleaning the mentor's wisdom. This wisdom is typically shared through listening, affirming, counselling, encouraging, and seeking input from the novice (Creasia & Parker, 1996).

LITERATURE APPLICATION

Citation: DiBartola, L. (2001). Listening to patients and responding with care. *Joint Commission Journal on Quality Improvement, 27*(6), 315–323.

Discussion: Clinicians who want to improve their listening skills benefit from identifying the way in which clients are most comfortable interacting. A tool for assessing the client's preference is demonstrated. After the client's interaction style has been identified, the clinician uses this information to move closer to the way in which the client is most comfortable communicating. This article discusses a communication model for improving client communication. Figure 6-3 describes behavioural characteristics of the four communication modes.

The framework for this model is the continuum of two intersecting axes. The horizontal axis poles are inquisitive and assertive. The vertical axis poles are objective and subjective. People who are most comfortable communicating in an inquisitive way and tend to be objective are called investigators. Those who are most comfortable communicating in an inquisitive way but are subjective in nature are called unifiers. People who are most comfortable communicating in an assertive way and favour subjectivity are called energizers. Those who are most comfortable communicating in an assertive way and tend to be objective are called enterprisers. Behavioural markers can be used to identify someone's preferred communication mode (see Figure 6-4).

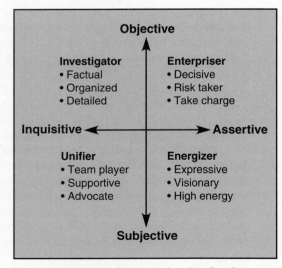

Figure 6-3 Behavioural Characteristics of the Four Communication Modes

Source: DiBartola, L (2001, June). Listening to Patients and Responding with Care. *Joint Commission Journal on the Quality Improvement*, 27(6), 322. Reprinted with Permission.

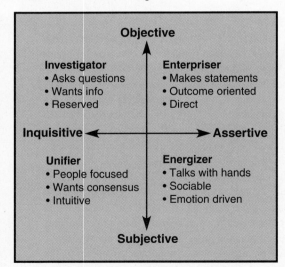

Figure 6-4 Behavioural Markers for the Four Communication Modes

Source: DiBartola, L (2001, June). Listening to patients and responding with Care. *Joint Commission Journal on the Quality Improvement*, 27(6), 319. Reprinted with Permission.

(*Continued*)

LITERATURE APPLICATION (CONTINUED)

Using your observation skills, determine where your client is on the inquisitive–assertive scale. Typical markers that would identify someone who is close to the inquisitive side are asking questions, attending carefully to detail, listening carefully to what the other person is saying, showing caution in making a decision without having adequate time to think about it, and preferring facts over intuition. On the other side of the scale, markers for someone who prefers to communicate in an assertive way are showing concern about wasting time, being quick to make a decision, being more interested in outcomes than in process, being willing to take risks, and making strong statements rather than asking questions.

In addition, you will want to make observations about the client's preference for objectivity or subjectivity. Whereas people with an objective preference are more interested in facts than intuition and in the project outcome than the process, people who are more subjective show more interest in the people who are working on the project than the project itself, are more willing to trust intuition than the facts, and show greater interest in being satisfied than in being right.

Nonverbal cues include the use of gestures or hands while talking for those on the assertive side, reserve and control for those on the inquisitive side, and high energy and expressiveness for those on the subjective side. To apply this model, think of an interaction that did not go well. Consider where both parties fit on the scale. The closer both parties are on the scale, the easier it will be for them to communicate.

Implications for Practice: After you understand the way in which both you and your client are most comfortable communicating, you can decide to communicate in a way that may be more comfortable for your client. You are not expected to change who you are; the goal of this approach is to know yourself, understand the client, and then move closer to the client. This approach will build trust and respect, and will result in the client feeling satisfied by the interaction.

LITERATURE APPLICATION

Citation: Nembhard, I. & Edmondson, A. (2006). Making it safe: The effects of leader inclusiveness and professional status on psychological safety and improvement efforts in healthcare teams. *Journal of Organizational Behaviour*, 27, 941–966.

Discussion: As today's health care institutions strive to include quality as part of their daily agenda, its health care leaders have the challenging responsibility to develop and sustain the processes that would support any quality improvement efforts. As a result, many of today's health care institutions have begun to use cross-disciplinary teams as a means to remain competitive. With that said, important considerations must be given to the pivotal influence that leaders have on the dynamics of a team, which greatly affects the team climate and orientation. Health care leaders must be inclusive in their approach to advancing any quality improvement initiatives within their organization. These leaders will be responsible for inviting and appreciating the input of their colleagues, as well as creating a team climate that is conducive to safe discussion, that questions current systems and practices, and that will yield provocative ideas leading to innovative solutions and outcomes.

Implications for Practice: Active and inclusive behaviours must be demonstrated by the health care leader to facilitate engagement and contribution of other team members to any team-based quality improvement initiatives.

Mentoring is facilitated by the novice and the mentor sharing the same work schedule. The novice is then exposed to the mentor, which allows for sharing and shadowing opportunities. The mentor can also anticipate added challenges with increasing responsibility that will likely occur. Outlining these challenges with suggestions for how to manage them prepares the novice for the expanding responsibilities. Role-playing, in which the expert preceptor nurse describes a theoretical situation and allows the novice to practise a response to new and sometimes challenging situations, is another helpful strategy.

REAL WORLD INTERVIEW

A 16-year-old, first-time expectant mother presented to the labour and delivery department in labour, anticipating an uncomplicated delivery. The admitting nurse completed normal admissions information and, because of the client's age, assessed whether a social service consult was needed. The delivery commenced uneventfully, and a healthy baby girl was born. Since the mother indicated on admission that she wanted to breastfeed, the nurse assisted the mother to breastfeed during the immediate postpartum period prior to the baby being taken to the nursery.

In this clinical situation, because hospital stays are short, communication is critical for comprehensive and quality care to occur. Numerous health care providers are responsible for ensuring quality care in this setting. Nurses play a central role in coordinating communication between the client and her family; other nurses; the physician or nurse midwife; and other health care providers, such as the lactation consultant or the social worker. For example, a social worker could be contacted for challenging social situations identified during the admitting assessment, such as a report of physical abuse, incest, or active alcohol or substance use. The nurse also identifies potential teaching needs during the antepartum period, such as breast-feeding. These needs are communicated to the appropriate caregiver when responsibility for care is transferred between members of the health care team. The admitting nurse focuses on the client's immediate needs during labour. This client's age required specific attention to adolescent developmental needs. As with all clients, the nurse assesses readiness to learn. Whenever possible, she communicates using the client's preferred communication style, for example, video, reading material, or demonstration.

During labour, the nurse explained what to expect, encouraged the client and her support person through the stages of labour, and constantly reassured the client and her support person using verbal and nonverbal modes. She used multiple communication skills, that is, attending, responding, and clarifying. A team of health care workers was involved in this delivery. The nurse often functions as informer, recorder, and coach. She communicates labour progress to the physician or midwife and documents the progress while simultaneously supporting the client. Following delivery, communication with the client and her family continues. The nurse's responsibilities include ongoing assessment of the client's postpartum status and the initial assessment of the baby's status. The nurse is responsible for communicating to the nursery or postpartum nurse details of the pregnancy, the delivery, and the baby's initial status. The nurse may also prepare the mother for transfer to a postpartum combined care unit where other nurses will assume responsibility for care. Once again, communication regarding the multifaceted concerns of the new family unit is necessary in order to ensure quality care. Nurses' attention to accurate verbal reports and written records facilitates communication among the client, the client's family, co-workers, and physicians while maintaining confidentiality.

Kay Kember, RN

CASE STUDY 6-1

A s a new graduate, you have finished your orientation and received notice that you have passed your CRNE (Canadian Registered Nurse Exam). The nursing care manager is relieved because two of the other regular nurses, one of whom is your preceptor, are pregnant and will soon be off on maternity leave. These absences will create a staffing crunch. Therefore, the nursing care manager is anxious to acclimatize you to the role of team leader because you will soon be expected to assume those responsibilities.

How can your preceptor help you to take on this additional responsibility? What techniques will you use to enhance your communication with subordinates?

KEY CONCEPTS

- Nurses rely on basic principles of communication to facilitate interactions with clients and their family members, peers, and practitioners in other disciplines.

- Principles of communication allow nurses to adapt to trends that affect the profession of nursing and its practice, such as increasing diversity, an aging population, and computer technology.

- Nurses follow a process of communication that is more universal than unique to nursing. At the most basic level, this process involves a sender, a message, a receiver, and feedback. The input comes from visual, auditory, and kinesthetic stimuli, which are delivered using verbal and nonverbal modes. Nurses engage in three levels of communication: intrapersonal, interpersonal, and public.

- Nurses participate in upward, downward, lateral, and diagonal communications that are typically defined by their organization. Additionally, nurses may take part in informal exchanges using the grapevine.

- Nurses rely on communication skills, such as attending, responding, clarifying, and collaborating, to effectively promote client care and professionalism in a variety of settings.

- Barriers of gender, culture, conflict, and incongruent responses exist.

- Communication in the workplace involves many different relationships that shift the focus of effective communication. These relationships include communicating with superiors, co-workers, subordinates, physicians and other health care workers, and mentors.

KEY TERMS

accommodating	interpersonal communication
attending	intrapersonal communication
auditory	kinesthetic
avoiding	message
clarifying	nonverbal communication
collaborating	public communication
competing	receiver
compromising	responding
confronting	sender
feedback	verbal communication
grapevine	visual

REVIEW QUESTIONS

1. Which of the following is a trend in society that affects communication?
   A. decreasing interest in technology
   B. increasing diversity among Canadians
   C. increasing proportion of younger Canadians
   D. decreasing need for writing skills

2. What element of the communication process returns input to the sender?
   A. feedback
   B. message
   C. receiver
   D. sender

3. Which of the following characteristics pertains to verbal communication?
   A. eye contact
   B. nodding
   C. smiling
   D. tone

4. Which of the following skills involves active listening and is an important skill used by nurses to gain an understanding of the client's message?
   A. attending
   B. clarifying
   C. confronting
   D. responding

5. Why must nurses be concerned about barriers to communication?
   A. because they enhance interactions
   B. so they can use them when communicating
   C. so they can compensate for them
   D. They don't need to be concerned.

REVIEW ACTIVITIES

1. You have recently been asked by your nurse manager to join a committee that is developing educational materials and programs for your client population, mainly newcomers to the country. What cultural considerations might you have when developing the educational program?

2. The charge nurse apologizes as she informs you that your assignment includes the "problem client" on the unit. What communication skills will you use to enhance communication with this client? How will you avoid barriers of communication with this client?

3. You found out that you passed your registration exams last month. When you report for your evening shift, you discover you are assigned to be the team leader. What considerations will be given as you communicate with subordinates?

EXPLORING THE WEB

- What sites would you consider to improve your communication skills? It depends on what aspect of communication you want to improve. By using the Google search engine *http://www.*

google.ca and searching for the phrase *communication + skills,* more than 38 million sites were identified. Try it and look at the incredible online possibilities.

- Keep up with what is happening in the field of nursing and technology. Visit *http://www.cnia.ca/.* What did you find?

- Are you curious how effectively you communicate? Take an online communication test at *http://www.queendom. com/tests/take_test.php.*

REFERENCES

Baker, C., Beglinger, J., King, S., Salyards, M., & Thompson, A. (2000). Transforming negative work cultures. *JONA, 30*(7/8), 357–363.

Creasia, J., & Parker, B. (1996). *Conceptual foundations of professional practice* (2nd ed.). St Louis, MO: Mosby.

DiBartola, L. (2001). Listening to patients and responding with care. *Joint Commission Journal on Quality Improvement, 27*(6), 315–323.

Ellis, A. (1997). *Anger: How to live with it and without it.* New York: Citadel Press, Kensington.

Grohar-Murray, E., & DiCroce, H. (2003). *Leadership and management in nursing* (3rd ed.). Upper Saddle River, NJ: Pearson Education Inc.

Hall, P. (2005). Interprofessional teamwork: Professional cultures as barriers. *Journal of Interprofessional Care, 19,* 188–196.

Institute for Healthcare Communication Canada website. (2007). Retrieved from http://www.ihcc.ca/about.asp

Jeans, M. E., & Rowat, K. M. (2005). *Leadership objective C: Competencies required of nurse managers.* Ottawa: Canadian Nurses Association.

Laswell, H. D. (1948). The structure and function of communication in society. In L. Bryson (Ed.), *The communication of ideas* (pp. 37–51). New York: Institute for Religious and Social Studies.

Lingard, L., Espin, S., Rubin, B., Whyte, S., Colmenares, M., Baker, G.R., et al. (2005). Getting teams to talk: development and pilot implementation of a checklist to promote interprofessional communication in the OR. *Quality and Safety in Health Care, 14,* 340–346.

Longest, B., Rakich, J., & Darr, K. (2000). *Managing health services organizations and systems* (4th ed.). Baltimore: Health Professions Press.

Malone, G., & Morath, J. (2001). Pro-patient partnerships. *Nursing Management, 32,* 46–47.

Narasimhan, M., Eisen, L., Mahoney, C., Aceerra, F., & Rosen, M. (2006). Improving nurse-physician communication and satisfaction in the intensive care unit with a daily goals worksheet. *American Journal of Critical Care, 15*(2), 217–222.

Nembhard, I., & Edmondson, A. (2006). Making it safe: The effects of leader inclusiveness and professional status on psychological safety and improvement efforts in healthcare teams. *Journal of Organizational Behaviour, 27,* 941–966.

Peach, C. (2005). The mosaic versus the melting pot and the USA. *Scottish Geographical Journal, 121*(1), 3–27.

Poole, V. L., Davidhizar, R. E., & Giger, J. N. (1995). Delegating to a transcultural team. *Nursing Management, 26*(8), 33–34.

Potter, P., & Perry, A. (2001). *Canadian fundamentals of nursing* (2nd ed.). Toronto: Harcourt Canada Ltd.

Raso, R. (2010). Social media for nurse managers: What does it all mean? *Nursing Management, 41*(8), 22–25.

Shaffer, B., Tallarica, B., & Walsh, J. (2000). Win-win mentoring. *Nursing Management, 31*(1), 32–34.

Shortell, S., & Kaluzny, A. (2006), *Health care management: Organizational design and behaviour* (5th ed.). Clifton Park, NY: Delmar Learning.

Simms, L. M., Price, S. A., & Ervin, N. E. (2000). *The professional practice of nursing administration* (3rd ed.). Clifton Park, NY: Delmar Learning.

Sobo, E. J., & Sadler, B. L. (2002). Improving organizational communication and cohesion in a health care setting. *Human Organization, 61*(3), 277–287.

Statistics Canada. (2010). *Population projections for Canada, provinces and territories, 2009 to 2036.* Catalogue No. 91-520-X.

Tija, J., Mazor, K., Field, T., Meterko, V., Spenard, A., & Gurwitz, J. (2009). Nurse-physician communication in long-term care setting: Perceived barriers and impact on patient safety. *Journal of Patient Safety, 5*(3), 145–152.

Valentine, P. E. B. (2001). A gender perspective on conflict management strategies of nurses. *Journal of Nursing Scholarship, 33*(1), 69–74.

Yogo, Y., Hashi, A. M., Tsutsui, S., & Yamada, N. (2000). Judgments of emotion by nurses and students given double-blind information on a patient's tone of voice and message content. *Perceptual and motor skills, 90,* 855–863.

SUGGESTED READINGS

Bellack, J. P., & O'Neil, E. H. (2000). Recreating nursing practice for a new century. *Nursing and Health Care Perspectives, 21*(1), 15–21.

Gray, J. (1992). *Men are from Mars, women are from Venus.* New York: HarperCollins.

Heller, B. R., Oris, M. T., & Durney-Crowley, J. (2000). The future of nursing education: 10 trends to watch. *Nursing and Health Care Perspectives, 21*(10), 9–13.

Hibberd, J., & Smith, D. (2006). *Nursing leadership and management in Canada* (3rd ed.). Toronto: Elsevier Mosby.

Johns, G., & Saks, A. (2008). *Organizational behaviour: Understanding and managing life at work.* Toronto: Pearson Prentice Hall.

Malloch, K., Sluyter, D., & Moore, N. (2000). Relationship-centered care: Achieving true value in healthcare. *JONA, 30*(7/8), 379–385.

Sherman, R. O. (2006). Leading a multigenerational nursing workforce: Issues, challenges, and strategies. *The Online Journal of Issues in Nursing, 11*(2). Retrieved from http://www.nursingworld.org/MainMenuCategories/ANAMarketplace/ANAPeriodicals/OJIN/TableofContents/Volume112006/No2May06/tpc30_216074.aspx

Shortell, S., & Kaluzny, A. (2006). *Health care management: Organizational design and behaviour* (5th ed.). Clifton Park, NY: Thomson Delmar Learning.

CHAPTER ENDNOTES

1. Institute for Healthcare Communication Canada website. (2007). "About us—Who we are." Retrieved from http://www.ihcc.ca/about.asp

2. Ibid.

CHAPTER 7

Politics and Consumer Partnerships

Terry W. Miller, PhD, RN
Adapted by Heather Crawford, BScN, MEd, CHE
Pat Frederickson, Former Executive Director/Registrar,
College of Licensed Practical Nurses of Alberta
Rita McGregor, Former Director of Professional Practice, College
of Licensed Practical Nurses of Alberta

We also worked hard to engage Canadians in our consultations, because medicare ultimately belongs to them. ... Strong leadership and the involvement of Canadians is key to preserving a system that is true to our values and is sustainable.

(Commission on the Future of Health Care in Canada, 2002)[1]

OBJECTIVES

The purpose of this chapter is to enable the reader to

- describe how politics defines health care services and affects nursing practice;
- recognize the need for nurses to be politically involved with the consumer movement in health care;
- describe the role of a nurse as a consumer advocate and political force;
- propose a political strategy for strengthening nurse–consumer relationships;
- articulate a service-oriented plan for providing nursing services to a selected consumer interest group; and
- describe how demographic changes are affecting nurses and nursing services.

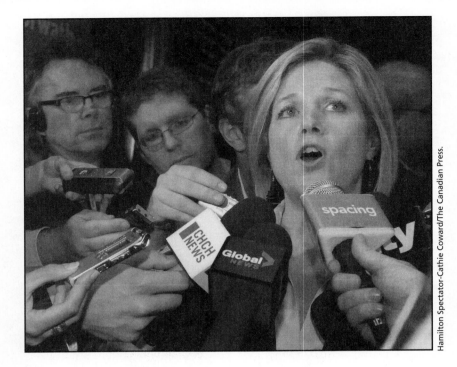

Hamilton Spectator-Cathie Coward/The Canadian Press.

The elderly man lying in a nursing home bed, pushing a call button and waiting for a nurse, is not thinking about anything other than the fact that he is not getting the service or care that he expected. He doesn't know whether the nursing shortage is affecting his care. He doesn't know the financial situation of the nursing home itself. He doesn't know the standards that the nursing home is expected to achieve.

> *Can we expect to improve the care of this elderly man given this scenario?*
>
> *Does politics play a role in this elderly man's care?*
>
> *Should nurses work with other consumer groups to improve care for elderly patients?*

Politics is predominantly a process by which people use different methods to achieve their goals. These methods inherently involve some level of competition, negotiation, and collaboration. Politics involves using power to influence, persuade, or change—it is the activity in which conflicting interests struggle for advantage or dominance in the making and execution of public policies (Rand Dyck, 2012, p. 17). Nurses who can effectively compete, negotiate, and collaborate with others to acquire what they either want or need have developed strong political skills. They have the greatest ability to build strong bases of support for themselves, clients, and the nursing profession.

Politics exists because resources are limited and some people control more resources than others. **Resources** include people; money; facilities; technology; and rights to properties, services, and technologies. Individuals,

groups, or organizations that have the ability to provide or control the distribution of desirable resources are politically empowered. The consumer movement in health care is a political movement about health care resources.

The purpose of this chapter is to support the need for nurses to be politically active for the good of both clients and the health care system. A major focus is how the consumer movement in health care creates new opportunities for nurses to advance nursing services by giving clients, including all people who receive health care, a stronger voice in their health care as consumers. Nurses are encouraged to develop a stronger political position by partnering with consumer groups instead of waiting for others to take the lead.

STAKEHOLDERS AND HEALTH CARE

Control of health care resources is spread among a number of vested interest groups called **stakeholders.** Everyone is a stakeholder in health care at some level, but some people are far more politically active about their stake in health care than others. See Table 7-1 for a list of some of Canada's most influential interest and lobbying groups. Many of these groups, as well as others, such as insurance companies, consumer groups, professional organizations, health care providers, and educational groups, exert political pressure on health policymakers—municipal, provincial, territorial, and federal legislative bodies—in an effort to make the health care system work to their advantage.

TABLE 7-1	**SOME OF CANADA'S INTEREST AND LOBBY GROUPS**

1. The Consumers' Association of Canada
2. The National Citizens Coalition
3. The Health Action Lobby
4. Canadian Health Coalition
5. Canadian Centre for Policy Alternatives

6. C. D. Howe Institute
7. Fraser Institute
8. Canada's Association for the Fifty-Plus
9. Greenpeace Canada
10. Aboriginal Youth Network

LITERATURE APPLICATION

Citation: Canadian Nurses Association. (2006). Celebrating international nursing partnerships. *Canadian Nurse, 102*(6), 15–17.

Discussion: The purpose of this article was to demonstrate the commitment of the Canadian Nurses Association to work in cooperation with nurses around the world to promote global health and equity, and to advance the nursing profession for the benefit of all. Since 1976, the Canadian Nurses Association has worked with national nursing associations (NNAs) in Africa, the Americas, Asia, and Eastern Europe, as well as with funding organizations in Canada and overseas. These organizations have built alliances to increase the NNAs' ability to strengthen the nursing profession and improve the quality of health services and nursing delivered in partner countries. The article describes specific efforts to improve health care, strengthen nursing organizations, collaborate with other nursing leadership, and build gender equity. Finally, partnerships for today and the future are identified, including the Canada–Russia Initiative in Nursing, the Canada–South Africa Nurses HIV/AIDS Initiative, and the Strengthening Nurses and Nursing Associations Program.

Implications for Practice: Significant success has been made in the last 30 years to strengthen international nursing partnerships and improve health systems. Further work is required in the area of global health, and it is incumbent on all nurses and nursing associations to work collaboratively to build alliances that will strengthen health systems around the world.

Nurses should be interested in influencing governments because politicians pay attention to the health-related issues and concerns raised by their constituents and the organizations within their electoral boundaries. If the governments don't pay attention, they will not be re-elected. If nurses do not speak both individually and collectively, the voices of others will be heard by government, and the priorities and potential solutions posed by nurses will not be heard. Not all stakeholders in health care support the consumers' potentially dominant role in health care politics. Some contend that consumers do not necessarily know what is best for them. Instead, they support the idea that health care experts, such as physicians, are better able to direct health care policy. Others maintain that only those directly paying for the services should make policy decisions

and that health care is not necessarily a right because services should be based on an individual's ability to pay.

To effectively influence governments and politicians, nurses need at least a basic awareness of the political structures in Canada. Canada's Parliament consists of three parts: the Queen, who is the head of state and is represented by the governor general; the appointed Senate; and the elected House of Commons. The governor general calls Parliament together after every general election, and reads the speech from the throne, outlining the government's objectives, and approves all bills passed by the Senate and the House of Commons. Senators are appointed by the governor general on the advice of the prime minister. The House of Commons has 308 elected members, who represent the individuals in their ridings.

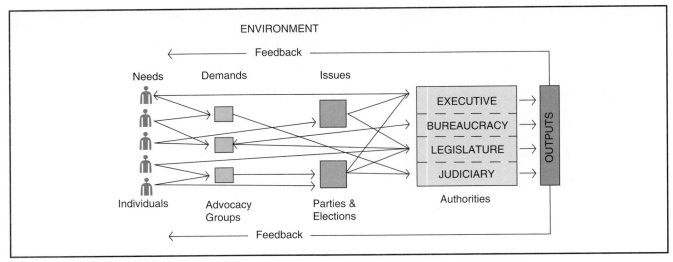

Figure 7-1 A Model of the Political System
Source: From DYCK. *Canadian Politics*, 5E. © 2012 Nelson Education Ltd. Reproduced by permission. www.cengage.com/permissions

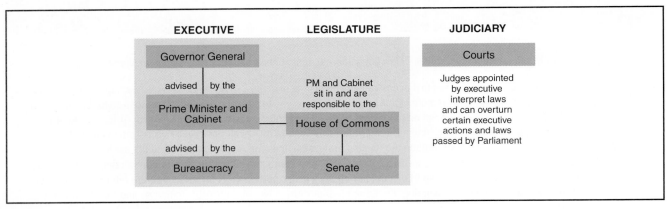

Figure 7-2 An Outline of Canadian Political Institutions
Source: From DYCK. *Canadian Politics*, 5E. © 2012 Nelson Education Ltd. Reproduced by permission. www.cengage.com/permissions

See Figure 7-1 for a model of the political system in Canada, and Figure 7-2 for an outline of Canadian political institutions.

The growing cost of health care has led to increasing political activism by nurses, other health care providers, and also as consumers. As noted in *Building on Values: The Future of Health Care in Canada*—the Romanow Report— "Canadians want and need a more accountable health care system (Commission on the Future of Health Care in Canada, 2002, p. xix). Nurses have come to understand how the control and distribution of resources in health care can dramatically affect their incomes, workloads, work environments, and clients. Nurses across the country have reported that the client load per nurse provider has increased significantly. However, without political influence, simply voicing these concerns does little to change health care at any level.

Nursing has a long history of uniting the various stakeholders and coordinating health care services around clients to ensure that clients obtain the health services they need; but, as pointed out by Ogren (2001), "many nurses have little knowledge about their history" (p. 7). Nurses who recognize they have a critical role in addressing the major issues in health care delivery at the bedside will ensure that nursing enters into discussions or partnerships with individuals and organizations that have control in the wider health care system. As partners, they will be able to compete, negotiate, and collaborate with other stakeholders at the system level to effect political change. These nurses are concerned with the price of health care at the system level and understand that resources are controlled and distributed through health policy decisions.

Many authors of nursing articles, some books, and a few research studies support nurses' involvement in public policy and health care politics (Fagin, 1998; Mason & Leavitt, 1999; Milstead, 1999; Williams, 1998). Several other authors promote greater inclusion of policy content and political process in nursing curricula (Brown, 1996; Gebbie, Wakefield, & Kerfoot, 2000; Jones, Jennings, Moritz, & Moss, 1997; Provost & Van Herk, 2006). Nurses' involvement in policy arenas, such as policy-making committees and institutional boards, includes advocating both for recipients of health care who are in need and have little or no voice and for those who need a stronger voice. Any professional nurse should understand and be able to articulate the relevance of politics to nursing practice. Making a difference in health care arenas is an outcome of involvement in policymaking. As Margaret Mead said, "never doubt that a small group of thoughtful committed citizens can change the world, indeed it's the only thing that ever has."

CRITICAL THINKING

Have you ever organized a local committee meeting, or a Nurses' Week event? Have you ever contacted your provincial member of Parliament or your local councillor regarding a provincial bill that affects health care or a safety issue in your neighbourhood? Have you ever been exhausted at the end of a busy day, after having managed complex client needs? Have you ever participated in an informational picket? If you have engaged in any of these activities, then you have been involved in politics and the early stages of political action.

REAL WORLD INTERVIEW

Nurses generally associate being political with politics, and don't consider themselves in that realm. Being political has a much broader context; it means being an advocate for your beliefs. Every day nurses play an advocacy role, most often for client care, but that role can extend to advocating for change in the workplace or, in a much broader context, change in the health care system, or in professional or labour legislation.

Pat Frederickson
Former Executive Director/Registrar, College of
Licensed Practical Nurses of Alberta

THE POLITICS AND ECONOMICS OF HUMAN SERVICES

Many nurses want to avoid the political nature of their work because they believe that human services should not be politically motivated. They also may ignore the business aspects of health care until they find themselves responsible for a budget. Yet all health care is inextricably linked to politics and economics and to the availability and services of providers. As a human service, health care has yielded remarkable returns in terms of improving overall quality of life and extending life spans. As a business, health care has afforded millions of people, including nurses, with economic opportunities and lifelong careers.

Health care in Canada depends heavily on a continuous supply of resources from both public and private sectors. These resources include people, such as the providers of health care services, and the money to educate and pay these providers. Buildings, technology, administration, and equipment are just some of the other resources needed for the health care system to be serviceable. With health care requiring so many resources on such a large economic scale, thousands of people are directly involved in the allocation of those resources; hence, the politics of health care. Most of those people have good intentions, but they often

REAL WORLD INTERVIEW

This morning I met with three very dedicated nurses from my riding. ... [and] spoke about the vital role of nurses in the field of mental health services. Because of the stigma attached to mental illness, this is not always a very high profile area—some would say it's the silent health issue. ... The nurses pointed out that four of five people in Ontario are affected at some level by mental illness. Our meeting this morning was a reminder of the far-reaching impact of the work done by Ontario's nurses in all aspects of health and wellness. Citizens of Durham riding are proud of the care and professionalism shown daily by nurses in our communities.

John O'Toole
MPP, Durham

Source: Registered Nurse Journal, May/June 2005, p. 27
(Adapted from *Hansard Issue* L142A). Reprinted with Permission.

disagree about how the resources can best be used to support health care.

Many consumers are aware that the ongoing redistribution of health care resources may not meet their health care needs, especially as they age and become more dependent upon related services. They are frightened by media reports of increasing national health care expenditures. Although most consumers do not directly pay for the majority of their health care, their individual portions of expenses incurred are rapidly increasing. Health policy is formulated, enacted, and enforced through political processes at the local, regional, provincial, territorial, and federal levels. For example, at the local or regional level, individual hospital boards or regional health authorities establish and implement policies regarding the availability of flu injections to high-risk populations in their area. At the provincial or territorial level, policies govern nurses within a province or territory by defining nursing practice, nursing education, and nursing registration. These policies are often governed by a provincial or territorial nurse practice act that designates a provincial or territorial nursing regulatory college or association as the authority for enforcing the policies. Federal policies are evident in the principles, rules, and regulations governing medicare, such as the Canada Health Act (1984). When bills affecting health care are being developed in provincial, territorial, and federal legislative bodies, nurses need to be aware of those actions and obtain copies of those bills, thus adding to their political knowledge base.

Ultimately, health care will be defined and controlled by those wielding the most political influence. If nurses fail to exert political pressure on the health policymakers, they will lose ground to others who are more politically active. It is unrealistic to believe that other stakeholders will take care of nursing while the competition for health care resources increases. Historically, some stakeholders in health care have never supported nursing as a profession or acknowledged professional roles for nurses. Nurses, like other health care providers, must compete, negotiate, and collaborate with others to ensure their future in health care.

CULTURAL DIMENSIONS OF PARTNERSHIPS AND CONSUMERISM

Data from the 2006 Census showed that the proportion of Canada's population who were born outside the country reached its highest level in 75 years.[2] The 2006 Census enumerated that there were 6.2 million immigrants from around the world, and most came from Asia. Most of these immigrants settled in the three largest metropolitan areas—Toronto, Montréal, and Vancouver. At that time, the total population of Canada was approximately 30 million (Statistics Canada, 2010). By July 1, 2009 the population had grown to over 33.7 million.[3] On January 1, 2011 the population was 34.3 million.[4] The most recent Census was performed on May 1, 2011. Even if immigrants are highly educated, they tend to have lower employment rates and lower salaries than individuals who were born in Canada. Leddy and Pepper (1998) recognized that "people's habits of promoting health, their ways of behaving when sick, their ways of recognizing and responding to illness, and their ways of defining health are strongly determined by their sociocultural background" (p. 35). Increasing racial and cultural diversity is indicated in the census data. Canada's Aboriginal population is much younger that the non-Aboriginal population. The median age of the Aboriginal population in 2006 was 27, which was 13 years younger than the median age of the non-Aboriginal population. About 71 percent of the country's entire Aboriginal population lived in urban areas (Statistics Canada, 2010).

If nurses intend to form partnerships with consumer groups distinguished by cultural heritage, racial makeup, or ethnic background, they must understand and value diversity. Strong partnerships will frame nursing services in ways that respect cultural differences.

POLITICS AND DEMOGRAPHIC CHANGES

Certainly not all consumers agree about what health care should be, who should provide it, or how it should be paid for. The social, cultural, economic, psychological, and demographic characteristics of consumers largely determine their attitudes and inclination toward the health care system, its providers, and its services. Consumers also recognize some level of personal risk when changes are made in the system, especially involving access and wait times. If consumers, such as retired people, perceive that their out-of-pocket costs for health care (e.g., for medication) either extends beyond their capacity to pay or will increase in the future, they are highly motivated to exert political pressure on their legislators to reverse the perceived trend.

The fastest growing consumer group for years to come is the elderly—people 65 years and older—due to lower fertility and higher life expectancy. During the period from 2009 to 2036, the entire baby boom generation turns 65. Canada's population will age rapidly until 2031, by which time the entire baby boom generation will have turned 65. This population will continue aging after 2031, but at a less rapid pace. By 2036 the number of seniors is projected to reach between 9.9 million and 10.9 million, more than double the level of 4.7 million in 2009. Between 2015 and 2021 they will surpass the number of children aged 14 or under for the first time.

CASE STUDY 7-1

Jillian is a registered nurse who visits newborns and their moms in their home, as part of the Healthy Babies, Healthy Children program. She also belongs to the Childbirth Nurses Interest Group. The Canadian Pediatric Society, the American Academy of Pediatrics, and the United Kingdom's Foundation for the Study of Sudden Infant Death have released guidelines that encourage parents to sleep in the same room as their infant, but do not advocate parents and infants sleeping in the same bed. However, parents are still encouraged to breastfeed and cuddle their babies in bed. Jillian knows that many new moms have difficult initiating breastfeeding or require encouragement when the baby is fussy and doesn't latch on to the breast easily. Jillian has just heard that the local hospital's breastfeeding clinic is about to close due to lack of financial resources.

What would you do if you were Jillian?

LITERATURE APPLICATION

Citation: Ferguson, S. L. (2001). An activist looks at nursing's role in health policy development. *Journal of Obstetric, Gynecologic, and Neonatal Nursing, 30*(5), 546–551.

Discussion: Nurses play a critical role in determining, developing, implementing, and evaluating health policies because of their knowledge of health care. A conceptual model (Longest, 1998) is useful to illustrate the public policy-making process. The model illustrated in this article depicts three phases: policy formulation, implementation, and modification.

Implications for Practice: Nurses will find the model illustrated in this article useful to influence public policy.

LITERATURE APPLICATION

Citation: McNeill, T. (2010). Family as a social determinant of health: Implications for governments and institutions to promote the health and well-being of families. *Healthcare Quarterly*, 14(Sp): 60–67.

Discussion: A growing appreciation of the impact of the social determinants of health, particularly the negative impact of poverty on health, is driving the need for a re-evaluation of the role of governments and institutions such as hospitals in the lives of children and families. As a **result**, there is a growing need for re-visioning priorities for health and social policies. Implications for families, governments, and institutions are explored in this paper.

Implications for Practice: Nurses and health are leaders must reflect on their role in the next evolution of the health care field. We cannot provide health care for children in a vacuum. We need to ask ourselves which political parties are advancing policies that will support families to care effectively for their children, and prepare them to be productive contributors to society in the future. Hospitals must do their part to address the social injustice of health inequalities and recast themselves as advocates of change within an expanded vision of health.

CRITICAL THINKING

How do you see the aging nursing workforce and the aging population affecting health care and your nursing practice? What are the political implications for health care providers with proportionally fewer people in the workforce and more people requiring health care services related to aging?

By 2036 the median age of the population will range between 42 and 45 years, compared with the current median of 39.5 (Statistics Canada, 2010).

Without doubt, this aging of the Canadian population profoundly affects health care at every level. The dramatic increase in the number of elderly people in the Western world means that about one-half of all people who have ever reached age 65 are alive today (Roszak, 1998).

Many seniors are joining consumer groups to have a greater political voice, influence health policy decisions, and ensure that they receive the health care services they will need for years to come. A growing number are bridging the gap of social isolation that characterized the past by using the Internet and becoming involved in consumer groups. They are establishing closer contact with the outside world and are managing to successfully strengthen their relationships with other stakeholders in health care.

Canada's Association for the Fifty-Plus (CARP), with more than 400,000 members, constitutes a growing influential advocacy group for the 50-plus age group, and an ideal consumer partner for nursing in many ways. A large percentage of nurses are 45 years of age or older and within 5 years of qualifying for membership in the CARP. Few other consumer groups appear to have the potential that CARP has for defining the health care system of the future.

NURSE AS POLITICAL ACTIVIST

Because of nurses' knowledge and expertise regarding the determinants of health, they are key informants when it comes to health and health care issues. Nurses have both a desire and a need to have meaningful involvement in decision making and informing decision makers at various levels in health care organizations and in government when decisions affect nurses, their work life, and client care. Nurses have a valuable role in policy development and, increasingly, are finding the need to become more politically active. They have long felt that changes in the health care system were having a negative impact on their work life, their working conditions, and client care, especially during the 1990s when cutbacks in health care led to the layoffs of nurses throughout the country. A serious negative impact affected the morale of nurses and ultimately client care: nurses were of the opinion that decisions had been made based on economics and that they were not being valued for their contribution to client care. That discontent lead to the formation of several studies, such as the Canadian Nursing Advisory Committee's (2002) *Our Health, Our Future: Creating Quality Workplaces for Canadian Nurses* and, a few year later, the National Nursing Sector Study Corporation (2005), *Building the Future: An Integrated Strategy for Nursing Human Resources in Canada.* Research conducted for these two projects provided detailed information on the work life, education, practice, and administration of nurses. This research provided valuable information so nurses could raise the awareness of issues affecting nurses and lobby for change.

Nurses have always enjoyed a high level of public trust, and they have leveraged this trust to their advantage. Over the past few years the Canadian Nurses Association (CNA) has increasingly provided support for registered nurses to convey their messages to politicians, particularly during election campaigns. CNA encourages nurses to ask political candidates what they will do to improve the health of Canadians. This strategy is a very effective way of bringing the issues of nurses and health care to the attention of politicians and requiring politicians make a public statement on their position.

Practical nurses, psychiatric nurses, nurse educators, nursing students, and nursing administrators have national organizations on a much smaller scale, but they have been able to make their voices heard. Nurses have successfully lobbied for a nursing voice at the federal level. In 1999 their successful lobbying resulted in Health Canada creating the Office of Nursing Policy. The purpose of this new office is to help Canadians maintain and improve their health through the development of policy that integrates the views of nurses and the nursing profession. This office advises Health Canada on various policy issues and programs and presents its perspective in various fora; as a result, this office contributes to health policy formulation and program development and works closely with the nursing community in developing advice for the minister of health and long-term care and Health Canada.[5] The functions of the Office of Nursing Policy include identifying and synthesizing issues, enhancing the evidence base for policy development, brokering knowledge, and creating opportunities for government and health care leaders to link with each other in policy meetings.[6] Priorities include health care access through workforce stability, health care quality through workforce development and capacity building, and health care sustainability through system transformation.[7]

Nurses who are politically active have a definitive voice in their work environments for client welfare as well as for themselves. In addition to studying issues and voting, politically active nurses directly contact policymakers, such as the chairperson of the hospital board or legislators, through phone calls, letters, and emails. Politically active nurses join professional organizations and actively participate to ensure a more collective, unified voice supporting health care issues and policies that have value for consumers and nursing. Nurses who are most involved will be seen running for office, supporting political activities and candidates, assisting during campaigns, and helping to draft legislation.

As nurses develop politically, they come to understand the need for political strategy. The purpose of developing political strategies is to understand different ways to achieve one's goals, or the goals one is advocating for, while identifying the other stakeholders and their goals. Political strategy attempts to persuade the people supporting an issue, formulating a policy, or taking an action to take the position that supports those using the political strategy. To be feasible, a political strategy requires commitment by those using it, as well as their awareness of the other stakeholders. Effective political strategy implies considerable forethought and clarity of purpose even in the most ambiguous situations. Nurses who are most likely to wield political influence operate with strategy in mind before taking political action, voicing concerns, making demands, or even advocating for others. Unfortunately, some nurses may become involved in political issues or take over political stands before adequately studying the political issue or the major stakeholders' positions regarding the issue.

Every nurse should be aware of the position of other involved groups regarding any relevant political health issue. Nurses need to listen to other policy perspectives and understand as many facets of the issue as possible when making health policy proposals. Proposals need to include a rationale. This will neutralize opposing views and ensure that unnecessary political fights can be avoided and that more collaboration will occur prior to submitting any policy proposal to policy-making bodies, such as hospital boards or provincial legislatures. The more support obtained from the various stakeholders in any policy arena, the better the chance for a workable policy to be developed and implemented.

To be most politically effective, nurses need an ability to clearly articulate at least four dimensions of nursing to any audience or stakeholder: what nursing is, what distinctive services nurses provide to consumers, how nursing benefits consumers, and what nursing services cost in relation to other health care services. Although anecdotal stories and emotional appeals may be effective with certain audiences, research-based evidence that supports the political position of the nursing profession exerts far more power.

POLITICS AND ADVOCACY

For several decades, the nursing profession has embraced client advocacy, even though nurses risk compromising their employment positions when they advocate for clients. However, some concern has been voiced that the restructuring of health care is eroding the advocacy role of nurses (O'Connell, 2000). Part of the problem is that nurses doubt that they have the ability to advocate for their clients. They are not comfortable with the level of risk they associate with being a client advocate. The greatest nurses throughout the profession's history have been strong advocates for clients and have taken far greater risks than the potential loss of a particular job.

Interestingly, some clients have begun advocating for nurses, a role reversal. Those clients perceive nurses as overextended by the nature of their work environment and contend that something must be done to improve nurses' working conditions.

ADVOCACY AND CONSUMER ALLIANCES

Nurses must understand the political forces that define their relationships with consumers. Consumers expect the best people to be health care providers, but they are confused about the roles and responsibilities of professional nurses. Informed consumers understand how health policy directly affects them but are less likely to recognize how health policy affects nurses. Consumers may expect nurses to be their advocates only in the context of providing direct client care.

Working through their professional organizations, nurses can collaborate with consumer groups by creating alliances, which serve to promote the role of nurses as consumer advocates in health policy arenas and to strengthen the political position of both partners. These alliances create a stronger political voice than either group has alone. The partners gain power when interacting with any policy-making body because they represent (1) a larger **voting block**—a group that represents the same political position or perspective; (2) a broader funding base—a source of financial support; and (3) a stronger **political voice**—an increase in the number of voices supporting or opposing an

TABLE 7-2	STEPS IN ESTABLISHING AN ALLIANCE WITH A CONSUMER GROUP
Listen	Become sensitized to the health care needs and political nature of the potential consumer ally.
Study	Seek both representative and opposing perspectives from consumer group meetings, focus groups, relevant literature, and interviews.
Assess	Determine the need, value, context, and boundaries for establishing the alliance.
Focus	Mutually identify the purpose and articulate the goals and specific, realistic objectives for the alliance.
Compromise	Work through nonessential and noncritical points and issues.
Negotiate	Agree on one's position and responsibilities in the alliance.
Plan	Develop a political strategy for achieving the goals and fulfilling the objectives.
Test	Test the political waters. Gather feedback on the plan from key people before taking action.
Model	Model the political work. Define the structure for working the political strategy with partners.
Direct the political action	Understand the bigger picture and concentrate on what can be changed.
Implement	Line up political support and take action.
Network	Be committed to the mutually recognized goal and consistently work to have an adequate base of support in terms of people, money, and time.
Build political credibility	Participate in local, provincial, and federal policy-making efforts that support the alliance and its political agenda.
Soothe and bargain	Downplay rivalry and address conflict in a timely, constructive manner.
Report, publicize, lobby	Report, publicize, and lobby the group's political cause, and draw public attention to the needs of the consumer group.
Reaffirm, redefine, or discontinue	Regularly evaluate work with consumer group.

issue—to any policy-making body. Increasingly, professional organizations in nursing recognize the value of partnering with consumers to build a better health care system. See Table 7-2 for steps in establishing an alliance with a consumer group.

CONSUMER DEMANDS

As recipients of health care, consumers demand to be treated as something more than passive recipients of health care. They are vocal in their requests that providers and organizations be more consumer-friendly and service-oriented, and they are seriously requesting a voice in how health care is delivered.

Nurses, working through professional organizations, such as the Canadian Nurses Association (CNA), have been strong supporters for clients' rights; however, other professional groups, such as the Canadian Medical Association (CMA) and the Canadian Healthcare Association (CHA), have received far more media recognition for their support of clients' rights, particularly regarding safety. This situation may be an indication that the CMA and CHA are better funded, wield more political power, and do a better job of presenting their positions on consumer issues to the media than the CNA.

Any political vision to make health care more consumer-friendly and service-oriented must address cost, access, choice, and quality. Perhaps the vision starts with a formula: the highest quality of care for all people at the least cost. Yet, defining—much less evaluating—quality is culturally bound and very complicated. A vision for high-quality, low-cost care will require multiple stakeholders collaborating to develop a workable philosophy, including a mechanism for checks and balances to minimize abuse and misuse and to encourage intelligent, ethical decisions by those wielding the most political power.

TURNING A CONSUMER-ORIENTED VISION INTO REALITY

Nurses have opportunities to be more than simply supporters of a consumer-oriented vision for health care; they can be co-creators. To make this vision real, nurses will need to be more educated and articulate about the value they add to the overall health care system. Encouraging other stakeholders and the policymakers to understand and promote the value of nursing to consumers will take considerable political work. This work will have to be more than anecdotal pleas, arguments in support of some consumer cause, or reactions to some particular health care issue or workplace injustice. Believing in a vision and working hard are not enough. Nurses must have a clear image of the vision; develop a sound philosophy; demonstrate intelligent, strategic thinking; and wield more political influence.

Although nurses may think they are the ones primarily affected by the changes in health care, a more powerful and, therefore, strategic position is to understand that everyone is affected, especially consumers. Doris Grinspun, Executive Director of the Registered Nurses Association of Ontario, suggests that a "working framework" is essential for shaping policy and transforming nursing into a social force. She believes four key tools—evidence, politics, communication, and media—are required throughout the policy process; from framing an idea, to promoting awareness, to securing uptake and sustaining change. These new directions may include the strategies outlined in Table 7-3.

CRITICAL THINKING

Carling Provost and Kim Van Herk (2006) in their article, "Political Activism and Nursing," suggest that nursing students need to be more aware of how health policies affect both themselves as health professionals and society as a whole. According to Provost and Van Herk, nursing students need to become more involved in political organizations to have a positive impact on their level of political activity, and they need to be formally educated to be politically active. They suggest that nurses can overcome barriers to being politically active by becoming aware of how policies are made and implemented within the Canadian system; for this to happen, opportunities for students to observe the policy-making process need to be built into nursing curricula. They also suggest incorporating political activity hours into clinical placements, and exposing students to health policy education, such as writing a paper about a nurse who is a political leader.

What recommendations could you make to prepare students and nurses to be more politically aware and politically active in the health care system?

TABLE 7-3	POLITICAL STRATEGIES FOR MOUNTING CONSUMER CAMPAIGNS

1. Lobbying at provincial and federal levels for health care regulations and guidelines that serve a consumer group's interest

2. Consulting with representatives from a consumer group when health care regulations and guidelines are being debated or written

3. Monitoring the enforcement of health care regulations and exacting corrective or punitive action when non-compliance occurs

4. Encouraging providers to make changes in delivery of services voluntarily to meet changing consumer demands

5. Changing consumer perceptions and behaviours through the distribution of educational materials or other media

THE CONSUMER DEMAND FOR ACCOUNTABILITY

When stakeholders are motivated and directed solely by their own perceived needs, competitive political strategies replace more collaborative approaches to addressing the consumer's health care needs. Accountability becomes a serious issue because the goal of pleasing stakeholders may supersede the goal of offering the highest quality services. People who will own the future of health care must address this growing problem of accountability. They will need to establish and sustain their credibility during a time when more people are distrustful of the health care system and legislators.

Most people comprehend that being accountable requires being held responsible for one's behaviour, decisions, and affiliations with others. Notwithstanding, some nurses claim they are not culpable for their actions because they are merely doing what they must do as defined by their employer or some other larger entity. These nurses fail to understand that professional accountability goes beyond responsibility in a particular employment situation. Accountability means that nurses will actively participate in risk identification and

management, problem solving, and implementation of any changes that are required. It is not acceptable to identify that a risk exists, and then sit back and expect others to correct the situation. If there are risks for our clients, ultimately our care providers are also at risk. The Canadian Nurses Association and each of the provincial and territorial regulatory bodies have statements related to accountability.

Increasingly, consumers are demanding positive results and are holding those in the health care system accountable for better health care outcomes. Many organizations have ethics committees or statements related to ethics within their mission statements, but the existence of committees and statements will not satisfy the consumer who experiences negative outcomes. The strongest potential for litigation in health care comes from too few health care professionals accepting personal responsibility for ensuring that health care services are provided in a safe, competent manner at a system level as well as at a personal level. Health care professionals, including nurses, depend upon each other to ensure the quality, consistency, and overall effectiveness of health care within their work environments.

CREDIBILITY AND POLITICS

To have credibility, nurses must demonstrate professional competence and a degree of professional accountability that exceeds consumers' expectations. Nurses who are most able to successfully overcome these challenges assert their professional credibility in several ways. They are lifelong learners and demonstrate professional growth throughout their careers in nursing. They approach their career as a service to the public and to the nursing profession and as an honourable way to make a living. They take ownership of the situations in which they find themselves

REAL WORLD INTERVIEW

Question: What role have civil servants played in your success?

Answer: During the formative years of the College of Licensed Practical Nurses of Alberta, we engaged the services of a consultant who had previously been a member of the Legislative Assembly (MLA). He provided us with some of the most valuable advice in developing government relationships. Although legislation and policy come from the elected officials, civil servants are the ones who have the ear of the ministers to provide them with advice and information. Therefore, it is essential to have a collaborative working relationship with the key government departments.

(*Continued*)

REAL WORLD INTERVIEW (CONTINUED)

For us, they are primarily the departments of Health and Wellness and Advanced Education. We have worked with staff in the Health and Wellness Department to develop legislation and make amendments over the years. Sometimes, recommendations for legislation come from the profession and sometimes they come from government. In our time with the College, we have gone through two complete writes of the regulations that govern our profession and the development of new umbrella legislation for all health professions. We have a very positive rapport with the staff in the department and always work through the process in a collaborative way. We would present our needs and suggestions for the legislation and our rationale, and work together to ensure a positive outcome for all, representing not only what is good for the profession but also what is in the best interest of public safety.

Question: Where else have you been able to succeed with that kind of attitude?

Answer: We have used the same attitude with employers when working towards common goals, and working with other health care professions. Many barriers were removed in legislation, and the education greatly improved for LPNs (licensed practical nurses), with tremendous results in increased value and utilization of LPNs. There has been a return of the LPN to settings such as obstetrics and pediatrics, where they had previously been eliminated. We have also seen many new opportunities for LPNs in settings where they were not traditionally a part of the care team, such as public health and as team leaders in long-term care.

This positive and solution-oriented attitude has gained us the respect of other health disciplines, and allowed us to be agents of change, not only for the LPN but also for the betterment of all nurses and the health care system. We are now welcomed at all tables where decisions that affect nurses and health care are made, both provincially and nationally. Our motto is to work *with* the system, never against it.

Pat Frederickson
Former Executive Director/Registrar, College of Licensed Practical Nurses of Alberta

Rita McGregor
Former Director of Professional Practice, College of Licensed Practical Nurses of Alberta

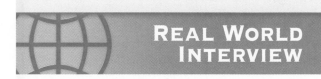

REAL WORLD INTERVIEW

In a recent issue of *Healthcare Executive*, Maureen Bisognano, president and CEO of the Institute for Healthcare Improvement, said, "Nurse involvement is essential to any significant healthcare improvement initiative, and it is fundamental to fulfilling the promise of healthcare reform, regardless of what shape that reform takes." I couldn't agree more.

Hugh MacLeod
CEO of the Canadian Patient Safety Institute

Source: MacLeod, H. (2010). A healthier health system is ours to create. *Canadian Nurse*, 106(9), p. 56. Reprinted with permission.

and work to resolve problems and overcome obstacles to providing the best care possible. Nurses strengthen their political position by taking ownership of their problems in serving consumers.

Nursing ownership, however, is not enough to guarantee the political credibility of nursing in the future because others see the political gains to be made from identifying themselves as consumer advocates.

A clear image of the vision you want to achieve and a sound philosophy for change are essential. Although it is always easy to bring problems forward, a far more effective approach is to clearly articulate the problem and present potential solutions. Consideration must be given to the options that are available and the most viable solutions. Seek out alliances with others who have the same vision and goals. Always maintain a consistent message and articulate it clearly, together with the benefits that can be expected. Persistence and patience are key when attempting to influence change, particularly through politics and political activity.

KEY CONCEPTS

- Individuals or groups take political action to achieve what they want or to prevent others from achieving a goal they do not agree with.

- Politics are inherent in any system in which resources are absolutely or relatively scarce and in which opposing interests compete for those resources.

- Nurses have a critical role in addressing the major system-level issues in health care delivery.

- Political, economic, and social changes in Canada are transforming the health care system.

- Nurses need to articulate what nursing is, the distinctive services nursing provides, how these services benefit consumers, and the cost of these services in relation to other health care services.

- If nursing is defined through politics to be less than critical or professional, nurses will be less empowered and paid less.

- The aging of the Canadian population constitutes a growing political issue and affords nursing with an opportunity to become stronger in health policy arenas.

- To be politically effective, consumer alliances are critical for all stakeholders in health care.

- When a consumer group forms a political coalition with other groups, such as nurses, the political influence of both groups is strengthened.

KEY TERMS

political voice
politics
resources
stakeholders
voting block

REVIEW QUESTIONS

1. Why does politics exist?
   A. It is required by law.
   B. Resources cannot be limited by political process.
   C. Some people control more resources than others.
   D. Resources must be equally distributed among stakeholders.

2. Which of the following describes the consumer movement in health care?
   A. a socialist movement about health care resources
   B. a growing movement because of the Internet and organizations such as the CARP

C. a movement supported by all stakeholders in the health care system
   D. a movement that's losing momentum

3. Which of the following describes the immigrant population in Canada?
   A. It includes 1.8 million racially and ethnically diverse people.
   B. It will surpass the white majority in another 10 years.
   C. It has resisted the consumer movement.
   D. It is a well-organized, cohesive group of consumers.

REVIEW ACTIVITIES

1. Identify your local, provincial, and federal politicians. Write a letter or e-mail them to learn which health care legislation they support.

2. Research whom is supporting current health care legislation. Are consumer protections being emphasized in any proposed legislation?

3. Identify a consumer group in which you are interested. Use the steps identified in Table 7-2 to establish an alliance with the group. What did you learn?

EXPLORING THE WEB

- Identify some websites for consumer groups.

  - Canada's Association for the Fifty-Plus: *http://www.carp.ca/*

  - The Health Action Lobby: *http://www.physiotherapy. ca/HEAL/english/index.htm*

  - National Citizens Coalition: *http://nationalcitizens.ca/*

- Note consumer tips at this site: *http://tips.blogs.cnn.com/*

- Note Health Canada's information on consumer participation and citizen engagement: *http://www.hc-sc.gc.ca/index-eng.php*

- Note this site for consumer reports: *http://www.consumer.ca/1652*

- Identify some sites for government bodies and health care agencies.

  - Parliament of Canada: *http://www.parl.gc.ca/ common/index.asp?Language=E*

  - Health Canada: *http://www.hc-sc.gc.ca/*

REFERENCES

Brown, L. D. (1996). *Health policy in the United States: Issues and options.* New York: The Ford Foundation.

Canadian Nurses Association. (2006). Celebrating international nursing partnerships. *Canadian Nurse,* 102(6), 15–17.

Canadian Nursing Advisory Committee. (2002). Our health, our future: Creating quality workplaces for Canadian nurses: Final report of the Canadian Nursing Advisory Committee. Ottawa: Advisory Committee on Health Human Resources.

Commission on the Future of Health Care in Canada. (2002). *Building on values: The future of health care in Canada.* Saskatoon: Author. Commissioner: Roy J. Romano.

Dyck, R. (2012). *Canadian Politics: Concise* (5th ed.). Toronto: Nelson Education Ltd.

Fagin, C. (1998). Nursing research and the erosion of care. *Nursing Outlook,* 46(6), 259–261.

Ferguson, S. L. (2001). An activist looks at nursing's role in health policy development. *Journal of Obstetric, Gynecologic, and Neonatal Nursing,* 30(5), 546–551.

Gebbie, K. M., Wakefield, M., & Kerfoot, K. (2000). Nursing and health policy. *Image: Journal of Nursing Scholarship,* 32(3), 307–314.

Jones, K., Jennings, B. M., Moritz, P., & Moss, T. M. (1997). Policy issues associated with analyzing outcomes of care. *Image: Journal of Nursing Scholarship,* 29(3), 251–276.

Kerfoot, K. (2000). On leadership—"Customerizing" in the new millennium. *MedSurg Nursing: The Journal of Adult Health,* 9(2), 97–99.

Leddy, S., & Pepper, J. M. (1998). *Conceptual bases of professional nursing* (4th ed.). Philadelphia: Lippincott.

Longest, B. (1998). *Health policymaking in the United States* (2nd ed.). Chicago: Health Administration Press.

MacLeod, H. (2010). A healthier health system is ours to create. *Canadian Nurse,* 106(9), 56.

McIntyre, M., & Thomlinson, E. (2003). *Realities of Canadian nursing: Professional, practice, and power issues.* Philadelphia: Lippincott Williams & Wilkins.

McNeill, T. (2010). Family as a social determinant of health: Implications for governments and institutions to promote the health and well-being of families. *Healthcare Quarterly,* 14(Special issue), 60–67.

Milstead, J. A. (1999). Health policy & politics: A nurse's guide. Gaithersburg, MD: Aspen.

Nursing Sector Study Corporation. (2005). *Building the future: An integrated strategy for nursing human resources in Canada.* Ottawa: Author.

O'Connell, B. (2000). Research shows erosion to advocacy role. *Reflections on Nursing Leadership,* 26(2), 26–28.

Ogren, K. E. (2001). The risk of not understanding nursing history. In E. C. Hein (Ed.), *Nursing issues in the 21st century: Perspectives from the literature* (pp. 3–9). Philadelphia: Lippincott.

Provost, K. & Van Herk, K. (2006). Political activism and nursing. *Registered Nurse Journal,* 18(2), 22–23.

Registered Nurses Association of Ontario. (2005). Policy at work. *Registered Nurse Journal,* 17(3), 27.

Registered Nurses Association of Ontario. (2006). Using evidence, politics, communication and media to shape healthy public policy. *Registered Nurse Journal, November–December 2006.*

Registered Nurses Association of Ontario. (2011a). Make your voice heard. *Registered Nurse Journal,* 23(2), 12–16.

Registered Nurses Association of Ontario. (2011b). Talking politics. *Registered Nurse Journal,* 23(2), 18–20.

Rehtmeyer, C. M. (2000). Seeing change as an opportunity. In F. L. Bower (Ed.), *Nurses taking the lead: Personal qualities of effective leadership* (pp. 173–198). Philadelphia: Saunders.

Roszak, T. (1998). *The longevity revolution and the true wealth of nations.* Boston: Houghton Mifflin.

Statistics Canada. (2006). *Canada year book 2006.* Ottawa: Author.

Statistics Canada. (2010). *Canada year book 2010.* Ottawa: Author.

Williams, R. P. (1998). Nursing leaders' perceptions of quality nursing: An analysis from academe. Nursing Outlook, 46(6), 262–267.

SUGGESTED READINGS

Abeln, S. H. (1994). Quality as a risk management tool. *Rehab Management,* 7(2), 105–106.

Alberta Association of Registered Nurses. (2004). *Turn up the heat! Political action and advocacy guide.* Edmonton: Alberta Association of Registered Nurses.

Anderson, E. T., & McFarlane, J. M. (2000). *Community as partner: Theory and practice in nursing.* Philadelphia: Lippincott, Williams & Wilkins.

Baird, K. (2000). *Customer service in health care: A grassroots approach to creating a culture of service excellence.* San Francisco: Jossey-Bass.

Buerhaus, P. I., Staiger, D. O., & Auerbach, D. I. (2000). Implications of an aging registered nurse workforce. *Journal of the American Medical Association,* 283, 2948–2954.

Canadian Nurses Association. (2005). Position statement. *Accountability: Regulatory framework.* Ottawa: Author.

DiCenso, A., Bryant-Lukosius, D., Martin-Misener, R., Donald, F., Abelson, J., Bourgeault, I., et al. (2010). Factors enabling advanced practice nursing role integration in Canada. *Nursing Leadership,* 23(Special issue), 211–238.

Edwards, T. (2000). *Contradictions of consumption: Concepts, practices, and politics in consumer society.* Buckingham: Open University Press.

Jones, K., Jennings, B., Moritz, P., & Moss, M. (1997). Policy issues associated with analyzing outcomes of care. *Image: Journal of Nursing Scholarship,* 29, 261–268.

Kaasalainen, S., Martin-Misener, R., Kilpatrick, K. Harbman, P., Bryant-Lukosius, D., Donald, F., et al. (2010). A historical overview of the development of advanced practice nursing roles in Canada. *Nursing Leadership,* 23(Special issue), 35–60.

Mason, D., & Leavitt, J. K. (1998). *Policy and politics in nursing and health care.* Philadelphia: Saunders.

Miller, T. W. (1996). Health policy, politics, and community health advocacy. In B. W. Spradley & J. A. Allender (Eds.), *Community health nursing: Concepts and practices* (pp. 635–657). Philadelphia: Lippincott.

O'Reilly, P. (2000). *Health care practitioners: An Ontario case study in policy making.* Toronto: University of Toronto Press.

Pope, T. (2000). The rising tide of consumerism: How will it affect long-term care decision making? *Long-Term Care Interface,* 1(1), 36–40.

Shaw, J. (2005). RNs lead by example. *Registered Nurse Journal,* 17(6), 23.

Sherman, S. G., & Sherman, V. C. (1998). *Total customer satisfaction: A comprehensive approach for health care providers.* San Francisco: Jossey-Bass.

Smith, S., Heffler, S., & Freeland, M. (1999). The next decade of health spending: A new outlook. *Health Affairs,* 18(4), 86–95.

Spradley, B. W., & Allender, J. A. (1996). *Community health nursing: Concepts and practice.* Philadelphia: Lippincott.

Strasen, L. (1987). *Key business skills for nurse managers.* Philadelphia: Lippincott.

Wojner, A. W. (2001). *Outcomes management: Applications to clinical practice.* St. Louis, MO: Mosby.

World Health Organization. (1978). *Declaration of Alma Ata: Report of the International Conference on Primary Health Care.* Alma-Ata, USSR, September 1978. Geneva: WHO. Retrieved from http://www.who.int/hpr/NPH/docs/declaration_almaata.pdf

CHAPTER ENDNOTES

1. Commission on the Future of Health Care in Canada. (2002). *Building on values: The future of health care in Canada* (p. xv.) Saskatoon: Author. Commissioner: Roy J. Romano.

2. Statistics Canada, "Immigration in Canada: A portrait of the foreign-born population 2006 Census." Retrieved from http://www12.statcan.ca/census-recensement/2006/as-sa/97-557/p2-eng.cfm

3. Statistics Canada. (May 26, 2010). The Daily, "*Population projections: Canada, the provinces and territories.*" Retrieved from http://www.statcan.gc.ca/daily-quotidien/100526/dq100526b-eng.htm

4. Statistics Canada. (March 24, 2011). The Daily, "*Canada's population estimates.*" Retrieved from http://www.statcan.gc.ca/daily-quotidien/110324/dq110324b-eng.htm

5. Health Canada, "About Health Canada, Office of Nursing Policy." Retrieved from http://www.hc-sc.gc.ca/ahc-asc/branch-dirgen/spb-dgps/onp-bpsi/overview-apercu-eng.php

6. Health Canada, "About Health Canada, Functions." Retrieved from http://www.hc-sc.gc.ca/ahc-asc/branch-dirgen/spb-dgps/onp-bpsi/overview-apercu-eng.php

7. Health Canada, "About Health Canada, Priorities." Retrieved from http://www.hc-sc.gc.ca/ahc-asc/branch-dirgen/spb-dgps/onp-bpsi/overview-apercu-eng.php

CHAPTER 8

Nursing Leadership and Management

Linda Searle Leach, PhD, RN, CNAA

Adapted by Heather Crawford, BScN, MEd, CHE, and John P. Angkaw, MBA(c), MEd, BScN

Nursing is a practice discipline and it is a political act. Nursing leadership is about critical thinking, action and advocacy—and it happens in all roles and domains of nursing practice. Nursing leadership plays a pivotal role in the immediate lives of nurses and it has an impact on the entire health system and the [Ca]nadians it serves. Therefore, Canada's health system requires a steady supply of visionary and energetic leaders across the domains of the discipline who are credible, courageous, visible and inspiring to others and who have [t]he authority and resources to support modern, [i]nnovative and professional nursing practice.

(Canadian Nurses Association, 2009)

OBJECTIVES

The purpose of this chapter is to enable the reader to

■ define management;

■ describe the management process;

■ explain management theories;

■ discuss motivation theories;

■ define leadership and nursing leadership and explain their importance for organizations;

■ differentiate between leadership and management;

■ describe characteristics of effective leaders;

■ identify factors that influence nursing leadership;

■ identify leadership styles;

■ explain Hersey and Blanchard's situational theory of leadership and its application in nursing leadership practice;

■ identify Kouzes and Posner's five leadership practices;

■ discuss transformational leadership theory; and

■ examine the link between nursing leadership and management.

photos.com

participated in code arrests a few times, she had never witnessed one right before her eyes. Her knowledgeable action saved this client's life. The next morning Julie was assigned to work a day shift in the CCU. Julie entered Gary's room as the sun was rising. As he awoke, she spent some quiet time with him. While he embraced the start of a new day, his thoughts must have been intense. What he chose to share was this acknowledgment: "You saved my life. Thank you." This precious moment was a celebration of both of their lives

Do all of these nurses exhibit leadership qualities? What does it mean to be a nursing leader? Was Julie a leader in delivering client care? What leadership characteristics do these nurses demonstrate? Why are each of them considered leaders, even though they are not necessarily in formal positions of authority?

Leadership can be demonstrated by any nurse in any setting. Consider the following scenarios:

Cindy is an experienced nursing director who is currently mentoring a newly hired unit manager, Jeff, at their institution. She has spent the last several weeks coaching and mentoring Jeff through the initial challenges he faced. Although not formally asked to assume this role, Cindy is aware of her corporate and professional responsibility to develop the next generation of nursing leaders.

Sally is a professor at a local university and has extensive research experience. She is currently supervising a group of five graduate students. She meets with the group twice a month to discuss their progress with their own research and coursework. Sally understands that it takes time to develop great researchers, and she had made a commitment to mentor these graduate students, because they represent the next generation of nursing researchers who will advance the knowledge in the profession.

Bradley is a new nurse on a busy medical unit and has recently grown accustomed to working with unregulated care providers. He understands that to accomplish his daily role and responsibilities he has to rely on the assistance of colleagues on the unit. As a result, he has paid attention to developing his communication, time management, and delegation skills.

Gary, a 45-year-old father of three, was admitted to the cardiac observation unit earlier in the day. He had been diagnosed previously with heart disease and had experienced episodes of ventricular arrhythmias. That evening, while Gary was talking to his family on the phone, he suddenly stopped talking and went into ventricular tachycardia and cardiac arrest. Julie, his nurse, reacted immediately, by giving a precordial thump to his chest. Normal sinus rhythm appeared on the monitor before anyone else could respond to the code. Gary was then transferred to the coronary care unit (CCU).

Julie has been a registered nurse (RN) in the cardiac observation unit less than one year, and although she had

Nursing professionals use their specialized knowledge, judgment, skills, and clinical experience to perform leadership roles. Many people think leaders are corporate executives, political representatives, military generals, or those who head organizations. However, effective nursing leadership is important in all nursing roles at all levels within an organization and across all domains of practice: direct practice, education, research, and administration. In today's world, nurses are called on to be leaders within their respective fields, thereby contributing to excellence in nursing and ensuring that quality client outcomes are achieved (Registered Nurses Association of Ontario, 2006). In their position statement on nursing leadership, the Canadian Nurses Association (CNA) states,

> Nursing leadership is about nurses who understand that the development of nursing leaders must begin at the outset of every nursing education program and continue throughout the career of every nurse…about the competent and engaged practice of nurses who provide exemplary care…about nurses who create and use research and who ask the kinds of questions and seek the kinds of answers that can shape healthy public policy…about nurses who develop, analyze and interpret policy…and about innovative and visionary administrators from the first level to the most senior nurse executives (2009).

The Academy of Canadian Executive Nurses (ACEN) and American Organization of Nurse Executives (AONE) believe that nursing leadership is important to the safety and reliability of the health care system.

Nurses have the potential to make a critical difference every day in the lives of their clients and their clients' families and in their practice environments.

However, many nurses believe those critical differences are part of their ordinary work. Nurses are leaders, and by using their expert knowledge and leadership, they provide knowledgeable care that is extraordinary. Because rapid, dramatic change will continue in nursing and the health care industry, it is increasingly important for nurses to develop skill in leadership roles and management functions (Marquis & Huston, 2006). Nurses must ensure that they incorporate leadership into their daily agenda as there is a need to maximize nursing leadership at all levels and across all domains of practice (clinical, education, research, and administration). Bednash (2003) suggests that "old conversations about entry to practice must be abandoned for a new conversation about how to best educate nurses for the dynamic world of health care in which health care therapeutics, technology and science are creating a complex and startlingly different practice reality" (p. 257). This chapter introduces the process of management and explains management theories and functions. Management will be defined, and current trends will be discussed. This chapter also discusses leadership and provides a framework to differentiate leadership and management. Leadership characteristics, styles of leadership, and leadership theories are described. In examining management and leadership, it will become evident that a symbiotic or synergistic relationship exists between the two concepts. The challenge for leaders and managers in today's complex practice settings is the integration of leadership and management skills to facilitate positive outcomes for clients, nurses, and the organization.

DEFINITION OF MANAGEMENT

Management can be defined as the systematic process of planning, organizing, leading, and controlling actions and resources to achieve organizational goals. Descriptive research about what managers do (Hales, 1986; McCall, Morrison, & Hanman, 1978; Mintzberg, 1973) has been a helpful way to expand our understanding of management. Managers often seem to work at a hectic pace and sustain that effort through long hours, frequently working without breaks. According to Yukl (1998), this practice reflects a preference by people in management positions; they become adept at continuously seeking information and are constantly engaged in interactions with others who need information, help, guidance, or approval. The typical manager is on the go.

Research by McCall et al. (1978) shows that the daily activities of managers are diverse and fast paced, with regular interruptions. Priority activities are integrated among inconsequential tasks. In the scope of one morning, a manager may engage in serious and far-reaching decisions about downsizing personnel, respond to a client complaint, problem-solve a sick call, and participate in a celebration for an employee. Managerial work is driven by problems that emerge in random order and that have a range of importance and urgency. These circumstances create an image of the manager as a fire-fighter, involved in immediate and operational concerns. The loss of so many Canadian managerial positions in the 1990s and beyond has left current managers with a large span of control, often spread across multiple units, sites, and professions. Canada's first-line managers average 71 direct reports, far exceeding the benchmark found in other work settings.[1]

A landmark paper by Bruch and Ghoshal—who studied busy managers in nearly a dozen large companies—found that "fully 90% of managers squander their time in all sorts of ineffective activities. In other words a mere 10% of managers spend their time in a committed, purposeful and reflective manner" (2002, p. 64). Effective managers need to balance both focus and energy. Focus is described by Bruch and Ghoshal as concentrated attention, or the ability to zero in on a goal and see the tasks through to completion. This description suggests that skilled managers have the wisdom to choose what to respond to and maintain active suppression to environmental distractions that can sidetrack the focused effort. Energy is described as the vivacity that is fuelled by intense personal commitment. Disequilibrium in focus and energy results in ineffective management.

THE MANAGEMENT PROCESS

In the early 1900s the study of management, as a discipline, emerged with a focus on the science of management. In 1924 Mary Parker Follet wrote about management as an art of accomplishing things through people. Henri Fayol, a manager, wrote a book in 1916 called *General and Industrial Management*, in which he described the functions of planning, organizing, coordinating, and controlling as the **management process** (Fayol, 1916/1949). His work has become a classic in the way that we define the process of managing. Two other individuals, Gulick and Urwick, in some part as a result of their esteemed status as informal advisers to President Franklin D. Roosevelt, served to define the management process according to seven principles (Henry, 1992). Their principles form the acronym POSDCORB, which stands for planning, organizing, staffing, directing, coordinating (CO), reporting, and budgeting (Gulick & Urwick, 1937; Henry, 1992). Their work is also considered to be a classic description of management and remains a relevant description of how management is carried out today.

I have always wondered what makes a nurse a "leader." I slowly began to realize that becoming a leader isn't necessarily confined to the formal position or title that one holds within the organization, but it is more linked with the individual intentions and actions. I believe that nurse leaders are people who go "above and beyond" in their daily work to make a difference for their clients, colleagues and organization. They instil confidence and empowers those around them, to improve client outcomes and to increase satisfaction. The leader is able to see the health care system as a whole, and realize that each contribution, whether large or small, is a step forward for the profession and the entire health care community, including the client. The leader is able not only to manage and maintain the status quo but also to lead and navigate in times of change and uncertainty. I believe nurse leaders are not only concerned with today, but also have an appreciation of the future, and they know how to get us there.

Rachel Wilson, RN, MScN
Professional Practice Leader

One of the most frequently referenced taxonomies of managerial roles is from an in-depth, month-long study of five chief executives by Henry Mintzberg. Taxonomy is a system that groups or classifies principles. Mintzberg's observations led to the identification of three categories of managerial roles: (1) information processing roles, (2) interpersonal roles, and (3) decision-making roles (Mintzberg, 1973). A role includes behaviours, expectations, and recurrent activities within a pattern that is part of the organization's structure (Katz & Kahn, 1978). The information processing roles identified by Mintzberg (1973) are those of monitor, disseminator, and spokesperson, and they are used to manage people's information needs. The interpersonal roles consist of figurehead, leader, and liaison, and each of these roles is used to manage relationships with people. The decision roles are entrepreneur, disturbance handler, allocator of resources, and negotiator. Managers take on these roles when they make decisions.

More recently, Yukl (1998) and colleagues (Kim & Yukl, 1995; Yukl, Wall, & Lepsinger, 1990) described 13 managerial role functions for managing the work and for managing relationships. The role functions for managing the work are planning and organizing, problem solving, clarifying roles and objectives, informing, monitoring, consulting, and delegating. The role functions for managing relationships are networking, supporting, developing and mentoring, managing conflict and team building, motivating and inspiring, and recognizing and rewarding.

The amount of time a manager spends in particular roles varies by the manager's position in the organization, ranging from the lowest level manager, to the middle-level manager, to the highest or executive-level manager. However, in health care environments, this generalization needs to be tempered with an understanding of the impact on hospital restructuring, complexity of service delivery, client acuity, and the ever-growing span of control for the nurse manager. Again, nursing managers need to be cognizant of the required balance between focus and energy to maintain effectiveness.

Typically, a low-level managerial job is the first-line manager, and in health care organizations that position is the typical role of the nurse manager. Ideally, the nurse manager spends most of her time in the clinical area, supervising, leading, and coaching staff as they deliver care, as well as maintaining active surveillance of the quality of care given. This means that managers are often less accessible due to the nature of their involvement on project teams, taskforces, and committees, and their competing priorities in balancing the costs and quality of health care. The next highest percentage of this manager's time is spent in planning, where other responsibilities—such as coordinating, evaluating, negotiating, and serving as a multi-specialist and generalist—each require less than 10 percent of the nurse manager's time. In contrast, the middle-level manager, often called a director (e.g., the director of critical care nursing), spends less time supervising and more time in each of the other assignments, particularly planning, monitoring, and delegating. At the highest level of the organization, usually described as the executive level, planning and serving as a generalist are greatly expanded role functions, whereas monitoring is not the primary role function as it is for the other two levels. Nurses in executive-level roles in health care organizations usually have the title of chief nursing officer; in acute care hospitals, their title is often vice president and chief nursing officer.

MANAGEMENT THEORIES

The current theories of management practice have evolved from earlier theories. Management practices were actually a part of the governance in ancient Samaria and Egypt as far back as 3000 B.C. (Daft & Marcic, 2001). Most of our current understanding of management, however, is based on the classical perspective of management or the classical theories of management that were introduced in the 1800s, during the industrial age, as factories developed.

CLASSICAL VIEWPOINT

The **classical viewpoint** prescribed a high degree of specialization of labour and a very high degree of coordination among staff. Some of the advocates of the classical viewpoint were Henril Fayol, James, Mooney, and Lyndall Urwick (Wren, 1987). The decision making was centralized and the decisions that came from upper management coordinated the efforts. The classical perspective includes three subfields of management: scientific management, bureaucratic theory, and administrative principles (Daft & Marcic, 2001; Wren, 1979).

SCIENTIFIC MANAGEMENT

While practising managers, such as Fayol, who was mentioned earlier, were describing the functions of managers, a man named Frederick Taylor was focusing his attention on the operations within an organization by exploring production at the workers' level. Taylor is acknowledged as the father of scientific management for his use of the scientific method and as the author of *Principles of Scientific Management* (1911). Taylor, an engineer, introduced precise procedures based on systematic investigation of specific situations. The underlying point of view is that the organization is a machine to be run efficiently to increase production. **Scientific management** is a management theory that is primarily concerned with improving productivity through the optimization of work processes and tasks. It emphasizes an analysis of labour division, standardization of work and work measurement.

Currently in Canada, the definition of nursing productivity/utilization is "workload over worked hours" (Canadian Institute for Health Information, 1999). Many nursing leaders recognize that this simple calculation does not account for the quality and outcomes of care delivered for the impact of length of stay on total cost (O'Brien-Pallas et al., 2004). In a dynamic state, such as a care delivery setting, the individual and collective capacity of the nursing personnel (i.e., their scope, competence, experience, and their physician and psychosocial status) must be balanced against client needs and system characteristics (i.e., census, type of client mix, staff mix, and occupancy). The maximum work capacity of any employee is 93 percent, because 7 percent is allocated in paid breaks during which no work is contractually expected (O'Brien-Pallas et al., 2004). O'Brien-Pallas and colleagues found that significant benefits, both fiscal and human, can be achieved by moderating productivity/utilization levels within a range of 85 percent, plus or minus 5 percent. This level suggests productivity targets may not be appropriate for specialty units, such as emergency departments or labour and delivery units, since their work flow demands can be variable.

Working independently of Taylor, Frank and Lillian Gilbreth also contributed significantly to the study of scientific management. They pioneered studies of time and motion that emphasized efficiency and culminated in "one best way" of carrying out work. Frank Gilbreth (1912) revolutionized surgical efficiency in the operating room, resulting in operations of shorter duration that substantially reduced risks from surgery for clients at that time.

BUREAUCRATIC THEORY

The beliefs of Max Weber, the German theorist recognized for the organizational theory of bureaucracy, were in stark contrast to the typical European organization that was based on a family-type structure in which employees were loyal to an individual, not to the organization, and resources were used to benefit individuals rather than to advance the organization. Weber, however, believed efficiency was achieved through impersonal relations within a formal structure, competence should be the basis for hiring and promoting an employee, and decisions should

LITERATURE APPLICATION

Citation: Casida, J., & Pinto-Zipp, G. (2008). Leadership-organizational culture relationships in nursing units of acute care hospitals. *Nursing Economics*, 26(1): 7–15.

Discussion: Nursing managers who exhibit transformational leadership are more likely to influence the culture of their units, in that their staff is more flexible and less resistant to change. This is especially important in a time when changes are frequent and unpredictable. Moreover, their staff will also have a better understanding of the direction of the organization. They will all share a common focus and vision during times of constant challenge, particularly when nursing managers are to maintain a healthy work environment and a high level of job satisfaction among nurses. A nursing unit that is more flexible and focused will be better able to adapt to the health care climate and meet the demands of the clients and their families.

Implications for Practice: The leadership style that a nurse manager chooses to apply relates to the organizational culture of the unit. Nursing managers must be aware of their leadership style and the influence it has on the culture of their unit. When used by nursing managers, transformational leadership has a positive impact at the unit level.

be made in an orderly and rational way, based on rules and regulations. The **bureaucratic organization** was a hierarchy with clear superior-subordinate communication and relations, based on positional authority, in which orders from the top were transmitted down through the organization via a clear chain of command.

ADMINISTRATIVE PRINCIPLES

Administrative principles are general principles of management that are relevant to any organization. In addition to some of the principles described as comprising the management process (e.g., planning, organizing, directing, coordinating, and controlling), principles such as unity of command and direction were identified. Unity of command and direction refers to a worker receiving orders from only one supervisor, and related work being grouped under one manager. These are examples of general principles generated during the early 1900s, which were useful and relevant to all organizations (Fayol, 1916/1949).

Another key aspect of this perspective is attributed to Chester Barnard. Barnard (1938) is associated with the concept of the informal organization. The informal organization consists of naturally forming social groups that can become strong and powerful contributors to an organization. Barnard understood that these informal forces can be valuable in accomplishing the organization's goals and should be managed properly. He is also credited with the acceptance theory of authority, which identified people as having free will and being able to choose to comply with orders they are given (Daft & Marcic, 2001). This view of people as making a difference in organizations was a precursor to the human relations movement that emerged from experiments at a Chicago electric company, discussed in the next section. See Table 8-1 for an overview of management theories.

TABLE 8-1	MANAGEMENT THEORIES	
Management Theory	**Main Contributors**	**Key Aspects**
Scientific management	Frederick Taylor (1856–1915) Frank Gilbreth (1868–1924) Lillian Gilbreth (1878–1972)	Machinelike focus Analysis of elements of an operation Training of the worker Use of proper tools and equipment Use of incentives Use of time and motion studies to make the work easier
Bureaucratic theory	Max Weber (1864–1920): German sociologist	Division of labour, hierarchy of authority, and chain of command Rationality, impersonal management Use of merit and skill as basis for promotion and reward Use of rules and regulations, focus on exacting work processes Career service, salaried managers
Administrative principles	Mary Parker Follet (1868–1933): Trained in philosophy and political science at Radcliffe	The science of management Principles of organization applicable in any setting
	Henri Fayol (1841–1925): French mining engineer, head of major mining company	Fayol's principles: unity of command, division of work, unity of direction, scalar chain, and management's principle functions—planning, organizing, coordinating, and controlling

(Continued)

TABLE 8-1	MANAGEMENT THEORIES (CONTINUED)	
Management Theory	**Main Contributors**	**Key Aspects**
	Chester Barnard (1886–1961): Harvard economics, president of New Jersey Bell Telephone	Concerned with the optimal approach for administrators to achieve economic efficiency
	Luther Gulick and Lyndal Urwick (1937): *Papers on the Science of Administration*	Planning, organizing, supervising, directing, controlling, organizing, reviewing, and budgeting = POSDCORB
	James Mooney (1939): *Principles of Organization*	Four principles: coordination, hierarchical structure (scalar), functional (division of labour), staff/line principle
Human relations (replaced later by the term *organizational behaviour*)	Elton Mayo (1933) Fritz Roethlisberger (1939): Harvard University	Hawthorne studies led to the belief that human relations between workers and managers and among workers were the main determinants of efficiency. The Hawthorne effect refers to change in behaviour as a result of being watched.

HUMAN RELATIONS

The next focus in the development of management theory is the human relations movement. The **human relations movement** espoused the individual worker as the source of control, motivation, and productivity in organizations. This is in sharp contrast to the science of exact procedures, rules and regulations, and formal authority that characterized scientific management. During the 1930s labour unions became stronger and were instrumental in advocating for the human needs of employees. During this time, experiments conducted at the Hawthorne plant of the Western Electric Company in Chicago led to a greater understanding of the influence of human relations in organizations.

Electricity had become the preferred power source over gas; the Hawthorne plant experiments were run to show that more light than was used before in the plant was necessary to increase productivity. This approach was designed to increase the use of electricity. Researchers Mayo (1933) and Roethlisberger and Dickson (1939) measured the effects on production when the intensity of lighting was altered. They found that with more and brighter light, production increased as expected. However, production also increased each time they reduced the light, even when the light was extremely dim. Their research findings led to the conclusion that something else besides the light was motivating these workers.

The notion of social facilitation, or the idea that people increase their work output in the presence of others, was a result of the Hawthorne experiments. They also concluded that the effect of being watched and receiving special attention could alter a person's behaviour. The phenomenon of being observed or studied—resulting in changes in behaviour—is now called the **Hawthorne effect** (Hughes, Ginnet, & Curphy, 1999). Emerging from this study was the concept that people benefit and are more productive and satisfied when they participate in decisions about their work environment. This concept introduced the next phase in the evolution of management, called human relations management. In addition, social groupings, people's feelings, and their motivations became a focus of interest for future studies.

MOTIVATION THEORIES

The human relations perspective in management theory grew from the conclusion that worker output was greater when the worker was treated humanistically. This theory spawned a human resources point of view and a focus on the individual as a source of motivation. **Motivation** is not explicitly demonstrated by people but rather is interpreted from their behaviour. Motivation is the incentive that influences our choices and creates direction, intensity, and persistence in our behaviour (Hughes et al., 1999; Kanfer, 1990). Motivation is a process that occurs internally to influence and direct our behaviour in order to satisfy needs (Lussier, 1999). Motivation theories are not management theories per se; however, they are frequently included along with management theories.

There are two types of motivation theories: content motivation theories and process motivation theories (Lussier, 1999). The process motivation theories are expectancy theory and equity theory. The content motivation theories include Maslow's needs hierarchy and Herzberg's two-factor theory. These two theories are presented here along with Theory X, Theory Y, and Theory Z (see Table 8-2).

Motivation theories help explain why people act the way they do and how a manager can relate to individuals as human beings and workers. When you are interested in creating change, influencing others, and managing performance and outcomes, it is helpful to understand the motivation that is reflected in a person's behaviour. Motivation is a critical part of leadership because, to be good leaders and good followers, we need to understand each other. Covey (1990), in his national bestseller, *The Seven Habits of Highly Effective People*, defines habit number five as

"Seek first to understand, then to be understood," which is a practice focused on the importance of empathetic communication, which is critical to effective leadership.

MASLOW'S HIERARCHY OF NEEDS

One of the most well-known theories of motivation is Maslow's hierarchy of needs. Maslow (1970) developed a hierarchy of needs that shows how an individual is motivated. Figure 8-1 applies Maslow's hierarchy of human needs to how organizations motivate employees. Motivation, according to Maslow, begins when a need is not met. For example, when a person has a physiological need, such as thirst, this unmet need has to be satisfied before a person is motivated to pursue higher level needs. Certain needs have to be satisfied in a certain order: first, physiological needs, then safety and security needs, followed by belonging social needs, and then esteem and ego needs; after these needs are fulfilled an individual can be motivated by the needs at the next level. The need for self-actualization drives people to the pinnacle of performance and achievement.

HERZBERG'S TWO-FACTOR THEORY

Frederick Herzberg (1968) contributed to research on motivation and developed the two-factor theory of

TABLE 8-2	MOTIVATION THEORIES	
Motivation Theory	**Main Contributors**	**Key Aspects**
Selected content of motivation theories	Abraham Maslow (1908–70)	Hierarchy of satisfaction of physiological, safety, belonging, ego, and self-actualization needs
Two-factor theory	Frederick Herzberg (1968)	Hygiene-maintenance factors = prevention of job dissatisfaction: provide adequate salary and supervision, safe and tolerable working conditions
		Motivators = job satisfaction: satisfying and meaningful work, development opportunities, responsibility, and recognition
Theory X	Douglas McGregor (1906–64)	Theory X: Leaders must direct and control as motivation results from reward and punishment.
Theory Y		Theory Y: Leaders remove obstacles as workers have self-control, self-discipline; their reward is their involvement in work.
Theory Z	William Ouchi (1981)	Theory Z: Collective decision making, long-term employment, mentoring, holistic concerns, and use of quality circles are used to manage service and quality; a humanistic style of motivation is based on Japanese organizations.

motivation. He analyzed the responses of accountants and engineers, and concluded that two sets of factors were associated with motivation. One set of motivation factors must be maintained to avoid job dissatisfaction: salary, job security, working conditions, status, quality of supervision, and relationships with others. These factors have been labelled **maintenance or hygiene factors.** Factors such as achievement, recognition, responsibility, advancement, and the opportunity for development also contribute to job satisfaction. These factors are intrinsic and serve to satisfy or motivate people. Herzberg proposed that when these **motivation factors** are present, people are motivated and satisfied with their job. When these factors are absent from a work setting, people have a neutral attitude about their organization. In contrast, when the maintenance factors are absent, people are dissatisfied. Herzberg believed that by providing the maintenance factors, job dissatisfaction could be avoided, but that the presence of these factors will not motivate people.

New graduate nurses can use Herzberg's theory by evaluating the maintenance factors present in a health care organization when they apply for a job. The pay, working conditions, and the beginning relationship that has been established with the nurse manager are aspects of the job that the nurse should consider. If these maintenance factors are not adequate to begin with, then the nurse may become easily dissatisfied with the job. The higher level needs that Herzberg describes as motivation factors should also be evaluated by the nurse before joining an organization. Are opportunities available for the nurse to achieve professional growth, to take on new responsibilities, to advance, and to be recognized for one's contributions?

McGregor's Theory X and Theory Y

Continuing the emphasis on factors that stimulate job satisfaction and that motivate people to be involved and contribute productively at work, McGregor capitalized on his experience as a psychologist and university president to

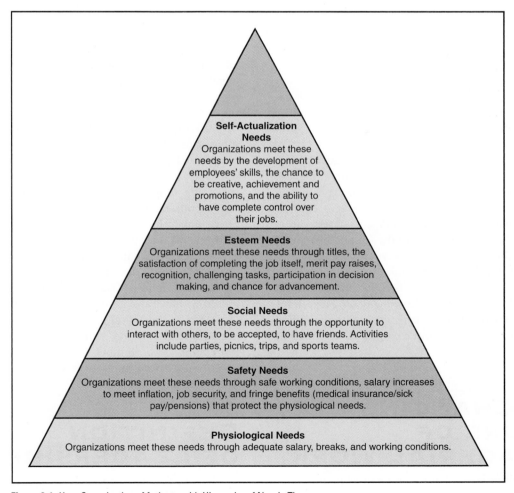

Figure 8-1 How Organizations Motivate with Hierarchy of Needs Theory
Source: From LUSSIER/ACHUA. *Leadership*, 4E. © 2010 South-Western, a part of Cengage Learning, Inc. Reproduced by permission. www.cengage.com/permissions

develop Theory X and Theory Y (McGregor, 1960). Theory X and Theory Y describe two different ways to motivate or influence others based on underlying attitudes about human nature. Each view reflects different attitudes about the nature of people. The **Theory X** view is that in bureaucratic organizations, employees prefer security, direction, and minimal responsibility. Coercion, threats, or punishment are necessary because people do not like the work that needs to be done. These employees are not able to offer creative solutions to help the organization advance. McGregor's beliefs about Theory X were related to the classical perspective of organizations that included scientific management, bureaucracy theory, and administrative principles.

The assumptions of **Theory Y** are that, in the context of the right conditions, people enjoy their work; can show self-control and discipline; are able to contribute creatively; and are motivated by ties to the group, the organization, and the work itself. In essence, this view espouses the belief that people are intrinsically motivated by their work. Theory Y was a guide for managers to take advantage of the potential of each person, which McGregor thought was being only partially used, and to provide support and encouragement to employees to do good work (McGregor, 1960).

OUCHI'S THEORY Z

Theory Z was developed by William Ouchi (1981) based on his years studying organizations in Japan. He identified that Japanese organizations had better productivity than organizations in the United States and that they were managed differently, through their use of quality circles, to pursue better productivity and quality. Theory Z focuses on a better way of motivating people through their involvement. Collective decision making is a hallmark of Theory Z, as is a focus on long-term employment that involves slower promotions and less direct supervision. The organization and the worker are viewed more holistically. Through progressive development, the organization will be productive, and quality goals will be achieved. The organization invests in its employees and addresses both home and work issues, creating a path for career development. Democratic leaders, who are skilled in interpersonal relations, foster employee involvement (Ouchi, 1981).

THE CHANGING NATURE OF MANAGERIAL WORK

Current trends indicate that the number of managers in an organization, particularly at the middle level, is being reduced and that downsizing of staff has been a common phenomenon in most health care institutions across Canada. Hospitals are increasingly adopting structures with wider managerial spans of control (Pillai & Meindl, 1998; Spence Laschinger, Sabiston, Finegan, & Shamian, 2001), creating dramatic changes in the work environment and significantly affecting the relationship between nurses and managers. Blythe, Baumann, and Giovannetti (2001) found that as a result of an increased span of control, relations between managers and nurses became distant, and communications became less frequent and more formal. After reorganization, those left in management positions are fewer in number and have taken on more responsibility over more areas, thereby increasing their respective spans of control.

As individual nurses become more involved in managing consumer relations and consumer care, managers will become managers of systems rather than managers of nurses per se. As the role of the direct practice nurse evolves to integrate the managing of consumer relations and care, a significant shift will occur in training and coaching. The nurse manager will be key as a change agent in managing the change process and sustaining the outcomes. As system managers, nurses will manage clinical systems, cost information systems, and data systems on consumer satisfaction and feedback.

Leadership responsibilities will be integrated among all organizational participants who function as **knowledge workers** and provide their professional expertise. This vision of true interprofessional practice will require all practitioners "to operate from a framework of trust, respect, authenticity, collaboration and common interest problem solving to effect positive outcomes for our mutual clients and our community of practitioners" (Doucette, 2006). Knowledge workers are those involved in serving others through their specialized knowledge. Among nurses, this specialized knowledge is the science of nursing, which is transacted via practice and art to serve clients and their families. Porter-O'Grady (2003) hypothesizes that knowledge has become the new currency, changing the traditional relationship between worker and employer, and between what people know and how they translate it into innovations and practices of work that are critical to the continuing viability of the organization. For now and for the immediate future, leadership responsibilities need to be dispersed among all nurses, who are knowledge workers by virtue of their professional nursing expertise.

DEFINITION OF LEADERSHIP

Leadership is commonly defined as a process of influence in which the leader influences others toward goal achievement (Yukl, 1998). Influence is an instrumental part of leadership and refers to a leader's ability to affect others, often by inspiring, enlivening, and engaging them to participate. The process of leadership involves the leader and the follower in interaction, which implies that leadership is a reciprocal relationship. Leadership can occur between the leader and another individual; between the leader and a group; or between a leader and an organization, a community, or a society. Defining *leadership* as a process helps us understand leadership more than the traditional view of a leader as a person in a position of authority who exerts command, control, and power over subordinates.

As professionals, nurses function as leaders when they influence others toward goal achievement. Nurses are leaders. There are many more leaders in organizations than those people who are in positions of authority. Each person has the potential to serve as a leader. In the nursing literature, definitions of the term *nursing leader* are highly varied. Definitions tend to centre on either the process or the individual leader. Dunham and Klafehn (1990) define a leader as an individual with decision-making capacity, shared values with nurses, a vision, and the ability to inspire others to work toward this vision. McCloskey and McCain (1987) and Huber et al. (2000) define leadership as a process whereby the leader's role is to influence nurses to accomplish the goals of the organization. Fagin (1996) contends that nursing leaders are people who (1) have demonstrated skill in managing, (2) influence others in the advancement of the profession, (3) possess interpersonal skills within and outside the discipline, (4) have impressive publications, and (5) maintain an imposing reputation. Edwards (1994) saw nursing leadership as playing a central role in spearheading changes, and predicted: "Two of the foremost tasks of a new nursing leadership will be to raise the consciousness of nurses through an ongoing critique of the present system and to offer philosophical and practical rationales for fundamental change based on nursing values and the central role that nursing plans in the health care process" (Edwards, 1994).

Leadership in nursing can take two forms: namely, formal and informal leadership. **Formal leadership,** describes a person in a position of authority or a sanctioned, assigned role within an organization that connotes influence, such as a clinical nurse specialist (Northouse, 2001). Other formal leadership roles are nurse managers, nurse practitioners, and professional practice leaders. As advanced practice nurses, nurse practitioners also provide leadership, act as consultants, researchers, and educators, and incorporate new knowledge from research studies and other sources into their practice. Nurse practitioners play a key role in community organizational development and capacity building, as well as health policy development.[2]

An **informal leader** is an individual who demonstrates leadership outside the scope of a formal leadership role or as a member of a group, rather than as the head or leader of the group. The informal leader is considered to have emerged as a leader when she is accepted by others and is perceived to have influence.

It is important to understand that not all leaders are managers, but Manthey (1990) asserts that all managers need to be leaders. Another way to define leadership is through the differentiation of leadership and management (Zalenik, 1977). Bennis's work on differentiating the characteristics of managers versus leaders popularized the phrase "Managers are people who do things right and leaders are people who do the right thing" (Bennis & Nanus, 1985, p. 21).

Kotter (1990a) describes the differences between leadership and management in the following way: Leadership is about creating change, and management is about controlling complexity in an effort to bring order and consistency. According to Kotter, leading change involves establishing a direction, aligning people through empowerment, and motivating and inspiring them toward producing useful change and achieving the vision. On the other hand, *management* is defined as planning and budgeting, organizing and staffing, problem solving, and controlling complexity to produce predictability and order (Kotter, 1990b).

LEADERSHIP CHARACTERISTICS

According to Bennis and Nanus (1985), effective leaders share three fundamental qualities. The first quality is a guiding vision. A vision statement outlines what an organization wants to be and focuses on tomorrow (i.e., the preferred future); it is inspirational (i.e., it has reach) and provides a reference point to guide the nature of all decision making (Industry Canada, 2004). Nursing leaders focus on a professional and purposeful vision that provides direction toward the preferred future. The second quality is passion. Passion, as expressed by the leader, involves the ability to inspire and align people toward the promises of life. The third quality, integrity, is based on knowledge of self, honesty, and maturity, which is developed through experience and growth. McCall (1998) describes how self-awareness—knowing our strengths and weaknesses—can allow us to use feedback and learn from our mistakes. Daring and curiosity are also basic ingredients of leadership. Leaders draw on these capacities when they take risks, and they learn from what works as much as from what doesn't work (Bennis & Nanus, 1985).

A requirement for all nursing leaders is Olympic thinking, which requires all nursing leaders to nurture an inspiring vision of the preferred future, maintain a burning desire (i.e., a passion), and implement purposeful action towards achieving their vision. To be a leader who lacks any one of these Olympic thinking elements is to be a leader who daydreams of the preferred future. Kraus (2006) asserts that research in sports psychology has shown that visualization can enhance success and

REAL WORLD INTERVIEW

In our organization, we believe that nurses are critical to successful client-centred care, positive client outcomes, and effective interprofessional practice. As a result, we are committed to leadership development for nurses. With financial support from the Hospital Foundation, we have designed and implemented an internship program for our new graduate nurses. This six-month preceptor program provides opportunities for general and specialized clinical knowledge transfer regarding the complexities of acute care and professional practice. A preceptor for each new graduate provides leadership, support, and guidance for being a professional and competent nurse. This new program is positioned for success as it is focused on socializing, educating, and developing competencies among our nursing graduates to help them to succeed and advance in our organization.

Anne-Marie Clayton
Vice President Clinical Services and
Chief Nursing Executive

performance (i.e., achievement of vision), and parallel research in positive psychology has confirmed that visualization can enhance success in everyday life, making it a valuable tool for those interested in motivation, self-help, and self-improvement. Kraus reports that visualization enhances confidence, boosts motivation, and engages the individual in a practice or discipline that keeps the leader focused on achieving a vision.

Certain desirable characteristics are commonly attributed to leaders, including intelligence, self-confidence, determination, integrity, and sociability (Stodgill, 1948, 1974). Research among 46 hospitals designated as magnet hospitals— due to their success in attracting and retaining registered nurses— emphasized the value of leaders who are visionary and enthusiastic, supportive and knowledgeable, have high standards and expectations, value education and professional development, demonstrate power and status in the organization, are visible and responsive, communicate openly, and are active in professional associations (Kramer & Schmalenberg, 1988; McClure, Poulin, Sovie, & Wandelt, 1983; Scott, Sochalski, & Aiken, 1999). Research findings from studies of nurses reveal that a caring nature, respectability, trustworthiness, and flexibility are the most valued leader characteristics. In one study, nurse leaders identified leadership characteristics as managing the

dream, mastering change, designing organization structure, learning, and taking initiative (Murphy & DeBack, 1991). Research by Kirkpatrick and Locke (1991) concluded that leaders are different from non-leaders across six traits: drive, the desire to lead, honesty and integrity, self-confidence, cognitive ability, and knowledge of the business. Although no set of traits is definitive and reliable in determining who is a leader or who is effective as a leader, many people still rely on personality traits to describe and define leaders.

Another important leadership trait is surfacing in the nursing literature: **emotional intelligence,** or EI. Salovey and Mayer (1990) describe EI as the ability both to recognize the meaning of emotions and their relationships and to reason and solve problems on the basis of emotions. Goleman (2006) further explored the concept of EI and hypothesized that EI can be learned and improves with age. Current studies consistently demonstrate that EI is the common trait or factor that distinguishes individuals as leaders, innovators, and effective managers.

The emotionally intelligent nurse will be obvious in the practice environment as the nurse who can identify, use, and regulate emotions to maximize critical thinking. This results in sound decisions that support both positive outcomes and interprofessional collaboration in client care. As the complexities in practice and the delivery of care intensify, nursing leaders will need to guide with their heads and heart and to foster interprofessional practice, which is underpinned with teamwork, collaboration, high-quality **client-centred care**, and positive outcomes for clients. This requirement of all nursing leaders amplifies the need for all nurses to maintain emotional awareness to develop and maintain emotional intelligence.

Huston (2008) believes it is important for nursing to pay attention to the following eight skills, which she suggests will be "essential nurse leaders' competencies for 2020:

1. a global perspective regarding healthcare and professional nursing issues
2. technology skills which facilitate mobility and portability of relationships, interactions and operational processes
3. expert decision-making skills rooted in empirical science
4. the ability to create organization cultures that permeate quality healthcare and client/worker safety
5. understanding and appropriately intervening in political processes
6. highly developed collaborative and team building skills
7. the ability to balance authenticity and performance expectations; and
8. being able to envision and proactively adapt to a healthcare system characterized by rapid change and chaos."[3]*

*Huston, C. (2008). Preparing nurse leaders for 2020. *Journal of Nursing Management,* 16: 905–911. Reprinted by permission of John Wiley.

FACTORS THAT INFLUENCE THE QUALITY OF NURSING LEADERSHIP

Nursing history, education, use of self, organization structure and power, and organizational redesign are all factors that have contributed to the evolution of nursing leadership. Each will be examined briefly for its major contribution to the evolution of nursing leadership.

Nursing leadership has a strong and rich history with deep roots in both religious and military ground (Girvan, 1996). Meighan (1990) describes the influence that nursing's military roots played in the continuation of a command-and-control approach to achieve conformity in practice. The cost of this approach, however, was the further distancing of frontline nurses from decision making related to client care. Although the paradigm has shifted from controlling to empowering nurses to practise to their full scope, the change has not been a simple undertaking and has evolved in the face of hospital restructuring, new program reporting structures, and a mismatch between the demand and supply of nurses.

Nursing leaders must be lifelong learners with a thirst for knowledge and a desire to maintain and enhance leadership competencies. To effectively manage in chaotic and complex practice environments, leaders must be comfortable with and aware of the constant need for change, possess budget and financial skills, and remain committed to team building through effective management of personal growth (Gelinas & Manthey, 1997). The concept of future professional growth and mentoring of nurse leaders has been the centrepiece in a number of continuing educational programs. Stordeur, Vandenberghe, and D'hoore (2000) investigated the idea that role modelling of transformational leadership behaviour would have a cascading effect on lower level managers. However, the study did not hold this hypothesis to be true, and Stordeur suggested that purposeful and coordinated effort was needed to provide leadership development and education to potential future nurse leaders. Dunham-Taylor (1995) found the idea that leadership competencies could be learned, and suggested that preceptorship, mentoring, and education are key strategies for the development of future nursing leaders.

A strong factor that influences the quality of leadership is use of the self. Upenicks (2003) argues that some specific leader attributes may be more effective than others in creating environments that lead to positive outcomes for nurses. In a study conducted with senior nurse executives, Upenicks concludes that a passion for nursing and the ability to articulate this passion to nurses and other members of the administration are coupled with leadership effectiveness and support of nursing. Nursing research has also demonstrated a strong link between the emotional intelligence (EI) of leaders and the success of an organization. The concept of EI was explored in the leadership characteristics discussed earlier in this chapter. The concept of self and the ability to transact self in an effective and authentic manner directly contributes to the quality of leadership.

Leaders must function in various practice environments where the characteristics of structure and power play a role in the quality of leadership. Variation of leadership styles is affected by the organizational structure and culture (i.e., the context) of the organization (Stordeur et al., 2000). Upenicks's study (2003) of nurse leaders from magnet and non-magnet hospitals confirms that access to power, opportunity, information, and resources create an empowered environment with a climate that fosters leadership success and enhanced levels of job satisfaction among nurses. Upenicks also suggests that nurse leaders could have more power and credibility among peer executives if they learned how to think as professionals do in the business world.

Organizational redesign has been a major influence on the quality of nursing leadership. Nursing leaders have not only been changed by redesign but in the process of changing they have also had to lead the redesign of clinical care, delivery systems, and integrated care (Gelinas & Manthey, 1997). Leatt and Porter (2003) describes the need for nursing leaders to have an ability to work effectively across disciplines given the increased emphasis on interprofessional team-based care, which is prevalent in organizational redesign of health care. Tim Porter-O'Grady (2003) asserts that a new leadership role requires new skill sets. In our progress towards the preferred future, Porter-O'Grady espouses a need for leaders who are able to help others, see the need for change, challenge past practices, create a vision for the future, and construct new models for service delivery. Smith et al. (1994) describe the need for nurse leaders to have knowledge of nursing practice, but also to understand regulatory issues and business skills, and to have an understanding of risk, liability, strategic planning, and political acumen.

Nurses don't tend to leave their place of employment; nurses leave their managers, according to Bernard Bass's transformational leadership theory (Ribelin, 2003). Transformational leaders tend to engage the emotions of their followers, which leads to trust in the leader's mission, and a sense of empowerment to follow it (Jung & Avolio, 2000). This trusting relationship is developed through four leadership strategies, including charismatic role modelling, individualized consideration, inspirational motivation, and intellectual stimulation (Gumusluoglu & Ilsev 2009). Robbins and Davidhizer (2007) maintain that educating nurse managers in these strategies increases the job satisfaction of staff and leads to a reduction in staff turnover and improved retention. For leaders to be a truly transformational one, they need excellent communication skills and an ability to effectively communicate with a multigenerational workforce. See Table 8-3 for suggestions related to generational leadership strategies.

TABLE 8-3	GENERATIONAL LEADERSHIP STRATEGIES

Leadership Strategies for the Baby Boomers	Leadership Strategies for Generation X	Leadership Strategies for Generation Y (Millennials)
Implement a shared governance model where staff members can contribute to decision making (Malleo & Fusilero, 2008)	Implement a shared governance model where staff members can contribute to decision making (Carver & Candela, 2008)	Implement a shared governance model where staff members can contribute to decision making (Weingarten, 2009)
Provide mentorship or committee head positions that recognize their expertise (Weingarten, 2009)	Cast an exciting vision that motivates (Cordeniz, 2002)	Motivate these nurses with a compelling mission that is inspirationally conveyed and modelled (Piper, 2008)
Offer shorter shifts or part-time work (Carver & Candela, 2008)	Allot generous amounts of one-on-one time (individualize attention) (Weston, 2001)	Foster and environment of teamwork and interdisciplinary care (Piper, 2008; Wieck, Prydun, & Walsh, 2002)
Increase the ergonomic support for aging staff (Carver & Candela, 2008)	Charismatic role modelling as a credible, competent manager (Kupperschmidt, 2000)	Coach rather than direct them towards success (Piper, 2008)
Provide tangible recognition strategies, such as monthly Tim Horton's gift certificates	Provide opportunities for education (Carver & Candela, 2008)	Review their learning needs and ensure that they are met (Piper, 2008)
Expect and articulate benchmarks of performance (Weston, 2001)	Take care not to publicly criticize their performance (Cordeniz, 2002)	

Source: Lobo, V. M. (2010). Transformational leadership to promote cross-generational retention. *Canadian Journal of Nursing Leadership*, 23(2), 21–31.

LEADERSHIP THEORIES

Many believe that the critical factor needed to maximize human resources is leadership (Bennis & Nanus, 1985). A more in-depth understanding of leadership can be gleaned from a review of leadership theories. The major leadership theories can be classified according to the following approaches: behavioural, contingency, and contemporary.

LITERATURE APPLICATION

Citation: Allen, D. W. (1998). How nurses become leaders: Perceptions and beliefs about leadership development. *Journal of Nursing Administration*, 28(9): 15–20.

Discussion: This article presents the factors that influence the development of leadership skills in nurses and the successful transition from a staff nurse role to a leadership role. Twelve registered nurses who had been in leadership positions for 9 to 29 years were interviewed. A core set of questions was used as a guide, followed by additional questions that helped to clarify misunderstanding of the answers provided. The article identifies five dominant factors that greatly influence the nurses' leadership development: (1) self-confidence, (2) innate leader qualities/tendencies, (3) progression of experiences and success, (4) influence

(Continued)

of significant others, and (5) personal life factors. For most of the nurses, at least one individual fostered a sense of self-confidence through reinforcement and positive feedback. Education provided the participants with skills and knowledge that also contributed to their self-confidence. Innate leader qualities, going back as far as childhood, also contributed significantly to their leadership development. For example, most of the interviewed nurses, at some point in their life, were team captains or class officers. According to the author, a pattern of progressively successful experiences also emerged as a significant factor in leadership development. Education, especially when focused on leadership and management, provided the participants with new skills useful in their advancement. Mentors who recognized the strengths of the participants were able to improve their self-confidence and create opportunities for learning. Personal life factors, such as needing to work during the day shift or not being able to perform physically strenuous activities, led some of the participants to pursue nursing leadership and management. The factors that contributed to the development of these nurses were interconnected and promoted their gradual development as leaders.

Implications for Practice: Although many individual and environmental factors contribute to leadership development, each nurse can actively participate in designing and implementing a leadership development plan that facilitates development and enhancement of competence (i.e., from novice to expert). An important avenue of growth involves acquiring a mentor. This is someone who can help create a progression of experiences that develop leadership skills and judgment in working with other people and who can coach a nurse about the importance of examining "the self" aspect of leadership quality. Coaching provides a powerful space between two individuals (i.e., the coach and the coachee), where an honest exploration of needs, motivations, desires, skills, and thought processes can be examined through the use of questioning techniques that facilitate critical thinking. Ultimately, coaching encourages commitment to action and the development of lasting personal growth and change. Pursuing education to learn new skills that involve leadership behaviours and management practices is another excellent way to develop into a nurse leader. Nursing associations, unions, specialty nursing groups, and the Canadian Nursing Students' Association are valuable training grounds for leadership. Nationally, the Canadian Nurses Association (CNA) has facilitated the exchange of knowledge through discussion papers, policy statements, think tanks, and its co-sponsorship of two national conferences: the Nursing Leadership Conference and the Health Care Middle Management Conference. The International Council of Nurses (ICN) also supports leadership development through projects such as its Leadership for Change program. The Dorothy Wylie/Health Leaders Nursing Leadership Institute is a two-part, 7-day interprofessional, residential leadership institute with a variety of speakers, including Barry Posner, and the Five Practices of Exemplary Leaders. These observations suggest the profound importance of leadership training and the need for a multi-level approach, beginning with the individual nurse and moving to a global commitment, such as spearheaded by the ICN. Sharing a desire to change and improve nursing practice with others, through participation in professional nursing associations, is another important vehicle for development as a leader and a professional.

BEHAVIOURAL APPROACHES

Leadership studies from the 1930s by Kurt Lewin and colleagues at Iowa State University conveyed information about three leadership styles that are still widely recognized today: autocratic, democratic, and laissez-faire leadership (Lewin, 1939; Lewin & Lippitt, 1938; Lewin, Lippitt, & White, 1939). **Autocratic leadership** involves centralized decision making, with the leader making decisions and using power to command and control others. **Democratic leadership** is participatory, with authority delegated to others. To be influential, the democratic leader uses expert power and the power base afforded by having close, personal relationships. The third style, **laissez-faire leadership,** is passive and permissive, and the leader defers decision making. Lewin (1939) contrasted these styles and concluded that autocratic leaders are associated with high-performing groups, but that close

supervision is necessary and feelings of hostility are often present. Democratic leaders engendered positive feelings in their groups, and performance was strong, whether or not the leader was present. Low productivity and feelings of frustration were associated with laissez-faire leaders.

Behavioural leadership studies from the University of Michigan and from Ohio State University led to the identification of two basic leader behaviours: job-centred and employee-centred behaviours. Effective leadership was described as having a focus on the human needs of subordinates and was called **employee-centred leadership** (Moorhead & Griffin, 2001). **Job-centred leaders** were seen as less effective because of their focus on schedules, costs, and efficiency, resulting in a lack of attention to developing work groups and high-performance goals (Moorhead & Griffin, 2001).

CRITICAL THINKING

Among the individuals commonly identified as leaders (Table 8-4), can you identify a set of traits that they all possess or traits that are associated with them? Are they perceived as leaders because they are characterized as having intelligence, self-confidence, determination, integrity, and charisma? What other traits do (did) they have?

The researchers at Ohio State focused their efforts on two dimensions of leader behaviour: initiating structure and consideration. **Initiating structure** involves an emphasis on the work to be done, a focus on the task and production. Leaders who focus on initiating structure are concerned with how work is organized and on the achievement of goals. This type of leader behaviour includes planning, directing others, and establishing the deadlines and details of how work is to be done. For example, a nurse demonstrating the leader behaviour of initiating structure could be a charge nurse who, at the beginning of a shift, sets up a client assignment.

The dimension of **consideration** involves activities that focus on the employee and emphasizes relating to and getting along with people. This leader behaviour focuses on the well-being of others. The leader is involved in creating a relationship that fosters communication and trust as a basis for respecting other people and their potential contribution. A nurse who demonstrates consideration takes time to talk with co-workers, be empathetic, and show an interest in others as people.

The leader behaviours related to initiating structure and consideration define leadership styles as follows:

■ low initiating structure, low consideration
■ high initiating structure, low consideration
■ high initiating structure, high consideration
■ low initiating structure, high consideration

The Ohio State University studies associate the high initiating structure–high consideration leader behaviours with better performance and higher satisfaction outcomes than the other styles. This leadership style is considered effective, although it is not appropriate in every situation.

Another model based on these two dimensions is the managerial grid developed by Blake and Mouton (1985). As demonstrated by leaders, five leadership styles identify the extent of structure—called concern for production—and the extent of consideration— called concern for people These styles are (a) the impoverished leader (1,1) for low production and low people concern; (b) the authority compliance leader (9,1) for high production concern and low people concern; (c) the country club leader (1,9) for high people concern but low production concern; (d) the middle-of-the-road leader (5,5) for moderate concern in both dimensions; and (e) the team leader (9,9) for high production and people concern. Figure 8-2 shows the leadership grid with the dimensions of people and production from low to high on a scale from 1 to 9. Team management (9,9) is usually a more effective leadership approach than an overemphasis on either concern for people or concern for production.

TABLE 8-4	LEADERS AMONG US: PAST AND PRESENT
Mother Teresa	Martin Luther King Jr.
Alexander Graham Bell	Sir John A. MacDonald
Chief Dan George	Mahatma Gandhi
Tiger Woods	Terry Fox
Roméo Dallaire	Florence Nightingale
Colin Powell	Pierre Elliott Trudeau
Pope John Paul II	Lester B. Pearson
Chris Hadfield	Joan of Arc
Frances Hesselbein	Julius Caesar
Margaret Thatcher	Alexander the Great
Henry Kissinger	Cleopatra
Nelson Mandela	The Queen
Barack Obama	Michaelle Jean

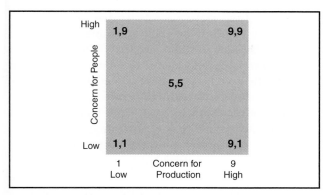

Figure 8-2 Blake, Mouton, and McCanse Leadership Grid
Source: From LUSSIER/ACHUA. *Leadership,* 4E. © 2010 South-Western, a part of Cengage Learning, Inc. Reproduced by permission. www.cengage.com/permissions

CONTINGENCY APPROACHES

Another approach to leadership is **contingency theory.** Contingency theory acknowledges that other factors in the environment influence outcomes as much as leadership style and that leader effectiveness is contingent upon, that is, depends upon, something other than the leader's behaviour. The premise is that different leader behaviour patterns will be effective in different situations. Contingency approaches include Fielder's contingency theory, the situational theory of Hersey and Blanchard, path-goal theory, and the idea of **substitutes for leadership**.

FIELDER'S CONTINGENCY THEORY

Fielder (1967) is credited with the development of the contingency model of leadership effectiveness. Fielder's theory of leadership effectiveness views the pattern of leader behaviour as dependent upon the interaction of the personality of the leader and the needs of the situation. The following factors are involved in the needs of the situation or how favourable the situation is toward the leader: leader–member relationships, degree of task structure, and leader's position of power (Fielder, 1967). **Leader–member relations** are the feelings and attitudes of followers regarding the acceptance, trust, and credibility of the leader. Good leader–member relations exist when followers respect, trust, and have confidence in the leader. Poor leader–member relations reflect distrust, lack of confidence and respect, and dissatisfaction with the leader by the followers.

Task structure refers to the degree to which work is defined, with specific procedures, explicit directions, and measurable goals. High task structure involves routine, predictable, clearly defined work tasks. Low task structure involves work that is not routine, predictable, or clearly defined, such as creative, artistic, or qualitative research activities.

Position power is the degree of formal authority and influence associated with the leader. High position power is favourable for the leader, whereas low position power

is unfavourable. When all of these dimensions—leader–member relations, task structure, and position power—are high, the situation is favourable to the leader. When these dimensions are low, the situation is not favourable to the leader. In both of these circumstances, Fielder showed that a task-directed leader concerned with task accomplishment was effective. When the range of favourableness is intermediate or moderate, a human relations leader who is concerned about people is most effective. These situations need interpersonal and relationship skills to foster group achievement. Fielder's contingency theory is an approach that matches the organizational situation to the most favourable leadership style for that situation.

HERSEY AND BLANCHARD'S SITUATIONAL THEORY

Situational leadership theory addresses follower characteristics in relation to effective leader behaviour. Whereas Blake and Mouton focus on leader style and Fielder examines the situation, Hersey and Blanchard consider follower readiness as a factor in determining leadership style. Rather than using the words *initiating structure* and *contingency*, they use *task behaviour* and *relationship behaviour.*

High task behaviour and low relationship behaviour is called a telling leadership style. A high task, high relationship style is called a selling leadership style. A low task and high relationship style is called a participating leadership style. A low task and low relationship style is called a delegating leadership style.

Nurse leaders assess follower-readiness: also called job maturity. Then it is possible for them to select from the four leadership styles the one that is appropriate for a given situation. Consequently, nursing leaders must be able to assess the job maturity levels of individual nurses and match the leadership style of the nurse to the context of the situation. Regardless of an individual staff member's maturity level, some situations require the leader to adopt a telling style, as is the case with situations involving client safety or significant infractions of professional standards or practice regulations. According to Hersey and Blanchard's situational leadership theory (2000), groups with low maturity, whose members are unable or unwilling to participate or are unsure, need a leader to use a telling leadership style to provide direction and close supervision. This same style serves preceptors well, as they take on largely instructional roles with new graduates who have a limited basis of clinical experiences and are still working to master clinical competencies.

The selling leadership style is a match for groups with a low to moderate level of maturity, specifically, those unable but willing and confident and need clear direction and supportive feedback to get the task done. This type of leadership style may serve nurse leaders well in their efforts to launch new programs or revamp care-delivery processes. The selling style serves the nurse leader well in promoting and developing professional practice among nurses at the advanced beginner or competent levels, as described by Benner (1984). Participating is the leadership style recommended for groups that have a moderate to high level of maturity, that are able—but unwilling or unsure—and that need support and encouragement. The leader should use a delegating style with groups of followers with high maturity who are able and ready to participate and can engage in the task without direction or support. Nurses who have developed their practice, within their chosen domain, to proficient and expert levels demonstrate both ability and willingness. They may benefit from a delegational leadership style from their nurse managers.

An additional aspect of this model is the idea that the leader not only changes leadership style according to the followers' needs but also develops followers over time to increase their level of maturity (Lussier & Achua, 2001). Use of these four leadership styles helps a nurse manager to appropriately assign work to others and provide a trajectory for individual professional development.

PATH-GOAL THEORY   In this leadership approach, the leader works to motivate followers and influence goal accomplishment. The seminal author on path-goal theory is Robert House (1971). By using the appropriate style of leadership for the situation (i.e., directive, supportive, participative, or achievement-oriented), the leader makes the path toward the goal easier for the follower. The directive style of leadership provides structure through direction and authority, with the leader focusing on the task and getting the job done. The supportive style of leadership is relationship-oriented, with the leader providing encouragement, interest, and attention. Participative leadership means that the leader focuses on involving followers in the decision-making process. The achievement-oriented style provides high structure and direction as well as high support through consideration behaviour. The leadership style is matched to the situational characteristics of the followers: for example, the desire for authority, the extent to which the control of goal achievement is internal or external, and the ability of the follower to be involved. The leadership style is also matched to the situational factors in the environment, including the routine nature or complexity of the task, the power associated with the leader's position, and the work-group relationship. This alignment of leadership style with the needs of followers is motivating and is believed to enhance performance and satisfaction. The path-goal theory is based on expectancy theory, which holds that people are motivated when they believe they are able to carry out the work, and when they think their contribution will lead to the expected outcome, and that the rewards for their efforts are valued and meaningful (Northouse, 2001).

SUBSTITUTES FOR LEADERSHIP   Certain variables may influence followers to the same extent as the leader's behaviour. Kerr and Jermier (1978) investigated situational variables and identified some substitutes that eliminate the need for leader behaviour and also neutralizers that nullify the effects of the leader's behaviour.

Some of these variables include follower characteristics, such as the presence of structured routine tasks, the amount of feedback provided by the task, and the presence of intrinsic satisfaction in the work; other variables include organizational characteristics, such as the presence of a cohesive group, a formal organization, a rigid adherence to rules, and low position power. For example, an individual's experience can substitute for task-direction leader behaviour (Kerr & Jermier, 1978). Nurses and other professionals with a great deal of experience already have knowledge and judgment and do not need direction and supervision to perform their work. Thus, their experience serves as a leadership substitute. Another substitute for leader behaviour is intrinsic satisfaction that emerges from just doing the work. Intrinsic satisfaction occurs frequently among nurses when they provide care to clients and their families. Intrinsic satisfaction substitutes for the support and encouragement of relationship-oriented leader behaviour.

CONTEMPORARY APPROACHES

Contemporary approaches to leadership address the leadership functions necessary to develop learning organizations and lead the process of transforming change. These approaches include charismatic leadership and transformational leadership theory.

CHARISMATIC THEORY   A charismatic leader has an inspirational quality that promotes an emotional connection from followers. House (1977) developed a theory of charismatic leadership that describes how charismatic leaders behave, their distinguishing characteristics, and situations in which such leaders would be effective. Charismatic leaders display self-confidence and strength in their convictions, and communicate high expectations and their confidence in others. They have been described as emerging during a crisis, communicating vision, and using personal power and unconventional strategies (Conger & Kanungo, 1987). One consequence of this type of leadership is a belief in the charismatic leader that is so strong it takes on an almost supernatural purpose, and the leader is worshipped as if superhuman. Worship can take both positive and negative forms. Examples of charismatic leaders who have been worshipped by some include Martin Luther King Jr., Sir Winston Churchill, and Jim Jones.

Charismatic leaders can have a positive and powerful effect on people and organizations. Lee Iacocca, former chief executive officer (CEO) of Chrysler Corporation, and Herb Kelleher, the former CEO of Southwest

Airlines, are described as effective charismatic leaders. This type of leader can contribute significantly to an organization, even though all the leaders in an organization are not charismatic leaders and effective leaders do not exhibit all the qualities associated with charismatic leadership. Charisma seems to be a special and valuable quality that some people have and some people do not. Whether charismatic or not, leaders must be self-confident, energetic, knowledgeable, articulate, passionate, and honest. These are just a few of the traits of charismatic leaders, and although not all effective leaders are charismatic, many have integrated various charismatic traits into their leadership style. This approach is critical to success, given today's complex and chaotic practice environments.

TRANSFORMATIONAL LEADERSHIP THEORY

Burns defined transformational leadership as a process in which "leaders and followers raise one another to higher levels of motivation and morality" (Burns, 1978, p. 21). Transformational leadership theory is based on the idea of empowering others to engage in pursuing a collective purpose by working together to achieve a vision of a preferred future. This kind of leadership can influence both the leader and the follower to a higher level of conduct and achievement that transforms them both (Burns, 1978). Burns maintained that there are two types of leaders: the traditional manager concerned with day-to-day operations, called the **transactional leader,** and the leader who is committed to a vision that empowers others, called the **transformational leader.**

Transformational leaders motivate others by behaving in accordance with values, providing a vision that reflects mutual values, and empowering others to contribute. Bennis and Nanus (1985) describe this new leader as a leader who "commits people to action, who converts followers into leaders, and who converts leaders into agents of change" (p. 3). According to research by Tichy and Devanna (1986), effective transformational leaders identify themselves as change agents; are courageous; believe in people; are value-driven; are lifelong learners; have the ability to deal with complexity, ambiguity, and uncertainty; and are visionaries. Transformational leadership may be demonstrated by anyone in an organization regardless of a person's position (Burns, 1978). The interaction that occurs between individuals can be transformational and motivate both the leader and the follower to a higher level of performance (Bass, 1985).

Significant, systemic change requires specific and intentional efforts from the leaders tasked with carrying out transformational activities.[4]

At the organizational level, transformational leadership is concerned with innovation and change. The transformational leader uses a vision based on shared values to align people and inspire growth and advancement. Both

LITERATURE APPLICATION

Citation: Raymond, G., & Walton, M. (2011). Enabling transformational change: The Ontario Shores experience. *Healthcare Quarterly*, 14(1): 56–61. Reprinted with Permission.

Discussion: This case study outlines key considerations for health care organizations experiencing significant transformational change, based on the experience of Ontario Shores Centre for Mental Health Sciences (Ontario Shores), formerly Whitby Mental Health Centre. Significant systemic change requires specific and intentional efforts from transformational leaders. This article presents the perspectives of leaders involved in the transformation of Ontario Shores as it moved from a government-based agency to a stand-alone specialty psychiatric hospital in 2006. During this time several conventional strategies were applied to manage the transition, but various critical approaches also emerged that assisted the organization to effect significant change and achieve marked improvements in key areas.

Implications for Practice: Significant systemic change requires specific and intentional efforts from the leaders who have to transform an organization. This case study demonstrated that Ontario Shores found great success in carrying out several conventional change management strategies to manage the transition. At the same time, other critical strategies were discovered to assist in making significant organizational change. This example demonstrates the importance of effective transformational leadership.

the inspiration and the empowerment aspects of transformational leadership lead to a commitment beyond self-interest, a commitment to a vision, and a commitment to action that creates change. Transformational leadership theory suggests that the relationship between the leader and the follower inspires and empowers an individual toward a commitment to the organization.

Nurse researchers have described nurse executives according to transformational leadership theory and have used this theory to measure leadership behaviour among nurse executives and nurse managers (Dunham & Klafehn, 1990; Dunham-Taylor, 1995, 2000; Leach, 2000; McDaniel & Wolf, 1992; McNeese-Smith, 1995; Trofino, 1995; Wolf, Boland, & Aukerman, 1994; Young, 1992). Additionally, transformational leadership theory has been the basis for nursing administration curricula and for investigation of relationships such as between a nurse's commitment to an organization and productivity in a hospital setting (Leach, 2000; McNeese-Smith, 1997; Searle, 1996). Cassidy and Koroll (1998) explore the ethical aspects of transformational leadership, and Barker (1990) comprehensively discusses nursing in terms of transformational leadership theory. Gullo & Gerstle (2004) co-authored a descriptive study of transformational leadership and hospital restructuring. Raymond and Walton (2011) describe a transformational change that occurred in the mental health hospital environment. Of the contemporary theories of leadership, transformational leadership is a popular approach in nursing.

KOUZES AND POSNER'S FIVE LEADERSHIP PRACTICES

Kouzes and Posner's five leadership practices continue to gain popularity as a leadership model that underpins many leadership development training programs. Kouzes has found that people look for four characteristics in a leader. "First, people want a leader who is honest, trustworthy and has integrity. Second, people also want a leader who is forward looking, who has a vision of the future, foresight and thinks about the long term. Third, people want a leader who is competent, has expertise, knows what they are doing and last, is inspiring, dynamic, energetic, optimistic and positive about the future" (Kouzes & Posner, 2002). The five practices defined by Kouzes and Posner are (1) model the way, (2) inspire a shared vision, (3) challenge the process, (4) enable others to act, and (5) encourage the heart. Modelling the way is about being authentic and true to your values and aligning actions with shared values. Inspiring a shared vision focuses the leader's attention to envision the future by imagining exciting and enabling possibilities and by enlisting others so that the vision becomes common to all and appeals to the notion of shared aspirations. Challenging the process calls upon and highlights the leader's sense of self, courage, risk-taking, and emotional intelligence, as the leader searches for ways to change, grow, and improve. Although difficult, it is necessary to challenge established processes, especially if that process is not in the best interests of professional practice and client-focused care. Enabling others to act is a transformational activity associated with quality leadership. This activity requires the manager to foster collaboration by promoting cooperative goals and building trust. In addition, the leader must strengthen individuals by sharing power and discretion (e.g., sharing decision making, delegating, critical thinking, and professional

judgment). This requirement is pivotal to the success of interprofessional practice teams.

Given the theories of motivation, Kouzes and Posner wrap up the five leadership practices with a commitment to encourage the heart. To create and sustain the effects of quality leadership, leaders must recognize the contributions of individuals by showing appreciation for individual excellence. Although many leaders ascribe to the current axiom, "there is no I in the word team," a fine balance exists between the need for individual and team recognition. Finally, encouraging the heart takes the form of celebrations of success and fostering a spirit of community. Collectively, these five practices comprise what Kouzes and Posner call the "leadership challenge."

NURSING LEADERSHIP AND OUTCOMES

Snow (2001) commented that nursing has not kept pace with other industries in exploring the relationship between leadership and performance. The complexity of client care environments, and the number of uncontrollable factors that exist, may affect the ability of nursing researchers to design quality research initiatives that examine true cause-and-effect relationships between leadership and outcomes.

George et al. (2002) examined how the implementation of a shared leadership model influenced staff leadership behaviours and autonomy, and improved client outcomes. The intervention took the form of an educational series called the shared leadership concept program (SLCP), which consisted of four 8-hour-day modules delivered over a period of two months. George and colleagues carried out three studies between 1995 and 1999 using different research designs; the final one used a qualitative design with key information interviews. Interviews were conducted at three, six, and twelve months following the SLCP. According to the three key findings (1) nurses saw that leadership behaviour improves their ability to meet client needs and promote faster recovery; (2) the barriers to using leadership skills include increased workloads, boring work, insufficient goal setting by managers, high turnover, and lack of responsibility; and (3) nurses were more assertive in addressing the barriers after they completed the program.

An important study described by Houser (2003) used both qualitative and quantitative approaches to examine the contextual factors influencing the delivery of nursing care. Thematic analysis of the interviews demonstrated that excellent communication skills, problem-solving skills, and an ability to articulate clear expectations are the most common desirable leadership traits. The most exciting findings derive from the quantitative component that used the Leadership Practices Inventory (LPI), developed by Kouzes and Posner. Key findings suggest a positive relationship between strong leadership and staff expertise and stability, and an inverse relationship between strong levels of expertise and negative client outcomes: such as hospital-acquired pneumonia and urinary tract infections, mortality, medication errors, and client falls. This study suggests strong committed leaders are required to develop professional leadership skills among staff and to guide professional development to impact positively on the expertise of staff.

Anderson, Issel, and McDaniel (2003) also made a significant contribution to the understanding of the relationship between leadership and client outcomes. Their research in a long-term care environment focused on perceptions of open communication and participation in decision making. The client outcomes measure the following: resident behaviour, immobility complications, fractures, and restraint use. Correlations existed between larger facilities with experienced directors of nursing (DONs) who had good communication skills and a lower use of restraints. Experienced DONs with more experience and greater relationship-oriented leadership had a lower prevalence of complications associated with immobility. Finally, organizations with a relationship-oriented leader had a lower prevalence of fractures. Based on the work of these three nursing researchers, a relationship between nursing leadership and client outcomes has been demonstrated. However, further research is required to fully appreciate the extent of the relationship.

The emergence of the magnet-hospital concept as originally described by Kramer and Schmalenberg (1988) has been significant in helping nurse researchers to examine the relationship between leadership and nurse outcomes. Nurse outcomes include control over practice, autonomy, a culture of valuing nurses, and job satisfaction. The relationship between leadership and nurse outcomes has been supported in research work in both magnet and non-magnet hospitals (Aiken et al., 2001). A significant positive relationship between head nurses exhibiting transformational leadership style and job satisfaction was demonstrated in a descriptive study by Medley and Larochelle (1995). Twenty-first century nurse administrators and executive leaders must expand their understanding of leadership to encompass the needs of large, multiprofessional teams that may include many categories of health professionals and other human resources working across multiple settings.[5] Aiken and colleagues noted that having fewer frontline nurse administrators significantly impacts frontline staff because there is no one to articulate and reinforce the mission of the organization, nor anyone to provide a timely response to concerns of frontline caregivers. Aiken's five-country study found that significant numbers of novice nurses under the age of

30 intended to leave their jobs the following year; intent to leave is associated with actual increases in turnover. As a result, the relationship between nursing administration and leadership and organizational outcomes can be profound. Laschinger et al. (1999) implemented a descriptive study in a recently merged health care facility and explored the link between leader-empowering behaviours and staff nurse perceptions of workplace empowerment. Results suggest that staff believed their sense of workplace empowerment, job tensions, and judgment of their ability to get their work completed were related to the manager's use of empowering behaviours.

Kouzes and Posner's five leadership behaviours and their impact on job satisfaction, productivity, and commitment were examined by Chiok Foong Loke (2001). Statistically significant differences were found between the managers' use of the five behaviours and employee outcomes of satisfaction, productivity, and organizational commitment. Kramer and Schmalenberg (2003) identified that clinical competence supports autonomous practice and that leadership is essential to facilitate personal growth opportunities, which enhance maintenance of competence. McGillis Hall et al. (2001) demonstrated a statistically significant positive relationship between leadership and job satisfaction and a statistically negative influence on nurses' perception of job stress, role tension, and job pressure.

Nursing needs to be led by nurse executives who sit at the highest decision-making tables and have fiscal authority over clinical programs. Otherwise, the collective voices of nurses are diminished, and clinical leadership is compromised even further.

A study by Laschinger et al. (2008) describes the profile of nursing leadership structures in Canada and assessed the relationships among structures, processes, and outcomes related to nurse leaders' work. The results of the study reveal that the then contingent of nursing leaders in Canada saw themselves as an empowered and influential group within their organizations. Although they had very large spans of control, the nurse leaders at all levels were positive about their work life and confident in their ability to provide effective nursing leadership in their facility. They averaged 49 years of age, highlighting the need for succession planning.

FUTURE DIRECTIONS

The organizations that nurses are a part of are constantly changing, and care delivery is increasing in its acuity and complexity. As a discipline, nursing is challenged to discover innovative and effective ways to plan, implement, and evaluate care. The promise of transformational leadership, new knowledge management, and clinical-care technologies will help us to perform our work both effectively and efficiently, and will result in positive client outcomes.

Peter Drucker (1994) identifies the organization of the future as a knowledge organization composed of knowledge workers. Knowledge workers are those people who bring specialized, expert knowledge to an organization, and are valued for what they know. The knowledge organization will share and provide the information necessary to work efficiently and effectively, and help it grow. Drucker says that knowledge organizations, in which the knowledge worker is on the front lines with the expertise and the information to act, will become the dominant organizational type (Drucker, 1994; Helgesen, 1995).

This description suggests that health care organizations are likely to be prime examples of knowledge-based organizations and will require a fundamental commitment to leadership development and knowledge management. In organizations such as these, the ideas that leadership is at the top and is equated with the power of a position are obsolete notions. Workers with the expertise and information to act are the organization's leaders. They provide the service, interact with the customer, represent the organization, and accomplish its goals. Effective nursing leadership is important in all nursing roles. Every worker will play a role in fulfilling the purpose of the organization and, in so doing, will be both a leader and a follower. This future direction will challenge all nurses to assess, develop, and continually appraise and enhance their personal leadership competencies, style, and effectiveness.

The expectation of clients and health care providers that care will be as safe as possible is not going away. Safety and reduction in adverse events are priorities of senior executive and information technology specialists. Both clients and health care providers will expect that data be readily shared across settings and be available at the point of care. Technology will prompt health care practitioners to do the right thing and help prevent mistakes. Public reporting will increase.

Cost pressures will force health care organizations to become more efficient. Organizations will need to find new ways of doing things. Leaders will have to address issues such as skill-mix change, the use of alternative roles in the delivery of health care (such as physician assistants, nurse practitioners, first assists), and new models of care delivery. Organizations will employ hospitalists to integrate consistency into the hospital. Clients themselves will become more involved in "self-care." New technology makes self-monitoring safe and effective for many diseases.

Cost and quality transparency will be demanded by all. Quality measures will increase and outcomes will be public. These demands require that leadership is transformational. It is unacceptable to constantly "put out fires." Proactivity is essential. Leaders need to continually "see the big picture," scan the environment, gather data by talking to people, recognize emerging trends, "connect the dots," strategize to shape and enable innovations or change, and test novel ideas (calculated risk-taking) (Shaver, 2005).

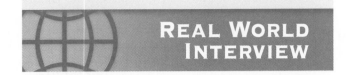

REAL WORLD INTERVIEW

Personal growth demands a lot of hard, conscious thinking. But it also involves the emergence of deeply buried feelings, revelations about oneself that are startling and unexpected. Know thyself is the name of the game, maturity is the result.

Betty Oliphant
Founder, National Ballet School of Canada

According to the Public Health Agency of Canada (PHAC), the state of rural health care is in sharp contrast to its urban counterpart. The health of rural Canadians has evidently reached a low status; overall, rural residents exhibit less healthy behaviours, such as smoking, reduced physical activity, shorter life expectancy, and higher mortality rates (PHAC, 2006). Nursing leaders need to be aware of rural health issues, and support increased access to health care for the rural communities.

THE NEW LEADERSHIP

Margaret Wheatley, in *Leadership and the New Science* (1992), says, "There is a simpler way to lead organizations, one that requires less effort and produces less stress than the current practices" (p. 3). She presents a new view of leadership, one encompassing connectedness and self-organizing systems that follow a natural order of both chaos and uncertainty, which is different from the linear order in a hierarchy. The leader's function is to guide an organization using vision, to make choices based on mutual values, and to engage in the culture to provide meaning and coherence. This type of leadership fosters growth within each of us as individuals and as members of a group. The notion of connection within a self-organizing system optimizes autonomy at all levels because the relationships between the individual and the whole are strong (Wheatley, 1992). Effective interprofessional collaboration in health care settings is essential. Federal policy and funding agencies have focused efforts on promoting interprofessional practice by using new technologies. A study by Russell et al. (2005) presented positive evidence of using computer technology to support teamwork and interprofessional collaboration in practice settings.

For nursing, such systems might be the infrastructure that will foster interprofessional decision making and strengthen the connection with non-professional workers. New possibilities may emerge that help nursing move away from dependence on numbers of staff, numbers of client care hours, cost and volume productivity

CASE STUDY 8-1

Sharon, a licensed practical nurse, was making rounds on her new client admitted to the continuing complex care unit. The client was a 95-year-old woman who had sustained a fall at home. Following three days of immobility on a hard surface, the client presented with a sacral pressure ulcer. On assessment of the client, Sharon noted the pressure ulcer was being managed with saline wet-to-dry dressings. On changing the dressing, Sharon found the ulcer was covered with necrotic tissue. Sharon immediately took a swab of the area, which returned positive for Methicillin-Resistant *Staphylococcus aureus* (MRSA) and *Streptococcus*. She contacted the most responsible physician and presented a clear picture of the wound, and recommended debridement of the wound and consideration of topical negative pressure. A surgical consult was ordered by the physician, and surgical debridement was completed on day 4 following admission. Topical negative pressure was applied following consultation with the enterostomal therapist. On day 6 post-intervention granulation tissue was reported in the wound, and by day 11, the wound length and width had decreased by more than half and the depth decreased by 1.0 cm. The client was discharged to a long-term care facility with a completely closed wound.

What leadership characteristics did this licensed practical nurse demonstrate?

Why is leadership important at all levels throughout a health care organization?

How can a nurse develop this type of leadership skill?

measures, and the tools of both an industrial age and Newton's physics toward the new science focused on naturally occurring events, wholeness, and interaction.

GENERATIONAL LEADERSHIP ISSUES

Organizations have become more complex, and nursing's systems and ways of leadership must keep pace with the

complexities and the advances of a highly technological, information-driven environment. Leadership will emerge from teams that self-organize and self-direct (Avolio, 1999). Organizational teams will become diverse, both racially and ethnically, but also because different generations will participate in the workforce simultaneously.

The generation known as the baby boomers, born between 1946 and 1964, will work with different

REAL WORLD INTERVIEW

Clinical nurses have a role to play in guiding corporate decision making related to clinical practice. We teach students to be critical thinkers and agents for change, and encourage each nurse to use leadership skills, yet we fail to take advantage of these skills. Even today, when we think of leadership, we refer mostly to formal positions. Strict procedures, such as those in program management models that emphasize the bottom line, risk turning nursing leaders into generic executives. We need to evolve a model that replaces top-down hierarchies and linear reporting structures with teams of individual professionals who work in a fluid matrix. All nurses need to play a role in interprofessional teams to keep the nursing profession visible and active in decisions for client care. Rethinking approaches to leadership also means thinking about how to prepare nurses for their roles as future leaders. Each one of us should engage in this kind of creative thinking and not just leave it to schools of nursing, health care agencies, or nursing associations and unions. By sharing and debating our ideas and bringing them into the policy arena, we can also demonstrate a vital aspect of leadership.

Dr. Ginette L. Rodger
Vice President Professional Practice and Chief Nursing Executive,
The Ottawa Hospital, Ottawa

Source: Dr. Ginette L. Rodger, Vice President Professional Practice and Chief Nursing Executive, The Ottawa Hospital, Ottawa age-related groups, such as the baby-buster generation—also known as Generation X or Gen-Exers—born between 1965 and 1981 (Moats Kennedy, 1998). According to Moats Kennedy, the boomers and busters exhibit different values about work, motivation, lifestyle, and communication. For example, boomers tend to demonstrate loyalty to an employer, whereas busters regularly change organizations to advance their development. Additionally, busters have a more individual approach to work and tend to value a balanced work–family lifestyle more than boomers, who tend to work hard and emphasize money and acquiring possessions. Such different styles reveal differences in how learning occurs, and also the methods best suited for busters, who are computer skilled and comfortable with high-tech tools, compared to boomers, who tend to prefer more personalized training methods.

Research among nurses reveals that contrasting feelings about work, job tenure, and work behaviours can generate conflict and stress across these generations. For example, some boomers hold negative views about the degree of commitment and the self-centred focus exhibited by busters (Santos & Cox, 2000). Within a team-based approach to organizational work, leadership development must embrace an understanding of generational differences and support the idea of maximizing the strengths of boomers, busters, and the most recent group, generation nexters, born between 1980 and 2000.

REAL WORLD INTERVIEW

Leadership in nursing is probably one of the more personal forms of leadership. Nursing is one of the most intimate leadership relationships because of the vulnerability the client brings to the relationship. For clients who are dying or in terrible situations, the nurse provides two vital leadership characteristics: optimism and courage. For clients who have lost their courage, it is the nurse who shows courage and strength that supports the client and their family. Optimism and courage are the trademarks of great leaders. Nurses lead the client, their family, their nurse colleagues, and other health care providers. They have the courage to care in the face of fear and uncertainty, and in the face of disability or in death. Caring, hope, and support are a source of optimism that nurses provide. There are very few professions where you touch an individual's life so profoundly.

Jay Conger, PhD
Author, Learning to Lead

NURSING LEADERSHIP AND MANAGEMENT: THE LINK

This chapter has set out a clear distinction between leadership and management and also provided an overview of the direct and proximate theories that underpin these concepts.

Over the past two decades nursing has responded to changing technological and social forces that affect health care organizations. The response has required managers to develop new competencies related to the business of health care, including financial and marketing skills.

Providing care in a situation of diminished resources has meant that managers need to possess excellent leadership skills, which are critical to effective team building in organizations. Successful team building is associated with successful recruitment, retaining a cohesive staff, and maintaining high-quality practice. Stout-Shaffer and Larrabee (1992) have identified the hallmarks of the new paradigm in health care organizations as semiautonomous work units, empowerment of all, trust, intuition and creativity, and planning with clients.

The relationship between management and leadership is a rich source for debate among theorists. Tranbarger (1998) asserts that leadership is one of many functions of the manager's role; however, the contrary view is expressed by Gardner (1986), who contends that leadership requires more skills and, as a result, management is but one role of leadership. The notion that a manager guides, directs, and motivates, and that leaders empower others was described by Manthey (1990), who claims that every manager should be a leader. Bennis and Nanus (1985) are well known for their differentiation between managers and leaders, as in their assertion that "managers are people who do things right and leaders are people who do the right thing," which has become a mantra in leadership and management development courses. Marquis and Huston (1996) contend that strong management skills have been valued more than strong leadership skills in health care, which may be in keeping with the shift to more business management models, such as program management. Marquis postulates that leadership and management have a symbiotic or synergistic relationship. The synergistic notion suggests that the two concepts must be integrated so that the effective application of both skill sets results in dynamic management and inspirational leadership. Both are required to steward professional development, job satisfaction, and navigate change. Gardner (1990) suggests that individuals who have integrated both skill sets can be distinguished from traditional managers. Following are their distinguishing traits: (1) they think longer term; (2) they look outward to the larger organization; (3) they influence others beyond their own group; (4) they emphasize vision, values, and motivation; (5) they are politically astute; and (6) they think in terms of change and renewal.

The fundamental challenge within nursing is to determine the entry-to-practice leadership and management competencies and then to ensure that basic undergraduate programs and continuing nursing education programs are focused on those competencies. At the end of the day, clients have a right to quality care, delivered within safe and effective care environments. Nursing leaders and managers have an obligation to create, maintain, and enhance those care environments. In pursing effective leadership and management, and achievement of a voice in strategic organizational planning, individual nurses and the discipline as a whole must persevere and remain determined.

Judith Shamian (2011) wrote in an article in *Nursing Leadership* that we are starting to see a new breed of leader: the clinician executive. These are individuals who have previously held leadership positions; have developed competencies that were not taught in their basic education, such as finance, economics, LEAN health care and project management; and whose career path has taken them to the top position in the organization—the CEO. She believes that this type of leader is best suited to lead the health system transformation in the future.

REAL WORLD INTERVIEW

Nothing in the world can take the place of persistence. Talent will not; nothing is more common than unsuccessful men with talent. Genius will not; unrewarded genius is almost a proverb. Education alone will not; the world is full of educated derelicts. Persistence and determination alone are omnipotent.

Calvin Coolidge
30th President of the United States

Client-centred care is a concept that clinician executives know well: they know the processes and issues that arise in the frontline world of the clinicians. They understand the "players" in the system. "Healthcare organizations have a duty to create professional development opportunities for those clinicians who are willing to take on the challenge of embarking on the executive track."[6]

KEY CONCEPTS

- Leadership is the fuel needed to sustain nursing through a constant evolution of care-delivery systems.

- Nurses are leaders and make a difference to health care organizations through their contributions of expert knowledge and leadership. Leadership development is critical to developing knowledge workers.

- Leaders provide vision, inspire, and encourage. Change in health care organizations occurs because leaders value creativity and innovation.

- Management is a process used to achieve organizational goals. It involves the management functions of planning, leading, organizing, and controlling.

- Motivation is an internal process that contributes to our behaviour in an effort to satisfy our needs. Maslow's hierarchy of needs reflects the belief that the needs that motivate us have an order, and lower-level needs have to be satisfied first or we will not be motivated to address higher-level needs. Herzberg's two-factor theory of motivation identifies maintenance factors, such as security and salary, which are needed to prevent job dissatisfaction; whereas motivators, such as development and opportunities to advance, contribute to job satisfaction.

- Leadership is a process of influence that involves the leader, the follower, and their interaction. Followers can be individual practitioners, professional groups, or interprofessional practice communities, and members of society in general. Leadership can be formal and informal, and occurs in a position of authority in an organization, such as the chief nursing officer, or outside the scope of a formal role, such as individual practitioners.

- Leadership and management are different. Management refers to the strategic actions used to achieve organizational goals; leadership is the effort to envision, inspire, and facilitate change. Current thinking suggests that individuals need to develop competencies in both leadership and management. The resulting synergy facilitates the promotion of professional practice and safe client care at the individual practitioner and discipline level.

- Future directions for nurses in organizations will be influenced by technology and by the need for communities of practice and effective knowledge-management structures and processes. Nursing leadership in the future will be needed at all levels within an organization, not just at the top or from managers. Every knowledge worker with specialized knowledge and expertise will be both a leader and a follower in knowledge organizations.

- Organizations are being viewed as self-organizing systems in which, initially, what looks like chaos and uncertainty is indeed part of a larger coherence and a natural order. Such a living system, when understood better by participants, will be a less stressful and more holistic environment in which to work.

■ Work teams are becoming generationally diverse as more baby boomers are working alongside younger generations, called baby busters or Gen-Exers. Busters are less concerned with loyalty to an organization but value balance in their personal and work life. Boomers show commitment to their employer, work hard, and are motivated by financial rewards. These differences can be a source of stress among nurses.

KEY TERMS

administrative principles	leader–member relations
autocratic leadership	leadership
bureaucratic organization	maintenance or hygiene
client-centred care	factors
consideration	management
contingency theory	management process
democratic leadership	motivation
emotional intelligence	motivation factors
employee-centred leadership	position power
formal leadership	substitutes for leadership
Hawthorne effect	task structure
human relations movement	Theory X
informal leader	Theory Y
initiating structure	Theory Z
job-centred leaders	transactional leader
knowledge workers	transformational
laissez-faire leadership	leader

REVIEW QUESTIONS

1. Why is leadership development important for nurses if they are not in a management or formal leadership position?
   A. It is not really important for nurses.
   B. Leadership is important at all levels in an organization because nurses have expert knowledge and are interacting with and influencing the client.
   C. Nurse leaders leave their jobs sooner for other positions.
   D. Nurses who lead are less satisfied in their jobs.

2. As a process used today by nurses or nurse managers in health care organizations, which of the following best describes management?
   A. scientific management
   B. decision making
   C. commanding and controlling others, using hierarchical authority
   D. planning, organizing, coordinating, and controlling

3. Motivation is related to whatever influences our choices. What factors did Herzberg say would motivate workers and lead to job satisfaction?
   A. being offered a substantial bonus when being hired
   B. realizing that no one ever gets fired from the organization and that job security is high
   C. having good relationships with colleagues and supervisors
   D. being offered opportunities for development and advancement

4. Which of the following defines leadership?
   A. being in a leadership position with authority to exert control and power over subordinates
   B. a process of interaction in which the leader influences others toward goal achievement
   C. managing complexity
   D. being self-confident and democratic

5. According to Hersey and Blanchard and House, a participative leadership style is appropriate for which of the following employees?
   A. those who are not able to get the task done and are less mature
   B. those who are able to contribute to decisions about getting the work done
   C. those who are unable and unwilling to participate
   D. those who need direction, structure, and authority

6. According to Kouzes and Posner's model, leadership is founded upon five practices.

   True or False

7. The quality of leadership is linked to nurse and client outcomes.

   True or False

8. Which of the following is *not* an example of emotional intelligence (EI)?
   A. appraising and expressing emotions in self and others
   B. integrating emotions into thought processes
   C. understanding emotions
   D. intelligence quotient

9. Which of the following is *not* a characteristic of growing nurse leaders?
   A. refraining from building strategic relationships
   B. seizing opportunities for change
   C. practising personal accountability
   D. advocating for safe, effective, and ethical client care

10. The Canadian Nurses Association's position statement on leadership emphasizes that nurses in all domains and at all levels must maximize their leadership potential.

    True or False

Very important 5		Somewhat important 3	Not important 1		
	4		**2**		

_____	1. an interesting job I enjoy doing
_____	2. a good manager who treats people fairly
_____	3. getting praise and other recognition and appreciation for the work I do
_____	4. a satisfying personal life at the job
_____	5. the opportunity for advancement
_____	6. a prestigious or status job
_____	7. job responsibility that gives me freedom to do things my way
_____	8. good working conditions (safe environment, nice office, cafeteria)
_____	9. the opportunity to learn new things
_____	10. sensible company rules, regulations, procedures, and policies
_____	11. a job I can do well and succeed at
_____	12. job security and benefits

Motivating factors	Maintenance factors
1. _____	2. _____
3. _____	4. _____
5. _____	6. _____
7. _____	8. _____
9. _____	10. _____
11. _____	12. _____
Totals _____	_____

Source: Lussier, R. N., & Achua, C. F. (2001). Lussier, R. N., & Achua, C. F. (2001). *Leadership: Theory, Application, Skill Development* (pp. 15–16). Cincinnati, OH: South-Western College Publishing.

REVIEW ACTIVITIES

1. Take the opportunity to learn about yourself by reflecting on the five predominant factors identified as being influential in a nurse's leadership development: self-confidence, innate leader qualities or tendencies, progression of experiences and success, influence of significant others, and personal life factors. Consider the factors that reinforce confidence in yourself. What innate qualities or tendencies do you have that contribute to your development as a leader? Consider what professional experiences, mentors, and personal experiences or events can help you influence and change nursing practice.

2. Describe the type of leader you want to be as a nurse in a health care organization. Identify specific behaviours you plan to use as a leader. In what way are the theories of transformational leadership and the charismatic leadership useful to your development as a leader?

3. Rate each of these 12 job factors that contribute to job satisfaction by placing a number from 1 to 5 on the line before each factor.

Write the number from 1 to 5 that you selected for each factor. Total each column for a score between 6 and 30 points. The closer to 30 your score is, the more important these factors (motivating or maintenance) are to you.

EXPLORING THE WEB

- Emerging Leader: *http://www.emergingleader.com*

- Leadership Directories: Who's who in leadership in Canada: *http://www.sources.com*

- National Quality Institute Leadership Excellence Program: *http://www.nqi.ca* (National Quality Institute became Excellence Canada in November 2011).

- Dorothy M. Wylie Nursing Leadership Institute: *http://dwnli.ca/*

- Indigenous Leadership Development Institute Inc.: *http://ildii.ca/*

- Registered Nurses' Association of Ontario: Best Practice Guidelines: *http://www.rnao.org/Page.asp?PageID= 861&SiteNodeID=133*

- The Canadian Leadership Institute: *http://www.cdnleadership.com*

REFERENCES

Aiken, L. H., Clarke, S. P., Sloane, D. M., Sochalski, J. A., Busse, R., Clarke, H., et al. (2001). Nurses' report on hospital care in five countries. *Health Affairs, 20*(3), 43–53.

Allen, D. W. (1998). How nurses become leaders: Perceptions and beliefs about leadership development. *Journal of Nursing Administration, 28*(9), 15–20.

American Organization of Nurse Executives. (2006). *Position statement: The role of the nurse executive in patient safety.* Washington, DC: Author.

Anderson, R. A., Issel, L. M., & McDaniel, R. R., Jr. (2003). Nursing homes as complex adaptive systems: Relationship between management practice and resident outcomes. *Nursing Research, 52,* 12–21.

Avolio, B. (1999). *Full leadership development: Building the vital forces in organizations.* Thousand Oaks, CA: Sage.

Barker, A. (1990). *Transformational nursing leadership: A vision for the future.* Baltimore: Williams & Wilkins.

Barnard, C. (1938). *The functions of the executive.* Boston: Harvard University Press.

Bass, B. (1985). *Leadership and performance beyond expectations.* New York: Free Press.

Bednash, G. P. (2003). Leadership defined. *Policy, Politics and Nursing Practice,* 4(4), 257–258.

Benner P. (1984). *From novice to expert: Excellence and power in clinical nursing practice.* Menlo Park, CA: Addison-Wesley.

Bennis, W., & Nanus, B. (1985). *Leaders: The strategies for taking charge.* New York: Harper & Row.

Blake, R. R., & Mouton, J. S. (1985). *The managerial grid III.* Houston, TX: Gulf.

Blythe, J., Baumann, A., & Giovannetti, P. (2001). Nurses' experiences of restructuring in three Ontario Hospitals. *Journal of Nursing Scholarship,* 33, 61–68.

Bruch, H., & Ghoshal, S., (2002) Beware the busy manager. *Harvard Business Review,* 80(2), 63–69.

Burns, J. M. (1978). *Leadership.* New York: Harper & Row.

Canadian Institute for Health Information. (1999). *MIS guidelines for Canadian healthcare facilities.* Ottawa: Author.

Canadian Institute for Health Information. (2004). *MIS Guidelines for Canadian health care facilities.* Ottawa: Author.

Canadian Nurses Association. (2009). *Position statement: Nursing leadership.* Ottawa: Author. Retrieved from http://www.cna-aiic.ca/CNA/issues/position/leadership/default_e.aspx

Carver, L., & Candela, L. (2008). Attaining organizational commitment across different generations of nurses. *Journal of Nursing Management,* 16(8), 984–991.

Cassidy, V., & Koroll, C. (1998). Ethical aspects of transformational leadership. In E. Hein (Ed.), *Contemporary leadership behavior: Selected readings* (5th ed., pp. 79–82). Philadelphia: Lippincott.

Chiok Foong Loke, J. (2001). Leadership behaviours: Effects on job satisfaction, productivity and organizational commitment. *Journal of Nursing Management,* 9, 191–204.

College of Nurses of Ontario. (1998). *Practice setting consultation program: An information guide.* Toronto: College of Nurses of Ontario.

Conger, J., & Kanungo, R. (1987). Toward a behavioral theory of charismatic leadership in organizational settings. *Academy of Management Review,* 12, 637–647.

Cordeniz, J. A. (2002). Recruitment, retention and management of generation X: A focus on nursing professionals. *Journal of Healthcare Management,* 47(4), 237–249.

Covey, S. R., (1990). *The seven habits of highly effective people* (1st ed.). New York: Simon & Schuster Inc.

Daft, R. L., & Marcic, D. (2001). *Understanding management* (3rd ed.). Philadelphia: Harcourt College.

Doucette, E. (2006). Role of the professional practice leader. *Brant Community Healthcare System What's Up Newsletter.* Brantford: Author.

Drucker, P. F. (1994). *The post-capitalist society.* New York: Harper & Row.

Dunham, J., & Klafehn, K. A. (1990). Transformational leadership and the nurse executive. *Journal of Nursing Administration,* 20(4), 28–34.

Dunham-Taylor, J. (1995). Identifying the best in nurse executive leadership: Part 2, interview results. *Journal of Nursing Administration,* 25(7/8), 24–31.

Dunham-Taylor, J. (2000). Nurse executive transformational leadership found in participative organizations. *Journal of Nursing Administration,* 30(5), 241–250.

Edwards, R. (1994). Image, practice and empowerment: A call to new leadership for the invisible profession. *Revolution,* 4(1), 18–20.

Fagin, C. M. (1996). Executive leadership: Improving nursing practice, education and research. *Journal of Nursing Administration,* 26(3), 30–37.

Fayol, H. (1916/1949). (C. Storrs, Trans.). *General and industrial management.* London: Pitman.

Fielder, F. (1967). *A theory of leadership effectiveness.* New York: McGraw-Hill.

Gardner, J. W. (1986). *The nature of leadership: Introductory considerations.* Washington, DC: The Independent Sector.

Gardner, J. W. (1990). *On leadership.* New York: The Free Press.

Gelinas, L. S., & Manthey, M. (1997). The impact of organizational redesign on nurse executive leadership. *Journal of Nursing Administration,* 27(10), 35–42.

George, V., Burke, L. J., Rodgers, B., Duthie, N., Hoffman, M. L., Koceja, V., et al. (2002). Developing staff nurse shared leadership behaviour in professional nursing practice. *Nursing Administration Quarterly,* 26(3), 44–59.

Gilbreth, F. (1912). *Primer of scientific management.* New York: Van Nostrand.

Girvan, J. (1996). Leadership and nursing: Part 1: History and politics. *Nursing Management,* 3(1), 10–12.

Goleman, D. (2006). *Emotional intelligence: Why it can matter more than IQ.* New York: Bantam Books.

Gulick, L., & Urwick, L. (Eds.). (1937). *Papers on the science of administration.* New York: Institute of Public Administration.

Gullo, S., & Gerstle, D. (2004). Transformational leadership and hospital restructuring: A descriptive study. *Policy, Politics and Nursing Practice,* 5(4), 259–266.

Gumusluoglu, L., and Ilsev, S. (2009). Transformational leadership and organizational innovation: The roles of internal and external support for innovation. *Journal of Product Innovation Management,* 26, 264–277.

Hales, C. P. (1986). What managers do: A critical review of the evidence. *Journal of Management Studies,* 23, 88–115.

Helgesen, S. (1995). *The web of inclusion: A new architecture for building organizations.* New York: Doubleday Currency.

Henry, N. (1992). *Public administration and public affairs* (5th ed.). Englewood Cliffs, NJ: Prentice Hall.

Hersey, P., & Blanchard, K. (2000). *Management of organizational behavior* (8th ed.). Englewood Cliffs, NJ: Prentice Hall.

Herzberg, F. (1968). One more time: How do you motivate employees? *Harvard Business Review, January/February,* 53–62.

House, R. H. (1971). A path-goal theory of leader effectiveness. *Administrative Science Quarterly,* 16, 321–338.

House, R. H. (1977). A 1976 theory of charismatic leadership. In J. Hunt & L. Larson (Eds.), *Leadership: The cutting edge* (pp. 21–26). Carbondale, IL: Southern Illinois University Press.

Houser, J. (2003). A model for evaluating the context of nursing care delivery. *Journal of Nursing Administration,* 33(1), 39–47.

Huber, D. L., Maas, M., McCloskey, J., Scherb, C. A., Goode, C. J., & Watson, C. (2000). Evaluating nursing administration instruments. *Journal of Nursing Administration, 30*(5), 251–272.

Hughes, R. L., Ginnett, R. C., & Curphy, G. J. (1999). *Leadership: Enhancing the lessons of experience* (3rd ed.). San Francisco: Irwin McGraw-Hill.

Huston, C. (2008). Preparing nurse leaders for 2020. *Journal of Nursing Management, 16*, 905–911.

Industry Canada. (2004). *Steps to competitiveness: Explanation step one—Defining vision and mission.* Ottawa: Author. Retrieved from http://strategis.ic.gc.ca/epic/site/stco-levc.nsf/en/qw00046e.html

Jung, D. I., & Avolio, B. J. (2000). Opening the black box: An experimental investigation of the mediating effects of trust and value congruence on transformational and transactional leadership. *Journal of Organizational Behaviour, 21*(8), 949–964.

Kanfer, R. (1990). Motivation theory in industrial and organizational psychology. In M. D. Dunnette & L. M. Hough (Eds.), *Handbook of industrial and organizational psychology: Vol. 1* (pp. 53–68). Palo Alto, CA: Consulting Psychologists Press.

Katz, D., & Kahn, R. L. (1978). *The social psychology of organizations* (2nd ed.). New York: John Wiley.

Kerr, S., & Jermier, J. (1978). Substitutes for leadership: Their meaning and measurement. *Organizational Behavior and Human Performance, 22*, 374–403.

Kim, H., & Yukl, G. (1995). Relationships of self-reported and subordinate-reported leadership behaviors to managerial effectiveness and advancement. *Leadership Quarterly, 6*, 361–377.

Kirkpatrick, S. A., & Locke, E. A. (1991). Leadership: Do traits matter? *The Executive, 5*, 48–60.

Kotter, J. (1990a). *A force for change: How leadership differs from management.* Glencoe, IL: Free Press.

Kotter, J. (1990b). What leaders really do. *Harvard Business Review, 68*, 104.

Kouzes, J. M., & Posner, B. Z. (2002). *The leadership challenge* (3rd ed.). San Francisco: Jossey-Bass Inc.

Kramer, M., & Schmalenberg, C. (1988). Magnet hospitals: Part II institutions of excellence. *Journal of Nursing Administration, 18*(2), 11–19.

Kramer, M., & Schmalenberg, C. (2003). Securing "good" nurse/physician relationships. *Nursing Management, 34*(7), 34–38.

Kraus, S. (2006). Success lessons from the Winter Olympics: Visualization. Retrieved from http://ezinearticles.com/?Success-Lessons-from-the-Winter-Olympics:-Visualization&id=148344

Kupperschmidt, B. R. (2000). Multigenerational employees: Strategies for effective management. *Health Care Manager, 19*(1), 65–76.

Laschinger, H., Wong, C., Ritchie, J., D'Amour, D., Vincent, L., Wilk, P., et al. (2008). A profile of the structure and impact of nursing management in Canadian hospitals. *Healthcare Quarterly, 11*(2), 85–94.

Leach, L. S. (2000). *Nurse executive leadership and the relationship to organizational commitment among nurses* (Unpublished doctoral dissertation). University of Southern California, Los Angeles.

Leatt, P., & Porter, J. (2003). Where are the healthcare leaders? The need for investment in leadership development. *Healthcare Papers, 4*(1), 14–31.

Levi, P. (1999), Sustainability of healthcare environments. *Image: Journal of Nursing Scholarship, 31*(4), 395–398.

Lewin, K. (1939). Field theory and experiment in social psychology: Concepts and methods. *Journal of Sociology, 44*, 868–896.

Lewin, K., & Lippitt, R. (1938). An experimental approach to the study of autocracy and democracy: A preliminary note. *Sociometry, 1*, 292–300.

Lewin, K., Lippitt, R., & White, R. (1939). Patterns of aggressive behavior in experimentally created social climates. *Journal of Social Psychology, 10*, 271–299.

Lobo, V. M. (2010). Transformational leadership to promote cross-generational retention. *Nursing Leadership, 23*(2), 21–31.

Lussier, R. N. (1999). *Human relations in organizations: Applications and skill building* (4th ed.). San Francisco: Irwin McGraw-Hill.

Lussier, R. N., & Achua, C. F. (2001). *Leadership: Theory, application, skill development.* Cincinnati, OH: South-Western College.

Malleo, C., & Fusilero, J. (2008). Shared governance: Withstanding the test of time. *Nurse Leader, 7*(1), 32–36.

Manthey, M. (1990). The nurse manager as leader. *Nursing Management, 21*(6).

Marquis, B. L., & Huston, C. J. (1996). *Leadership roles and management functions in nursing* (2nd ed.). Philadelphia: J.B. Lippincott.

Maslow, A. (1970). *Motivation and personality* (2nd ed.). New York: Harper & Row.

Mass, H. (2008). ACEN and the health of Canadians. *Canadian Journal of Nursing Leadership, 21*(4), 24–28.

Mayo, E. (1933). *The human problems of an industrial civilization.* New York: Macmillan.

McCall Jr, M. W. (1998). *High flyers: Developing the next generation of leaders.* Boston: Harvard Business School Press.

McCloskey, J. C., & McCain, B. E. (1987). Satisfaction, commitment and professionalism of newly employed nurses. *Image, 19*(1), 20–24, 178.

McClure, M., Poulin, M., Sovie, M., & Wandelt, M. (1983). *Magnet hospitals: Attraction and retention of professional nurses.* Kansas City, MO: American Nurses Association.

McDaniel, C., & Wolf, G. (1992). Transformational leadership in nursing service. *Journal of Nursing Administration, 12*(4), 204–207.

McGillis Hall, L., Doran, D., Baker, G. R., Pink, G. H., Sidani, S., O'Brien-Pallas, L., et al. (2001). *A study of the impact of nursing staff mix models and organizational change strategies on patient, system and nurse outcomes.* Toronto: Faculty of Nursing, University of Toronto and Canadian Health Research Foundation.

McGregor, D. (1960). *The human side of enterprise.* New York: McGraw-Hill.

McNeese-Smith, D. (1995). Job satisfaction, productivity, and organizational commitment: The result of leadership. *Journal of Nursing Administration, 25*(9), 17–26.

McNeese-Smith, D. (1997). The influences of manager behavior on nurses' job satisfaction, productivity, and commitment. *Journal of Nursing Administration, 27*(9), 47–55.

Medley, F., & Larochelle, D. R. (1995). Transformational leadership and job satisfaction. *Nursing Management, 26*(9), 64JJ-64NN.

Meighan, M. (1990) The most important characteristics of nursing leaders. *Nursing Administration Quarterly, 15*(1), 63–69.

Mintzberg, H. (1973). *The nature of managerial work.* New York: Harper & Row.

Moats Kennedy, M. (1998). Boomers versus busters: Addressing the generation gap in healthcare management. *Healthcare Executive,* 13(6), 6–10.

Mooney, J. (1939). *Principles of organization.* New York: Harper.

Moorhead, G., & Griffin, R. W. (2001). *Organizational behavior: Managing people in organizations* (6th ed.). Boston: Houghton Mifflin.

Murphy, M., & DeBack, V. (1991). Today's nursing leaders: Creating the vision. *Nursing Administration Quarterly,* 16(1), 71–80.

Northouse, P. (2001). *Leadership: Theory and practice* (2nd ed.). Thousand Oaks, CA: Sage.

O'Brien-Pallas, L., Thomson, D., McGillis Hall, L., Pink, G., Kerr, M., Wang, S. et al. (2004). *Evidence-based standards for measuring nurse staffing and performance.* Toronto: Faculty of Nursing, University of Toronto and Canadian Health Services Research Foundation.

Ouchi, W. (1981). *Theory Z: How American business can meet the Japanese challenge.* Reading, MA: Addison-Wesley.

Pillai, R., & Meindl, J. (1998). Context and charisma: A "meso" level examination of the relationship of organic structure, collectivism, and crisis to charismatic leadership. *Journal of Management,* 24, 643–671.

Piper, L. E. (2008). The generation Y workforce in health care: The new challenge for leadership. *Health Care Manager,* 27(2), 98–103.

Porter-O'Grady, T. (2003). A different age for leadership, Part 2. *Journal of Nursing Administration,* 33(3), 173–178.

Public Health Agency of Canada. (2006). How healthy are rural Canadians? An assessment of their health status and health determinants. Summary Report. Retrieved from http://www.phac-aspc.gc.ca/publicat/rural06/pdf/rural_Canadians_2006_report_e.pdf-PDF_file

Registered Nurses Association of Ontario. (2006). *Developing and sustaining nursing leadership (Healthy work environments best practice guidelines).* Toronto: Author.

Ribelin, P. (2003). Retention reflects leadership style. *Nursing Management,* 34(8), 18–19.

Robbins, B., & Davidhizer, R. (2007). Transformational leadership in healthcare today. *Healthcare Manager,* 26(3), 234–239.

Roethlisberger, J. F., & Dickson, W. J. (1939). *Management and the worker.* Cambridge, MA: Harvard University Press.

Russell, A., Campbell, H., Scardamalia, M., Lamon, M., Melnick, B., Henderson, J., et al. (2005). Collaborating to innovate and improve patient-centred care at Hamilton Health Sciences. *Healthcare Quarterly,* online case study. Retrieved from http://www.long-woods.com/content/17724

Salovey, P., & Mayer, J. (1990). Emotional intelligence. *Imagination, Cognition and Personality,* 9, 185–211.

Santos, S. R., & Cox, K. (2000). Workplace adjustment and intergenerational differences between matures, boomers, and Xers. *Nursing Economics,* 18(1), 7–13.

Scott, J. G., Sochalski, J., & Aiken, L. (1999). Review of magnet hospital research: Findings and implications for professional nursing practice. *Journal of Nursing Administration,* 29(1), 9–19.

Searle, L. (1996). 21st century leadership for nurse administrators. *Aspen's Advisor for Nurse Executives,* 11(4), 1, 4–6.

Shamian, J. (2011). Clinician executives: A new breed of leader. *Nursing Leadership,* 23(4), 22–27.

Shaver, J., (2005). Focus on leaders: Joan Shaver on nurturing leaders. *Nursing Leadership,* 18(2), 25–27.

Smith, P. M., Parsons, R. J., Murray, B. P., Dwore, R. B., Vorderer, L. H., & Wallock Okerlund, V. (1994). The nurse executive, an emerging role. *Journal of Nursing Administration,* 24(11), 56–62.

Snow, J. L. (2001). Looking beyond nursing for clues to effective leadership. *Journal of Nursing Administration,* 31(9), 440–443.

Spence Laschinger, H., Sabiston, J. A., Finegan, J., & Shamian, J. (2001). Voices from the trenches: Nurses' experiences of hospital restructuring in Ontario. *Canadian Journal of Nursing Leadership.* 14(10), 6–13.

Spence Laschinger, H., Wong, C., McMahon, L., & Kaufmann, C. (1999). Leader behavior impact on staff empowerment, job tension and work effectiveness. *Journal of Nursing Administration,* 29(5), 28–39.

Stodgill, R. M. (1948). Personal factors associated with leadership, A survey of the literature. *Journal of Psychology,* 25, 35–71.

Stodgill, R. M. (1974). *Handbook of leadership: A survey of theory and research.* New York: Free Press.

Stordeur, S., Vandenberghe, C., & D'hoore, W. (2000). Leadership styles across hierarchical levels in nursing departments. *Nursing Research,* 49, 37–43.

Stout-Shaffer, S., & Larrabee, J. (1992). Everyone can be a visionary leader. *Nursing Management,* 23(12), 54–58.

Taylor, F. (1911). *Principles of scientific management.* New York: Harper & Row.

Tichy, N., & Devanna, D. (1986). *Transformational leadership.* New York: Wiley.

Tourangeau, A., Lemonde, M., Luba, M., Dakers, D., & Alksnis, C. (2003). Evaluation of a leadership development intervention. *Canadian Journal of Nursing Leadership,* 16(3), 91–104.

Tranbarger, R., (1998). The nurse executive in a community hospital. In M. Johnson (Ed.), *Series on nursing administration* (Vol. 1). Menlo Park, CA: Addison Wesley.

Trofino, J. (1995). Transformational leadership in health care. *Nursing Management,* 26(8), 42–47.

Upenicks, V. (2003). Nurse leader's perceptions of what comprises successful leadership in today's acute care environment. *Nursing Administration Quarterly,* 27, 140–152.

Weingarten, R. M. (2009). Four generations, one workplace: A gen X-Y staff nurse's view of team building in the emergency department. *Journal of Emergency Medicine,* 35(1), 27–31.

Weston, M. (2001). Coaching generations in the work place. *Nursing Administration Quarterly,* 25(2), 11–21.

Wheatley, M. J. (1992). *Leadership and the new science: Learning about organization from an orderly universe.* San Francisco: Berrett-Koehler.

Wieck, K. L., Prydun, M., & Walsh, T. (2002). What the emerging workforce wants in its leaders. *Journal of Nursing Scholarship,* 34(3), 283–288.

Wolf, G., Boland, S., & Aukerman, M. (1994). A transformational model for the practice of professional nursing. Part 1. *Journal of Nursing Administration,* 24(4), 51–57.

Wren, D. (1987). *The evolution of management thought* (3rd ed.). New York: Wiley

Young, S. (1992). Educational experiences of transformational nurse leaders. *Nursing Administration Quarterly,* 17(1), 25–33.

Yukl, G. (1998). *Leadership in organizations* (4th ed.). Upper Saddle River, NJ: Prentice Hall.

Yukl, G., Wall, S., & Lepsinger, R. (1990). Preliminary report on validation of the managerial practices survey. In K. E. Clarke & M. B. Clark (Eds.), *Measures of leadership* (pp. 223–238). West Orange, NJ: Leadership Library of America.

Zalenik, K. A. (1977). Managers and leaders: Are they different? *Harvard Business Review,* 55(5), 67–80.

SUGGESTED READINGS

Avolio, B. J., Zhu, W., Koh, W., & Bhatia, P. (2004) Transformational leadership and organizational commitment: Mediating role of psychological empowerment and moderating role of structural distance. *Journal of Organizational Behaviour,* 25(8), 951–968.

Bass, B. (1998). *Transformational leadership: Industrial, military, and educational impact.* Mahwah, NJ: Erlbaum.

Bauman, A., O'Brien-Pallas, L., Armstrong-Stassen, M., Blythe, J., Bourbonnais, R., Cameron, S., et al. (2001). *Commitment and care: The benefits of a healthy workplace for nurses, their patients and the system.* Ottawa: Canadian Health Research Foundation and the Change Foundation.

Bower, F. L. (2000). *Nurses taking the lead: Personal qualities of effective leadership.* Philadelphia: Saunders.

Buerhaus, P. I. (2000). Implications of an aging registered nurse workforce. *Journal of the American Medical Association,* 283, 2948–2954.

Cadman, C., & Brewer, J. (2001). Emotional intelligence: A vital prerequisite for recruitment in nursing. *Journal of Nursing Management,* 9(6), 321–324.

Canadian Nursing Advisory Committee. (2002). *Our health, our future: Creating quality workplaces for Canadian nurses: Final report of the Canadian Nursing Advisory Committee.* Ottawa: Advisory Committee on Health Human Resources.

Canadian Nurses Association. (2009). *The next decade: CNA's vision for a healthy tomorrow.* Ottawa: Author.

Collins, D., & Holton, E. (2004). The Effectiveness of managerial leadership development programs: A meta-analysis of studies from 1982 to 2001. *Human Resources Development Quarterly,* 15(2), 217–248.

Cronin, S. N., & Bechere, D. (1999). Recognition of staff nurse job performance and achievements: Staff and manager perceptions. *Journal of Nursing Administration,* 29(1), 26–31.

Evans, M. G. (1996). R. J. House's "A path-goal theory of leader effectiveness." *Leadership Quarterly,* 7(3), 305–309.

Ferguson-Paré, M., Mitchell, G., Perkin, K., & Stevenson, L. (2002). Academy of Canadian Executive Nurses (ACEN) background paper on leadership. *Canadian Journal of Nursing Leadership,* 15(3), 4–8.

Goleman, D. (1998). *Working with emotional intelligence.* New York: Bantam Books.

Gordon, S. (1997). *Life support: Three nurses on the front lines.* New York: Little, Brown.

Herbert, R., & Edgar, L. (2004). Emotional intelligence: A primal dimension of nursing leadership? *Canadian Journal of Nursing Leadership,* 17(4), 56–63.

Hesselbein, F., Goldsmith, M., & Beckhard, R. (Eds.). (1996). *The leader of the future: New visions, strategies, and practices for a new era.* San Francisco: Jossey-Bass.

Jeans, M., & Rowat, K. (2005). *Competencies required of nurse managers: Identifying the skills, personal attributes and knowledge required of nurse managers, and the enablers and barriers for nurse managers to acquire and sustain these competencies. The pulse of renewal: A focus on nursing human resources. May, 2005. Special report.* Toronto: Canadian Journal of Nursing Leadership.

Kanges, S., Kee, C. C., & McKee-Waddle, R. (1999). Organizational factors, nurses' job satisfaction and patient satisfaction with nursing care. *Journal of Nursing Administration,* 29(1), 32–42.

Kohles, M. K., Baker Jr, W. G., & Donoho, B. (1995). *Transformational leadership: Reviewing fundamental values and achieving new relationships in health care.* Chicago: American Hospital.

Kramer, M. (1990). The magnet hospitals: Excellence revisited. *Journal of Nursing Administration,* 20(9), 35–44.

Kramer, M., & Schmalenberg, C. (1990). Fundamental lessons in leadership. In E. Simendinger, T. Moore, & M. Kramer (Eds.), *The successful nurse executive: A guide for every nursemanager* (pp. 42–56). Ann Arbor, MI: Health Administration Press.

Laborde, A. S., & Lee, J. A. (2000). Skills needed for promotion in the nursing profession. *Journal of Nursing Administration,* 30(9), 432–439.

Laschinger, H., Finegan, J., & Shamian, J. (2001). The impact of workplace empowerment, organizational trust on staff nurses' work satisfaction and organizational commitment. *Health Care Management Review,* 26(3), 7–23.

Lemire Rodger, G. (2005). Leadership challenges and directions. In J. M. Hibberd & D. L. Smith (Eds.), *Nursing leadership and management in Canada* (3rd ed.). Toronto: Elsevier Canada.

Luthans, S. F., Hodgetts, R., & Rosenkratz, S. (1988). *Real managers.* Cambridge, MA: Ballinger.

O'Neil, E., & Coffman, J. (Eds.). (1998). *Strategies for the future of nursing: Changing roles, responsibilities, and employment patterns of registered nurses.* San Francisco: Jossey-Bass.

Parse, R. (1997). Leadership: The essentials. *Nursing Science Quarterly,* 10(3), 109.

Porter-O'Grady, T., & Wilson, C. K. (1995). *The leadership revolution in health care: Altering systems, changing behaviors.* Gaithersburg, MD: Aspen.

Rosenbach, W. E., & Taylor, R. L. (1998). *Contemporary issues in leadership* (4th ed.). Boulder, CO: Westview Press.

Senge, P. M. (1990) *The fifth discipline. The art and practice of the learning organization.* London: Random House

Storr, L. (2004). Leading with integrity: a qualitative research study. *Journal of Health Organization & Management,* 18, 415–434.

Urwick, L. (1944). *The elements of administration.* New York: Harper & Row.

Villeneuve, M., & MacDonald, J. (2006). *Toward 2020: Visions for nursing.* Ottawa: Canadian Nurses Association.

CHAPTER ENDNOTES

1. Laschinger, H., & Wong, C. (2007). A profile of the structure and impact of nursing management in Canadian hospitals. *Healthcare Quarterly*. 11(2), 85-94.

2. Canadian Nurses Association. (2009). *Position statement: The nurse practitioner*. Ottawa: Canadian Nurses Association. Retrieved from http://www.cna-aiic.ca/CNA/issues/position/leadership/default_e.aspx

3. Huston, C. (2008). Preparing nurse leaders for 2020. *Journal of Nursing Management*, 16, 905.

4. Raymond, G., & Walton, M. (2011). Enabling transformational change: The Ontario Shores experience. *Healthcare Quarterly*, 14(1), 56–61.

5. Canadian Nurses Association. (2009). Position Statement: Background. Retrieved from http://www.cna-aiic.ca/CNA/issues/position/leadership/default_e.aspx

6. Shamian, J. (2011). Clinician executives: A new breed of leader. *Nursing Leadership*, 23(4), 22–27.

CHAPTER 9

Effective Team Building

Karin Polifko-Harris, PhD, RN, CNAA
Adapted by Heather Crawford, BScN, MEd, CHE

Exemplary leaders enable others to act. They foster collaboration and build trust. This sense of teamwork goes far beyond a few direct reports or close confidantes. They engage all those who must make the project work. (Kouzes & Posner, 2002)[1]

OBJECTIVES

The purpose of this chapter is to enable the reader to

- identify the differences among groups, teams, and committees;
- discuss the stages of group development;
- review key concepts of effective teams; and
- discuss ways in which a nurse manager can create an environment conducive to team building.

Jim Parkin/Shutterstock

As a new nurse, you are making the day's assignments for a 34-bed medical-surgical unit. Working with you today will be another two registered nurses, two licensed practical nurses, and one unregulated care provider. You graduated only months ago but were recently promoted to the role of charge nurse. Today, one of the licensed practical nurses and the unregulated care provider are challenging your client care assignments, suggesting that you do not have enough experience to make a fair assignment, and they are trying to get the two registered nurses to side with them. The two registered nurses often work together, as do the two licensed practical nurses. You know you made the best assignment given the staff available, yet you are wondering whether there is a better solution.

What are your thoughts on how to proceed?

What would be the best way to address their concerns?

How could you more actively involve them in the client assignment responsibility?

The essential leadership and management skills in nursing always include some element of effective teamwork. Working together in a successful team requires more than good luck or chance. As the health care delivery system continues to increase in complexity, issues such as span of control, more seriously ill hospitalized clients, and a move from acute health care to non-acute health care delivery challenge nurse managers to alter how they provide nursing care to clients. A critical trend in human resource development is team training. Whereas Canadian business culture emphasizes the role of the individual in achieving success, the nursing profession has begun refocusing on teamwork and team building as a method for meeting the needs of a changing health care delivery model. Nurses generally do not work in isolation but provide

care that is interdependent and interprofessional, providing a level of expertise to help the client achieve optimal wellness. Initially implemented at the beginning of the 20th century to coordinate work, teams are now an integral feature of health care delivery in acute, long-term, and primary care settings (Lemieux-Charles & McGuire, 2006). This chapter discusses the key factors that contribute to a successful nursing team, including team building. It also discusses characteristics and skills of an effective team leader.

DEFINING TEAMS AND COMMITTEES

Clements, Dault, and Priest (2007) define a **team** as "something that exists any time two or more people are working together with a shared purpose...team members have particular responsibilities that relate to their own specific skills and knowledge. One individual is always the leader, and this is agreed upon by the team or those who created it" (p. 28). Teamwork requires an explicit decision by the team members to cooperate in meeting the shared objective. Consequently, team members need to lose their autonomy, which means allowing their own activity to be coordinated by the team, either through decisions by the team leader or through shared decision making.[2] On some teams, all members may have similar backgrounds and abilities, such as a nursing policy and procedure team. Other teams may consist of members who have a variety of skills and talents; this provides different perspectives and ideas on how to solve problems.

The members of an **interprofessional team** have a range of clinical expertise. An advantage of an interprofessional team is the different strengths and viewpoints the team members contribute. All team members, such as nurses, physicians, social workers, dieticians, case managers, have had specialized training and so they each look at care delivery with a different focus. Having so many viewpoints can be difficult sometimes, especially if a single decision is needed and everyone has a different opinion. The best way to work with an interprofessional team is to allow everyone to be heard, and to entertain various problem-solving methods and potential solutions. The team leader's role is to ensure that all members have the opportunity to participate and accomplish the work of the team.

Multiple committees may develop to complete the work of an organization and assist in communication. A **committee** is a work group with a specific task or goal to be accomplished. An ad hoc committee is generally temporary and formed for a specific purpose, for a specific time frame, or to accomplish a certain short-term goal. For example, an ad hoc committee may be the bed utilization committee that meets only until flu season is over. By contrast, standing committees may be an integral component of the organizational structure: for example, a board's client care and quality committee that meets on a monthly basis. Standing committees may be mandated through organizational bylaws, such as medical staff meetings. Other committees exist because a formal process is needed for decision making, as in the Critical Care Committee. Regardless of the purpose of the committee, after the work has been completed, the group should be disbanded. Individuals are far too busy to continue to attend committee meetings after the mandate of the committee has been fulfilled.

A committee may also be advisory, such as a committee that meets to discuss the concerns of the professional nursing staff—for example, a professional practice council—and then reports back to the chief nurse executive (CNE).

STAGES OF TEAM PROCESS

All teams progress through predictable phases of development, much like people do, as they evolve from an immature stage to (one hopes!) a mature stage. However, it is critical to note that not all teams reach maturity for a variety of reasons, such as perhaps there is ineffective leadership, problematic members, unclear goals and directives, or lack of focus or energy. Similar to individuals on a continuum of maturity, some teams may become fully functional and mature quickly, bypassing a stage or two along the way. High-functioning teams, whose members are familiar with one another, are usually able to make decisions quickly and accurately; it may take longer for other teams, whose members need to get to know and trust one another before the actual work can take place.

Tuckman and Jensen (1977) identified five stages that a group normally progresses through to reach maturity. These stages, known as **group development,** consist of forming, storming, norming, performing, and adjourning (see Table 9-1). They are built on the classic work by Tuckman, first described the four stages of group development in 1965. The stage of adjourning was added ten years later. Lacoursiere (1980) identified these same developmental stages as orientation, dissatisfaction, production, and termination.

In the first stage, called **forming,** several critical phases begin: the expectation phase, the interaction phase, and the boundary formation phase. The expectation phase starts when the first meeting begins. Everyone is curious, wanting to know what the group is

all about—how it will meet their needs, what they will need to do to fit in, and what they can gain from group membership. During the interaction phase the group takes shape, opinions begin form, and expectations and boundaries become more clearly defined. The group establishes its identity, with the help of the group leader who provides the team with information on the purpose of the group and the vision and boundaries of what the group is expected to accomplish.

During the second stage of group development, called **storming,** everyone begins to feel more comfortable in the group setting. As certain feelings and statements occur, members may find a position within the group to which they can contribute. The storming phase is generally difficult because of conflict that may, at times, be quite apparent. Differences among group members—even possibly the group leader—become obvious, and people often take sides on certain concerns or issues. Although this phase can be confrontational full of tension, a group often needs to journey through the storming phase to encourage resolution of the emerging problems and actively solve the issues at hand.

Stage three, called **norming,** follows the conflict and confrontation of the storming stage. Although the problems are not yet solved, and decisions may

CRITICAL THINKING

You are the nurse who is working with Mr. Ward, a 76-year-old male who was admitted for congestive heart failure and chronic kidney disease. Mr. Ward is well known to the staff at Memorial Hospital for his multiple admissions. During this admission, his blood pressure was unusually high and he appeared sluggish. His wife is visiting her relatives out of town, and he is by himself. When you attend the daily client care conference, you note most of the interprofessional team is present: the community nurse case manager, the social worker, the nurse caring for him, the hospital chaplain, the dietician, the pharmacist, and his primary care physician.

What key issues are concerning you? What perspective does each of the team members bring to the discussion on the care of Mr. Ward? How would you proceed to develop or alter Mr. Ward's plan of care? Are there any other team members who may be able to assist you with Mr. Ward's care?

TABLE 9-1	STAGES OF GROUP PROCESS (DRAWING ON TUCKMAN & JENSEN, 1977; LACOURSIERE, 1980)			
Forming	**Storming**	**Norming**	**Performing**	**Adjourning**
■ Expectations	■ Tension	■ Positioning	■ Actual work	■ Closure
■ Interactions	■ Conflict	■ Goal setting	■ Relationships	■ Evaluation
■ Boundary formation	■ Confrontation	■ Cohesiveness	■ Group maturity	■ Outcomes review

not have been made, members have a general understanding of the issues are and will be progressing toward solving them. Positions within the group are now established, and members having a sense both of belonging and of setting goals to meet the expectations outlined in the forming stage. Conflict has converted into cohesiveness.

The fourth stage in the maturity of a group, called **performing,** is probably the most enjoyable phase. Interdependence is the foremost activity—members know what their role is and what they are supposed to do—and obvious progress is made toward achieving the overall goal of the team. The group is considered mature at this stage, and the individual members are now ready to focus on the actual work that will meet the group's objectives. Another strength of the performing stage is the emphasis placed on maintaining effective relationships with group members, as the individual members function as a whole (Tappen, 2001).

During the final stage, called **adjourning,** the primary focus is closure activities and the termination of team relationships. The group has met its objectives, and the team members review the team's progress. Were the goals and objectives of the team met? Would anything have been done differently if the team were to start over? During the final stage, the group should evaluate whether the stated purpose was accomplished. What were the outcomes of both the group process and the individuals' participation? Groups are often disbanded without this closing review, leaving some members feeling empty and without a feeling of accomplishment.

GROUP ROLES

As in any gathering, when people come together in a group, everyone takes on a different role. Some may want the role to be self-serving, as with the person who wants

to be the centre of attention and insists on being the dominant force in any decision. Others play a role that is clearly supportive: they are there to contribute in any way they can to the betterment of the whole, but do not need or want to be in the limelight. People may take on numerous other roles, though some roles are not always clearly defined.

FUNCTIONAL VERSUS DYSFUNCTIONAL MEMBERS

A team can have participants who are functional and those who are somewhat dysfunctional in their behaviours. Sometimes the behaviours are unconsciously acted out—perhaps in the form of a defence mechanism, such as denial. At other times a group member is quite clear and focused about the role being played, such as the antagonizer. In any case, the astute group leader needs to be aware of everyone's roles to facilitate the optimal group process possible.

So what role would a functional group member perform? Several roles are critical to the successful meeting of a group's goal (Bradford, 1978). When a project first begins, a group member is needed to fill the role of initiator—the person who gets the ball rolling and defines the group's problem. A role complementary to the initiator is that of coordinator—the person who is aware of the project flow and who keeps it moving in the right direction. Likewise, the team needs a mobilizer, whose job is to keep things energized and who provides the spark needed to keep team members interested in the project. Other functional roles include the questioner, who asks the questions that are on everyone's mind; the antagonist, who looks at the situation in an opposite manner to everyone else; and the recorder, who chronicles the details of the group meeting and process. It is not necessary to have all the roles filled at all times in functional groups.

What makes a good team? I think a team is effective when everyone is able to contribute to the goals and objectives without fear of being "put down." Everyone's contribution is valued. The decision of the group, and the conflicts that may have occurred, stay within the confines of the group. However, if you are talking about the clinical unit, a good team is everyone working well together—nurses assisting each other without being asked, no gossip about members of the team, answering the call light regardless whether the client was assigned to you.

Heather Jones, BScN
Team Leader

What are the dysfunctional roles that hinder the progress of a group? Unfortunately, numerous personality types can be difficult, especially during the group's formative stages. Criticizers find fault with everything and everybody, yet seldom contribute positively when asked. Everything is a strong "No!" and if it is not done their way, they believe it will not be done correctly. Passive members will rarely take a stand on anything. Their passivity and inability to make a decision is often frustrating. They will not say a word for fear of rebuttal.

Detailers get so caught up with the facts that it is hard for them to see the big picture or to keep heading toward the goal. Likewise, controllers monopolize the group discussion—no one else can be heard. The only opinion that matters is theirs. They need constant refocusing by

the leader to keep them on track. Finally, pleasers want to do just that—please. They will not make a comment or decision that may be unfavourable to anyone else. Refer to Table 9-2 for suggestions on how to cope with difficult personalities.

KEY CONCEPTS OF EFFECTIVE GROUPS

A familiar saying is that "the whole is greater than the sum of the parts." An effective group is one in which all members are equally important, everyone's voice and opinions are heard, and progress is made toward the stated goal on a steady basis. How does one encourage the energy that comes from placing people of different

TABLE 9-2	STRATEGIES FOR COPING WITH DIFFICULT PERSONALITIES
Personality Type	**Coping Strategies**
Criticizer	Do not argue—it will only add fuel to the fire! Ask for input and practise active listening by reflecting on what you hear. Give criticizers a project to which they can directly contribute.
Passive one	Engage in communication, ask direct questions, ask for direct responses.
Detailer	Allow the detailer to give details at certain points in the meeting. Begin with the objective for the session, repeat information when necessary, and summarize.
Controller	Keep focused on the task at hand; note any inconsistencies in the controller's conversation.
Pleaser	Let pleasers know that their comments are safe from attack and that their opinions are valued.

backgrounds and specialties together to mutually solve problems and make decisions? What are the necessary skills to work with interdisciplinary team members in an increasingly complex health care delivery system?

GREAT TEAM GUIDELINES

An assumption is often made that any group of people who come together will inevitably become a team. This assumption is not necessarily true. Some groups will just remain work groups, whereas most teams will initially function as effective working groups. A **group** is a collection of individuals who are in an interdependent relationship with one another. A team, on the other hand, goes beyond that; as shown in Table 9-3, team members share the ownership of the team's function and direction to increase their confidence and commitment (Mears, 1994).

Great teams don't just happen; before anyone even meets, behind-the-scenes planning, preparation, and forward thinking have already taken place. For several decades theories of effective teams have been discussed in the literature: Lewin (1951), McGregor (1960), Argyris (1964), Burns (1978), Bennis (1989), and Senge (2006). What are the guidelines for encouraging great teams? A great team accomplishes what it sets out to do, with everyone on the team participating to achieve the desired outcomes. See Figure 9-1 for great team guidelines.

CASE STUDY 9-1

Your nurse executive has assigned you as the new team leader of the task force on client falls. This task force has been meeting for almost a year without making much progress. At your first meeting, you note that there are several challenging personalities in the group and wonder whether they will ever be able to work together effectively.

Jamie is a new graduate nurse and volunteers for everything so that he will be liked. Angela is the detailer, often asking everyone to repeat what they said so that she can get more information on the topic. Samantha is the passive one and just looks annoyed at having to be there. You noticed she was doing some of her client charting during the meeting. Annabelle attempts to keep the team on track, but with her soft-spoken voice, she is not well heard. Finally, no matter what anyone says, Beth is critical and comes up with a reason why something will not work.

Where do you begin?

How would you deal with the five group members?

What is your primary focus at the beginning of your time as team leader and why?

TABLE 9-3   TEAM VERSUS GROUP

Team	Group
Decisions are made by consensus with all inputs heard and valued	Groups tend to have majority and minority opinions
Disagreements are carefully examined and resolution is sought	Criticism tends to be destructive and disagreements are not effectively dealt with
Objectives are well understood and accepted by the team	Group members do not necessarily accept common objectives
Free expression of ideas occurs and others listen to what is said	Personal feelings are hidden

(Continued)

TABLE 9-3	TEAM VERSUS GROUP (CONTINUED)
Self-examination of how the group is functioning frequently occurs	Discussions are avoided regarding how the group is functioning
Roles are understood by all members	Individuals tend to protect their role and their niche in the group
Shared leadership occurs on an as-needed basis	Leadership is appointed

Source: Mears, P. (1994). *Healthcare Teams Building Continuous Quality Improvement.* Florida: St. Lucie Press Inc. Reprinted with Permission by the author.

First and foremost, the team must have a clearly stated purpose: what are the goals, what are the objectives, and how long and how often will the team meet? What is the vision of the team? What does the leader see the team accomplishing? An effective team keeps the larger organization's mission in mind as it progresses; otherwise, its goals will be inconsistent with those of the parent organization. Second is an assessment of the team's composition: what are the team members' personal strengths and weaknesses? How do the team members see themselves—all as individuals? Do they see themselves as part of a cohesive team? Are any additional members needed? What are the roles of each team member?

Third is the communication link. Are effective communication patterns in place? Is there a need to improve communication, either in written or verbal format? Does the team work well with email and voice mail, or does it need the traditional paper trail to stay connected? Is communication open, with minimal hidden agendas by the members? Can the truth be told in order to reach a difficult decision, in a compassionate and sympathetic manner?

Active participation by all team members is a critical fourth item. Does everyone have a designated responsibility? Do people listen to one another, or is everyone trying to be heard at the same time? What are

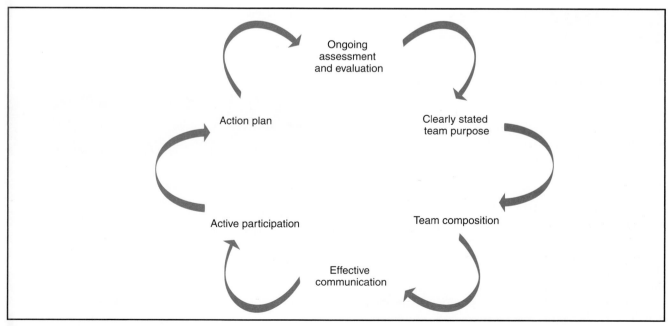

Figure 9-1 Great Team Guidelines

the relationships of the team members? Is there mutual trust and respect for members and their decisions, however unpopular? Are there turf issues that must be resolved before proceeding? The climate of the team should be relaxed but supportive, especially during brainstorming of new ideas or discussion of problems and problem solving. In health care, entrenched attitudes about scopes of practice, professional "turf," and historical power structures can sabotage the essence of teamwork. The providers need to address the power issues, adopt common goals, break down hierarchies, and educate clients about how each team member contributes to their care.[3]

Is there a clear plan for how to proceed? This fifth element leads to an action plan that everyone agrees with early on and that is revisited at designated times. To maintain the group's focus, feedback is necessary from team members and others affected by the team's decisions. The sixth guideline is actually ongoing, in that assessment and evaluation are continuous throughout the team's history. Outcomes have to be consistent and related to the expectations of the organization. Creativity is also encouraged at the team level; perhaps a member has an idea for solving a problem, a solution that no one has ever tried. In a supportive environment, pros and cons of all reasonable ideas should be freely discussed. A team needs to periodically assess its progress.

CREATING AN ENVIRONMENT CONDUCIVE TO TEAM BUILDING

Before any members can be effective in a team, whether the team is a committee or is part of the staff on a nursing unit, a team leader needs to ensure that the environment is conducive to team building. The attitudes, organizational culture, policies, and procedures all help to determine how successful the team will be in accomplishing its directives. Developing an environment that is supportive and exciting to work in is an ongoing process rather than a one-shot event.

Many hospitals employ authoritarian styles of management and leadership rather than true participatory or democratic styles. If the team members work in an authoritarian environment, they may be hesitant or uncomfortable in making decisions for themselves and may prefer the leader to make clear the parameters for decision making. Creativity and creative solutions to problems may be a challenge in this environment—but creativity is critical for progress to occur. Organizational hierarchy

needs to be carefully looked at. Is it a formal or informal hierarchy? Who has the power to make decisions or to derail solutions? Having a top-heavy organizational structure and power base may discourage a team from being effective—too many people need to be informed of all the team's steps, decisions, and solutions, and some may actually thwart progress from occurring.

Resources must be made available to the team to carry out its work. Is there a meeting space that is conducive to conversation and available on a regular basis? Is

CRITICAL THINKING

The chief nurse executive has asked your nurse manager to initiate a new committee to review client safety issues in the hospital. She has asked you to join the committee. Although you are a nurse on a stroke rehabilitation unit, you know that challenging client safety issues are everywhere in the hospital. So far, no one else has volunteered to be on the committee, even though the nurse manager posted the request for members several weeks ago.

Who are you interested in having on the committee? Are they all registered nurses? Why or why not? How will you encourage people to join the committee? How will the nurse manager initiate the group process? Discuss several types of staff that you have worked with who were either functional or dysfunctional in a group and why.

REAL WORLD INTERVIEW

When you start working with a team, it is really important to understand everyone's perspective—what their experiences are, where they work, what is important to them. You need to be observant and pay attention to both verbal and nonverbal communication. You need to be able to read between the lines.

John Fielding, RN
Risk Manager

necessary secretarial support available to set up the meetings and to record and distribute the minutes? Is there adequate staffing to allow team members the time to meet? Are the communication systems reliable?

Are the administrators supportive of the team's efforts? For example, is there a problem in having key members attend meetings, is it lack of commitment or other conflicting duties, will the administrator support efforts to change this situation? Often, a staff nurse is assigned to a team that is focused on solving an institutional problem, such as use of restraint, but another nurse may not have been assigned to take care of the staff nurse's clients during the committee meetings.

Team members need to see that progress is being made, especially consistent progress. Does the environment reward team members' contributions? Is team membership an expectation? Can the team's work be linked to a continuous process of improvement so that members can see they are making a difference? Specifically, can they see the difference their efforts make to the client's care, the client's families, or community they serve; system enhancement; or overall improvement of the quality of the organization? Continuous improvement is a process in which the status quo is never accepted and in which the care delivered is always being reviewed for better ways to improve satisfaction, decrease errors, or smooth the care-delivery processes. Likewise, the administration must be notified if the team is not progressing as expected. Better to share the unfavourable news as soon as it is discovered, unless there's a good chance the team's direction may change with time or other changes. Involving others early in the process may deflect more serious issues later on, because other people may be able to offer additional resources or information that team members may not have access to.

Table 9-4 offers a team evaluation checklist to evaluate whether your team environment is healthy and receptive. Any areas checked *no* may be opportunities for further improvement. There is also a web-based application called Rypple (www.rypple.com), which allows team members to provide anonymous, rapid-fire feedback on team processes and performance. Plaza et al. (2011) describe how the University Health Network's Centre for Innovation in Complex Care uses this web-based application for their team feedback tool.

TEAMWORK ON A CLIENT CARE UNIT

The role of the nurse is multifaceted. Depending on the scenario, a nurse may work directly or indirectly with a wide variety of staff on the health care team. A registered nurse (RN) is directly responsible for the care of the client. That care encompasses both ensuring that physician orders and nursing orders are carried out and that documentation is completed accurately and appropriately for the shift. The RN makes sure that all ordered treatments and procedures have been completed; discharge planning is coordinated with the social worker, the community case manager, and the pharmacist; the client's family understands how to dress the client's wound; and finally, the client understands the discharge instructions. The role of the RN team leader incorporates the entire spectrum of care provided to the family by many people. The

TABLE 9-4	TEAM EVALUATION CHECKLIST		
Question		**Yes**	**No**
1. Is the environment or climate conducive to successful team building?			
2. Do the team members have mutual respect and trust of one another? Are the team members honest with one another?			
3. Does everyone actively participate in the decision making and problem solving of the team?			
4. Are the purpose, goal, and objectives of the team obvious to all participants?			
5. Are creativity and mutual support of new ideas encouraged by all team members?			
6. Is the team productive and does it see actual progress toward goal attainment?			
7. Does the team begin and end its meetings on time?			
8. Does the team leader provide vision and energy to the team?			

effective nurse possesses excellent communication skills, both written and verbal; communicates in a manner sensitive to others' cultural and value differences; is aware of others' abilities; and shows genuine interest in the team members. An open and objective communication style is needed, and communication should be carried out in an unbiased, constructive manner.

EFFECTIVE TEAM MEETINGS

To run an effective team meeting, the team leader needs to plan and coordinate the work of the team. The leader needs to have a clear understanding of the purpose and goals of the team, which facilitates members' full participation. People are more apt to accomplish objectives when the vision is clearly stated and mapped. The leader should embrace and understand the change process and be able to teach staff members and inspire followers toward participative management according to how they work and communicate in groups (Marquis & Huston, 2012). Another critical function of the leader is to prepare the team members ahead of time, perhaps meeting with them individually to fully engage them in the team. This time spent between the nurse leader and the team member is critical. Table 9-5 outlines new perspectives on the assumptions of working with teams and the involvement of effective followers.

When the team meeting is in session, the leader will often be (1) the time keeper, ensuring that the meeting begins and ends when stated; (2) the coordinator, making sure that necessary items and information are available to the team; (3) the peacemaker, tempering opposite viewpoints that are discussed in meeting sessions; (4) the delegator, assigning tasks as needed, such as appointing someone to research a particular perspective of the problem being investigated, or ensuring that the minutes are available; (6) the feedback loop, providing information on the status of goals; and (7) the role model, inspiring others on the team to continue their focus on the goals of the team, especially when performance does not show progress.

| TABLE 9-5 | THE USE OF TEAMS: WORKING WITH FOLLOWERS |

Conventional Assumptions	New Perspectives
Followers are expected to commit to and accept decisions made by others.	Effective followers delay commitment to and acceptance of decisions until they have been able to assess the long- and short-term implications of their decisions and their value for realizing the group's vision.
The role of followers in decision making is to help gather necessary information.	Effective followers help the organization "unlearn" and then relearn.
Followers are valuable because the help create order in organizations.	Effective followers help create disorder so that groups and organizations continue to grow.
Followers enable execution of the organization's strategy.	Effective followers help decide the strategy of the group or organization.
Followers support and reinforce the hierarchy that is essential for goal achievement.	Effective followers reduce the hierarchy by questioning the effectiveness and efficiency of rigid structures.
All followers are guided by the organization's beliefs, more so than their own.	Effective followers challenge the beliefs of the group or organization.
Followers are empowered by leaders or managers.	Effective followers empower themselves.

Source: D. Ashmos (1998) from "Building effective healthcare teams" in W.J. Duncan, P.M. Ginter and L.E. Swayne (eds), *Handbook of Healthcare Management* (p. 313–337). Copyright © 1998 John Wiley & Sons Ltd. Reproduced with permission of John Wiley & Sons Ltd. Adapted by: Grossman, S.C., & Valiga, T.M. (2009). *The new leadership challenge: Creating the future of nursing.* Third edition. Philadelphia: FA Davis Co.

One thing I always try to keep in mind is that one can never over communicate. I try to communicate both up and down the ladder with different modalities, such as direct email, communiqués, open forums, newsletters, and voice mail messages to groups. The message always needs to be delivered in a positive way. People are more likely to eagerly anticipate further updates if your message is delivered positively, succinctly, and important to them.

Leanne Danford, MScN
Director of Nursing

An effective team does not attain results on its own. In addition to providing a supportive environment that nurtures success for its members, an effective team has a leader with vision. This leader has a clear idea of the team's strategic plan and will help others see the plan clearly and understand its place in the institution. The leader readily inspires trust and respects all members of the team, regardless of their status in the organization. Ross, Wenzel, and Mitlyng (2002) offer the following suggestions for building a successful team through effective leadership:

■ Identify with a mission—value the contributions of all team members. All members are critical to the success of the team regardless of their position on the team. Recognize that the mission of the organization is more important than personal ambition.

■ Build confidence and trust—team members cross traditional organizational lines because there is a high level of interpersonal confidence and trust. Encourage interaction among group members. Know when verbal and nonverbal behaviour is appropriate and inappropriate, and keep the flow of communication going. Minimize turf issues.

■ Promote debate—discourage "we versus they" thinking. Build teamwork that encourages inter-team participation and relationships. Team members are able to disagree with each other and debate issues from varying viewpoints. After a decision is made, the entire team supports one another and the decision, and moves the issues forward.

■ Identify with team success—acknowledge and celebrate team accomplishments. Publicly and frequently acknowledge positive contributions by team members, and keep the team members abreast of

the positive changes they are actively involved in making. Team members share the limelight and share credit for success with their colleagues.

■ Evaluate the effectiveness of all team members—regardless of each one's role. Are you carrying your weight, or are you expecting others to carry out your directives?

INTERPROFESSIONAL HEALTHCARE TEAMS

Interprofessional Care: A Blueprint for Action in Ontario defines interprofessional care (IPC) as "the provision of comprehensive health services to clients by multiple health caregivers, who work collaboratively to deliver quality care within and across settings... It is a collaborative, team-based approach to providing optimal client care, given the systemic demands and unprecedented challenges in health care" (Healthforce Ontario, 2010, p. 7).

The work of interprofessional health care teams can result in more effective and efficient client care. Clients benefit from the specific expertise of individual health professionals who provide individual care according to their problems. Teamwork can provide coordination, which can prevent any aspect of the client's care from being overlooked. There is also the potential to more fully understand how the health professions can work together to enhance health promotion, public health, prevention, interprofessional research, and many other health-related but not specifically client care oriented activities.

The National Interprofessional Competency Framework of the Canadian Interprofessional Health Collaborative describes the following six national interprofessional core competencies:

■ interprofessional communication
■ patient/client/family/community-centred care
■ role clarification
■ team functioning
■ collaborative leadership
■ interprofessional conflict management

Figure 9-2 shows the configuration of the competencies and highlights the three considerations that influence how the competency framework may be applied in different situations.

For teams to function effectively, collaboration is essential. Collaborative working among different individuals or groups may enable professionals to achieve cost-effective, client-focused care, regardless of where the care is delivered—that is, in institutions or in the community. At a practice level, professional identities and traditional roles are no longer prescribed, but are actively negotiated among those who are involved in client care. Traditional care delivery practices have been challenged.

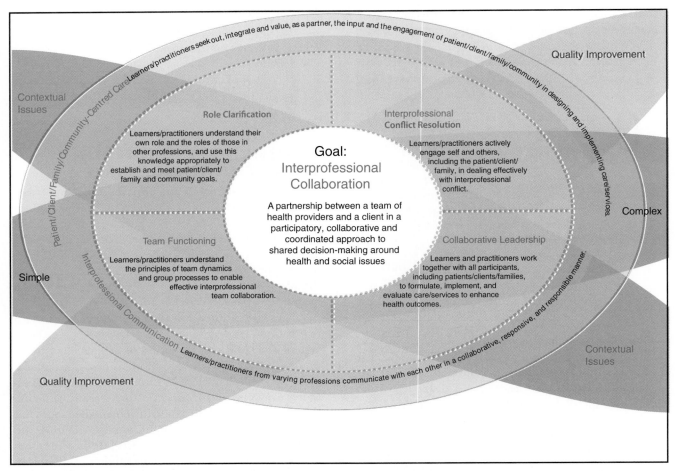

Figure 9-2 National Interprofessional Competency Framework

Source: College of Health Disciplines University of British Columbia. (2010). *Canadian interprofessional health collaborative: A national interprofessional care competency framework.* Vancouver, British Columbia.

DEVELOPING DECISION-MAKING AND PROBLEM-SOLVING SKILLS

Huber (2000) discusses a range of decision-making approaches that assist in accomplishing the stated goals and objectives of a particular nursing team. Knowing when to have the entire team participate in the decision-making process or when to have only the leader make the decision varies depending on the situation and the desired outcome. A leader uses the *autocratic* decision process in the following situations: (1) the task or outcome is relatively simple (e.g., finding space to meet); (2) most team members would agree with the decision and provide consensus; and (3) a decision has to be made promptly.

In the *consultative* decision process, the leader will ask the opinions of the entire team, but the final decision lies with the leader. A fully developed team may use the *joint* decision process, in which team members and the leader are involved in mutual decision making, and everyone has an equal vote. This process encourages everyone to fully accept the team's conclusion. The joint decision

process is also the most creative because everyone has the opportunity to provide input and differing perspectives into the decision.

On the opposite end from the autocratic decision process is the *delegated* decision process, in which the leader is not involved with the final verdict. Instead, the team is truly self-governed and accountable for its decisions. An example of a delegated decision process is the setting up of a unit orientation program for new graduate nurses. After the leader provides the necessary parameters, the team develops its own orientation program and merely reports its decision to the nurse executive.

What are some common problems teams have when charged with decision making and problem solving? A primary issue is that of actually coming to a decision. An autocratic decision is made by one person, regardless of input from others. A joint decision is made together by everyone, with some members winning (i.e., those whose idea was chosen) and some losing (i.e., those whose idea was not chosen). Another common style of decision making is that of consensus: in decisions by consensus, everyone must agree with the final outcome, or else everyone must agree to work together until an acceptable decision is made.

Teams must also grapple with the issue of low productivity, or minimal results. People sometimes cannot focus in the right direction; if a team meets infrequently, an entire year can pass without the team accomplishing anything of significance. In contrast, some teams believe that group members do not have any other commitments except to work on their team's goals and objectives. These high-powered teams expect team members to devote a fair amount of non-meeting time to writing, researching, and producing results for the next team meeting, regardless of other organizational obligations.

SUCCESSFUL TEAM MEMBERSHIP

Within any group, some members are productive, results-oriented team players, and other members are perfectly content to let others do the work. Some members may

LITERATURE APPLICATION

Citation: Oandasan, I., Barker, K., Bosco, C., D'Amour, D., Jones, L., et al. *Teamwork in Healthcare: Promoting Effective Teamwork in Healthcare in Canada: Policy Synthesis and Recommendations (2006)*. Canadian Health Services Research Foundation.

Discussion: Teamwork and collaboration in health care are priority issues for Canadians and their decision makers, with many reports calling for improved collaboration as a key strategy in health care renewal. Effective teamwork can improve the quality of client care, enhance client safety, and reduce workload issues for health professionals. This report was commissioned to answer three questions: What are the characteristics of an effective team, and how do you measure its effectiveness? What interventions have been successful in implementing and sustaining teamwork in health care, and what can we learn from other countries? To what extent has teamwork been implemented in Canadian health care settings, and what are the barriers to implementation? The report was completed by an interprofessional research team that conducted interviews and completed an in-depth review of "team" literature. They identified the challenges of building and maintaining effective teamwork, which included lack of common definition of teams and teamwork, organizational factors that affect teamwork, and the implication of current policy and legislation on teams. Collaboration is needed to support teamwork. Leadership and commitment at all levels of the health care system are required.

Implications for Practice: To foster effective teamwork and collaboration, leadership and commitment are needed from all levels of the health care system. Turf battles have to be eliminated. A common definition for health care teams, teamwork, and team effectiveness is imperative. In all domains—leadership, education, practice, and research—more work is needed to create effective teams and inspire collaborative efforts.

LITERATURE APPLICATION

Citation: Moe, J.S.E., Bailey, A. L., Kroeker, S., & Moe, G. (2010). An interprofessional collaborative practice model: Primary-care clinical associates at the family practice setting. *Healthcare Management Forum*, 23: 159–163.

Discussion: The Alberta Westview Primary Care Network (WPCN) introduced the Primary Care Clinical Associate (CA) program in 2005. This interprofessional collaborative practice model recruits non-physician health professionals from different disciplines as autonomous, independent practitioners. They become associates of the family physician and use their full scope of practice to jointly care for a panel of clients in a family practice setting. The present direction of Canadian primary health care reform is towards team approaches.

Implications for Practice: This knowledge transfer will enable replication of the WPCN CA model in other jurisdictions.

be destructive, exhibiting such behaviour as being the aggressor, the disapprover, or the blocker of others' suggestions; being a recognition seeker; being a self-confessor of personal, non-group-oriented feelings or comments; being a playboy or playgirl; being a group dominator or help seeker; or using the group to meet personal needs or plead special interests (Northouse & Northouse, 1992).

If a team is to work successfully toward a common goal, it is important to have the right blend of personalities, experience, and temperaments. For example, if a new graduate nurse is placed on a critical committee responsible for developing a new sick call policy, senior staff nurses should also be included for their experience.

If an entire team is composed of aggressive, visionary members who are not detail-oriented, many fine points may be missed. However, if a team is predominantly composed of people who get caught up with specific issues, the team members may miss the overall goal, because they get bogged down in details.

For a team to have positive outcomes, an astute team leader will keep in mind that some personality types complement others. One tool that some organizations use to assist them in devising effective work teams and team building is the Myers-Briggs Type Indicator, a psychological instrument that identifies different personality types. Successful teams are those that use the right blend of personalities to achieve their goals.

KEY CONCEPTS

- Teams, groups, and committees are essential to the effective functioning of any health care organization.

- Teams may be formed for a variety of reasons, including the need for professional affiliation, the need for socialization, and the need for psychological fulfillment.

- Teams, groups, and committees consist of people who come together for a common purpose and who need each other's contributions to achieve the overall goal.

- Each group goes through defined stages of increasing maturity.

- Group members can perform functional or dysfunctional roles, which may ultimately enhance or hinder the group's progress toward goal attainment.

- Great teams have clearly stated purposes, effective communication, an action plan, and continuously evaluate their progress.

- The team leader has certain designated responsibilities and tasks to ensure team productivity.

- An environment conducive to team building should be in place for maximum success.

- Interprofessional teams and collaborative practices are the future in health care.

KEY TERMS

adjourning	interprofessional team
committee	norming
forming	performing
group	storming
group development	team

REVIEW QUESTIONS

1. When forming a group, the leader should keep which of the following thoughts in mind?
   A. The group should decide the goals and objectives.
   B. The group is responsible for developing its vision.
   C. The group should be constructed of similar personality types.
   D. The group should encourage active participation by all members.

2. Which is the normal sequencing of group development?
   A. forming, norming, storming, performing, adjourning
   B. norming, forming, storming, performing, adjourning
   C. forming, storming, norming, performing, adjourning
   D. forming, storming, conforming, norming, adjourning

3. Which of the following group roles is considered functional?
   A. initiator
   B. detailer
   C. pleaser
   D. controller

4. Which of the following is a primary duty of an effective team leader?
   A. ensuring that all the details are taken care of all the time
   B. enabling the team to envision their goals and objectives
   C. taking effective minutes of the meetings
   D. allowing everyone a chance to participate, even if the meeting goes longer than expected

5. Which of the following is important in maintaining an environment conducive to team building?
   A. having leaders with an autocratic management style.
   B. encouraging creativity within the organization.

C. rewarding employees who consistently revise the team's objectives.
D. holding an evaluation session at the completion of the team's duration.

REVIEW ACTIVITIES

1. You are the manager of a 36-bed medical surgical unit. In light of recognition of scope of practice, you have hired three licensed practical nurses to fill positions in which only registered nurses worked before.
    ■ How would you plan for the LPNs to become part of the team?

    ■ What are some important considerations for you, your established staff, and the new employees?

    ■ What are some things you can do to assist them in becoming members of your team?

2. Because of the increase in client complaints about the quality of care, you have been asked to develop a team to address these client care issues.
    ■ What are your expectations of the five stages of group development?

    ■ How will you encourage the group members to progress though each stage?

3. On the unit on which you work as a registered nurse, the team is interprofessional in nature: you work directly with licensed practical nurses, unregulated care providers, a unit clerk, one physiotherapist, one respiratory therapist, one community nurse case manager, and one clinical nurse specialist.
    ■ What are some of the advantages of working with inter-professional teams?

    ■ What are some of the challenges of working with inter-professional teams?

    ■ How does one best communicate with an interprofessional team?

EXPLORING THE WEB

Where would you find additional information on effective team building on the Internet?

■ http://www.cihc.ca/

■ http://erc.msh.org/quality/ittools/ittipstm.cfm

What type of leadership style do you have in a team situation?

■ http://www.nwlink.com/~donclark/leader/leadstl.html and http://www.mindtools.com/pages/article/newLDR_84.htm

REFERENCES

Argyris, C. (1964). *Integrating the individual and the organization.* New York: Wiley.

Ashmos, D. (1998) from "Building effective healthcare teams" in W.J. Duncan, P.M. Ginter and L.E. Swayne (eds), *Handbook of Healthcare Management* (p. 313–337).

Bennis, W. (1989). *Why leaders can't lead.* San Francisco: Jossey-Bass.

Bradford, L. P. (1978). *Group development.* La Jolla, CA: University Associates.

Burns, J. M. (1978). *Leadership.* New York: Harper & Row.

Campbell, B., Fryers, M., Devitt, R., & Vestal, K. (2009). Towards a collaborative model of care. *Healthcare Management Forum,* 22(3), 27–31.

Clements, D., Dault, M., & Priest, A. (2007). Effective teamwork in healthcare: Research and reality. *Healthcare Papers,* 7(Special issue), 26–34.

College of Health Disciplines, University of British Columbia. (2010). Canadian interprofessional health collaborative: A national interprofessional care competency framework. Vancouver, BC.

Cziraki, K., Lucas, J., Rogers, T., Page, L., Zimmerman, R., Hauer, L. A., et al. (2008). Communication and relationship skills for rapid response teams at Hamilton Health Sciences. *Healthcare Quarterly,* 11(Special issue), 66–71.

Drew, P., Jones, B., & Norton, D. (2010). Team effectiveness in primary care networks in Alberta. *Healthcare Quarterly,* 13(3), 33–37.

Gardner, D. (2005). Ten lessons in collaboration. *OJIN: The Online Journal of Issues in Nursing,* 10(1), manuscript 1.

Grossman, S. C., & Valiga, T. M. (2009). *The new leadership challenge: Creating the future of nursing* (3rd ed.). Philadelphia: FA Davis Company.

Healthforce Ontario. (2010). Implementing Inter-professional Care in Ontario: The Final Report of the Inter-professional Care Strategic Implementation Committee.

Huber, D. (2000). *Leadership and nursing care management* (2nd ed.). Philadelphia: W. B. Saunders.

Husting, P. M. (1996). Leading teams and improving performance [Electronic version]. *Nursing Management,* 27(9), 35.

Katzenbach, J. R., & Smith, D. K. (1993). *The wisdom of teams: Creating the high-performance organization.* New York: Harper Business.

Kouzes, J. M., & Posner, B. Z. (2002). *The leadership challenge* (3rd ed.). San Francisco: Jossey-Bass/A Wiley Company.

Lacoursiere, R. B. (1980). *The life cycle of groups: Group development stage theory.* New York: Human Sciences Press.

Lemieux-Charles, L., & McGuire, W. (2006). What do we know about health care team effectiveness? *Medical Care Research and Review,* 63(3), 263–300.

Lewin, K. (1951). *Field theory in social sciences.* New York: Harper & Row.

Marquis, B. L., & Huston, C. J. (2012). *Leadership roles and management functions in nursing: Theory and application* (7th ed.). Philadelphia: Lippincott, Williams, & Wilkins.

McGregor, D. (1960). *The human side of enterprise.* New York: McGraw-Hill.

Mears, P. (1994) *Healthcare teams: Building continuous quality improvement.* Orlando, FL: St. Lucie Press.

Moe, J. S. E., Bailey, A. L., Kroeker, S., & Moe, G. (2010). An interprofessional collaborative practice model: Primary-care clinical associates at the family practice setting. *Healthcare Management Forum,* 23, 159–163.

Northouse, P. G., & Northouse, L. L. (1992). *Health communication: Strategies for health professionals* (2nd ed.). Norwalk, CT: Appleton & Lange.

Oandasan, I., Baker, G. R., Barker, K., Bosco, C., D'Amour, D., Jones, L., et al. (2006). *Teamwork in healthcare: Promoting effective teamwork in healthcare in Canada: Policy Synthesis and Recommendations*. Ottawa: Canadian Health Services Research Foundation.

Plaza, C., Beard, L., Di Fonzo, A., Di Tommaso, M., Mujawaz, Y., Serra-Julia, M., & Morra, D. (2011). Innovation in healthcare team feedback. *Healthcare Quarterly, 14*(2), 61–68.

Ragaz, N., Berk, A., Ford, D., & Morgan, M. (2010). Strategies for family health team leadership: Lessons learned by successful teams. *Healthcare Quarterly, 13*(3), 39–43.

Ross, A., Wenzel, F. J., & Mitlyng, J. W. (2002). *Leadership for the future: Core competencies in healthcare*. Chicago: Health Administration Press.

Senge, P. M. (2006). *The fifth discipline: The art & practice of the learning organization*. New York: Doubleday/Currency.

Tappen, R. M. (2001). *Nursing leadership and management: Concepts and practice* (4th ed.). Philadelphia: F. A. Davis.

Tuckman, B. W., & Jensen, M. A. C. (1977). Stages of small group development revisited. *Group and Organizational Studies, 2*(4), 419.

SUGGESTED READINGS

Abrahamsen, C. (2003). Patient safety: Take the informatics challenge. *Nursing Management, 34*(4), 48–52.

Bellack, J., & O'Neil, E. (1999). Recreating nursing practice for a new century: Recommendations and implications of the Pew Health Professions Commission's final report. *Nursing & Health Care Perspectives, 21*(1), 14–21.

Farrell, M. P., Schmitt, M. H., & Heinemann, G. D. (2001). Informal roles and the stages of interdisciplinary team development. *Journal of Interprofessional Care, 15*(3), 281–295.

Henderson, E. (2003). Communication and managerial effectiveness. *Nursing Management—UK, 9*(9), 30–35.

Kennedy, M. M. (2001). What do you owe your team? Survival tips for people who dread teamwork. *Physician Executive, 27*(4), 58–60.

Leeseberg Stamler, L., & Yiu, L. (2005). *Community health nursing: A Canadian perspective*. Toronto: Pearson/Prentice-Hall.

Lengacher, C. A., Mabe, P. R., VanCott, M. L., Heinemann, D., & Kent, K. (1995). Team-building process in launching a practice model. *Nursing Connections, 8*(2), 51–59.

Leppa, C. J. (1996). Nurse relationships and work groups disruption. *Journal of Nursing Administration, 26*(10), 23–27.

Morand, D. A. (2001). The emotional intelligence of managers: Assessing the construct validity of a nonverbal measure of people skills. *Journal of Business and Psychology, 16*(1), 21–33.

Myers, I. B. (1995). *Introduction to type*. Palo Alto, CA: Consulting Psychologists Press.

Opt, S. K., & Loffredo, D. A. (2000). Rethinking communication apprehension: A Myers-Briggs perspective. *Journal of Psychology, 134*(5), 556–570.

Prager, H. (1999). Cooking up effective team building. *Training & Development, 53*(12), 14.

Shope, T. C., Frohna, J. G., & Frohna, A. Z. (2000). Using the Myers-Briggs Type Indicator (MBTI) in the teaching of leadership skills. *Medical Education, 34*(11), 956.

Stein, S., & Book, H. (2000). *The EQ edge: Emotional intelligence and your success*. Toronto: Stoddart Publishing Company Limited.

Woolf, R. (2001). How to talk so people will listen. *Journal of Nursing Administration, 31*(9), 401–402.

CHAPTER ENDNOTES

1. Kouzes, J. M., & Posner, B. Z. (2002). The leadership challenge (3rd ed., p. 18). San Francisco: Jossey-Bass/A Wiley Company.

2. Clements, D., Dault, M., & Priest, A. (2007). Effective teamwork in healthcare: Research and reality. *Healthcare Papers*, 7(Special issue), p. 28.

3. Ibid., p. 31.

CHAPTER 10

Budget Concepts for Client Care

Corinne Haviley, RN, MS

Adapted by Heather Crawford, BScN, MEd, CHE

There is nothing more difficult to take in hand, more perilous to conduct, or more uncertain in its success than to take the lead in the introduction of a new order of things.
(Jean-Jacques Rousseau, 1712–1778)

OBJECTIVES

The purpose of this chapter is to enable the reader to

- describe the budget preparation process for health care organizations;
- define commonly used budgets for planning and management;
- describe key elements that influence budget preparation;
- identify services and products that generate revenue; and
- identify expenses associated with the delivery of service.

Jacqueline Shaw/Shutterstock

You are assigned to a new unit for your clinical experience. You wonder what types of services are provided to clients on this unit. You talk with your instructor and, if appropriate, the nursing manager of the unit to review the unit's budget. You review the unit's scope of service and budget.

What kinds of clients are cared for on this unit?

What kinds of services are provided to clients on this unit?

How does the unit's budget help ensure provision of care for clients on this unit? A key factor that influences client care is the cost involved in the delivery of service. Resources—people, equipment, and time—are required to support the services delivered by nurses. These resources cost money. The economic success of a health care organization depends on those who are involved with service delivery. The decline in health care funding, as well as escalating costs and increasing demands, have required hospitals to improve operational efficiency and to make economically sound decisions. The challenge in health care is to ensure that the quality of care and the calibre of the staff are not compromised in this ever-changing, cost-controlled environment.

Nurses need to understand how to manage the cost of client care as it relates to their own clinical practice. Nurses are accountable for the distribution and consumption of resources, whether those resources are time, supplies, drugs, or staff. It is essential that appropriate decisions be made regarding cost-effective practices. Cost containment affects the financial viability of a nursing department or unit. Hence, nurses need to be informed and partner with the management team to control expenses in relation to client care. Including staff input is good management practice when budget variances are analyzed and ideas are generated for saving money on medical-surgical supplies.

The purpose of this chapter is to provide an overview of the operating budget process, including budget development, implementation, performance, and evaluation.

Common financial language and tools are discussed so nurses can understand the process involved in cost-effective care.

TYPES OF BUDGETS

Hospitals use several types of budgets to help with future planning and management, including operating, capital, and construction budgets.

OPERATING BUDGET

An **operating budget** accounts for the income and expenses associated with day-to-day activity within a department or organization. The expenses associated with equipment, supplies, staffing, and other indirect costs, and having the correct accommodation for clients is the basis of revenue generation. If a client stays in the wrong accommodation revenue may be reduced. For example, if a client has semi-private insurance, and is in a standard ward room, the organization loses the revenue from the insurance company for the accommodation.

CAPITAL BUDGET

A **capital budget** accounts for purchases of new or replacement major pieces of equipment. This equipment typically has a longer operating life (greater than 5 to 7 years) and is more expensive than the operating supplies. Equipment is purchased when new technology becomes available or when older equipment becomes too expensive to maintain. Age-related equipment problems include inefficiencies related to the speed of the equipment or downtime (i.e., the amount of time equipment is out of service for repairs). Sometimes either the expense or the scarcity of replacement parts makes it prohibitive to maintain equipment. In addition, old equipment may become unable to deliver service consistently, meet industry or regulatory standards, or provide high-quality outcomes.

Because a significant expense is associated with equipment acquisition, organizations want to make the best and most economical and informed decisions. Staff members from a variety of areas, including materials management, clinical specialties, the legal department, biomedical engineering, information technology, finance, and management can contribute important input when plans are being made for equipment purchases. A team of staff members must understand the equipment features, benefits, and limitations in relation to the specific needs and goals of a department or institution. Substantial analysis is required because multiple vendors or companies often sell similar or varying products with different terms, conditions, and warranty and maintenance agreements all of which can have short- and long-term effects.

Health care organizations classify specific value amounts as capital purchases. That amount may vary from one organization to another, but usually is in the range of $2,000 to $10,000, depending on the size of the organization and the concomitant size of the operating budget. For example, in one organization, a stent costing $2,000 is a supply item used during a surgical procedure. This supply is considered an operational expense because its life expectancy is two years. On the other hand, a computed tomography (CT) scanner that costs more than $100,000 and has a life expectancy of seven years is considered a capital expense.

CONSTRUCTION BUDGET

A **construction budget** is developed when renovation or new structures are planned. The construction costs generally include labour, materials, building permits, inspections, equipment, and contingency dollars. Expenses may be shifted to another department that absorbs the services on a temporary basis.

BUDGET OVERVIEW

An operating budget is a financial tool that outlines anticipated revenue and expenses over a specified period. Managers engage in a process called **accounting** to record and report financial transactions and data, which assist with budget documentation. The budget translates operating plans into financial and statistical terms so that the budget can be calculated. Budgets serve as standards to plan, monitor, and evaluate the performance of a health care system. Budgetary details relate to specific areas. In contrast to the expenses needed to deliver the service, budgets account for the income generated. Budgets connect the

operating plans and the allocation of resources; this is especially important because health care organizations measure multiple key indicators of overall performance. For example, along with financial performance, organizations routinely evaluate quality client outcomes and customer and staff satisfaction. All these indicators are intertwined and hold value in terms of client care. Collectively, they reflect organizational success.

A **balanced scorecard** is a documentation tool that provides a snapshot of pertinent information and activity at a particular point in time. A balanced scorecard identifies any of four perspectives about an organization: finances, customer satisfaction and services, internal operating efficiency, and learning and growth (Norton & Kaplan, 2001). Figure 10-1 shows the Neonatal Intensive Care Unit patient care team's balanced scorecard at the Winnipeg Health Sciences Children's Hospital, Winnipeg Regional Health Authority. This scorecard displays the indicators of neonatal transport team response times, pain assessment, parent satisfaction, radiology results communicated to parents, central line infection rates, access to appropriate ventilators, continuity of nursing care, and staff satisfaction. Figure 10-2 shows a balanced scorecard with a variety of indicators that illustrate the connectivity between performance and quality outcomes. During the past decade substantial progress has been made towards developing performance measurement and quality improvement frameworks associated with the delivery of health care. Efforts have focused on responsiveness to client demands,

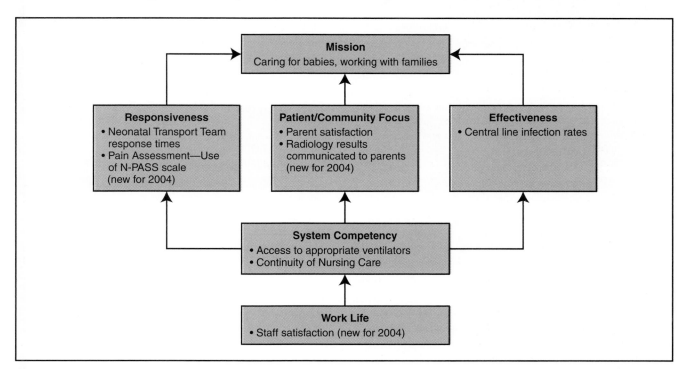

Figure 10-1 NICU (Neonatal Intensive Care Unit) Patient Care Team's Balanced Scoreboard

Source: Sawatzky-Dickson, D. (2004). "A Balance with the NICU Quality Team". Child Health Quality Team. *Quality for Kids Newsletter,* 3(2): 2. Reprinted with permission of Winnipeg Regional Health Authority.

while simultaneously improving quality and efficiency; increasingly, to quantify the profession's contribution to quality and safety, efforts are focusing on nursing-specific or nursing-sensitive outcomes.[1] Figure 10-3 outlines Bridgepoint Health's Nursing Balanced Scorecard, which consists of 22 strategic objectives and aligned indicators.

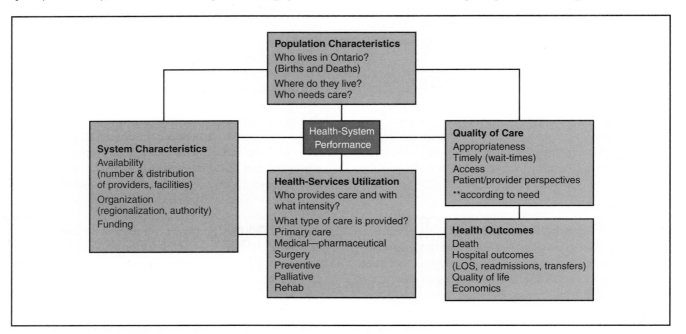

Figure 10-2 Characteristics for Examining Health-system Performance: A Balanced Scorecard Approach

Source: Iron, K. (2006). ICES Report: Health Data in Ontario: Taking Stock and Moving Ahead. *Healthcare Quarterly*, 9(3): 24–26. Reprinted with Permission.

1. Nursing Resource Management Domain	
Strategic Objective	Indicators
Attract and retain the best nursing professionals	Nurse Retention Index External turnover rate Attrition rate Nurse Recruitment Index Nurse satisfaction survey results
Build and optimize nursing resource allocation and services	Efficiency Index RN-worked hours per patient day RN-worked hours per patient day (agency, sick time and overtime)

2. Nursing internal processes: care delivery and clinical practice domain	
Strategic Objective	Indicators
Implement the Chronic Care Model and the Live Well philosophy	Continuity and transition, % positive scores
Leverage information and apply knowledge for best care and service	Electronic clinical documentation Sustainability Plan achievement
Put quality and safety first every day	Quality Index Falls Infection rates Medication incidents Pain assessment compliance Pressure ulcers

(Continued)

Strengthen our academic and clinical education infrastructure	Peer-reviewed papers Peer-reviewed conference abstracts
Develop advanced nursing knowledge in specialty areas and chronic disease prevention and management	Specialty Certification Index Nursing expertise
Generate, disseminate and apply new knowledge at the point of care	Falls prevention strategy plan implementation
Cultivate discovery and innovations in care	Advanced practice nurse recruitment rate
Set the standards and models for healthcare in the 21st century	Implementation of Royal Bank of Canada (RBC) grant
Enable inspired and proactive nursing leadership	% completion of performance appraisals Practice Environment Scale
Influence health system priorities and decisions	No. of nurses on academic and hospital-related external boards/committees/Local Health Integration Network (LHIN) committees
Be accountable	% compliance with clinical documentation audits Staff response time to patient call

3. Outcomes domain

Strategic Objective	Indicators
Safe reliable patient-centred/partnership-oriented care	Patient satisfaction
Efficient care processes	Sick time Overtime Agency time
Knowledge generation and enactment	Intravenous insertion competency
Nurses leading change	Staff RN committee participation

4. Nursing organizational capabilities domain

Strategic Objective	Indicators
Implement the nursing service delivery model	Clinical model of care Clinical skill mix
Enable nursing leadership development and succession planning	RN leadership training
Create communities of nursing practice	Number of mentors
Build professional practice infrastructure	Unit councils
Foster inter-professional care and partnerships	RN academic appointments Nursing student hours Pre-graduate placements

Figure 10-3 Bridgepoint Health's Nursing Balanced Scorecard

Source: Jeffs, L., Merkley, J., Richardson, S., Eli, J., & McAllister, M. (2011). Using a nursing balanced scorecard approach to measure and optimize nursing performance. *Nursing Leadership*, 24(1): 51–53. Reprinted with permission.

Similar to controlling personal funds— such as managing one's chequing or savings account—budgeting helps to define services. This is done by projecting how much cash will be generated (i.e., revenue) and how much services will cost to operate (i.e., expenses). Budgeting requires forward thinking so that problems and obstacles can be anticipated and planned for. Budgets also serve as a benchmark to measure whether the planning expectations are being met. Typically, budgets are monitored monthly. If deficiencies arise, financial improvement plans can be instituted early. Corrective action is often initiated to prevent long-term effects in a particular area, such as waste or loss of supply items. The budget functions as a tool to foster collaboration because individuals within a department must work together to achieve its goals.

BUDGET PREPARATION

Formulating a budget involves a systematic approach that begins with preparation (Grohar-Murray & DiCroce, 1997). Budgets are generally developed for a 12-month period. The yearly cycle is based on a fiscal year as determined by the province or territory (e.g., April 1 through March 31) Short- or long-term budgets may also be developed depending upon the organizational planning process.

Before the beginning of the budget year, most organizations devote approximately six months to preparing and developing the operating budget. To prepare a budget, organizations gather fundamental information about a variety of elements that influence the organization, including demographic information, volume and cost increases or decreases, regulatory influences, and strategic plans. Additionally, it is helpful to review the department's scope of service, goals, and history.

DEMOGRAPHIC INFORMATION

Pulling together demographic information related to the population that the organization serves is most helpful. This information makes it possible to identify unique demographic characteristics such as age, race, sex, and income that influence client behaviour. For example, an obstetrics practice would expect to attract women of childbearing age rather than an older male population. Therefore, understanding the demographics and market share (i.e., the percentage of the population living in the area that uses the organization's services) helps paint a clear picture regarding the client population.

REGULATORY INFLUENCES

Accreditation Canada (AC) accredits health facilities to ensure that organizations meet specific standards. In addition, AC can make recommendations that will affect the capital or operating budget of the facility.

REAL WORLD INTERVIEW

Staff nurses need to understand their own department's client volume, the nature of their case load, the effects of client acuity, and how it may change. As client acuity changes, so does client care delivery. We may be able to anticipate the services that will be needed based upon client acuity and how those services will affect the client's stay. Communicating this information to management is most helpful. Remember that the budget process is fluid and not stagnant. Situations change and can alter the budget over time. A budget is not made in stone; it is only a guideline. Nurses can have an impact upon cost by understanding, through cost accounting, which supplies are being used with different types of admissions or procedures. Once calculated, this data can be shared with physicians. The use of standardized products can be compared when analyzing procedures or admissions by physicians and nurses. This process should assist in understanding both practice patterns and costs related to client care. Physicians and nurses control major costs.

Nurses need to be stewards in recognizing expenses. For example, nurses are key to the client's length of stay and when and how resources are allocated during a client's stay. Nurses need to act on issues before they become critical. Wastage is a good area to focus on because it adds to the cost of a client's stay. If a nurse wastes four gloves, the cost may be only $10 to cover the cost of the gloves. But think further about additional costs, such as packaging, shipping, stocking, charging the unit, and tracking, which may inflate the cost to $30. If this expense occurs during all 3 shifts multiplied by 30 beds, then the dollar amount adds up considerably. This cost in turn cuts into the ability of the unit to balance its budget.

Barb Seeley, BScN
Surgical Unit Manager

Regulatory requirements may change regarding who may deliver a specific service and in what type of setting. For example, a procedure may have to be performed in a hospital rather than in a physician's office if it is to be reimbursed by the insurance company. Similarly, reimbursement may depend on whether a nurse practitioner or a physician is consulted.

Revenue is also affected by consumers' willingness to pay out of pocket when they are not covered by insurance. For example, the cost of circumcision is no longer covered by health insurance, and if someone requires a cast, the cost of a plaster of Paris cast is covered, but a fibreglass cast is not.

STRATEGIC PLANS

Generally, hospitals have strategic plans that map out the direction for the organization over several years. Strategic plans guide the staff at all levels so that the entire organization can have a shared mission and vision, with clearly defined steps to meet the goals.

Each department develops unit-specific plans to help the organization follow its overall strategic plan. For example, an organization's goal may be to become the centre of excellence for gastroenterology endoscopy laboratories for the surrounding region. To meet the goal, one department may focus on client satisfaction and room turnaround time for a certain procedure to increase the volume and decrease client wait times for their appointments. This goal is part of the organization's overall plan.

SCOPE OF SERVICE AND GOALS

During the budget preparation phase, individual departments or sections need to be thoroughly examined. For organizational purposes, hospitals frequently compartmentalize their systems, that is, divide them into sections, departments, or units. These sections or units, commonly called **cost centres,** are used to track financial data.

Each department or cost centre defines its own scope of service (Figure 10-4 and Figure 10-5 provide examples of scopes of service). The scope of service provides helpful information related to the types of service and the sites at which services are offered, including the usual treatments and procedures, hours of operation, and the types of client and customer groups.

Departmental goals may include the introduction of new technology or treatments, client education, and the creation of a special client care environment. Staff members are generally questioned to determine whether they have any proposed quality initiatives that should be included in the plans for the upcoming year. Generally,

The gastrointestinal endoscopy suite may be defined as a specialized department that performs major procedures that are both diagnostic and therapeutic in nature, such as upper GI endoscopies, colonoscopies, flexible sigmoidoscopies, and endoscopic retrograde cholangiopancreatography (ERCP). Conscious sedation is typically delivered to clients to provide comfort during the procedures. The endoscopy suite is open Monday through Friday from 0700–1700 hours, and provides after-hours service for emergent cases. Pre-procedure, intra-procedure, and post-procedure care, including full recovery, is provided on site. Services are provided to critical in-house clients at the bedside via the staff assigned to travel to inpatient units. The department employs nurses, technicians, and receptionists, who work with gastroenterologists and surgeons to provide care. The unit is equipped with 10 procedure rooms, 25 recovery bays, and a gastrointestinal scope cleaning facility on site.

Figure 10-4 Endoscopy Suite Scope of Service

A medical nursing unit provides primarily inpatient care to clients with acute or chronic medical problems, such as congestive heart failure, diabetes, pulmonary disease, and cancer. The unit, equipped with 30 private and semi-private beds, a lounge, and conference/consultation rooms, is operational 24 hours per day, 7 days per week. Client education and support groups are held routinely in the library located on the unit. Team nursing is employed as the model of care. Nurses, licensed practical nurses, unregulated care providers, and unit clerks are employed, with a social worker and diabetes educator providing additional client support. Clients admitted to the unit for longer than 48 hours are discussed during daily multidisciplinary rounds. The rounds include community nurse case managers; psychosocial counsellors; and nutrition, nursing, and medical staff. Staff discusses client problems to facilitate future care, including discharge planning.

Figure 10-5 Medical Nursing Unit Scope of Care

new treatments, client education materials, and documentation tools require different types or amounts of supplies. Technically trained staff members are often needed to implement new services. Both the staff and supplies can have varying costs during the early induction phase through full implementation. Additional funding, which must be identified early in the planning stages, may be needed to create a new environment or provide an "evidence-based best practice" experience. The manager is responsible for identifying the expenses associated with client care upfront so that they are budgeted.

The manager from an inpatient unit asks for staff input to identify ways to decrease the use of medical supplies and paper items. These items have been identified as exceeding the budget by 10 percent to 20 percent during the past three months. This is the first time that the staff members have been involved in helping with cost containment. Clinical nurses and assistants have been invited to participate.

When approaching an analysis of medical supply use, what might be the first step in the process? If you were to divide the staff into work groups, which members should be chosen to analyze the use of clerical supplies? How would you proceed if you were trying to determine the supply costs associated with starting an IV with continuous infusion?

HISTORY

Organizations typically use history or past performance as a baseline of experience and data to better understand activity in a department or unit. These data are used to assist in interpreting associated expenses with staff productivity and unit performance. Most often adjustments are made to planned budgets because of the ever-changing cost of products and supplies. Bulk contracts are negotiated so that predetermined reduced rates can be realized when organizations purchase large quantities of supplies. For example, if a hospital purchases a large quantity of one product, the vendor may reduce the price as an incentive. Additionally, knowledge about historical volume (e.g., procedures, admissions, or client visits and average length of stay) provides a perspective on how a department has grown or declined over time. This information may help with anticipating future demand and capacity. The story behind a unit and how the department developed is equally important because the financial numbers are tracked over time. Often the culture and complexity of a unit unfold during interviews of staff who were involved in the unit in the past, including physicians, nurses, technologists, assistants, housekeeping, and nutritionists. This information may provide further insight into why and how past decisions were made. Hence, multiple phases of data gathering are essential for budget development.

BUDGET DEVELOPMENT

After background data have been gathered, the development of the budget can follow, including the projection of revenue and expenses.

REVENUE

Revenue is income generated through a variety of means, including billable client services, investments, and donations to the organization. Specific unit-based revenue is generated through billing for services such as special accommodation. In preparing a budget, the specific number and types of services and procedures have to be projected. Each type of service may have a different volume of activity associated with it. For example, projections for the volume and type of procedures conducted in a gastrointestinal laboratory are based on feedback from the referring physicians and technical staff, as well as conclusions from historical data.

Similarly, the same types of projections occur for inpatient units, including the anticipated number of clients to be admitted, the average length of stay (e.g., three to five days), and the projected occupancy rate. The type and amount of services and patient days can be measured. The number of patient days or the service delivered is tracked from a productivity and efficiency perspective.

It is important to note that the reimbursement rates of third-party payers affect revenue and can change from year to year. For example, the rate for semi-private accommodation may increase from $150 to $200 per day. Uniform rates are often used. Insurance companies dictate or negotiate rates with health care organizations on an annual basis, depending on whether they notice particular trends occurring, such as a hospital that offers only semi-private or private accommodation.

EXPENSES

Expenses are determined by identifying the costs associated with the delivery of service. Expenditures are resources used by an organization to deliver services and may include supplies, labour, equipment, utilities, and miscellaneous items.

LITERATURE APPLICATION

Citation: Barnardo, C., & Jivanni, A. (2009). Evaluating the Fraser Health balanced scorecard – A formative evaluation. *Healthcare Management Forum*, 22(2): 49–60.

Discussion: Fraser Health is a large, Canadian, integrated health care network in British Columbia. It adopted the balanced scorecard approach to monitor organizational performance in 2006. This article reports on the results of a formative evaluation that was conducted in April 2008 to assess the usefulness of the balanced scorecard as a performance-reporting system and a performance management tool. The results indicate that the balanced scorecard was useful for reporting performance but was not currently used for performance management in a substantial way in that organization.

Implications for Practice: A balanced scorecard is strategic management tool that helps the organization focus on strategies and improvement activities. To realize its benefits, a balanced scorecard must be used for more than a reporting system. This means that performance information must be embedded into the decision-making process at all levels of the organization. In addition, accountabilities for performance improvement need to be assigned. Organizations need to develop new or improved data collection processes and systems that can capture relevant and timely information efficiently and effectively.

REAL WORLD INTERVIEW

It is not just my job to be responsible for the budget. I encourage my staff to know the costs of supplies and to understand the rationale behind transferring clients to the correct accommodation. In addition, I teach them about patient days, and hours per patient day, so that they understand how the budget is formulated. I don't think the staff realize how something simple can negatively affect our bottom line. For example, the nurses will stockpile such items as face cloths or incontinence pads in the client's bedside table. Admittedly, this practice saves some time for the nurse, but if the client is discharged prior to these items being used, the linen is returned to the company for re-laundering, and the incontinence pads are discarded. Both will cost our unit precious dollars. I have asked the staff for suggestions on how to save money and supplies, and they have some very creative solutions. In addition, they are more aware of wasteful activity, and our collective endeavour has helped reduce our supply usage.

Maureen Shaughnessy, MSN
Unit Manager, Cardiology

Understanding what it takes to deliver client care services helps to ensure that appropriate budgets are in place to pay for the services. Expenses are commonly separated into line items, representing specific categories that contribute to the cost of the procedure or activity, such as paper supplies, medical supplies, drugs, and so on. This arrangement helps identify a service's significant expenses. For example, a colonoscopy may have a high medical supply cost, whereas chemotherapy administration may be associated with a high drug cost.

SUPPLIES

As new procedures are introduced, or when a manager wants to assess the actual cost of supplies associated with a procedure or activity, an organization may institute zero-based budgeting. This is a process used to drill down into expenses, which means that every supply item and the quantity of items typically used is listed in detail.

Someone develops a list of supplies, including large and small items, and their expenses. Supplies are often packaged in bulk and sold in quantity. Hence, the expense of each item has to be calculated—rather than derived from the bulk figure—to accurately depict the expense.

Figure 10-6 illustrates the zero-based budgeting that may be needed to account for all of the expenses associated with delivering a procedure. The budgeting in this example can be expanded to further calculate the total expense associated with the anticipated number of procedures. This calculation can be achieved by multiplying the number of anticipated procedures by the total expense per procedure, which leads to authentic projections.

HUMAN RESOURCES

Human resources represent a significant expense in the field of medical and nursing care. Health care services are very labour intensive. An estimated 80 percent of operating costs go toward salaries and benefits. Therefore, it is very important to calculate the amount of time that all staff members—professional, technical, and support staff—are involved with the service. For example, the time that it takes to schedule an appointment, register a client, and escort a client to a procedure room or unit needs to be calculated into the overall cost of care for the client.

General Supplies	Quantity	Price	Drugs	Quantity	Price
4 Chux	4	$ 3.00	Fentanyl	1	$ 0.25
Tri Pour Container	1	$ 0.20	Versed	1	$ 2.10
Sterile Water 1,000 ml	1	$ 0.40		Total	$ 2.35
Normal Saline Vial	2	$ 0.10			
Cannister/Lid	2	$ 3.25			
Tubing	2	$ 0.50			
02 Cannula	1	$ 0.05	Printed Forms	Quantity	Price
Suction Catheter	1	$ 0.02			
Disposable Gowns	2	$ 3.80	Hospital Consent	1	$ 0.10
Gloves	6	$ 0.35	Procedure Consent	1	$ 0.75
4X4's	10	$ 0.25	Nursing Form	1	$ 0.75
Surgilube	2 oz.	$ 0.15	Vital Sign Sheet	1	$ 0.05
Photos	2	$ 4.30	Doctors Orders	1	$ 0.15
Syringe 10cc	2	$ 0.15	History/Physical	1	$ 0.10
Syringe 60cc	1	$ 0.35	Discharge Instruction	1	$ 0.20
Emesis Basin	1	$ 0.10	Education Sheet	1	$ 0.80
Denture Cup	1	$ 0.15	Charge Voucher	1	$ 0.10
Recording Paper	1	$ 0.05	Procedure Education	1	$ 0.10
Alcohol Pads	2	$ 0.05		Total	$ 3.10
Slippers	1	$ 0.75			
Mask	2	$ 0.25			
Goggles/Face Shield	1	$ 1.20	Clerical Supplies	Quantity	Price
Cetacaine Spray	1	$ 0.10			
Bite Block	1	$ 2.00	Patient File	1	$ 0.80
Patient Bag	1	$ 0.20	Labels	2	$ 0.05
Cleaning Brush	1	$ 2.20	Xerox Paper	6	$ 0.05
	Totals	$23.92	Pen	1	$ 0.05
			Pencil	1	$ 0.05
			Marker	1	$ 0.05
IV Start	Quantity	Price	Highlighters	1	$ 0.05
				Total	$ 1.10
Tourniquet	1	$ 0.15			
Alcohol Wipes	2	$ 0.05			
Angiocath	1	$ 0.05			
IV Solution	1	$ 0.60			
IV Primary Set	1	$ 4.00			
Tegaderm	1	$ 0.15			
Tape	6 inches	$ 0.05	Grand Total		
Band-Aid	1	$ 0.05			
4X4	4	$ 0.10			
	Totals	$ 5.20			

Figure 10-6 Zero-Based Budgeting for GI Lab

Source: Adapted with permission of Northwestern Memorial Hospital, Chicago, IL.

In the ambulatory area, staff time is calculated relative to the delivery of a specific procedure, including preparation for the procedure, intra-procedure care, and post-procedure care. Pre-procedure preparation entails gathering of supplies, assembling equipment, and preparing the environment. Preparing the client may involve taking a history, completing a physical, administering medication or taking specimens, placing tubes or establishing an intravenous line, and positioning the client. Intra-procedure care is the actual care delivered after the procedure has been initiated. Post-procedure care may require educating and discharging a client, or extensive recovery activity requiring several hours of direct nursing care and removal of equipment and supply items. Refer to Table 10-1 for a sample time analysis related to labour.

STAFFING

The number of staff and the types of staff are often accounted for in a staffing model. This model outlines the number of staff required based upon the primary statistic, such as procedures or clients. An outpatient model may focus on the number of procedure rooms

CRITICAL THINKING

The staff who handle client care activities on a day-to-day basis are in the best position to identify where practices can improve efficiency and cost-effectiveness. Managers can consult with staff and then organize processes to assist with unit-based improvement. Think back on the steps taken by a nurse during the first hour of a shift. Reflect on the communication process and how the information is received. Examine the amount of time spent in client care versus other activities. Create a journal of activity for different time increments during a shift. Discuss your observations with your co-workers and manager. What problems in flow of activity and gaps in communication or efficiency did you find? How can you drill down further to understand how the unit operates and how productivity can be increased? How could you improve your team's functioning?

TABLE 10-1	TIME ANALYSIS PER PROCEDURE

Pre-Procedure Care	Time (minutes)		Intra-Procedure Care	Time (minutes)
Appointment schedule	5		Positioning	5
Registration	10		Initiation of conscious sedation	10
Escort to change room	5		Procedure	10
Subtotal	20		Subtotal	25
Direct Client Preparation			**Post-Procedure Care**	
History	5		Recovery	120
Client education and consent	10		Education	10
IV initiation	10		Changing and discharging	10
Subtotal	25		Subtotal	140

Grand total = 210 minutes per procedure

that require staff. One nurse may be needed to staff a gastrointestinal laboratory procedure room, and one shared technician may staff two procedure rooms.

Models can help in analyzing productivity, as illustrated in the following:

1. Scenario 1: One nurse is assigned to a procedure room during a 4-hour period, during which 8 clients are treated.
2. Scenario 2: One nurse and a technical assistant are assigned to a procedure room for 4 hours, and 16 clients are treated.

The second scenario depicts greater productivity because the number of procedures delivered doubled by using two staff, recognizing that the assistant staff member will cost the organization less in terms of salary expense. Because labour is one of health care's greatest operational costs, enhancing productivity will likely produce savings.

For an inpatient unit, nurses may be assigned to a fixed number of clients during all three shifts. The ratios vary depending upon the shift and client acuity. The nurse-to-client ratio on a medical nursing unit may be one nurse to five (1:5) clients during the day and evening shift, whereas it may be 1:10 during the night shift. The nurse-to-client ratio may be 1:1 for all shifts on a critical care unit. Chapter 11 deals with effective staffing in more depth.

CRITICAL THINKING

"Staying in the loop" is key to becoming energized and feeling engaged as a part of the client care team and as a vital part of the organization (Nelson, 1997). When you walk onto a unit, ask a staff member what key quality initiatives the unit is working on to reflect continuous quality improvement. Ask what the unit's goals are and how staff participate in decisions so that the goals may be achieved. Think about how these initiatives may increase productivity, or staff or client satisfaction, or decrease expenses. Ask the staff what impact their efforts are having. How is the staff involved in helping the organization to meet its goals?

BUDGET APPROVAL AND MONITORING

Once developed, budgets are submitted to administration for review and final approval. The approval process may take several weeks because the unit budgets are combined to determine the overall budget for the health care organization. Senior management, representing finance and operations, often makes the final decisions regarding acceptance of a budget.

The unit or department manager is responsible for controlling the budget. Budget monitoring is generally carried out on a monthly basis to ensure that revenue is generated consistent with projected productivity and standards. Organizations often recognize a flexible budget, which allows for adjustments if the volume or census increases or decreases. If the volume increases, expenses will likely increase. If the volume decreases and expenses increase, then the manager needs to determine what actions are necessary to control or reduce costs. Many organizations require managers to complete a budget variance report, which identifies when categories are out of line and corrective action is needed. Figure 10-7 illustrates a variance report. The entire health care team is responsible for ensuring that expenses are kept within the budgeted amount and that the volume or census is maintained. The manner in which these controls are accomplished depends on the organization. Some institutions request that balanced scorecards be developed to reflect departmental activity at a glance. Variance reports or scorecards may be posted so that all staff members have an opportunity to review the budget and participate in any improvement needed.

Staff can meet to discuss implementation or reinforcement of strategies that can positively affect the budget (Elser & Nipp, 2001; Yoder-Wise, 1998). The following are some examples of such strategies:

1. Analyze time efficiency of staff involved in client care.
2. Plan for supplies needed for every client encounter and consciously eliminate unnecessary items.
3. Learn how a department is reimbursed for services delivered, identifying covered and excluded expenses.
4. Discuss quality and cost differences in supplies with other staff and management.
5. Evaluate staff and equipment downtime.
6. Analyze the causes of schedule delays, cancelled cases, and extended procedure times.
7. Explore new products with vendor representatives and network with colleagues who have tried both new and modified products.
8. Reduce the length of client stays by troubleshooting early.
9. Assist staff in organizational planning.
10. Enhance productivity through rigorous continuous quality improvement.

	Budget	Actual	% Variance	Comments/Action
Revenue				
Inpatient				
Outpatient				
Other				
	List all line items over or under budget			
Expenses				
Salary				
Full-time equivalent employees (FTEs)				
Medical supplies				
Clerical supplies				
Purchased service				
Maintenance				
Miscellaneous				

Figure 10-7 Variance Report per Cost Centre

11. Post overtime and high/low productivity analysis.
12. Explore how time and motion studies may increase efficiencies by identifying gaps or duplication in effort.
13. Ensure that staff has the right tools and that the tools are ready when needed.
14. Analyze client supplies and review costs per client encounter (e.g., chemotherapy administration, dialysis, insertion of indwelling or peripheral catheter).
15. Track various steps in client care that are time consuming or problematic for a unit (e.g., communication from front desk to recovery room, staff response to client call lights, number of staff responding to an emergency code).
16. Acquire a working knowledge of how a department/unit monitors financial and quality indicators, and participate in the development of action plans to increase client satisfaction or to create the "best client experience."

KEY CONCEPTS

- Nurses play an integral role in the development, implementation, and evaluation of a unit or department budget.

- If nurses are not aware of revenue and expenses, then financial performance will deviate from the financial plan.

- Overall, organizational performance is dependent upon the insight and skills of staff members regarding client care quality and financial outcomes.

- Hospitals use several types of budgets to help with future planning and management, including operating, capital, and construction budgets.

- During budget preparation, data are gathered on factors that influence an organization, including demographic information, regulatory influences, and strategic initiatives. It is also helpful to understand the department's scope of service, goals, and history.

- Hospital systems are divided into cost centres, that is, sections, departments, or units, to track financial data, and these need to be thoroughly examined during budget preparation.

- Organizations typically use history or past performance as a baseline of experience and data to better understand activity in a department or unit.

- The development of the budget, including the projection of revenue and expenses, follows the gathering of background data.

- Expenses are determined by identifying the cost associated with the delivery of service. Expenditures are resources used by an organization to deliver services and may include labour, supplies, equipment, utilities, and miscellaneous items.

- After budgets are developed, they are submitted to administration for review and final approval. The approval process may take several weeks because the unit budgets are combined to determine the overall budget for the health care organization.

KEY TERMS

accounting
balanced scorecard
capital budget
construction budget

cost centres
operating budget
revenue

REVIEW QUESTIONS

1. An operating budget accounts for which of the following?
   A. the purchase of minor and major equipment
   B. construction and renovation
   C. income and expenses associated with daily activity within an organization
   D. applications for new technology

2. How can revenue be generated?
   A. client accommodation
   B. donations to service organizations
   C. use of generic drugs
   D. messenger and escort activities

3. Which of the following describes the function of cost centres?
   A. They develop historical and demographic information.
   B. They track expense line items
   C. They plan for strategic growth and movement
   D. They track financial data within a department or unit

4. What is the purpose of monitoring a budget?
   A. to keep expenses above budget
   B. to maintain revenue above the previous year's budget
   C. to ensure revenue is generated monthly
   D. to generate revenue and control expenses within a projected framework

5. Productivity can be measured by which of the following factors?
   A. the number of beds in a hospital
   B. the cost for services rendered
   C. past performance and history regarding revenue
   D. the volume of services delivered

REVIEW ACTIVITIES

1. Look around your clinical agency. Do you see any balanced scorecards? What do they reveal about your agency?

2. Using the zero-based budgeting figure in this chapter, construct an analysis of one of the clinical procedures in your agency.

EXPLORING THE WEB

Go to the site for Accreditation Canada. What information do you find there?

- *http://www.accreditation.ca/en/default.aspx*

Review the site for the Academy of Canadian Executive Nurses. Is the information helpful?

- *http://www.acen.ca/*

Review the following sites for helpful information. What do you find there?

Canadian College of Health Leaders

- *http://www.cchse.org/default1.asp?active_page_id=&action=login*

Health Canada

- *http://www.hc-sc.gc.ca/*

REFERENCES

Albanese, M. P., Evancs, D. A., Schantz, C. A., Brown, M., Disbot, M., Moffa, J. S., et al. (2010). Engaging clinical nurses in quality and performance improvement activities. *Nursing Administration Quarterly*, 34(3), 226–245.

Barnardo, C., & Jivanni, A. (2009). Evaluating the Fraser Health balanced scorecard – A formative evaluation. *Healthcare Management Forum*, 22(2), 49–60.

Cholewa, S., Moran, K., & Cheung, Y. (2010). Evaluation of the consensus-building process to develop a balanced scorecard for York Region public health. *Healthcare Quarterly*, 13(2), 55–59.

Clancy, C. (2007). The performance of performance measurement. *Health Services Research*, 42(5), 1797–1801.

Doran, D., & Pringle, D. (2011). Patient outcomes as an accountability. In D. Doran (Ed.), *Nursing outcomes* (2nd ed.). Sudbury, MA: Jones & Bartlett Learning, LLC.

Elser, R., & Nipp, D. (2001). Worker designed culture change. *Nursing Economics*, 19(4), 161–163, 175.

Escaf, M., McGrath, P., & Costello, J. (2009). An innovative approach to goal setting and reporting in a complex organization. *Healthcare Management Forum*, 22(3), 15–19.

Frith, K. H., Anderson, F., & Sewell, J. P. (2010). Assessing and selecting data for a nursing services dashboard. *Journal of Nursing Administration*, 40(1), 10–16.

Grohar-Murray, M. E., & DiCroce, H. R. (1997). *Leadership and management in nursing*. Stamford, CT: Appleton & Lange.

Iron, K. (2006). ICES report: Health data in Ontario: Taking stock and moving ahead. *Healthcare Quarterly*, 9(3), 24–26.

Jeffs, L., Merkley, J., Richardson, S., Eli, J., & McAllister, M. (2011). Using a nursing balanced scorecard approach to measure and optimize nursing performance. *Nursing Leadership*, 24(1), 47–58.

Kaplan, R. S., & Norton, D. P. (2004). *Strategy maps: Converting intangible assets into tangible outcomes*. Boston: Harvard Business School Press.

Klassen, A., Miller, A., Anderson, N., Shen, J., Schiarti, V., & O'Donnell, M. (2010). Performance measurement and improvement frameworks in health, education and social services systems: A systematic review. *International Journal for Quality in Health Care*, 22(1), 44–69.

McGillis Hall, L. (2002). Report cards: Relevance for nursing and patient care safety. *International Nursing Review*, 49(3), 168–177.

McGillis Hall, L., Doran, D., Laschinger, H. S., Mallette, C., Pederson, C., & O'Brien-Pallas, L. (2003). A balanced scorecard approach for nursing report card development. *Outcomes Management*, 7(1), 17–22.

Naranjo-Gil, D. (2009). Strategic performance in hospitals: The use of the balanced scorecard by nurse managers. *Health Care Management Review*, 34(2), 161–170.

Nelson, B. (1997). *1001 Ways to energize employees*. New York: Workman Publishing.

Norton, D., & Kaplan, R. (2001). *The strategy-focused organization: How balanced scorecard companies thrive in the new business environment*. Boston: Harvard Business School Press.

Sawatzky-Dickson, D. (2004). A balance with the NICU quality team. Child Health Quality Team. *Quality for Kids Newsletter*, 3(2).

Yoder-Wise, P. (1998). *Leading and managing in nursing* (2nd ed.). St. Louis, MO: Mosby.

SUGGESTED READINGS

Baker, G. R., & Pink, G. H. (1995). A balanced scorecard for Canadian hospitals. *Healthcare Management Forum*, 8(4), 7–13.

Carruth, A., Carruth, P., & Noto, E. (2000). Nurse managers flex their budgetary might. *Nursing Management*, 31(2), 16–17.

DiJerome, L., Dunham-Taylor, J., Ash, K., & Brown., R. (1999). Evaluating cost center productivity. *Nursing Economics*, 117(6), 334–340.

Dixon, N. M., (2000). *Common knowledge: How companies thrive by sharing what they know*. Boston: Harvard Business School Press.

Garvin, D. (2000). *Learning in action: A guide to putting the learning organization to work*. Boston: Harvard Business School Press.

Iowa Intervention Project. (2001). Determining cost of nursing instrumentations: A beginning. *Nursing Economics*, 19(4), 146–160.

Keeling, B. (2000). How to establish a position and hours budget. *Nursing Management*, 31(3), 26–27.

Macdonald, M. (1998). Using the balanced scorecard to align strategy and performance in long term care. *Healthcare Management Forum*, 11(3), 33–38.

CHAPTER ENDNOTES

1. Jeffs, L., Merkley, J., Richardson, S., Eli, J., & McAllister, M. (2011). Using a nursing balanced scorecard approach to measure and optimize nursing performance. *Nursing Leadership*, 24(1), p. 48.

CHAPTER 11

Effective Staffing

Anne L. Bernat, RN, BSN, MSN, CNAA
Adapted by John P. Angkaw, MBA (c), MEd, BScN
Jeanne Besner, RN, PhD
Heather Crawford, BScN, MEd, CHE

Nurses will be more satisfied in the workplace if staffing and scheduling policies and procedures are thoughtfully developed, fairly applied, and clearly communicated to all employees. (Marquis & Huston, 2012)

OBJECTIVES

The purpose of this chapter is to enable the reader to

- ■ discuss utilization of workload measurement systems data by the staff nurse and the nurse manager;
- ■ develop a staffing pattern for a critical care unit with 22 clients;
- ■ evaluate staffing effectiveness on an inpatient unit using two client outcomes;
- ■ compare and contrast models of care delivery; and
- ■ discuss the role of a case manager versus a unit staff nurse.

You are a new nurse manager of a 28-bed surgical unit that uses total client care as the care delivery model. You have 15 full-time employees and 20 part-time employees, with vacancies for an additional four full-time staff. The current schedule utilizes eight-hour shifts, but the majority of full-time staff would like to work 11-hour shifts. However, the most experienced nurses on the unit threaten to retire if you implement 12-hour shifts. Recent graduates will only work for you if you offer 12-hour shifts.

> *How can you accommodate the needs of both groups of nurses?*

> *What effect will the 12-hour shifts have on your care delivery model?*

The ability of a nurse to provide safe and effective care to a client is dependent on many variables, including the knowledge and experience of the staff, the severity of illness of the clients, the amount of nursing time available, the **care delivery model**, care management tools, and organizational supports in place to facilitate care. Changes associated with staffing levels of nurses have been demonstrated to have an impact on client outcome (Thungjaroenkul, Cummings, & Embleton, 2007). It is important that managers consider matching staffing with the care needs of the client (Rothberg, Abraham, Lindenauer, & Rose, 2005). This chapter will explore these factors, how they affect planning for staffing, and the results of staffing plans. By the end of this chapter, you will understand how to plan staffing and how to measure the effectiveness of a staffing plan. You will also be able to articulate the models of care delivery that are applicable to your environment and client population.

DETERMINATION OF STAFFING NEEDS

Nurse staffing has ranged widely since the inception of nursing as a profession. In Florence Nightingale's time, nursing staffing was one nurse for many soldiers. Today you may see one nurse working with one client in a critical care area. To determine nurse staffing requirements for today's rapidly changing health care environment, many variables must be considered. The effectiveness of the staffing pattern is only as good as the planning that goes into its preparation. The following key budget concepts and issues need to be reviewed and assessed when building or assessing a staffing pattern.

CORE CONCEPTS

To understand staffing patterns you need to be familiar with the following key terms—full-time equivalents (FTEs), worked hours, benefit hours, paid hours, direct and indirect care, and nursing hours per patient day (NHPPD).

RESOURCE AND FTE REQUIREMENTS

FTEs

A **full-time equivalent (FTE)** is a measure of the work commitment of a full-time employee. A full-time employee typically works 5 days a week, or 37.5 hours per week for 52 weeks a year, which amounts to 1,950 hours of work time (see Figure 11-1).

A full-time employee who works 37.5 hours a week is referred to as 1.0 FTE. A part-time employee who works five days in a two-week period is considered a 0.5 FTE. The FTE calculation is used to mathematically describe how much an employee works (see Figure 11-2). Understanding FTEs is essential when moving from a staffing pattern to the actual number of staff required.

FTE hours are a total of all paid hours: worked hours plus benefit hours. Worked hours refer to the number of hours an employee provides direct care to clients or participates in indirect care such as documentation.

Benefit hours include the number of hours spent on vacation, sick time, education time, statutory holidays, orientation, and paid leave such as bereavement. When considering the number of FTEs you need to staff a unit, you must count only the worked hours available for each staff member. Available productive time can be easily

---

| 5 days per week | × 7.5 hours per day | = 37.5 hours per week |
| 37.5 hours per week | × 52 weeks per year | = 1,950 hours per year |

Figure 11-1 Calculation of Full-Time Equivalent Hours

> 1.0 FTE = 37.5 hours per week or five 7.5-hour shifts per week
>
> 0.8 FTE = 30 hours per week or four 7.5-hour shifts per week
>
> 0.6 FTE = 22.5 hours per week or three 7.5-hour shifts per week
>
> 0.4 FTE = 15 hours per week or two 7.5-hour shifts per week
>
> 0.2 FTE = 7.5 hours per week or one 7.5-hour shift per week

Figure 11-2 FTE Calculation for Varying Levels of Work Commitment

Vacation hours	20 days	or	150 hours
Sick time (average)	6 days	or	45 hours
Statutory holidays	12 days	or	90 hours
Education	2 days	or	15 hours
Total benefit hours		=	300 hours

1,950 − 300 = 1,650 worked hours available for each staff member with these benefits

Figure 11-3 Calculation of Worked and Benefit Hours

calculated by subtracting benefit time from the time a full-time employee would work (see Figure 11-3).

In this case, a full-time registered nurse (RN) would have 1,650 worked hours per year available to care for clients.

Employees who work with clients can be classified into two categories: those who provide direct care and those who provide indirect care. **Direct care** is time spent providing hands-on care to clients. **Indirect care** is the amount of time spent on activities that are client related but do not involve hands-on client care, such as documentation, consulting with other health care disciplines, and following up on outstanding issues. Even though RNs, licensed practical nurses (LPNs), and unregulated care providers (UCPs) engage in indirect care activities, the majority of their time is spent providing direct care. Therefore, they are classified as direct care providers, and are considered **unit producing.** Nurse managers, clinical specialists, unit clerks, and other support staff are considered **non-unit producing** because most of their work is indirect in nature and supports the work of the direct care providers.

NURSING HOURS PER PATIENT DAY

Nursing hours per patient day (NHPPD) is a standard measure that quantifies the nursing time available to each client by available nursing staff. For example, a nursing unit that has 20 clients at a given point during a 24-hour period, usually the midnight census, and five nursing staff each shift would calculate into 5.6 nursing hours per patient day. NHPPD reflect only worked hours available (see Figure 11-4). In quantifying nursing care, this measure is useful for both nurses and the financial staff in an organization.

WORKLOAD MEASUREMENT SYSTEMS

To assess staff needed at any given time, it is necessary to determine the clients' needs. Workload measurement systems first appeared during the 1960s. At the time, they were called patient classification systems. Today, they are often referred to as the **workload measurement system,** which is a measurement tool used to articulate the nursing workload for a specific client or

> 20 clients on the unit
>
> 5 staff × 3 shifts = 15 staff
>
> 15 staff each working 7.5 hours = 112.5 hours available in a 24-hour period
>
> 112.5 nursing hours ÷ 20 clients = 5.6 NHPPD
>
> FTE = 7.5 hours per week or one 7.5-hour shift per week

Figure 11-4 Calculation of Nursing Hours per Patient Day (NHPPD) group of clients over a specific period of time. It identifies direct and indirect nursing care requirements and also unit activities that are not related to client contact. Nurse managers must consider its results as a guide when they generate a staffing plan to best meet the client care needs. The measure of nursing workload that is generated for each client is called the **client acuity.** Classification data can be used to predict the amount of nursing time needed based on the client's acuity. As a client becomes sicker, the acuity level rises, which means the client requires more nursing care. As a client acuity level decreases, the client requires less nursing care. In most patient classification systems, each client is classified using weighted criteria that are used to predict the nursing care hours needed for the next 24 hours. The criteria reflect the nursing care hours for such activities as bathing, mobilizing, and eating; supervision; assessment; and frequent observations. In most cases, clients are classified once a day. The ideal workload measurement system produces a valid and reliable rating of individual client care requirements, which is matched to the latest clinical technology and caregiver skill variables (Malloch & Conivaloff, 1999). These systems are generally applied to all inpatients in an organization. Systems to classify outpatients have been less prevalent because outpatients tend to be more stable and similar in care needs. There are two different types of classification systems: factor and prototype.

FACTOR SYSTEM

The factor system uses units of measure that equate to nursing time. Nursing tasks are assigned time or are weighted to reflect the amount of time needed to perform a task. These systems attempt to capture the cognitive functions of assessing, planning, intervening, evaluating client outcomes, and preparing written documentation. Many factor systems have been homegrown or built for a specific organization, and many other factor systems are available for purchase on the open market. The factor system is the most popular type of classification system because it can project care needs for individual clients as well as client groups. The time assigned or the weighted factor for different nursing activities can be changed over time to reflect the changing needs of the clients or the hospital system.

ADVANTAGES AND DISADVANTAGES In the factor system, data are generally readily available to managers and staff for day-to-day operations. These data provide a base of information against which one can justify changes in staffing requirements.

The disadvantages of this type of system include the nurse's ongoing workload in classifying clients every day. Other documented problems include "classification creep," which means acuity levels rise as a result of the

misuse of classification criteria. Another disadvantage is that these systems do not holistically capture the client's needs for psychosocial, environmental, and health management support. Finally, these systems calculate the needed nursing time based on a typical nurse. A novice may take longer to perform activities than the average or the more experienced nurse. If most staff are novices, the recommended nursing times will be longer than the actual time needed, based on the actual expertise of the staff.

PROTOTYPE SYSTEM

The prototype system allocates nursing time to large client groups, but based on an average of similar clients. For example, specific **case mix groups (CMGs)** have been used as groupings of clients to which a nursing acuity is assigned based on past organizational experience. CMGs are client groupings established by the Canadian Institute for Health Information (CIHI), and they describe types of clients discharged from acute care hospitals. Based on U.S. charge data and Canadian length-of-stay data, CIHI developed weights, known as **resource intensity weights (RIWs),** to measure the expected use of hospital resources. Cost weights are relative resource values associated with specific grouping methodologies. In addition to CMGs and RIWs, day procedure group RIWs have been developed using the same scale as the in-resource allocation methodology developed for continuing care residents.[1]

Our hospital uses a workload classification system, and the nurses calculate the requirements daily, but we don't pay much attention to the data collected. Some of my colleagues deliberately "fudge" the numbers to determine if anybody is paying attention! The challenge with the system we use is that it doesn't anticipate demand, or adjust for the learning time necessary for new employees. In addition, it doesn't provide time for us to have relationships with our clients; it just gives us time to complete tasks. It also doesn't recognize the change in workload related to admissions and discharges throughout the 24 hours. Now, it isn't recognizing the fact that I am slower than I was 20 years ago!

Claire Stanfield, MScN
Prototype System

ADVANTAGES AND DISADVANTAGES The distinct advantage of the prototype system is the reduction of work for nurses who are not required to classify clients daily. A major disadvantage of this system is the lack of an ongoing measure of the actual nursing work required by individual clients. Also, no ongoing data is available to monitor the accuracy of the pre-assigned nursing care requirements. This type of system is much less common than the factor system.

UTILIZATION OF CLASSIFICATION SYSTEM DATA

A large body of literature is available on workload measurement systems, such as Baumann et al., (2001), Giovannetti (1994), O'Brien-Pallas (2007), Shamian and El-Jardali (2007), and the final report of the Canadian Nursing Advisory Committee in 2002 (Canadian Nursing Advisory Committee, 2002). Although managers cannot rely entirely on the workload measurement system to predict staff requirements and produce a staffing plan, this system provides some useful information related to client acuity. The review by McGillis Hall et al. (2006) provides extremely weak evidence in support of workload measurement systems. The authors concluded that most of these systems have never been used as intended and, therefore, are of little value. When nurses are asked to spend time collecting data that they know make no real difference to their workload or to improved client outcomes, the data collection soon becomes just an exercise performed without scrutiny ... "garbage in, garbage out."

CONSIDERATIONS IN DEVELOPING A STAFFING PATTERN

Developing a staffing pattern is a science and an art. The following sections present areas for consideration in addition to the acuity data and NHPPD just discussed. Each of these areas should be reviewed and the findings incorporated into development of the staffing pattern.

BENCHMARKING

Benchmarking is a management tool for seeking out the best practices in one's industry so as to improve performance (Swansburg, 1996). It can also serve as a reference point and signify a level of quality of goods or services. This provides a basis for comparing quality in similar organizations or situations (Schmele, 1996). When developing a staffing pattern that will lead to a budget, benchmark your planned NHPPD against other organizations with similar client populations. Workload measurement systems that can be purchased often offer as part of their system both acuity and NHPPD benchmarking data from across the country. Such data can help establish a starting point for a staffing pattern or help justify an increase or reduction in nursing hours. Use caution, however,

because each organization has in place at the unit level, varying levels of support for the nurse. For example, in a nursing unit where aides from the dietary department distribute and pick up meal trays, less nursing time is needed than in a unit that has no external support for this activity. Such factors contribute significantly to differences in hours of care from one organization to another.

REGULATORY REQUIREMENTS

In Canada, no regulatory requirements address staffing levels. However, in the United States the situation is changing as the nursing shortage heightens. California stipulates in law and regulation the required minimum nurse-to-client ratios that must be maintained at all times. In several other states hospitals must have staffing committees that are responsible for plans and staffing policy. Fifteen states plus the District of Columbia have enacted legislation or adopted regulations to address nurse staffing. Five states require some form of disclosure or public reporting related to staffing. In 2009 North Carolina studied the use of mandatory ratios as a staffing tool. Some nurses are adamant that they need to be protected by law with stipulated staffing levels. Some nurse leaders are concerned that the mandated staffing levels would soon become the maximum staffing levels rather than the minimum.

In the United States, the Joint Commission on Accreditation of Healthcare Organizations (JCAHO) surveys hospitals on the quality of care provided. The JCAHO does not mandate staffing levels but does assess an organization's ability to provide the right number of competent staff to meet the needs of clients served by the hospital (Joint Commission on Accreditation of Healthcare Organizations, 2000). Part of this assessment asks how often a unit is staffed to the level required by its staffing pattern and how the effectiveness of the staffing pattern is evaluated. If an organization's standard staffing pattern calls for four RNs for 20 clients—1:5 ratio—the JCAHO will assess how often the organization meets that standard. As a rule, nurses in the United States pay close attention to the state and federal regulations related to their client population for any regulated staffing requirements.

In Canada, a review of staffing ratios commissioned by the Canadian Federation of Nurses Unions (CFNU) and conducted by Dr. Gail Tomblin Murphy suggests that much more research is needed to determine what or whether staffing ratios should be implemented. Accreditation Canada surveys hospitals on the quality of care provided but does not mandate the staffing levels. The human resources team may identify the number of overtime hours provided for client care, or the number of illness-related absent days. Indirectly, the surveyors assess whether the organization has met its standards with respect to staffing.

SKILL MIX

Skill mix is another essential element in nurse staffing. **Skill mix** refers to the percentage of one type of staff to the total staff complement. For example, an RN skill mix represents the percentage of RN staff to all staff, including other direct care staff, LPNs, and unregulated care providers (UCPs). A professional skill mix represents the percentage of professional staff to all staff, including unregulated staff. In a unit that has 40 FTEs budgeted—20 FTE RNs and 20 FTEs of other skill types—the RN skill mix is 50 percent. If the unit had 40 FTEs—30 FTEs of RNs and LPNs, and 10 FTEs of unregulated providers—the professional skill mix would be 75 percent.

The skill mix of a unit should vary according to the care required and the care delivery model utilized. For example, in a critical care unit, the RN skill mix will be much higher than in a nursing home, where the skills of an RN have been required to a lesser degree. Today, the skills of the RN are probably required more often than is reflected in current staffing models. Although professional (RN and LPN) hours of care are more costly than those of unregulated providers, evidence shows that RNs and LPNs are a very productive and efficient type of labour. As nurses become scarcer, and clients are discharged earlier from acute care facilities, it will become even more important to evaluate the client care required and determine which care provider is the most appropriate for the situation. For instance, when many clients need assistance with daily living, an unregulated care provider may be most appropriate.

STAFF SUPPORT

Another important factor to consider when developing a staffing pattern is the kind of supports that are in place for the unit or department's operations. For instance, does your organization have a systematic process to deliver medications to the unit, or do unit personnel have to pick up client medications and narcotics? Does your organization have staff to transport clients to and from ancillary departments? Has your organization implemented a manager-on-call system so staff can have support for urgent issues "after hours"?

The less support available, the more nursing hours need to be built into the staffing pattern. The addition of a materials coordinator, who tracks and supplies a significant amount of equipment, may be beneficial in nursing areas, such as critical care. This kind of staff support allows nurses to spend the available precious time with clients, rather than looking for equipment or supplies.

An additional important unit-based need is clerical support. If the unit has admissions, discharges, and transfers, it makes sense to provide unit clerical support. In intensive care units (ICUs) and emergency departments (EDs), unit clerks are commonly scheduled around the clock to provide support for the unit staff as well as for other disciplines.

HISTORICAL INFORMATION

As you consider the many variables that affect staffing, it helps to ask the following questions: "What has worked in the past? Was the staff able to provide the care that was needed? How many clients were cared for? What kind of clients were they? How many staff was utilized, and what kind of staff were they?" This information can help to identify operational issues that would not be apparent otherwise. For example, an older part of a facility may not have a pneumatic tube delivery system, a system that is available in most other parts of the facility. Because this system is generally available, you may not notice its absence. However, the staffing pattern you develop will be affected because a significant amount of time will be required to collect the needed items. It is also important to review any data on quality or staff perceptions regarding the effectiveness of the previous staffing pattern. This information will allow you to calculate previous NHPPD and outcomes for comparison to your staffing plan. History is a valuable tool, often overlooked in planning for the future.

ESTABLISHING A STAFFING PATTERN

A **staffing pattern** is a plan that articulates how many and what kind of staff are needed per shift and per day to staff a unit or department. A staffing pattern can be developed

---

CASE STUDY 11-1

You are the manager of a 24-bed critical care unit. The nurse-to-client ratio is budgeted at one nurse to one client for 20 of the beds, and one nurse to two clients for four of the beds. Of the 24 clients in your unit, three are well enough to go to a general internal medicine unit and two can be discharged to the general surgery unit, where the respective nurse-to-client ratios are one to four. You are planning the staff requirements for the next 12 hours. What factors should you consider? After consideration of key factors, what is your plan for staffing? What would you communicate to your staff?

in two basic ways: by determining the required ratio of staff to clients and then calculating nursing hours and total FTEs; or by determining the nursing care hours needed for a specific client or group of clients, and then generating the FTEs and staff-to-client ratio required to provide that care. In most cases, you will use a combination of methods to validate your staffing plan. We will start with the development of a plan from the staff-to-client ratio.

INPATIENT UNIT

An **inpatient unit** is a hospital unit that provides care to clients 24 hours a day, 7 days a week. To establish a staffing pattern for an inpatient unit, you will use all the data discussed above. Considering the data from all your sources, you can build a staffing pattern that you believe will meet the needs of the clients, the staff, and the organization. Using a staffing pattern template, plot the number and type of staff needed during the week and weekend for 24 hours a day for the number of clients you expect to have (see Figure11-5). In this example, the number and type of staff are delineated as well the additional FTEs for weekend coverage, orientation and education, and benefit hours.

For example, on a 24-bed medical unit, you expect to have, on average, 22 clients per day. The ratio of one RN to five clients and one UCP for every 12 clients works well from 0700 to 1900 hours. From 1900 to 0700 hours, the ratio can go to one RN to eight clients. Two UCPs are needed from 1900 to 2300 hours, and then one UCP from 2300 to 0700 hours. A total of 131.25 staff hours per day are needed. The average number of clients on this unit is 22. To calculate the NHPPD see Figure 11-6. In this example, the number of care hours available would be six NHPPD.

As you can see, the staffing pattern drives the NHPPD: the more staff available for each client, the higher the NHPPD. Cost is associated with hours of care available and skill mix. Some staffing patterns have many hours of care available, but they may be lower-cost FTEs. The key is to have the right number and skill level of caregivers available to ensure safe, effective, and appropriate care.

To develop a staffing pattern using NHPPD, start with a target NHPPD. If your target NHPPD were 8, for example, and you expected to have 22 clients on your 24-bed unit, you would multiply 8 NHPPD times 22 clients to get 176 worked hours needed every day. Dividing 176 by 7.5-hour shifts worked by an FTE gives you 23.5 FTEs needed per day.

DETERMINING THE NUMBER OF FTES NEEDED TO MEET THE STAFFING PATTERN

You have determined a staffing pattern for your unit. The staffing pattern calculates the number of FTEs needed per day, but does not account for the benefit hours or replacement hours for staff days off. You must now calculate the number of additional staff that will be needed to provide for days off and benefit hours. Direct caregivers will need to be replaced, but the support staff may not need to be replaced for days off or benefit hours. Managers typically are not replaced on days off. Note that each 7.5-hour shift for a FTE is equal to 0.2 FTE; to provide coverage for two days off a week, multiply the number of staff needed per day by a 0.4 FTE. In the example in Figure 11-6, 17.75 FTEs per day multiplied by 0.4 FTE would be an additional 7.1 FTEs to cover two days off per week, for a total of 24.8 FTEs.

The next step is to provide additional FTEs to cover benefit hours, which include vacation, educational time, and orientation time. The amount of time away from work varies with each organization. If every employee receives four weeks of vacation a year and two educational days, the benefit hours would equate to 1,785 hours of worked time per FTE (1,950 possible hours minus 165 hours). Total FTE hours divided by 1,785 hours gives you the total FTEs needed to provide coverage. In the previous example, 24.8 FTEs multiplied by 1,950 hours equals 48,360 hours, and 48,360 hours divided by 1,785 would be 27.1 FTEs or 2.3 additional FTEs to ensure that there are staff available to work when other staff is taking benefited time off. Thus, a total of 27.1 FTEs are needed to staff this 24-bed unit.

DETERMINING THE FTES NEEDED TO STAFF AN EPISODIC CARE UNIT

An **episodic care unit** refers to a unit that sees clients for defined episodes of care: for example, a dialysis unit or an ambulatory care unit. In these units, clients tend to be more homogenous and have a more predictable path of care. To determine staffing needs for an episodic unit, start with an assessment of the hours of care required by the clients. Using a dialysis unit as an example, to care for 16 clients receiving treatments, you determine you need 4 RNs for all 12 hours the unit is open, or 48 hours of RN care per day. The unit is open 12 hours a day, 6 days a week, or 312 days a year; 48 hours per day multiplied by 312 days = 14,976 total hours. As in the previous example, the number of FTEs needed to provide coverage for worked hours can be calculated by dividing the total number of hours needed by the actual number of worked hours an employee would work. This method provides coverage for days off and benefit hours for direct caregivers. The worked FTE hours of 1,650 from Figure 11-3, divided into the 14,976 hours required gives a total of 9.1 RN FTEs.

The same calculation can be applied to other caregivers. In this same example, if two technicians were required for 12 hours a day of operation, that would mean 2 × 12 = 24 hours needed per day, and 24 × 312 days = 7,488 total hours needed.

Hospital Business Planning Brief/Accountability Agreement 2005/06

Hospital Site: Brantford General Site

Department Name:

Department No.:

NOTE: One shift equals 7.5 hours

WORKED TIME

Job Class-Descrip	Shifts	S	S	M	T	W	T	F	TOTAL
	D								
Job Code	E								
	N								

Weekly # of Shifts
F.T.E.'s (# Shifts divided by 5)
Paid Hours (FTE's X 1950 hours)

Worked Time

BENEFIT TIME

	F/T	# of Days	Total Days	Shifts Not Replaced	Shifts Replaced
Statutory Holidays	# of F.T. Staff	X			
Paid Sick (Average)	# of F.T. Staff	X			
Education Leave	# of F.T. Staff	X			
Inservice	# of Staff	X			
Orientation	# of New Staff	X			
Vacation	Total Weeks	X			

Total # of Shifts
F.T.E.'s (# Shifts divided by 260 days)
Paid Hours (FTE's X 1950 hours)

NOTE: Worked time plus benefit time replaced equals Total Staff F.T.E.'s

NOTE: Shifts not replaced and shifts replaced equals Benefit Hours

NOTE: Worked time less shifts not replaced equals Worked Hours

Benefit Time

For Premium Calculations Only

*Annual Shifts

	*Weekly Shifts
M.L.O.A. (# of Weeks)	Even. Prem.
O/T Shifts - Annual	Night Prem.
# Call Backs - Annual	Wkend Prem.
Stats Worked - Annual	In Charge
M.O.A. - U.I.C. Pymts.	Resp. Shifts
Other:	Resp. Shifts
Other:	Stdby. Shifts

TOTAL STAFFING REQUIREMENTS

Staff Ratio	TOTAL F.T.E.'s	F.T.E.'s		TOTAL PD. HRS	Paid Hours	
		Worked	Benefit		Worked	Benefit
Full-Time						
Part-Time						
TOTAL						

*STAFF COUNT	Full-Time	Part-Time

*Note: Staff Count should be actual number of bodies

*Note: Annual Shifts are calculated by taking the number of shifts per day and multiplying by 7 (number of Days in a week) then multiplying by 52 (number of weeks in a year)

*Note: Weekly Shifts are calculated by taking the number of shifts per day and multiplying by 7 (Number of days in a week)

Figure 11-5 Brant Community Healthcare System—Staffing Pattern Worksheet and Human Resources

Figure 11-5 (Continued)

Source: Brant Community Healthcare System, Brantford, ON. Reprinted with Permission.

Skill	Day	Evening	Night	Total
Direct				
UM				
RN	5.5	4.25	3	12.75
LPN				
Tech				
UCP	2	2	1	5
Subtotal				

12.5 staff   × 7.5-hour shifts   = 93.75 hours

5 staff   × 7.5-hour shifts   = 37.5 hours

Staff hours available per day   = 131.25 hours

131.25 hours ÷ 22 clients per day   = 6 hours of NHPPD

131.25 hours ÷ 7.5-hour shifts   = 17.5 FTEs to fill the staffing pattern

Figure 11-6 Staffing Plan for a 24-Bed Medical Unit

The benefit package for technical staff is not as rich as the RN package. Their vacation allotment is 10 days or 75 hours per year, which increases their productive time to 1,875 hours per year—7,488 divided by 1,875 = 4.0 technical FTEs. Any staff members who do not require coverage would simply be added to the overall FTEs for the unit as a 1.0 FTE. This situation might apply to a secretary, social worker, or nurse manager, all of whom support the unit, but their days off and benefited time off do not need to be replaced.

SCHEDULING

Scheduling of staff is the responsibility of the nurse manager, or staffing clerks or schedulers, who must ensure that the appropriate staffs are scheduled on each day and on each shift for safe, effective client care. Many issues need to be considered when you schedule staff: the client type and acuity, the number of clients, the care and services required by the client, the experience of your staff, and the supports available to the staff. The combination of these factors should guide the number of staff scheduled on each day and shift. These factors must be reviewed on an ongoing basis as client types and client acuity drive different client needs and staff expertise.

CLIENT NEEDS

Clients' nursing needs related to tasks or activities are measured by the workload measurement system. However, a client-centred needs assessment should be determined through assessment of the bio-psycho-social-spiritual needs of the client and family, which can only be

One of the things that always amazed me was that managers tended to use different figures and assumptions when planning their staffing needs. As a result, I formed a committee of nurse managers and directors to see whether or not we could develop a template for them to use, which would ultimately save time and frustration. The spreadsheet template we developed afforded the managers an opportunity to accurately project the number of FTEs needed to meet the staffing pattern. This template included worked and benefit hours. The benefit hours included vacation, statutory holidays, sick time, education days, orientation days, and paid leave. In addition, the template included opportunities to budget for maternity leaves of absence (MLOA). One of the biggest benefits for the managers is that the template allowed them to develop what-if scenarios for planning purposes.

Peter Exford, C.A.
Director of Finance

assessed with their input. This involvement of client and family is seldom included when workload measurement systems are applied. Workload measurement systems do not predict when, over the next 24 hours, the nursing activity will take place. In addition to planning for the acuity of the clients, the staffing pattern must support having staff at work when the work needs to be done. A good example is an oncology unit, where chemotherapy and blood transfusions typically occur on the evening shift. In this scenario, more staff may be needed in the evening to support these nurse-intensive activities. As client types change, so do clients' need for specific treatments and staffing requirements. Adding a population of step-down clients from the ICU would likely require additional FTEs on a medical-surgical unit. When client populations change, staffing and NHPPD need to be assessed.

EXPERIENCE AND SCHEDULING OF STAFF

Nurses differ regarding their knowledge base, experience level, and critical thinking skills. A novice nurse may take longer to accomplish a task than an experienced nurse. An experienced RN can handle more, in terms of workload and acuity of clients. If a particular unit or department requires special skills or competencies from the staff, consideration must be given to plan for additional

Citation: Health Canada "Our Health, Our Future: Creating Quality Workplaces for Canadian Nurses" <http://hc-sc.gc.ca/hcs-sss/pubs/nurs-infirm/2002-cnac-cccsi-final/index-eng.php>

Discussion: The Canadian Nursing Advisory Committee (CNAC) was created in 2001 in response to the National Nursing Strategy. Because of concerns regarding the nursing shortage in the Canadian nursing workforce in the late 1990s, the Conference of Deputy Ministers and Ministers of Health directed the Advisory Committee on Health Human Resources (ACHHR "to develop a pan-Canadian strategy for nursing" (ACHHR, 2000a, p. 2). The primary goal of the CNAC was to formulate recommendations "for policy direction to improve quality of nursing work life, which would provide a framework and context for work life improvement strategies at the provincial or territorial level" (ACHHR, 2000b). The committee made recommendations for changes in three key areas: (1) increasing the number of nurses, (2) improving the education and maximizing the scope of practice of nurses, and (3) improving working conditions of nurses.

Implications for Practice: It is clear that there is and will continue to be a nursing shortage for the next decade. In addition to devising global strategies to draw more people into the nursing profession, it is imperative for managers and nurse leaders to create environments that retain staff, including the planning of staff schedules that nurses find compatible with their personal lives. As the nursing workforce ages, we must also take measures to make accommodation for the older worker, including technology to simplify work and physical plant changes to make the work less physically taxing.

Citation: Thungjaroenkul, P., Cummings, G., & Embleton, A. (2007). The impact of nurse staffing on hospital costs and patient length of stay: A systematic review. *Nursing Economics*, 25(5): 255–265.

Discussion: Hospitals have been faced with limited funding and rising health care costs. As a result, they have reviewed their current operations and advanced solutions that would continue to meet the care needs of clients without decreasing quality of care. Staff scheduling has been affected, as managers have explored other opportunities to deliver client care, including increased use of unregulated care providers and decreased use of professional staff. The implications of reducing the number of registered nurses at the bedside include negative impacts on nurses' well-being and their ability to provide high-quality care. Evidence suggests that having adequate registered nurse staffing allows for better delivery of client care and decreased incidence of adverse events. The availability of registered nurses and their professional nursing skills may also influence client length of stay and hospital costs.

Implications for Practice: To optimize client outcomes and staff health, there need to be staffing complements that include the right skill mix, for the right client, at the right time, in the right place.

NEW OPTIONS IN STAFFING PATTERNS

As the nursing shortage deepens, schedules will need to be developed to meet the needs of both clients and workers. In recent years more new options in scheduling have been available to meet both these needs. Twelve-hour shifts have become very popular across the country. In future it might be possible for nurses to work fewer than 37.5 hours per week and still be able to obtain full-time benefits. Some schedules allow nurses to work a rotation of four shifts on, five shifts off. These new scheduling options require flexibility in the wording of union contracts.

A popular option in both Canada and the United States is to schedule shifts for workers who work only on weekends. Weekend program staff work 24 hours in two 12-hour shifts every weekend and are paid a rate equal to 40 hours of work during the week. Some of these programs include full-time benefits as well. Such

nursing hours. In this way, staff with the special skills are scheduled according to the likelihood that a particular skill will be needed. Remember, the underlying principle of good staffing is that those you serve come first. Following this principle may lead to some undesirable shifts, but your responsibility is to ensure both the appropriate number of staff and the appropriate mix of staff are on hand to provide the best quality care for the clients you serve. Figure 11-5 shows how the number of staff is plotted across a staffing sheet.

Weekend staff working at $35 an hour $\times$ 24 hours = $840 per weekend

Regular staff working at $20 an hour $\times$ 24 hours = $480 per weekend

Difference in cost = $360 per weekend

Six weekend staff members at $360 would cost $2,160 more than regular staff per weekend;

$2,160 for 52 weekends a year would cost $112,320 more than regular staff annually.

Figure 11-7 Annual Cost of a Weekend Program for One Nursing Unit

programs are designed to improve weekend staffing and to allow full-time staff members, who usually work 26 weekends a year, to work fewer weekends for staff retention purposes.

IMPACT ON CLIENT CARE

Any time you implement a scheduling plan, it is important to assess its effect on the care of clients. For example, workweeks made up of three 12-hour shifts have, in many units, disrupted the continuity of care, especially when the 12-hour shifts are not scheduled together. To mediate this impact, 12-hour staff can be paired so that the client has the same pair of nurses every day for three days, and then the client can be transitioned to a new pair of 12-hour staff. Units that have short client lengths of stay may have fewer continuity problems than units with longer lengths of stay. When implementing weekend programs, you must always ensure that the person who is scheduled is familiar with the clients and the events that have transpired.

FINANCIAL IMPLICATIONS

New staffing patterns or program changes may have significant financial implications. Because of the nursing shortage, a number of new programs are being initiated to recruit staff and to encourage staff to work more hours. Weekend programs are more expensive than traditional staffing patterns because of the high rate of hourly pay, but they are a recruitment and retention tool for nursing leadership. For example, see the financial impact of the weekend program referred to earlier (see Figure 11-7).

Before implementing a similar program or other new programs, collaboration with the finance and human resources departments is necessary. This collaboration is needed to develop a financial analysis that measures the dollar and human resource impact of the program.

CYCLICAL SCHEDULING

In **cyclical scheduling,** the nurse manager generates a schedule for a specified number of weeks at a time—with 6, 12, or 18 weeks as the typical time frame. This schedule repeats itself at the end of the cycle. An important consideration for cyclical scheduling is that it must adhere to collective agreement requirements. The staff is able to predict their time for weeks in advance and, as a result,

can schedule their personal time accordingly. Stability and predictability are its associated advantages. On the other hand, its structure doesn't allow for much flexibility and makes it difficult to switch work shifts among the different staff members (Dechant, 2006).

SELF-SCHEDULING

Self-scheduling is a process in which staff on a unit collectively decide and implement the monthly work schedule (Dearholt & Feathers, 1997). One of the issues that drives nurses from their place of employment is scheduling (Hill-Popper, 2000). Self-scheduling has been implemented to boost staff morale by increasing staff control over their work environment through self-governance activities (Dearholt & Feathers, 1997). This approach provides opportunities for staff to increase communication among themselves and promotes empowerment and professional growth. This form of scheduling provides maximum flexibility for staff and serves to increase their sense of ownership and shared responsibility in ensuring that their respective work areas are adequately staffed (Shullanberger, 2000). To ensure that client care needs are met, self-scheduling programs need to be structured.

BOUNDARIES OF SELF-SCHEDULING To implement self-scheduling, responsibilities and boundaries need to clearly state the expectations of staff. These guidelines are best established by the nurse manager or by a unit-based committee of staff that reports to the nurse manager. The roles and responsibilities should be spelled out for everyone—the unit-based committee, the chairperson if there is one, the staff, and the manager. Generic boundaries need to be established regarding fairness, fiscal responsibility, evaluation of the self-scheduling process, and the approval process. Table 11-1 spells out specific issues that must be addressed. During the self-scheduling process, the unit staff should be included and educated regarding the guidelines as they are being developed. For this process to be successful, all staff members must understand the process, their responsibilities, and the effect of their decisions on staffing. All personnel must also be committed to providing safe staffing on all shifts for their clients.

TABLE 11-1	ISSUES TO BE SPELLED OUT IN SELF-SCHEDULING GUIDELINES

1. Scheduling period: Is the scheduling period a 2-, 4-, or 6-week interval?

2. Schedule timeline: What are the time frames for staff to sign up for regular work commitments, special requests, and overtime?

3. Staffing pattern: Will 8- or 12-hour shifts be used, or a combination of both? What are the union contract requirements?

4. Nurse-to-client ratio: What is the expected nurse-to-client ratio for a day and/or night shift?

5. Weekends: Are staff expected to work every other weekend? If there are extra weekends available, how are they distributed?

6. Holidays: How will statutory holidays be allocated?

7. Vacation time: Are there restrictions on the amount of vacation during certain periods?

8. Unit vacation practices: How many staff from one shift can be on vacation at any time?

9. Requests for time off: What is the process for requesting time off and/or schedule changes?

10. Short-staffed shifts: How are short-staffed shifts handled?

11. On call, if applicable: How are staff assigned on-call time or how do they sign up for on-call time?

12. Cancellation guidelines: How and when are staff cancelled for scheduled time if they are not needed?

13. Sick calls: What are the expectations for calling in sick, and how are these shifts replaced?

14. Schedule changes: What is the process for changing one's schedule after the schedule has been approved?

15. Shifts defined: When do available shifts begin and end?

16. Committee time: When does the self-scheduling committee meet and for how long?

17. Seniority: How does seniority affect staffing and request decisions?

18. Staffing plan for crisis or emergency situations: What is the plan when staffing is inadequate?

EVALUATION OF STAFFING EFFECTIVENESS

Many client outcomes are driven by the available hours of care delivered and the competence of staff delivering the care. The nurse manager and the organizational nurse leader have the ongoing responsibility to monitor the effectiveness of the staffing pattern. To ensure objectivity, staffing outcomes must be delineated, measured, and reviewed.

CLIENT OUTCOMES AND NURSE STAFFING

The Canadian Nurses Association has summarized, on its website, numerous research studies that highlight relationships between nurse staffing and client outcomes. All these studies confirm that there is a relationship. The outcomes found to be affected by nurse staffing are length of stay, incidence of pneumonia, postoperative infections, medication errors, falls, client satisfaction, and nurse satisfaction. These outcomes are negatively affected when nurse staffing or the skill mix is inadequate (Aiken et al., 2002; Aiken et al., 2003; McGillis Hall, Doran, & Pink, 2004; O'Brien-Pallas et al., 2001, 2002; Sovie & Jawad, 2001). Tracking these outcomes over time will provide the data to judge whether your staffing pattern is adequate or inadequate. In addition to having the right number of the right type of provider (staffing), outcomes are influenced by the quality of the relationships among nurse providers, which is in large measure influenced by clear and distinct roles—and valuing the distinct but complementary roles of each category of worker.

NURSE STAFFING AND NURSE OUTCOMES

In the previous section, we reviewed outcome measures for clients directly affected by staffing. In addition to client outcomes, nurse outcomes should also be

REAL WORLD INTERVIEW

As a staff nurse of a busy surgical unit, I can say that self-scheduling has greatly increased the staff's satisfaction with their schedules. I think the biggest factor in the success of our process was the initial buy-in from the staff. The staff originally requested that they be responsible for the schedule. Following discussion, and lengthy literature review, the staff voted 100 percent to try self-scheduling. The next step was to establish an implementation committee made up of staff from the unit. One of the first tasks the implementation committee undertook was to establish clear guidelines for the process. These included timelines for how and when staff can sign up for time and how time off is prioritized.

During implementation, the staff learned many things. One key factor they had not anticipated was that confrontation and nego-tiation skills were required for this process to work. Inevitably, there were situations when staff had to change their schedule. When confrontation and negotiation didn't take place, there were periods of short-staffing and of client care needs not being met. They also learned that scheduling is a time-consuming process. It takes about 16 hours per month for the self-scheduling committee to put the schedule together.

Another key element was that the manager had to maintain accountability for staffing. She met with the scheduling committee regularly and provided any new staff with an orientation to the self-scheduling process. She approved and signed every schedule to ensure that the schedule maintained appropriate staffing levels at all times. She also needed to identify trends that may be affecting staffing and assist the staff to address those trends. Finally, the most important role she played was to be very clear about the expectations for all—the committee, the staff, and the manager. This scheduling process has been one of the most positive quality-of-work-life efforts for my staff.

Sharon Bilan, BScN
Staff Nurse, 3 West, Surgery

REAL WORLD INTERVIEW

In July of 2005 a practice change took place in the Children's Hospital Emergency Department (ED), which enabled nurses to order X-rays on children who presented with minor orthopedic injuries. Prior to this practice change, X-rays were exclusively ordered by physicians. A working group was established and after doing a process flowchart, it was hypothesized that if nurses could initiate X-rays before clients were seen by a physician, ED waiting times could be reduced. To determine whether this hypothesis was successful, a chart audit was conducted to compare waiting times before and after the practice change. Children with minor orthopedic injuries, prior to the practice change, waited an average of 1 hour, 22 minutes from the time they were triaged to the time they received an X-ray, whereas after the practice change, they waited an average of only 20 minutes. Having nurse-initiated X-rays also served to shorten the length of ED visits. Prior to the practice change, the average time bet-ween triage and discharge was 2 hours, 28 minutes. After nurse-initiated X-rays were implemented, the time between triage and discharge went down by 48.6 percent to 1 hour, 16 minutes. Statistical testing confirmed that the difference in ED waiting times between the sample of clients seen prior to the practice change and after the practice change was not due to chance alone. An audit has also shown that 55.5 percent of nurse-delegated X-rays indicate abnormalities, which suggests that this process change has not resulted in excessive use of X-rays.

Maggie Jugenburg, Quality Analyst
Child Health Quality Team, Winnipeg Health Sciences Centre

Source: Maggie Jugenburg, Quality Analyst, Child Health Quality Team, Winnipeg Health Sciences Centre measured. Nurses need to be able to communicate their staffing concerns in both written and verbal forms so that their perceptions of staffing adequacy can be tracked. Nurses have the obligation to report to their supervisor their concerns regarding staffing, and every manager has the responsibility to follow up on staffing issues identified by staff. Formalizing this communication process indicates that you take the issues seriously; you are also provided with data to act on. In addition, actual staffing levels compared to the recommended staffing levels should be tracked to identify changes in client acuity and clues to other possible staffing issues. Medication error is another measure that has been linked with inadequate NHPPD. When resources are scarce, data are necessary to drive the needed changes. The outcomes of ineffective staffing patterns and nursing care can be devastating to both clients and staff.

MODELS OF CARE DELIVERY

Nurse staffing and nurse and client outcomes influence and are influenced by the way in which the delivery of care is organized or structured. The growing shortage of health professionals, and the concurrent underutilization of many health care providers, is placing increasing pressure on the ability of health care agencies to provide timely access to needed services. Consequently, many organizations are exploring the implementation of new service delivery models based on the principles of collaborative practice. The aim is to achieve optimal use of the health workforce, strengthen the provision of safe and high quality care, improve retention, and enhance client and staff satisfaction. Collaborative practice is commonly defined as "an interdisciplinary process for communication and decision making that enables the separate and shared knowledge and skill of the care providers to synergistically influence the client/patient care provided."[2]

To achieve effective collaborative practice, each team member must have a strong sense of their own professional identity and confidence in their distinctive role in care delivery. Research examining role perception of nurses'—registered nurses (RNs), licensed practical nurses (LPNs), and registered practical nurses (RPNs)—and other providers has highlighted considerable role confusion within the three occupational nursing groups, as well as between nursing and other health care professionals. Most health care providers have a tendency to describe who they are as professionals (i.e., the role they are educated and authorized to perform) by reference to the tasks and activities they perform in enacting their respective roles.[3] Substantial overlap exists in the tasks or activities (e.g., medication administration, group

therapy, client assessment) performed by many health care providers. Therefore, this approach to discussing professionals' contribution to health care delivery results in significant role ambiguity and the perception by some providers of excessive duplication of effort. Few health care providers seem able to clearly articulate how differences in education, knowledge, or expertise across professional groups does or should influence decisions being made about the appropriate number and mix of personnel that are needed to optimize client health outcomes and to promote effective and efficient use of all health care providers. It is reasonable to assume that overcoming excessive role ambiguity could potentially help decrease inefficiency in service delivery. Ideally, all health care providers should be supported so they can fully perform the roles they are educated and legislated to perform. Models of care should therefore not only focus on the way in which care delivery is structured but also leverage the optimal use of every member of the care team (i.e., the functional aspect of delivery of care).

Over the history of nursing, many different models of care have been implemented; these represent diverse philosophies, strengths, and weaknesses. Elements of the most common staffing models are summarized in the following section.[4]

TOTAL PATIENT CARE

Total patient care is the oldest model of nursing care delivery, made prominent by Florence Nightingale during an era when most nursing was practiced in clients' homes and where nurses typically cared for a single client at a time. This model of nursing was dominant until the 1930s, reappeared again in the 1980s, and remains the predominant model of care in most acute care settings to this day. In the modern-day version of total patient care, a single registered nurse (or licensed practical nurse) provides all the direct care to his or her assigned clients (typically four or five) during a single shift. Unregulated providers may be available to provide support but are usually assigned to work with more than one nursing provider and group of clients.

ADVANTAGES AND DISADVANTAGES

Advocates of total patient care claim that this model promotes continuity and consistency of care, since the nurse caring for clients over an entire shift is able to establish a trusting relationship with the client and family. Although continuity of care may be assured within a shift, fragmentation inevitably occurs across shifts. Furthermore, the emergence of 12-hour shifts makes it difficult for the same nurse to be assigned to the same group of clients over their entire length of stay. Since a higher proportion of RNs, or LPNs, to unregulated providers is required, this model is not practical at times of cost constraint and nursing shortages. A major disadvantage of the total patient care model is its potential to limit RNs' ability to redistribute to other members of the health care team regulated work activities, such as routine medication administration or treatments, as well as unregulated activities—such as personal care—that could and, in many instances, should be done by others. When heavy workloads limit RNs' ability to perform essential role functions, such as comprehensive assessment, client and family teaching and support, discharge planning and coordination of care,[5] this model may be neither effective nor efficient.

FUNCTIONAL NURSING

Functional nursing emerged during World War II when a shortage of nurses led to the creation of auxiliary nursing roles, including practical nursing. In this model, a designated set of tasks or activities are assigned to specific team members according to their expertise and skill level. Registered nurses typically address the more complex needs of clients, while ancillary workers are assigned routine tasks. Each team member performs the same tasks for all clients, usually under the direction of a nurse manager or charge nurse (see Figure 11-8).

ADVANTAGES AND DISADVANTAGES

While this model maximizes the use of different skills, it contributes to ritualistic, task-focused practice that is heavily dependent on protocols, rules, and procedures, which diminish professional autonomy. Functional nursing was largely abandoned in the early 1970s, but vestiges remain in the form of "specialized" positions such as charge and resource nurses, discharge planners, chronic disease nurses, and nurse navigators. There is evidence to suggest that these functionally focused positions contribute to the underutilization of RNs involved in direct client care[6] and, to some extent, "explain" why the current

practice of registered nurses is so heavily focused on the performance of tasks and activities related to meeting clients' bio-medical needs.[7]

TEAM NURSING

In **team nursing** providers are jointly responsible for providing care to an assigned group of clients. The term **modular team nursing** is used to describe the assignment of team members to a group of clients who are clustered by geographic location on the unit. Team nursing also emerged in response to a shortage of nurses. Traditional forms of this model predominated when practical nursing was not a regulated occupation. Team nursing is differentiated from functional nursing in that the team usually involves a single registered nurse who assigns care for a defined group of clients; the RN divides tasks among team members (e.g., practical nurses and health care aides). The registered nurse team leader supervises and coordinates delivery of care and is responsible for coaching and mentoring other team members (see Figure 11-9).

ADVANTAGES AND DISADVANTAGES

Registered nurses often express concern with this model because they have to spend a significant amount of time coordinating team functions, which removes them from direct care of clients. Since registered nurses seldom provide "hands-on" care, more robust staffing is needed, and this can be quite costly. Team models of care are very dependent on the ability of the registered nurse team leader to delegate work and communicate effectively with other team members. Fragmentation of care across shifts occurs in team nursing, as it does in other models in which care for assigned clients is determined one shift at a time. Models of care in which responsibility for client care is jointly shared among team members can

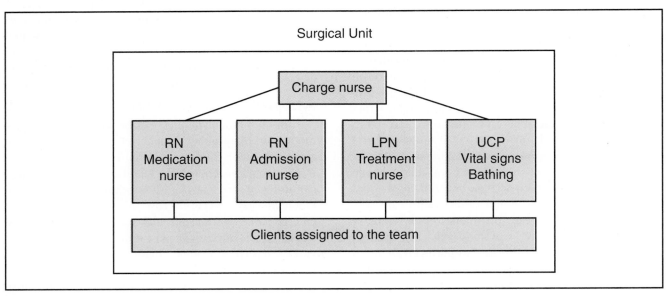

Figure 11-8 Functional Nursing Model

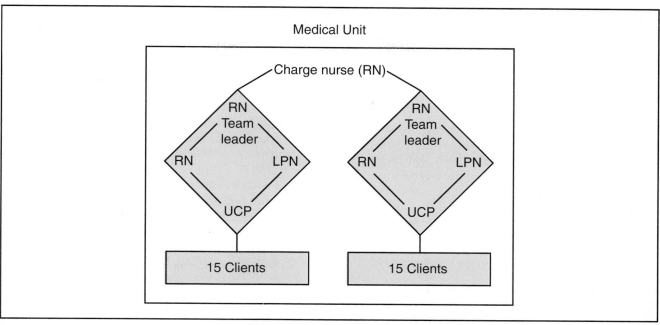

Figure 11-9 Team Nursing Model

be complex and confusing in the absence of effective communication and clear lines of accountability. For this reason, registered nurses often express dissatisfaction with these models.

PRIMARY NURSING

Primary nursing emerged in the 1960s in response to concerns about care fragmentation across shifts. In primary nursing, a single registered nurse is responsible for establishing a plan of care that guides the care delivered over the client's entire length of stay. The primary nurse (RN) is accountable for assessing, planning, organizing, implementing, coordinating, and evaluating care in collaboration with clients and families. All other nurses follow the care plan when the primary nurse is absent (see Figure 11-10). The primary nurse must be knowledgeable about both clients and unit staff, to ensure appropriate matching of a nurse's skill to client needs. Although work can be delegated to ancillary staff, it is often mistakenly assumed that this model requires a staff of all registered nurses.

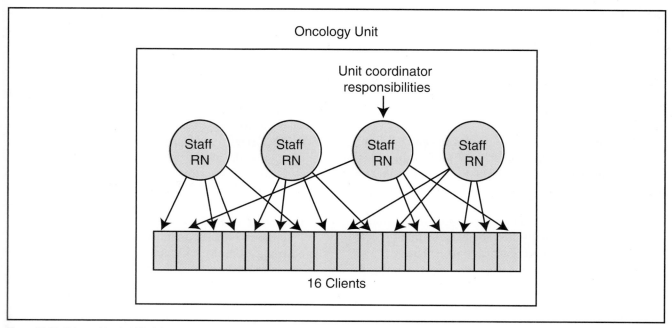

Figure 11-10 Primary Nursing Model

ADVANTAGES AND DISADVANTAGES

Primary nursing promotes the development of trusting relationships among the primary nurse, the clients and families; it also enhances continuity of care throughout the client's stay. Nurses find that having increased authority for decision making makes this model particularly rewarding professionally. This model does not easily accommodate 12-hour shift schedules or part-time work. Registered nurses working in this model frequently perform work that could be assigned to other team members, and, in the absence of adequate nurse-to-client ratios, workload pressures may preclude registered nurses from addressing comprehensive client-health needs. It is often assumed that this model requires all registered nurse staffing, which makes it costly and impractical during times of nursing shortage.

EMERGING MODELS OF CARE: CLIENT-CENTRED COLLABORATIVE PRACTICE

Action is required to deal with the emerging crisis in health human resources that is due in part to the aging of the population—including the health workforce—but largely attributable to poor workforce planning and decision making in the past. Health care is continually changing, and achieving a sustainable health system that provides timely access to quality health services requires modification of existing models of care and greater flexibility in the deployment and utilization of health professionals. Decision makers are responding by introducing innovative approaches to care delivery aimed at addressing current and future shortages not only of nurses but also of many types of allied health care providers. These new models underscore the essential role of clients and families in making decisions about their own care as they are able. They focus heavily on effective and efficient utilization of all members of the health care team and also emphasize the need to reduce fragmentation and duplication in care within and across the settings where clients and families interact with the health care system.

New models of care stress both the optimal application of the knowledge and skills of all care providers and also the shared responsibility for achieving health outcomes. These models are a hybrid of the traditional team and the total patient care models. They involve restructuring roles and differentiating practice among various members of the health care team, including registered nurses and licensed practical nurses. The goal is to ensure delivery of the right care, by the right provider, in the right setting. This requires that providers have a clear understanding of their own and other providers' roles.

Unfortunately, there is substantial evidence of role ambiguity within nursing occupational groups (e.g., registered nurses and licensed practical nurses) and between nurses and other professions. With the growing shortage of registered nurses that began in the mid-1990s, licensed practical nurses were reintroduced into acute care. Compared to earlier decades, both licensed practical nurses and also registered nurses have undergone substantial change in basic educational preparation, and licensed practical nurses have become regulated health care providers. Yet, in most organizations, little attention was paid to redesigning the work of registered nurses and licensed practical nurses as they began to work together again. The total patient care model continued to predominate, and, like registered nurses, licensed practical nurses were assigned to care for their own defined group of clients, albeit those generally considered stable and predictable. Both groups of nursing providers tended to focus on tasks and activities related to the bio-medical needs of clients, blurring the distinctiveness in their respective roles.

Since new collaborative models are still emerging, they have not been well studied. Early indications nonetheless suggest that where there has been investment in professional development to clarify roles and support effective team-based care, there are improved client outcomes, productivity, and job satisfaction among the care providers (see Figure 11-11).

CARE DELIVERY MANAGEMENT TOOLS

In the 1980s and 1990s, several initiatives were introduced to improve care and reduce costs, many of which had positive effects. The Canadian Institute for Health Information (CIHI) established case mix groups (CMGs) and resource intensity weights (RIWs). Case mix groups are groups of cases that are clinically similar with respect to resource use. The CMG is a way of relating the type of client a hospital treats to the resources used by the hospital. Cases are categorized by type of data, such as clinical (e.g., diagnosis, procedure); demographic (e.g., age, gender); or resource consumption (e.g., costs, length of stay [LOS]). CMGs are modelled after the DRG (diagnosis-related group) in the United States and were implemented in 1983.

Resource intensity weights or RIW values are calculated using exclusively Canadian data. The RIW system is a relative resource allocation method for estimating a hospital's inpatient specific costs for both acute care and day procedure care. RIWs are used to standardize the expression of hospital case volumes, recognizing that not all clients require the same health care resources.

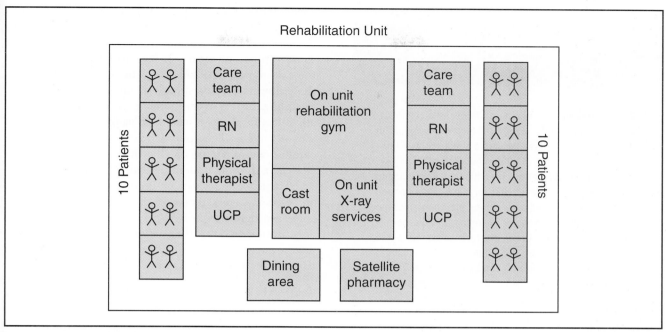

Figure 11-11 Patient-Centred Care Model

LITERATURE APPLICATION

Citation: McGillis Hall, L., Doran, D., & Pink, G. H. (2004). Nurse staffing mix models, nursing hours, and patient safety outcomes. *Journal of Nursing Administration*, 34(1): 41–45.

Discussion: This descriptive correlational study compares nursing staff-mix models with a higher proportion of RNs and their client outcomes. The sample was composed of 77 adult medical, surgical, and obstetrical units in 19 urban teaching hospitals in Ontario. Nurse staffing was categorized into four models: an RN/LPN mix, an all-RN mix, a proportion of regulated to unregulated mix, and an RN/LPN/UCP mix. Client safety outcomes included the rate of medication errors, urinary tract infections, wound infections, and client falls.

When the proportion of RNs and LPNs was lower, the number of medication errors and wound infections increased, and the number of nursing hours increased. The less experienced the RNs and LPNs were, the higher the number of wound infections. Older and more complex clients used more RN and LPN hours.

Implications for Practice: The underutilization of nurses is unacceptable at any time, but is particularly troublesome in the face of current nursing shortages and increasing cost pressures. Given the critical role that nurses play in promoting client safety and quality of care, every effort must be made to ensure that their ability to fully perform their respective roles in the health care system is supported. Although research to date has consistently demonstrated a relationship between the level of RN staffing and client outcomes, there has been no specific attention given to the model of care that has been linked to those outcomes. It is reasonable to predict negative outcomes if LPNs or HCAs are introduced into a new staffing model without due attention to the importance of continuing education to enhance skill in collaborative practice for all team members. As new models of collaborative practice are implemented, particular attention must be given to overcoming the relationship issues that may well account for the poorer outcomes observed in research that has examined the impact of reducing the proportion of RNs in the staffing mix. While it is much too soon to state with confidence that collaborative nursing practice is the "right" model of care in all settings of practice, it is also inappropriate to reject this model outright. Unless more conclusive evidence can be provided that client outcomes are positively or negatively impacted by introducing LPNs and HCAs into the staffing mix, collaborative nursing practice would appear to be a fiscally responsible approach to managing scarce nursing resources.

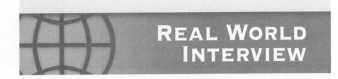

REAL WORLD INTERVIEW

In our organization, we have introduced a collaborative practice model of care delivery. It was important for our practitioners to practice to full scope. Therefore, it was important to differentiate the roles and responsibilities of the various practitioners. Performance expectations were developed for each classification of worker. In this model all nurses may participate in activities such as discharge planning, but the performance expectations for a master's prepared nurse would be different from the expectations of a baccalaureate prepared nurse. Practitioners work together, actively including the client and the family, in the care plan. Hourly "rounding" of the clients contributes to decreased adverse events and "noise" on the unit. Allied health professionals are also an integral component of the interprofessional team. The outcomes of this model have been improved job satisfaction, improved retention of staff, decreased sick time, and improved client outcomes. In addition, we have noticed that more staff have engaged in formal education and are accessing educational opportunities within the organization.

Trudy Fielding, RN, MSN
Chief Nursing Officer

RIWs are used for the following purposes:

- to translate case mix data into cost data
- to determine unit costs for atypical cases
- to identify priorities by CMG for utilization management
- to plan new programs
- to evaluate program efficiency[8]

As hospitals looked for opportunities to reduce costs through reduction in clients' length of stay, clinical pathways and case management surfaced as significant strategies.

CLINICAL PATHWAYS (CARE MAPS)

Clinical pathways were a major initiative to emerge from the efforts to reduce LOS and are widely used to enhance outcomes and contain costs within a constrained length of stay (Lagoe, 1998). **Clinical pathways** are care management tools that outline the expected clinical course and outcomes for a specific client type. Clinical pathways take a different form in each organization that develops them. Typically, they outline the normal course of care for a client. Pathways are often set up each day, when each day's expected outcomes are articulated. Client progress is then measured against the expected outcomes. In some setting, physician orders are incorporated into the pathway to facilitate care. In some organizations, the pathways include multidisciplinary orders for care, including orders from nursing, medicine, and other allied health professionals, such as physical therapy and dietary services. This approach serves to further expedite care for clients. Figure 11-12 provides an excerpt from a clinical pathway that identifies expected outcomes.

These pathways can be used by physicians, nurses, and case managers to care for the client and measure the client's progress against expected outcomes. Any variance in outcome can then be noted and acted upon to get the client back on track. Some organizations have up to 60 pathways implemented.

ADVANTAGES AND DISADVANTAGES

By articulating the normal course of care for a client population, clinical pathways are a powerful tool for managing care. They are very instructive for new staff, and they save a significant amount of time in the process of care. In most cases the implementation of a clinical pathway will improve care and shorten the length of stay for the population on the pathway. Pathways also allow for data collection of variances to the pathway. The data can then be used to look for opportunities to improve hospital systems and clinical practice.

An issue with development of pathways is that some physicians perceive pathways to be cookbook medicine and are reluctant to participate in their development; however, their participation is essential. Development of multidisciplinary pathways also requires a significant amount of work to gain consensus from the various disciplines on the expected plan of care. For client populations that are nonstandard, pathways are less effective because the pathway is constantly being modified to reflect the individual client's needs.

Clinical practice guidelines are evidence-based statements of best practice in the prevention, diagnosis, or management of a given symptom, disease, or condition for individual clients. The Canadian Medical Association (CMA) states that clinical practice guidelines provide better health care by clarifying which care is appropriate, promoting utilization or more beneficial care, and reducing liability. Clinical practice guidelines are an integral component of the CMA quality of care program. More than 40 organizations have been actively involved in guideline development, and Canada has more than 400 clinical practice guidelines.[9]

CASE MANAGEMENT

Case management is another accountability-based care delivery system that evolved in the late 1980s and early

**Clinical Pathway: Lower Extremity Revascularization
Page 21 of 22**

ADDRESSOGRAPH

DAILY ANTICIPATED OUTCOMES

POD2	Date/Time /Init When met	POD3	Date/Time /Init When met	POD4	Date/Time /Init When met	POD5	Date/Time /Init When met
Client rates pain 0-2 on pain scale 0-10 using po analgesia.		Graft signal present with doppler		Graft signal present with doppler		Graft signal present with doppler	
Graft signal present with doppler.		Incisional edges will be approximated without drainage.		Able to participate in self-care and adjunct therapies.		Ambulates independently	
Client will verbalize knowledge of plan of care, testing and treatment.		Site of invasive devices without signs of infection.		Patient viewed diet video.		Patient/significant other will verbalize understanding of activity/diet restrictions, medication use, wound management.	
Ambulate in hall Q I D		Ambulates in hall qid.				Completed nutrition post test.	
Tolerates po solids		Patient/significant other will describe appropriate problem solving skills to decrease anxiety.					
Voiding without difficulty		Rehab referral started: _yes _no					
		Family support available at discharge, specify _____					

TO BE KEPT IN PROGRESS NOTE SECTION OF CHART AT ALL TIMES.

Figure 11-12 Example of a Clinical Pathway (Excerpt)

Source: Courtesy of Albany Medical Center.

1990s in response to spiralling health care costs. The primary goal of case management is to deliver high quality client care in the most cost-effective way by managing both human and material resources. Other goals include managing the delivery of care within a given time frame, decreasing length of stay for inpatient care, ensuring appropriate use of services and resources, improving continuity of care, standardizing the care delivered for a given diagnosis, and improving client outcomes from a given episode of care (Satinsky, 1995). Nursing case management has used critical paths, care mapping (Zander, 1995), and interprofessional care protocols to achieve its objectives. The indicators of care embedded in these tools are used to measure the outcomes of care delivery.

Typically, a case manager is responsible for coordinating care and establishing goals from pre-admission through discharge (Del Togno-Armanasco, Hopkin, & Harter, 1995).

In the typical model of case management, a nurse is assigned to a specific high-risk client population or service, such as cardiac surgery clients. The case manager has the responsibility to work with all disciplines to facilitate care. For example, if a post-surgical hospitalized client has not met ambulation goals according to the clinical pathway, the case manager would work with the physician and the nurse to determine what is preventing the client from achieving this goal. If it turns out that the client is elderly and is slow to recover, they may

agree that physical therapy would be beneficial. In other models the case management function is provided by the staff nurse at the bedside. This approach works well if the client population requires little case management, but if this population requires significant case management services, sufficient RN time needs to be allocated for this activity. In addition to facilitating care, the case manager usually performs a data-collecting function to improve care. In this role, the case manager collects aggregate data on client variances from the clinical pathway. The data are shared with the responsible physicians and other disciplines that participate in the clinical pathway and are then used to explore opportunities for improvement in the pathway or in hospital systems.

KEY CONCEPTS

■ To plan nurse staffing, you must understand and apply the concepts of full-time equivalents (FTEs) and nursing hours per patient day (NHPPD).

■ Workload measurement systems predict the nursing time required for a specific client and then whole groups of clients; the data can then be used for staffing, budgeting, and benchmarking.

■ Determining the number of FTEs needed to staff a unit requires review of client classification data, NHPPD, regulatory requirements, skill mix, staff support, historical information, and the physical environment of the unit.

■ The number of staff and clients in your staffing pattern drives the amount of nursing time available for client care.

■ In developing a staffing pattern, additional FTEs must be added to a nursing unit budget to provide coverage for days off and benefit hours.

■ Scheduling of staff is the responsibility of the nurse manager, who must consider client need and intensity, volume of clients, and the experience of the staff.

■ When choosing a staffing variation, assessing the effect on client care and cost is essential.

■ Self-scheduling can increase staff morale and professional growth, but to be successful, it requires clear boundaries and guidelines.

■ Evaluating the outcomes of your staffing plan on clients, staff, and the organization is an essential activity that should be done daily, monthly, and annually.

■ Case management, clinical pathways, and clinical practice guidelines are care management tools that have been developed to improve client care and reduce hospital costs.

KEY TERMS

benchmarking
care delivery model
case management
case mix groups (CMGs)
client acuity
clinical pathways
clinical practice guidelines
cyclical scheduling
direct care
episodic care unit
full-time equivalent (FTE)
functional nursing
indirect care
inpatient unit

modular team nursing
nursing hours per patient day (NHPPD)
non-unit producing
primary nursing
resource intensity weights (RIWs)
self-scheduling
skill mix
staffing pattern
team nursing
total patient care
unit producing
workload measurement system

REVIEW QUESTIONS

1. Workload measurement systems assess the nursing workload needed by the client. The higher the client's acuity, the more care required by the client. Which of the following statements represents a weakness of workload measurement systems?
   A. Workload measurement data are useful in predicting the required staffing for the next shift and for justifying nursing hours provided.
   B. Workload measurement data can be utilized by the nurse making assignments to determine what level of care a client requires.
   C. Workload measurement systems typically focus on nursing tasks rather than a holistic view of a client's needs.
   D. Aggregate workload measurement data are useful in costing out nursing services and for developing the nursing budget.

2. To determine the number of FTEs required for a renal transplant unit, which of the following does *not* need to be reviewed?
   A. regulatory requirements from your government
   B. the client population care needs and the impact on your skill mix
   C. organizational structure or supports in place to enable care providers to care for clients
   D. the chief financial officer's opinion on the number of staff needed for your unit

3. In calculating the number of FTEs needed to staff your medical-surgical unit, which of the following does *not* require the scheduling of additional FTEs?
   A. benefit hours such as vacation and sick time
   B. educational time for staff, including orientation of new staff
   C. indirect client care staff that support the operation of the direct care staff 24 hours a day coverage for other departments that do not staff to cover their own benefit hours

4. If your RN staff members receive four weeks of vacation and six days of sick time per year, how many worked hours would each RN log in one year if all benefit hours were used?
   A. 1,950 worked hours
   B. 1,755 worked hours
   C. 1,905 worked hours
   D. 1,800 worked hours

5. In building your staffing plan, which of the following would *not* be a major consideration for determining how many staff you need each day and shift?
   A. the need for your staff to have more weekends off
   B. the volume of clients that you have at different times of the day
   C. the timing and volume of nurse-intensive activities such as administration of chemotherapy and blood
   D. the skill mix of your staff and the client care requirements throughout a 24-hour period

6. Client outcomes are the result of many variables, one being the model of care delivery that is utilized. From the following scenarios, select the worst fit between client needs and the care delivery model.
   A. cancer clients cared for in a primary nursing model
   B. rehabilitation clients cared for in a client-centred model
   C. medical intensive care clients being cared for in a team nursing model
   D. ambulatory surgery clients with a wide range of illnesses being cared for using a primary nursing model.

7. The care management tools of case management and clinical pathways have led to several improvements.

Which of the following would *not* be considered an outcome of these care management tools?
   A. increased public awareness of the nurse's role in health care
   B. length-of-stay reductions
   C. reduced cost of care in many populations
   D. identification of opportunities for improvement in care or in hospital systems

REVIEW ACTIVITIES

1. How do you know whether the outcomes of your staffing plan are positive? What measures do you have available in your organization to indicate your staffing is adequate or inadequate?

2. You are a nurse manager of a new unit for mental health clients. What would you consider in planning for FTEs and staffing for this unit?

3. You are the new nurse manager on a medical unit, and you are developing the schedule that will go from early October to late January. What factors do you consider when developing the staff schedule?

EXPLORING THE WEB

- To get more information on the American Nurses Association nurse staffing plans and ratios, go to *http://nursingworld.org/MainMenuCategories/ ANAPoliticalPower/State/StateLegislativeAgenda/ StaffingPlansandRatios_1.aspx*.

- Canada does not have mandated staffing levels; however, a recent Canadian Federation of Nurses Unions' position statement recommended a pilot project to test the use of standardized nurse-patient ratios in an appropriate setting. Read about it at *http://www.nursesunions. ca/publications/position-statements*

- The Canadian Nurses Association documents related to RN staffing and patient outcomes can be found at *http://www.cna-aiic.ca/CNA/issues/research_summaries/ default_e.aspx*

- Go to the magnet hospitals site (*http://nursingadvocacy. org/faq/magnet.html/*) and see whether the information there would help your organization foster professional nursing practice. Striving for magnet hospital designation increases an organization's ability to recruit and retain nurses.

REFERENCES

Advisory Committee on Health Human Resources. (2000a). *The Nursing Strategy for Canada*. Ottawa: Author. Retrieved from http://www.hc-sc.ca/english/nursing/

Advisory Committee on Health Human Resources. (2000b). *The Canadian Nursing Advisory Committee*. Retrieved from http://www.hc-sc.gc.ca/english/nursing/cnac.htm

Aiken, L. H., Clarke, S. P., Cheung, R. B., Sloane, D. M., & Silber, J. H. (2003). Educational levels of hospital nurses and surgical patient mortality. *Journal of the American Medical Association, 290*(12), 1617–1623.

Aiken, L. H., Clarke, S. P., & Sloane, D. M. (2002). Hospital staffing, organization and quality of care: Cross-national findings. *International Journal for Quality in Health Care, 14*(1), 5–13.

Anderson, R., & Kerfoot, K. (2009). The time has come for evidence-based staffing and scheduling. *Nursing Economics, 27*(5), 277–279.

Bailey, P., Jones, L., & Way, D. (2006). Family physician/nurse practitioner: Stories of collaboration. *Journal of Advanced Nursing, 53*(4), 381–391.

Baumann, A., O'Brien-Pallas, L., Armstrong-Stassen, M., Blythe, J., Bourbonnais, R., Cameron, S., et al. (2001). *Commitment and care: The benefits of a healthy workplace for nurses, their patients and the system*. Policy synthesis. Ottawa: The Change Foundation.

Besner, J., Doran, D., McGillis Hall, L., Giovannetti, G., Firard, F., Hill, W., et al. (2005). *A systematic approach to maximizing nursing scopes of practice*. Ottawa: Canadian Institutes of Health Research. Retrieved from www.cihr.gc.ca

Blastorah, M., Alvarado, K., Duhn, L., Flint, F., McGrath, P., & VanDeVelde-Coke, S. (2010). Development and evaluation of an RN/RPN utilization toolkit. *Nursing Leadership, 23*(Special issue), 33–50.

Campbell, B., Fryers, M., Devitt, R., & Vestal, K. (2009). Towards a collaborative model of care. *Healthcare Management Forum, 22*(3), 27–31.

Canadian Nursing Advisory Committee. (2002). *Our health, our future: Creating quality workplaces for Canadian nurses: Final report of the Canadian Nursing Advisory Committee*. Ottawa: Advisory Committee on Health Human Resources.

Canadian Nurses Association. (2003). *Staffing decisions for the delivery of safe nursing care*. Ottawa: Author.

Canadian Nurses Association. (2010). *Invitational round table nursing care delivery models and staff mix: Using evidence in decision-making*. Ottawa: Author.

Dearholt, S., & Feathers, C. A. (1997). Self-scheduling can work. *Nursing Management, 28*(8), 47–48.

Dechant, C. (2006). Human resource allocation: Staffing and scheduling. In J. Hibbard & D. Smith, *Nursing leadership and management in Canada* (3rd ed.). Toronto: Elsevier, Canada.

Del Togno-Armanasco, V., Hopkin, L. A., & Harter, S. (1995). How case management really works. *American Journal of Nursing, 5,* 24i, 24j, 24l.

Gilbert, J. H. V. (2005). Interprofessional education for collaborative, patient-centred practice. *Nursing Leadership, 18*(2), 32–38.

Hill-Popper, M. (2000, January). *Reversing the flight of talent*. Symposium at the Nursing Executive Center annual meeting, The Advisory Board Company, Washington, DC.

Joint Commission on Accreditation of Healthcare Organizations. (2000). *2000 hospital accreditation standards*. Oakbrook Terrace, IL: Author.

Lagoe, R. J. (1998). Basic statistics for clinical pathway evaluation. *Nursing Economics, 16*(3), 125–131.

Land, S., & Tiedeman, M. (2004). Traditional models of care delivery: What have we learned? *Journal of Nursing Administration, 34,* 291–297.

Marquis, B. L., & Huston, C. J. (2012). *Leadership roles and management functions in nursing: Theory and application* (7th ed.). Pennsylvania: Lippincott, Williams, & Wilkins.

McGillis Hall, L., Doran, D., & Pink, G. H. (2004). Nurse staffing mix models, nursing hours and patient safety outcomes. *Journal of Nursing Administration, 34*(1), 41–45.

McGillis Hall, L., Pink, L., Lalonde, M., Murphy, G., O'Brien-Pallas, L., Laschinger, H., et al. (2006). *Evaluation of nursing staff mix and staff ratio tools and models. Final report*. Ottawa: Canadian Nurses Association and Health Canada.

Moreau, K., Maxwell, H., Sorfleet, C., Ellis, J., Rashotte, J., Winsor-Stallan, B., et al. (2010). Innovative approaches to staffing and scheduling. *Nursing Leadership, 23*(Special issue), 138–139.

O'Brien-Pallas, L. (2007). Mapping out the territory. *Healthcare Papers, 7*(Special issue), 74–78.

O'Brien-Pallas, L., Doran, D. I., Murray, M., Cockerill, R., Sidani, S., Laurie-Shaw, B., et al. (2001). Evaluation of a client care delivery model, part 1: Variability in nursing utilization in community home nursing. *Nursing Economics, 19*(6), 267–276.

O'Brien-Pallas, L., Doran, D. I., Murray, M., Cockerill, R., Sidani, S., Laurie-Shaw, B., et al. (2002). Evaluation of a client care delivery model, part 2: Variability in client care outcomes in community home nursing. *Nursing Economics, 20*(1), 13–21, 36.

O'Brien-Pallas, L., Thomson, D., McGillis Hall, L., Pink, G., Kerr, M., Wang, S., et al. (2004). *Evidence-based standards for measuring nurse staffing and performance*. Report for the Canadian Health Services Research Foundation. Ottawa, ON.

Poochikian-Sarkissian, S., Hunter, J., Tully, S., Lazar, N.M., Sabo, K., & Cursio, C. (2008). Developing an innovative care delivery model: Interprofessional practice teams. *Healthcare Management Forum, 21*(1), 6–11.

Rothberg, M., Abraham, I., Lindenauer, P., & Rose, D. (2005). Improving nurse-to-patient staffing ratios as a cost-effective safety intervention. *Medical Care, 43*(8), 785–791.

Rothwell, D., Watson, A., & Payeur-Grenier, S. (2010). Utilizing a best practice staffing framework to promote interprofessional collaborative practice at the Niagara Health System. *Nursing Leadership 23*(Special issue), 126–127.

Satinsky, M. A. (1995). *An executive guide to case management strategies*. Chicago: American Hospital.

Schmele, J. (1996). *Quality management in nursing and healthcare*. Albany, NY: Delmar.

Shamian, J., & El-Jardali, F. (2007). Healthy workplaces for health workers in Canada: Knowledge transfer and uptake in policy and practice. *Healthcare Papers, 7*(Special issue), 6–25.

Shullanberger, G. (2000). Nurse staffing decisions: An integrative review of the literature. *Nursing Economics, 18*(3), 124–136.

Sovie, M. D., & Jawad, A. F. (2001). Hospital restructuring and its impact on outcomes: Nursing staff regulations are premature. *Journal of Nursing Administration, 31*(12), 588–600.

Suter, E., Arndt, J., Lait, J., Jackson, K., Kipp, J., Taylor, E., & Arthur, N. (2007). How can frontline managers demonstrate leadership in enabling interprofessional practice? *Healthcare Management Forum, 20*(4), 38–43.

Swansburg, R. C. (1996). *Management and leadership for nurse managers* (2nd ed.). Sudbury, MA: Jones & Bartlett.

Thungiaroenkul, P., Cummings, G., & Embleton, A. (2007). The impact of nurse staffing on hospital costs and patient length of stay: A systematic review. *Nursing Economics, 25*(5), 255–265.

White, D. et al. (2009). *Enhancing nursing role effectiveness through job redesign.* Ottawa: Canadian Institutes of Health Research. Retrieved from www.cihr.gc.ca

Zander, K. (1995). *Managing outcomes through collaborative care: The application of care mapping and case management.* Chicago: American Hospital.

SUGGESTED READINGS

Aiken, L. H., Sloane, D. M., & Sochalski, J. (1998). Hospital organization and outcomes. *Quality in Healthcare, 7*(4), 222–226.

American Hospital Association. (2002). *In our hands: How hospital leaders can build a thriving workforce.* Washington, DC: AHA Commission on Workforce for Hospitals and Health Systems.

Baker, C. M., Lamm, G. M., Winter, A. R., Robbleloth, V. B., Ransom, C. A., Conly, F., et al. (1997). Differentiated nursing practice: Assessing the state-of-the-science. *Nursing Economics, 15*(5), 253–261.

Buckingham, M., & Coffman, C. (1999). *First break all the rules: What the world's greatest managers do differently.* New York: Simon & Schuster.

Falco, J., Wenzel, K., Quimby, D., & Penny, P. (2000). Moving differentiated practice from concept to reality. *Aspen Advisor for Nurse Executives, 15*(5) 6–9.

Ferguson-Paré, M. (2004). ACEN position statement: Nursing workload: A priority for healthcare. *Canadian Journal of Nursing Leadership, 17*(2), 24–26.

Hay Group. (2001). *The retention dilemma: Why productive workers leave—Seven suggestions for keeping them.* Working Paper. Philadelphia: Hay Group

Leclerc, E., & Lavoie-Tremblay, M. (2007). Implementation of a nursing professional practice model. *Healthcare Management Forum, 20*(3), 24–26.

Lichtig, L. K., Knaug, R. A., Rison-McCoy, R., & Wozniak, L. M. (2000). *Nurse staffing and patient outcomes in the inpatient hospital setting.* Washington, DC: American Nurses Association.

Morash, R., Brintnell, J., & Rodger, G. L. (2005). A span of control tool for clinical managers. *Canadian Journal of Nursing Leadership, 18*(3), 83–93.

Nardone, P. L., Markie, J. W., & Tolle, S. (1995). Evaluating a nursing care delivery model using a quality improvement design. *Journal of Nursing Care Quality, 10*(1), 70–84.

Needleman, J., Buerhaus, P., Mattke, S., Stewart, M., & Zelevinsky, K. (2002). Nurse staffing levels and the quality of care in hospitals. *New England Journal of Medicine, 346*(22), 1715–1722.

Nelson, J. W. (2000). Consider this ... Models of nursing care: A century of vacillation. *Journal of Nursing Administration, 30*(4), 156, 184.

Priest, A. (2006). *What's ailing our nurses? A discussion of the major issues affecting nursing human resources in Canada.* Ottawa: Canadian Health Services Research Foundation.

Seago, J. A. (1999). Evaluation of hospital work redesign: Patient focused care. *Journal of Nursing Administration, 29*(11), 31–38.

Tourangeau, A. E., Giovannetti, P., Tu, J. V., & Wood, M. (2002). Nursing-related determinants of 30-day mortality for hospitalized patients. *Canadian Journal of Nursing Research, 33*(4), 71–88.

VanDerWal, R., & Globerman, J. (2008). Interventions that improved a practice environment: "Making a difference." *Healthcare Management Forum, 21*(3), 29–34.

VanDerWal, R., Globerman, J., Numata, Y., Schulzer, M., FitzGerald, M., & Yassi, A. (2008). Improving the practice environment: A pilot project in a critical care unit. *Healthcare Management Forum, 21*(2), 29–35.

Zander, K. (1996). The early years: The evolution of nursing case management. In D. L. Flarey, et al. (Eds.), *Handbook of nursing case management: Health care delivery in a world of managed care* (pp. 23–45). Gaithersburg, MD: Aspen.

CHAPTER ENDNOTES

1. Canadian Institute for Health Information, "Case Mix Groups." Retrieved from http://www.cihi.ca/CIHI-ext-portal/internet/EN/TabbedContent/standards+and+data+submission/standards/case+mix/cihi010690

2. Way & Jones. (1994). p. 29; as cited in Bailey, P., Jones, L., & Way, D. (2006). Family physician/nurse practitioner: Stories of collaboration. *Journal of Advanced Nursing, 53*(4), 381–391.

3. Besner, J., Doran, D., McGillis Hall, L., Giovannetti, G., Firard, F., Hill, W., et al. (2005). *A systematic approach to maximizing nursing scopes of practice.* Ottawa: Canadian Institutes of Health Research. Retrieved from www.cihr.gc.ca

4. Land, S., & Tiedeman, M. (2004). Traditional models of care delivery: What have we learned? *Journal of Nursing Administration, 34,* 291–297.

5. White, D., et al. (2009). *Enhancing nursing role effectiveness through job redesign.* Ottawa: Canadian Institutes of Health Research. Retrieved from www.cihr.gc.ca

6. Besner, J., Doran, D., McGillis Hall, L., Giovannetti, G., Firard, F., Hill, W., et al. (2005). *A systematic approach to maximizing nursing roles.* Ottawa: Canadian Institutes of Health Research. Retrieved from www.cihi.gc.ca

7. White, D. et al. (2009). *Enhancing nursing role effectiveness through job redesign.* Ottawa: Canadian Institutes of Health Research. Retrieved from www.cihr.gc.ca

8. Canadian Institute for Health Information, "Resource Intensity Weights and Expected Length of Stay." Retrieved from http://www.cihi.ca/cihi-ext-portal/internet/en/document/standards+and+data+submission/standards/case+mix/casemix_ri

9. CMA Infobase Clinical Practice Guidelines, "Foreward." Retrieved from http://mdm.ca/cpgsnew/cpgs/gccpg-e.htm

CHAPTER 12

Delegation of Nursing Care

Maureen T. Marthaler, RN, MS
Adapted by John P. Angkaw, MBA(c), MEd, BScN

Delegation is a formal process by which a regulated health professional who has the authority and competence to perform a procedure under one of the controlled acts delegates the performance of that procedure to others under certain conditions.[1]

OBJECTIVES

The purpose of this chapter is to enable the reader to

- review the history of delegation;
- define delegation, accountability, responsibility, authority, and assignment making;
- identify responsibilities the health team members can perform;
- list concepts associated with the delegation process;
- identify three potential delegation barriers;
- describe the five rights of delegation; and
- list six cultural phenomena that affect transcultural delegation.

A.G.E Foto Stock/First Light

Delegation to the appropriate personnel is an important responsibility in nursing. Inappropriate delegation can be life threatening, as illustrated in the following example.

A client was admitted to the hospital for asthma exacerbation. The client also had a history of chronic obstructive pulmonary disease (COPD). The client was receiving Ventolin every four hours and Atrovent therapy via inhalation every hour as needed. She required respiratory assessments to be performed at the onset of every shift and whenever necessary as indicated by a change in the client's condition. The night nurse assessed the client at the beginning of her shift, noting that her respiratory status was stable. The client did not appear to be in any respiratory distress. During the night, the nurse periodically checked on the client every two hours but did not awaken the client. A sitter was in the room with the client and had assured the nurse that the client was "doing fine." However, the sitter did not report to the nurse that she had been assisting the client to the washroom periodically throughout the night. Initially, the client had no difficulty. Upon assisting the client a second time, the sitter noted that the client became extremely short of breath and became weak and unstable. The sitter eventually required help from two unregulated care providers.

The incident and the change in the client's condition were not reported to the nurse. In the morning, the client's family became aware of the scenario and filed a formal complaint that their relative had not received any treatment during her distress.

How could this situation have been prevented?

Who is accountable?

What are the responsibilities of the nurse, the sitter, and the two unregulated care providers?

How could delegation have been appropriately performed in this situation?

E nsuring client safety is the most important priority for any care providers, including registered nurses (RNs), registered practical nurses (RPNs), registered psychiatric nurses (RPNs), licensed practical nurses (LPNs), and unregulated care providers (UCPs). On the Canadian Registered Nurse Examination (CRNE), students may encounter test questions that assess the ability of the nurse to delegate care. Safeguarding clients is a number-one care priority. To ensure that this responsibility is met, nurses are accountable under the law for care rendered by both themselves and other personnel.

Multiple levels of UCPs give care to clients, including nurse aides, personal support workers, health care aides, unit assistants, attendants, home support workers, homemakers, and other non-licensed personnel (College of Nurses of Ontario [CNO], 2005). This wide use of UCPs is part of a response to changes in the structuring of health care delivery. As a result of recent cost containment efforts, nurses are being given new and innovative job positions. Consequently, UCPs are often asked to consider performing duties that may not be within the scope of their education and abilities.

With increased opportunities to delegate care, nurses will be able to meet the duty of providing safe, quality care to their clients only by delegating properly. Without developing delegation skills, nurses caring for clients in today's health care community will not be able to complete the necessary duties, tasks, and responsibilities. They will find themselves stressed and exhausted by the many activities their nursing role requires. An inability to delegate can engender feelings of frustration, poor self-esteem, and lack of control. As nurses develop appropriate delegation skills, they become more productive and enjoy their work more.

PERSPECTIVES ON DELEGATION

As the history of nursing shows, Florence Nightingale had foresight regarding how nurses would function. Delegation in nursing was formally recognized in the 1800s, with Nightingale, and has continued to evolve as health care delivery models have developed.

Today, delegation is an essential skill for both the new nurse as well as the experienced nurse. Delegating to personnel with different educational levels from a variety of nursing programs requires nurses to be vigilant in ensuring that safety is maintained for the client.

According to Fisher (2000), delegation of certain tasks helps reduce health care costs by making more efficient use of nursing time and the facility's resources. Efficient delegation of care protects the client and provides desirable outcomes.

DELEGATION DEFINED

Different organizations and experts define delegation in different ways. According to the Canadian Nurses Association (CNA), delegation includes accepting accountability for actions and decisions when delegating, delegating health care activities to other health care providers consistent with their levels of expertise and education, and evaluating the outcome of delegated health care activities (CNA, 2009).

The CNO (2009) defines delegation as a formal process by which a regulated health professional, who is authorized and competent to perform a procedure under one of the controlled acts, delegates the performance of that procedure to someone—either regulated or unregulated—who is not authorized by legislation to perform it. The delegation process includes assessing competence and education, and establishing a process to evaluate ongoing competence.

Delegation in Saskatchewan is defined as the transfer of responsibility for a task when it is not part of the scope of practice of the care provider. The care provider performing the task must be accountable and competent in performing the delegated task. The safety of the client should not be compromised by substituting a less qualified worker to provide the care or perform the task (Saskatchewan Registered Nurses Association, 2004).

The Federation of Health Regulatory Colleges of Ontario developed their Interprofessional Guide on the Use of Orders, Directives and Delegation for Regulated Health Professionals in Ontario. The guide was developed to address questions about the use of orders and delegation to facilitate interprofessional care by health professionals practising in any setting across the province. It was developed as a consensus document and was designed to complement and assist with fulfilling guidelines, standards, and regulations developed by each health profession college.[2]

All delegation involves at least two individuals and specific duties to be accomplished with or through others via a transfer of authority. The authority needs to be delegated along with the ability to direct others. To be effective in accomplishing goals, the individual who is delegating must take on the leadership role. With successful delegation, the client's personal health needs are addressed and the nurse's professional goals are achieved. Communication techniques facilitate the delegation process for the registered nurse.

Registered nurses may be frustrated by having to accomplish all of their duties single-handedly. Many new graduate nurses become overwhelmed by the large number of duties to be learned and implemented. In nursing school, students typically perform total client care for one or two clients. Students might occasionally ask another student to help them, or they might pitch in to help others on their unit. Rarely will they have the opportunity to delegate to another nurse or to a UCP. Consequently, new nurses may be shocked to learn that delegation is now an expected part of their behaviour; however, delegation is required in the health care setting, and the CRNE tests nurse candidates on their ability to delegate.

Delegation is not meant to intimidate or isolate the new nurse. The sole purpose of delegation is to get the job done in the most efficient way, utilizing appropriate resources. The job must be delegated to staff who can handle it and who understand the goal. Delegation can spark interest and prevent individuals from becoming bored, non-productive, and ineffective. Identifying the most suitable duties or tasks can help others feel they are part of the team, regardless of their position. All staff want to feel they are making a difference in the well-being of the client, whether by giving a bath, dispensing medications, or simply sharing a smile. To delegate, the nurse takes into account other peoples' personal and professional positions within the health care team, including their abilities, education, and experience, and also the client's needs. Infection control and client safety are high priorities in making assignments.

To assist in delegation, the RN Delegation Decision-Making Framework is presented, which was originally adapted from the **National Council of State Boards of Nursing (NCSBN) (1995).** The framework can be viewed on the NCSBN website: https://www.ncsbn.org/delegationgrid.pdf. The NCSBN outlines five rights of delegation: the right task, the right circumstances, the right person, the right direction and communication, and the right supervision. The College of Nurses of Ontario has also developed a decision tree for teaching or delegating the performance of a procedure. It can be found on their website: http://www.cno.org/en/search/?q=decision+tree+for+delegation&p=1. In addition, the College of Nurses of Ontario provides guides to practise decision making; these are relevant for both entry-level licensed practical nurses and entry-level registered nurses.

ACCOUNTABILITY AND RESPONSIBILITY

Nurses are legally liable for their actions and are answerable for the overall nursing care of their clients. This is the definition of **accountability.** Accountability involves a retrospective review, which includes critical thinking to determine if the action was appropriate, and giving an answer for what has occurred.[3] Registered nurses and licensed practical nurses are accountable for their actions and the related consequences, including the initiation and follow-through of the nursing process. Nurses are also accountable for following their provincial and territorial standards of practice and legislation, the policies of their health care organization, and for demonstrating professional conduct as reflected by attitudes, beliefs, and values espoused in the CNA Code of Ethics for Registered Nurses (CNA, 2002). RNs and LPNs are accountable for monitoring changes in a client's status, noting and implementing treatment for human responses to illness, and assisting in the prevention of complications. The assessment, analysis, diagnosis, planning, teaching, and evaluation stages of the nursing process may not be delegated to UCPs. Delegated activities usually fall within the implementation phase of the nursing process.

Responsibility involves reliability, dependability, and the obligation to accomplish work. Responsibility also includes each person's obligation to perform at an acceptable level—the level to which the person has been educated. For example, a personal support worker (PSW) is expected to provide the client with a bed bath. The PSW does not administer pain medication or perform invasive or sterile procedures. After performing the assigned duties, the PSW provides, within a specified time frame, feedback to the nurse about the performance of the duties and the outcome of the actions. Note that feedback works two ways. The registered nurse has a responsibility to follow up with ongoing supervision and evaluation of activities performed by unregulated care providers. It is important to remember that although the nurse transfers responsibility and authority for the completion of a delegated task, the nurse retains accountability for the delegation process. Whenever nursing activities are delegated, the RN must follow the appropriate provincial or territorial nursing scopes of practices, nursing rules and regulations, and the policies and standards of the hospital or health facility.

AUTHORITY

The responsibility to delegate duties and give direction to UCPs places the RN and LPN in a position of authority. **Authority** refers to a person's right to delegate, based on the provincial or territorial nursing scope of practice, and based on that person also receiving official power from an agency to delegate. According to Ellis and Hartley (2000), the concept of authority is often associated with power because authority given by an agency legitimizes the right of a manager or supervisor to give direction to others and to expect that they will comply. The best working environment is one in which staff members view authority with respect.

ASSIGNMENT MAKING

Assignment making is the process of delegating the duties and all aspects of client care to individual staff, including giving clear, concise directions and delegating the responsibility and the authority for the implementation of the care. The RN or LPN retains accountability for the assignment, and must ensure that the education, skill, knowledge, and judgment levels of the personnel being assigned to a task are commensurate with the assignment. For example, administration of intravenous solutions to clients on a nursing unit would initially best be assigned to an RN or LPN who has received the appropriate education about intravenous solutions and who has acquired the experience performing these duties on a regular basis, rather than to someone who has little or no experience in administering intravenous solutions. When an assignment is made, the RN or LPN should specify the expected outcome of the assignment, the time frame for completion, and any limitations on the assignment.

RESPONSIBILITIES OF HEALTH TEAM MEMBERS

The new graduate nurse may feel overwhelmed by the amount of client care required and the lack of time to complete the care. The new graduate may also be consumed by feelings of inadequacy and failure. All of these feelings and behaviours may be a result of the challenge of attempting to accomplish a set of tasks and responsibilities without asking for help. New graduate nurses will quickly realize that if they do not delegate, the client's care will not be completed in a timely and effective manner.

Attention to the following six factors will improve both nursing delegation and nursing care:

1. The individual is adequately trained for the task.
2. The individual has demonstrated that the task has been learned.
3. The individual can perform the task safely in the given nursing situation.
4. The client's status is safe for the person to carry out the task.
5. Appropriate supervision is available during the task implementation.
6. The task is an established policy in the nursing practice setting, and policy is written, recorded, and available to all (Louisana State Board of Nursing [LSBN], 2009).

THE NURSE MANAGER'S RESPONSIBILITIES

The nursing manager is responsible for developing the staff members' ability to delegate. Guidance in this area is necessary because new graduates, who want to be regarded favourably, may not ask too much of other staff members. Delegation is a skill that requires practice and experience.

The nurse manager will determine the appropriate mix of personnel on a nursing unit. The nurse manager may have staff with a variety of skills, knowledge, and educational levels. The acuity and needs of the clients usually determine the personnel mix. From this personnel mix, the new graduate nurse will begin to identify who can best perform the assigned duties. The non-nursing duties are shifted toward other staff members such as clerical personnel, UCPs, or housekeeping staff; in this way their individual skill sets can be applied effectively.

THE NEW GRADUATE'S RESPONSIBILITIES

New graduate nurses need to focus on the duties for which they are directly responsible. In addition, they must also be aware of the duties they are able to delegate and to what extent. What do UCPs do? What do licensed practical nurses do? These questions need to be answered prior to the delegation of duties. Table 12-1 includes delegation suggestions for RNs.

THE REGISTERED NURSE'S RESPONSIBILITIES

The registered nurse is responsible and accountable for the provision of nursing care. According to the CNA (2002), the registered nurse is always responsible for client assessment, diagnosis, care planning, and evaluation. Nurses must ensure that the individual to whom they are delegating the authority to perform a controlled act has the knowledge, skill, and judgement to perform it safely and effectively for that client. Nurses must also ensure that the delegation is client-specific in that the procedure is appropriate for the client, and that the act is not performed on clients for whom it is not intended (CNO, 2009). Although unregulated care providers may measure vital signs, intake and output, or other client status indicators, the registered nurse or licensed practical nurse analyzes these data for comprehensive assessment, nursing diagnosis, and development of the plan of care. Unregulated personnel may perform simple nursing interventions related to client hygiene, nutrition, elimination, or activities of daily living, but the registered nurse or licensed practical nurse remains responsible for the client outcome. Having UCPs perform functions outside their scope of practice is a violation of provincial and territorial nursing practice acts and is a threat to client safety.

The misuse of UCPs is a practice common to many health care settings. According to the CNA (2002), the use of UCPs has a great impact on the care provided to the clients; therefore, several factors have to be considered. Primary considerations include the complexity of the care required and the safety of the client. Secondary considerations are respect for personal autonomy and the rights of clients to participate in decision making. Research indicates that the misuse of UCPs poses a risk to the public and, as a result, nurses must be alert to avoid such misuse of UCPs.

TABLE 12-1	**DELEGATION SUGGESTIONS FOR RNs OR LPNs**

1. Include all personnel in the delegation process when making assignments.

2. Assess which tasks are to be delegated and identify the staff to best complete the assignment.

3. Communicate the duty to be performed and identify the time frame for completion. The expectations for personnel should be clear and concise.

4. Avoid removing duties after they have been assigned. Removing duties should be considered only when the duty is above the level of the assigned staff member, such as when the client's care is in jeopardy because the client's status has changed.

5. Evaluate the effectiveness of the delegation of duties, check in frequently, and ask for a feedback report on the outcomes of care delivery.

6. Accept minor variations in the style in which the duties are performed. Individual styles are acceptable provided the duty is performed correctly within the scope of practice.

THE UCP'S RESPONSIBILITIES

The increase in the numbers of UCPs in acute care settings poses a degree of risk to the client. Many initiatives have been advanced to ensure safe staffing levels by using an appropriate skills mix. Ideally, UCPs become trained to perform duties such as bathing, feeding, toileting, and ambulating clients (see Figure 12-1). UCPs are also expected to document and report information related to these activities. The RN or LPN will delegate to the UCP and is liable for those delegations. According to the CNA (2002), if the RN or LPN knows or reasonably believes that the UCP has the appropriate training, orientation, and documented competencies, then the RN or LPN can reasonably expect that the UCP will function in a safe and effective manner.

Reasons for using UCPs in acute care settings include controlling costs, freeing RNs or LPNs from duties that are primarily non-nursing in nature, and allowing time for RNs or LPNs to complete the assessments of clients and their potential responses to treatments. UCPs cannot be assigned to assess or evaluate responses to treatment; this is the role of the RN or LPN. It is cheaper to have UCPs perform non-nursing duties than to have nurses perform them. UCPs can deliver supportive care, but they cannot practise nursing or provide total client care. The RN or LPN has an increased scope of liability when tasks are delegated to UCPs. The RN or LPN must be aware of the job description, skills, and educational background of the UCP prior to the delegation of duties.

Because the RN or LPN is accountable for the delegation of nursing care activities, the following questions need to be considered before using a UCP to deliver effective, safe, and ethical delivery of care:

- Is it appropriate that a UCP perform this activity, considering the client's condition, the associated risks, and the environmental supports?
- Is there a UCP available with the potential to perform the procedure?
- Is there a mechanism to determine the ongoing competence of the UCP?

THE LICENSED PRACTICAL NURSE'S RESPONSIBILITIES

Licensed practical nurses have a different scope of practice from registered nurses. Most provinces and territories differentiate the role of the licensed practical nurse from the role of the registered nurse. This distinction is based on the LPN's breadth and depth of knowledge and the stability of the client the licensed practical nurse cares for. LPNs are held to the same standard of care as registered nurses and, similarly, are responsible and accountable for their actions. LPNs commonly have the most responsibilities of all regulated care providers in care facilities, particularly in the long-term care sector. In that environment, the LPN is primarily responsible for overall client assessment, nursing diagnosis, planning, implementation, and evaluation of the quality of care delegated. The five rights of delegation, as highlighted in "Delegation: Concepts and Decision-Making Process," are identified in Table 12-2. These rights can be used as a mental checklist to clarify elements in the decision-making process (National Council of State Boards of Nursing, 1997).

When considering delegating the right task to the right person, check the applicable provincial or territorial nursing practice acts, the policies and procedures of the agency, and the job descriptions of all staff involved (e.g., LPNs, UCPs, RNs). Also consider the education and competence of all staff. What level of knowledge, skill, and judgment is required to perform the task? Does the individual have the ability to perform it? What are the risks involved? Is the task being delegated by the right person to the right person? Is it a task that can be delegated by a nurse? (CNO, 2009).

When considering the right circumstance, determine whether the staff members understand how to administer a procedure safely and correctly, and whether the action requires staff competency to be documented.

When considering the right person, ascertain whether the client is stable with predictable outcomes and whether it is legally acceptable to delegate to this person, keeping in mind the setting and available resources.

When considering the right direction and communication, ensure the RN communicates the task with clear directions and that the steps of the task and its expected outcomes are carefully outlined.

When considering the right supervision, ensure the RN answers all staff members' questions and is available to solve any problems that may arise. The UCP should report both task outcomes and the client's response to the RN who delegated the task. Thus, appropriate supervision and evaluation are maintained. The RN provides follow-up monitoring, intervention, feedback, evaluation, teaching, and guidance to the staff in an ongoing fashion.

DIRECT DELEGATION VERSUS INDIRECT DELEGATION

According to the CNA, direct delegation is usually verbal direction by the RN delegator regarding a procedure or task in a specific nursing care situation. Indirect delegation is performed using an approved list of activities or tasks that have been established in the policies and procedures of the health care institution or facility.

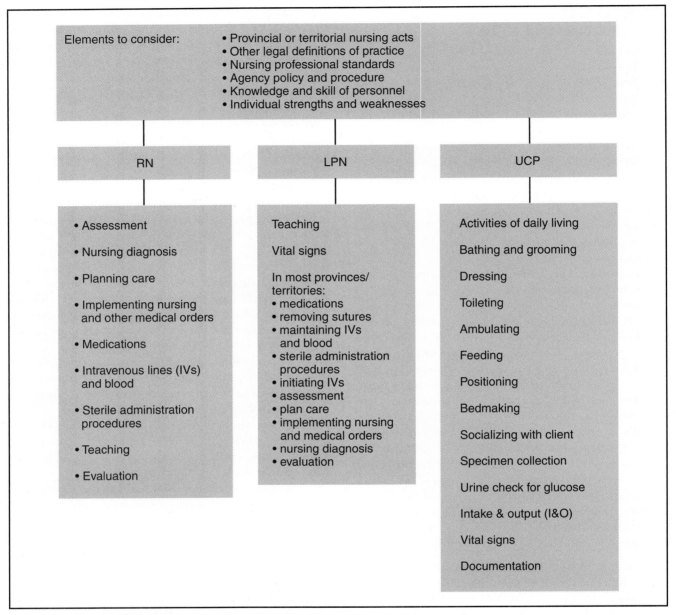

Elements to consider:
- Provincial or territorial nursing acts
- Other legal definitions of practice
- Nursing professional standards
- Agency policy and procedure
- Knowledge and skill of personnel
- Individual strengths and weaknesses

RN

- Assessment
- Nursing diagnosis
- Planning care
- Implementing nursing and other medical orders
- Medications
- Intravenous lines (IVs) and blood
- Sterile administration procedures
- Teaching
- Evaluation

LPN

Teaching

Vital signs

In most provinces/territories:
- medications
- removing sutures
- maintaining IVs and blood
- sterile administration procedures
- initiating IVs
- assessment
- plan care
- implementing nursing and medical orders
- nursing diagnosis
- evaluation

UCP

Activities of daily living

Bathing and grooming

Dressing

Toileting

Ambulating

Feeding

Positioning

Bedmaking

Socializing with client

Specimen collection

Urine check for glucose

Intake & output (I&O)

Vital signs

Documentation

Figure 12-1 Considerations in Delegation

The use of good professional judgment is vital when making the decision to delegate. Direct delegation gives the RN the opportunity to communicate clearly the duty to be completed, what to expect while completing the duty, and the expected outcome that the RN expects. The staff member then should have the opportunity to clarify the duty.

The process of indirect delegation begins at a variety of levels. The nurse manager prepares a list of duties that can be delegated, including those duties that are delegated from nurse manager to RN, RN to UCP, RN to LPN, LPN to UCP, nurse manager to unit clerk, RN to unit clerk, and so on. The duties are listed according to the hospital policy. The types of duties delegated reflect the ability of UCPs to complete the duties in a timely manner, according to their education and experience.

UNDERDELEGATION

People in a new job role, such as nurse manager, RN, LPN, or nursing graduate, often underdelegate. Believing that older, more experienced staff may resent having someone new delegate to them, new nurses may simply avoid delegation. Or, new nurses may seek approval from other staff members by demonstrating their capability to complete all assigned duties without assistance. In addition, new nurses may be reluctant to delegate because they do not know or trust individuals on their team or are not clear on the scope of the duties of the other staff or what they

REAL WORLD INTERVIEW

I use delegation now that I have completed school. I began working as a new graduate nurse immediately after graduating. Prior to graduation I worked as a personal support worker. I feel that I understand how it feels to be at both ends of the spectrum of client care delivery. I vowed that when I became a registered nurse, I would delegate appropriately and fairly to others.

As a registered nurse, I make it a point to delegate appropriately to personal support workers (PSWs). I delegate duties such as changing beds, bathing clients, feeding clients, and performing an accurate intake and output. I delegate these things after giving my PSW a complete report of my clients.

It is important to mention that I never delegate client assessments or client education. These duties are reserved for the registered nurse or licensed practical nurse. I will never delegate to a PSW to watch over clients while they take their medication. I never delegate the insertion or removal of Foleys. In short, I never delegate any tasks or responsibilities that are outside the PSW's scope of education and ability. I do believe my PSWs take me seriously as I do not delegate anything that I am not willing to do myself and have not done myself in the past. In essence, I do not give the impression that I am "beyond" or "better" than anyone else.

I am concerned when I see a nurse walk out of the room of a client who has just requested a bedpan and look for a PSW to get that bedpan. I would never make my client wait to perform such a necessary and often immediate task. Like I said earlier, I have been on both ends of client care delivery, and I know what it feels like to be neglected and unappreciated. So far, I have stuck to my promise to delegate appropriately and fairly. I strongly believe my PSWs would agree.

Shelly A. Thompson
New Graduate Nurse

TABLE 12-2	**FIVE RIGHTS OF DELEGATION**

1. the right task
2. under the right circumstances
3. using the right person
4. with direction and communication
5. with the right supervision

are allowed to do. New nurses can become frustrated and overwhelmed if they fail to delegate appropriately. They may fail to establish appropriate controls with staff or fail to follow up properly; they may fail to delegate the appropriate authority to go with certain responsibilities. Perfectionism and a refusal to allow mistakes can lead new nurses to be overburdened in client care responsibilities. Staff members with more experience can help new personnel by intervening early on and assisting in the delegation process, and by clarifying responsibilities.

INAPPROPRIATE DELEGATION

Inappropriate delegation of duties can place the client at risk. Delegating duties to others who lack the education and experience to carry out the task safely and competently is inappropriate and dangerous. The liability resting on the RN or LPN who has delegated professional duties to a UCP is clear. Although such inappropriate

REAL WORLD INTERVIEW

Upon evaluating delegation on several, varied nursing units, I arrive at one conclusion: we as professional nurses just do not do it well. There is the exception, of course, that being the individuals who have developed an outstanding ability to delegate nearly all of their responsibilities to others in an authoritative or diplomatic manner, with the recipients either loving or hating it.

On a nursing unit, the role of delegation and assigning tasks typically falls on the charge nurse. For this role, they are often criticized— most frequently behind the scenes— although at times, they are criticized openly. "What do you mean I am getting the next admission; I already have two!" One becomes apprehensive when assigning *anything*, from an admission to discharging a client. I wonder, if that is the fate of the charge nurse, just how well would one expect the staff RN to delegate?

I believe that the art of delegation and its related processes need to be taught and increasingly emphasized in nursing education, along with concepts of teamwork. The team becomes ineffective when proper delegation is neglected. The challenges in contemporary health care are tremendous and will only become even more challenging in the future. Professional nurses would benefit greatly by acquiring advanced skills in delegation, team building, and diplomacy; these are skills that will become essential tools to possess and utilize in the near future.

Andrea Chang, RN, MSN
Charge Nurse

REAL WORLD INTERVIEW

The concept of delegation was something that I had to adjust to as I transitioned from a nursing student to becoming a staff nurse. As a nursing student, tasks and procedures were often delegated to me by my nurse preceptor or other health care providers. There were a couple of times when I questioned whether the delegated task was within my scope of practice as a student. I had to consult my preceptor and faculty advisor from the university. I just wanted to make sure that I was only doing something that I was permitted to do.

When I became a staff nurse, it was expected that I would delegate tasks and procedures to other nurses and health care providers. This was quite an adjustment because my previous experience with delegation was being the one to receive the orders to carry out particular tasks. It was also a big learning curve for me because I had to familiarize myself with the organization's policies on delegation and the scope of practice of the other health care providers.

My biggest advice to a newly graduated nurse is to take the initiative to familiarize yourself with policies about delegation as articulated by your organization and by provincial and territorial regulatory colleges. Take the time to learn the culture of your unit, and the views of the staff with respect to delegation.

Sarah Jackson, BScN, RN
Staff Nurse, Transitional Care

delegation is against provincial and territorial nursing standards of practice, the reasons for it are numerous. Staff may feel uncomfortable performing a duty with which they are unfamiliar, or they may be unorganized or inclined either to avoid responsibility or to immerse themselves in trivia. The inappropriate delegation of duties can result in overwork for some staff and underwork for others, which creates resentment among colleagues.

LITERATURE APPLICATION

Citation: White, D., Oelke, N., Besner, J., Doran, D., McGillis-Hall, L., & Giovannetti, P. (2008). Nursing scope of practice: Descriptions and challenges. *Canadian Journal of Nursing Leadership*, 21(1): 44–57.

Discussion: The shortages of many healthcare providers, including nurses, have placed great challenges on organizations to effectively utilize the roles and skills sets of nurses and other health care providers. Before nursing skill sets can be most effectively used, it is important to consider the scope, boundaries, and potential overlap of knowledge and skills with other health care providers. Important questions need to be asked regarding clarification of roles, establishing boundaries of practice, levels of clinical autonomy, and educational preparation for these roles. To improve role distinction and client care outcomes, nursing leaders and educators must use a collaborative approach to articulate both the distinct and shared responsibilities of nurses and other health care providers.

Implications for Practice: It is important for nurses to consider the respective roles and scopes of practice that each member of the health care team contributes. Role differentiation must be established to best use the knowledge and skills of nurses and other health care providers.

LITERATURE APPLICATION

Citation: Weydt, A. (2010). Developing delegation skills. *OJIN: The Online Journal of Issues in Nursing*, 15(2).

Discussion: Delegation is a complex professional skill requiring sophisticated clinical judgment and final accountability for clients' care. This article discusses delegation and the related concepts of responsibility, accountability, and authority. Nursing judgment, interpersonal relationships, and assignment patterns are presented as additional factors to consider in the delegation process. The correlation between consistency of care givers and delegation potential is explored in the Work Complexity Assessment Program. Finally, the author concludes by sharing how to develop delegation skills.

Implications for Practice: Effective delegation is based on one's provincial or territorial nursing regulatory body standards. Concepts of responsibility, accountability, and authority are integral to each RN's understanding of professional nursing practice. This means that RNs must understand how to properly assume authority for the decisions and outcomes associated with client care, share the process of client care with other responsible members of the nursing team, and hold all members of the nursing team accountable for their responsibilities. To match staff expertise with client and family needs, RNs require critical thinking skills for effective delegation. Staff relationships also influence the delegation potential and the delegation process. When RNs do not effectively delegate to others, the quality of care can decrease and valuable resources can be mismanaged. Having clarity about what can be delegated helps to define quality professional practice not only for nurses but also for other team members, clients, and families.

TRANSCULTURAL DELEGATION

Nurses and clients come from diverse cultural backgrounds. Cultural diversity has increased significantly over the past decade in Canada. Transcultural delegation refers to the process of taking cultural diversity into consideration when determining which staff perform particular duties. Giger and Davidhizar (2002) suggest that six cultural phenomena need to be considered when delegating to a culturally diverse staff: communication, space, social organization, time, environmental control, and biological variations.

COMMUNICATION

Communication, the first cultural phenomenon, is greatly affected by cultural diversity in the workforce. Some of the characteristic elements of communication that differ among cultures include (1) communication patterns (i.e., the proximity of those communicating, such as different perceptions of personal space and tolerance of touching); (2) body movements; (3) paralanguage (i.e., inflections, silences, volume of voice, and pace of speaking); and (4) density of language. All these elements influence how messages are sent and received (Grohar-Murray & DiCroce, 2003). For example, if a nurse were talking to a UCP in a loud voice, it could be interpreted as anger. However, the nurse may be from a cultural background whose members always speak loudly—she may not be angry at all. Alternatively, a nurse, because of cultural upbringing, may speak in a quiet, nondirective way that could be wrongly perceived as lacking authority. All nursing programs teach fundamental communication skills, which are necessary for an effective process of delegation.

SPACE

Cultural background influences the space that individuals maintain between themselves when communicating. Some cultures prefer physical closeness, while other cultures prefer more distance to be maintained between people. Ineffective delegation can take place when an individual's space is violated. Some delegators stand too close when speaking, whereas some members of a group may feel isolated and disengaged if they are not sitting close to the delegator.

SOCIAL ORGANIZATION

In different cultures, the social support in a person's life varies from support in one's own family to support from collegial relationships with their co-workers. If a staff member looks to other staff for social support, those staff may have difficulty fulfilling any tasks delegated to them, which could threaten their social organization.

TIME

Another cultural phenomenon affecting delegation is the concept of time. How often have you heard people say, "They are on their own time schedule"? Some people tend to move slowly and are often late, whereas other people move quickly and are prompt in meeting deadlines.

Poole, Davidhizar, and Giger (1995) describe different cultural groups as being either past-, present-, or future-oriented. Past-oriented cultures focus on their tradition and its maintenance. For example, these cultures invest time in the preparation of food that is traditional even though prepared food can be bought in a store. Present-oriented cultures focus on day-to-day activities. For example, our present-oriented culture works hard for today's wages and does not plan for the future. Future-oriented cultures worry about what might happen in the future, and diligently prepare for possible financial- or health-related problems. A nurse delegator should always be aware of duties to be completed and their deadlines so that appropriate personnel can

CASE STUDY 12-1

A new nursing graduate, Melody, has been assigned to work with Patrick, who is a UCP, and six clients. Melody introduces herself to Patrick and asks him what types of client care he usually performs. He tells Melody that he gives baths and takes vital signs. Melody asks Patrick to get all of the vital signs and give them to her written on a piece of paper. She asks Patrick if he ever documents them. He replies that he does document them, and he will provide her with the set of vital signs as soon as he obtains them.

Later that morning, Dr. Parinas is making rounds on his clients, two of whom are Melody's clients. He asks Melody for their most recent vital signs. She then asks Patrick for the vital signs on all her clients. Patrick tells her he has not taken them yet as he was busy engaging in other client care activities. Dr. Parinas then asks Melody to obtain the vital signs herself. By the time Melody returns with the recorded vital signs, Dr. Parinas has gone and has left written orders that she cannot read.

Several factors in this delegation situation should have been handled differently. Can you name any?

Do you think the new graduate was ready to delegate to the UCP? Why?

Were the duties delegated appropriate for the UCP?

achieve their responsibilities in a timely fashion. Otherwise, the people who meet deadlines in a timely fashion may be frustrated by those who do not.

ENVIRONMENTAL CONTROL

Environmental control refers to people's perception of their control over their environment, which is also called internal locus of control. Some cultures place a heavier weight on fate, luck, or chance, believing, for example, that a client is cured from cancer based on chance. They may believe the health care treatment had something to do with the cure but was not the sole cause of the cure. The way in which staff members perceive their control of the environment may affect how they delegate and perform duties. Staff who have an internal locus of control are geared toward taking more initiative and not requiring assistance in decision making. They believe in taking action and not relying on fate. Staff with an external locus of control may wait for fate to determine their actions.

BIOLOGICAL VARIATIONS

The sixth and final cultural phenomenon is biological variations. Biological variations are the bio-psychological differences between racial and ethnic groups, which include physiological differences, physical stamina, and susceptibility to disease. Such factors need to be considered when delegating tasks. For example, it would be problematic if the care of a comatose client who weighs more than 135 kilograms and needs frequent turning were delegated to a small nurse who cannot physically handle the client. Perhaps this client should be assigned to two nurses. A nurse who is pregnant would not likely be assigned to this particular client because of the potential injury to the baby and nurse. Likewise, a pregnant nurse would not be assigned to a client with radium implants because of the risks that the radium poses to the baby and mother. Biological variations must be considered, for the sake of both the health care providers and the client.

KEY CONCEPTS

- Delegation is a practised and learned behaviour. It should not compromise client safety.

- The RN must have a clear definition of what constitutes the scope of practice of all personnel.

- The five rights of delegation are the right task, the right circumstance, the right person, the right direction and communication, and the right supervision and evaluation.

- Accountability refers to nurses' legal liability for their actions, being answerable for the overall nursing care of their clients.

- Responsibility involves reliability, dependability, and the obligation to accomplish work. Responsibility also includes each person's obligation to perform at an acceptable level.

- Authority refers to a person's right to delegate based on the provincial or territorial standards of practice and based on that person also receiving official power from an agency to delegate.

- The RN is accountable for the delegation and performance of all nursing duties.

- There are several potential barriers to good delegation.

- Transcultural delegation is encouraged to provide clients with optimal care.

KEY TERMS

accountability   delegation
authority   responsibility

REVIEW QUESTIONS

1. Which of the following elements should be considered when delegating a task?
   A. provincial or territorial nursing acts
   B. agency policy and procedures
   C. knowledge, skill and judgment of staff
   D. all of the above

2. If a nurse has difficulty completing nursing duties on schedule, which of the following transcultural phenomenon should be considered?
   A. biological variations
   B. time
   C. space
   D. social organization

3. Which element of delegation refers to an individual's reliability, dependability, and the obligation to accomplish work?
   A. responsibility
   B. accountability
   C. consistency
   D. authority

4. If a client being discharged requires teaching to be reinforced, who is the most appropriate caregiver to perform this task?
   A. a unit clerk
   B. an LPN
   C. a PSW
   D. a registered nurse

5. Which client is most appropriate to assign to the UCP for basic care?
   A. client with acute peritonitis
   B. client with stable congestive heart failure
   C. new post-op acute appendectomy client
   D. recent head injury client

REVIEW ACTIVITIES

1. To determine your scope of practice, contact your provincial or territorial nursing association for information on laws and regulations, or access the appropriate website. Does your agency have a policy on delegation and scope of practice?

2. Read the study in the April 14, 1999, *Journal of the American Medical Association*, by Dr. Peter Pronovost and colleagues at the John Hopkins University. They found that a decreased ICU nurse–client ratio during the day or evening was associated with increased ICU days and increased hospital length of stay. Could some of this high-acuity client care be safely delegated? Read the article, Clarke, S. P., & Aiken, L. H. (2006). More nursing, fewer deaths. *Quality and Safety in Health Care*, 15(1), 2–3. Is there an opportunity for unregulated care providers?

3. Observe delegation procedures at your institution. Is transcultural delegation considered? If so, which phenomena have you observed? Are the five rights of delegation being consistently considered? What are some of the challenges regarding delegation on your unit or agency?

4. Are UCPs used at your agency? Are the responsibilities of the UCPs consistent across all units? What duties are they assigned? What process does each unit use to delegate responsibilities to the UCP? Are there any duties the UCPs are not comfortable performing? Discuss your findings.

5. Have you had any clinical opportunities to delegate duties? To whom did you delegate, and what did you delegate? Discuss how your delegating of duties affected the client and your work. What would you do differently next time?

EXPLORING THE WEB

■ Log on to *http://www.cna-nurses.ca*. Note what policies or position statements, if any, consider delegation of care to UCPs and LPNs.

■ The College of Nurses of Ontario (2009) has two practice guidelines that discuss decision making and delegation: *Authorizing Mechanisms* and *Utilization of Unregulated Care Providers (UCPs)*. Log on to the College of Nurses of Ontario website at *http://www.cno.org* to view these practice guidelines.

REFERENCES

Anthony, M. K., & Vidal, K. (2010). Mindful communication: A novel approach to improving delegation and increasing patient safety. *OJIN: The Online Journal of Issues in Nursing*, 15(2), Manuscript 2.

Canadian Nurses Association. (2002). *Unregulated Health Care Workers Supporting Nursing Care Delivery*. Retrieved from http://www.cna-nurses.ca/CNA/documents/pdf/publications/PS38_Unregulated_HCW_Supporting_NCD_March_1995_e.pdf

Canadian Nurses Association. (2009a). *Issues discussion at annual meeting 2009: Increasing use of unregulated health workers*. Retrieved from http://www.cna-aiic.ca/cna/search/default_e.aspx?cx=017995081769602664776%3Amo7p1eqo4vc&cof=FORID%3A11&ie=UTF-8&q=Unregulated+Health+Care+Workers+Supporting+Nursing+Care+Delivery&sa=Search#1039

Canadian Nurses Association. (2009b). *Maximizing health human resources: Valuing unregulated health workers. Highlights of the 2009 Pan-Canadian symposium*. Retrieved from http://www.cna-aiic.ca/cna/search/default_e.aspx?cx=017995081769602664776%3Amo7p1eqo4vc&cof=FORID%3A11&ie=UTF-8&q=Unregulated+Health+Care+Workers+Supporting+Nursing+Care+Delivery&sa=Search#1039

Clarke, S. P., & Aiken, L. H. (2006). More nursing, fewer deaths. *Quality and Safety in Health Care*, 15(1), 2–3.

College of Nurses of Ontario (2009a). *Authorizing mechanisms. College of Nurses of Ontario: Compendium of Standards*. Toronto: Author. Retrieved from http://www.cno.org/en/learn-about-standards-guidelines/publications-list/list-of-all-publications/

College of Nurses of Ontario. (2009b). *Utilization of unregulated care providers (UCPs). College of Nurses of Ontario: Compendium of Standards*. Toronto: Author. Retrieved from http://www.cno.org/en/learn-about-standards-guidelines/publications-list/list-of-all-publications/

Ellis, J. R., & Hartley, C. L. (2000). *Managing and coordinating nursing care*. Philadelphia: Lippincott.

Federation of Health Regulatory Colleges of Ontario website. An interprofessional guide on the use of orders, direction and delegation for regulated health professionals in Ontario. Retrieved from http://www.regulatedhealthprofessions.on.ca/EVENT-SRESOURCES/medical.asp

Fisher, M. (2000). Do you have delegation savvy? *Nursing2000,* 30(12), 58–59.

Giger, J., & Davidhizar, R. (2002). The Giger and Davidhizar Transcultural Assessment Model. *Journal of Transcultural Nursing,* 13(3), 185–88.

Grohar-Murray, M., & DiCroce, H. (2003). *Leadership and management in nursing* (3rd ed.). Upper Saddle River, NJ: Prentice Hall.

Hansten, R., & Washburn, M. (2001, March). Delegating to UAPs: Making it work. *NurseWeek,* 21–23.

Louisana State Board of Nursing. (2009). Delegation Decision Making Process – Licensed –Tree Diagram. Retrieved from http://www.lsbn.state.la.us/Documents/delegation.asp

National Council of State Boards of Nursing. (1997). Delegation: Concepts and decision-making process. *Issues,* 1–2.

Poole, V., Davidhizar, R., & Giger, J. (1995). Delegating to a transcultural team. *Nursing Management,* 26(8), 33–34.

Saskatchewan Registered Nurses Association. (2004). Practice of Nursing: RN Assignment and Delegation. Retrieved from http://www.srna.org/search

Weydt, A. (2010). Developing delegation skills. *OJIN: The Online Journal of Issues in Nursing,* 15(2). Retrieved from http://www. nursing world.org/MainMenuCategories/ANAMarketplace/ ANsVol152010/No2May2010/Mindful-Communication-and-Delegation.aspx

White, D., Oelke, N., Besner, J., Doran, D., McGillis-Hall, L., & Giovannetti, P. (2008). Nursing scope of practice: Descriptions and challenges. *Nursing Leadership,* 21(1), 44–57.

SUGGESTED READINGS

American Nurses Association (ANA). (1996). *Registered professional nurses and unlicensed assistive personnel* (2nd ed.). Washington, DC: American Nurses Publishing.

Bellack, J. P., & O'Neil, E. H. (2000). Recreating nursing practice for a new century: Recommendations and implications of the Pew Health Professions Commission's final report. *Nursing and Health Care Perspectives,* 21(1), 14–21.

Benner, P. (1984). *From novice to expert: Excellence and power in clinical nursing practice.* Menlo Park, CA: Addison-Wesley.

Bernreuter, M. E., & Cardona, M. S. (1997). Survey and critique of studies related to unlicensed assistive personnel from 1975 to 1997, part I. *Journal of Nursing Administration,* 27(6), 24–29.

Bittner, N., & Gravlin, G. (2009). Critical thinking, delegation and missed care in nursing practice. *The Journal of Nursing Administration,* 39(3), 142–146.

Canadian Nurses Association. (2003). *Position statement: Staffing decisions for the delivery of safe nursing care.* Ottawa: Author.

Gordon, S., & Barry, C. (2009). Delegating guided by school nursing values: Comprehensive knowledge, trust, and empowerment. *The Journal of School Nursing,* 24(5), 352–360.

Hudson, T. (2008). Delegation: Building a foundation for our future nurse leaders. *MedSurg Nursing,* 17(6), 396–399.

McInnis, L., & Parsons, L. (2009). Thoughtful nursing practice: Reflections on nurse delegation decision-making. *Nursing Clinics of North America,* 44(4), 461–470.

Plawecki, L., & Amrheim, D. (2010). A question of delegation. *Journal of Gerontological Nursing,* 36(8), 18–20.

Potter, P., Deshields, T., & Kuhrik, M. (2010). Delegation practices between registered nurses and nursing assistive personnel. *Journal of Nursing Management,* 18(2), 157–165.

Snyder, D., Medina, J., Bell, L., & Wavra, T. (Eds.). (2004). Delegation Handbook. In *American Association of Critical Care Nurses* (2nd ed.). Baltimore: ACCN.

Standing, T., & Anthony, M. (2008). Delegation: What does it mean to acute care nurses? *Applied Nursing Research,* 21(1), 8–14.

CHAPTER ENDNOTES

1. College of Nurses of Ontario. (2009). *"Authorizing mechanisms." College of Nurses of Ontario: Compendium of Standards.* Toronto: Author. Retrieved from http://www.cno.org/en/learn-about-standards-guidelines/publications-list/list-of-all-publications

2. Federation of Health Regulatory Colleges of Ontario website. "An interprofessional guide on the use of orders, direction and delegation for regulated health professionals in Ontario." Retrieved from http://www.regulatedhealthprofessions.on.ca/EVENTSRESOURCES/medical.asp

3. Weydt, A. (2010). Developing delegation skills. *OJIN: The Online Journal of Issues in Nursing,* 15(2), Manuscript 1. Retrieved from http://www.nursingworld.org/MainMenuCategories/ANAMarketplace/ANAP.../OJIN/TableofContents/Vol152010/No2May2010/Delegation-Skills.aspx

UNIT IV
Managing Care

CHAPTER 13

Strategic Planning and Organizing Client Care

Amy Androwich O'Malley, RN, MSN
Ida M. Androwich, PhD, RNC, FAAN
Kathleen Fischer Sellers, PhD, RN
Adapted by Heather Crawford, BScN, MEd, CHE

Our moral responsibility is not to stop the future, but to shape it...to channel our destiny in humane directions to ease the trauma of transition.
(Alvin Toffler)

OBJECTIVES

The purpose of this chapter is to enable the reader to

- describe the importance of an organization's mission (purpose) and philosophy and their impact on the structure and behaviour of an organization;
- define the purpose of strategic planning and identify the steps in the strategic planning process;
- articulate the importance of aligning the organization's strategic vision both with the organization's own mission, philosophy, and values and also with the goals and values of the communities served by the organization;
- have a basic understanding of common organizational structures and a framework for examining their purposes, advantages, and disadvantages;
- discuss the elements of strategic planning—philosophy, mission, and vision;
- define nursing-shared governance;
- identify Benner's concepts of novice, advanced beginner, competent, proficient, and expert nursing practice; and
- identify measures of a unit's performance.

photos.com

You are a staff nurse in a hospital that has just celebrated its 50th anniversary. Your organization is about to merge with a facility that is only five years old. You have been asked to participate on a committee to develop a mission statement for the new merged facility.

What are your thoughts about the invitation to participate?

What information do you need to do your job well?

What resources do you need?

Is this situation unusual? How can it be meaningful for you?

There are increasing opportunities for nurses to become involved in strategic and tactical planning for the delivery of health care services in their organizations and communities. Yet, to be effective in leadership roles, nurses need a basic understanding of the way that organizations are structured, how organizational systems function, and how to engage in the strategic planning process. In the past many health care organizations were structured in a highly formal, top-down, militaristic manner. These bureaucratic organizations worked well in a relatively stable environment when communication channels could be hierarchical. However, these organizations are not useful in a dynamic health care system in which information is rapidly changing. Increasingly, managers recognize the importance of obtaining subordinate input from all levels of the organization, both to give strategic plans meaning and to increase the likelihood of implementation (Marquis & Huston, 2012). In addition, workers in today's health care systems are considered knowledge workers—professionals hired for their knowledge, skills, and expertise. They need a system that supports their ability to practise to the full extent of their professional accountability.

Leadership in the health care organizations of the 21st century demands competent nurses with different skill sets than in the past. Functioning in a leadership role in today's highly complex health care environment requires an understanding of how systems function and how to improve health care delivery. Yet, health care providers, including professional nurses, have been slow to integrate this information into their clinical practice. The ability to plan for continuous improvement of quality, service, and cost-effectiveness is a critical competency for successful 21st century health care organizations and nurses.

The Canadian Adverse Events Study in 2000 estimated that preventable adverse events cause between 9,000 and 24,000 deaths each year in Canada (Baker et al., 2004). In the United States in 2000, the National Advisory Council on Nurse Education and Practice and the Council on Graduate Medical Education concluded that client safety depends upon the implementation of an interdisciplinary system (1) that addresses the realities of practice and client care and (2) that emphasizes interdisciplinary approaches to education and service. Other studies stress that a major determinant of client welfare is the way that nurses' work is organized (Havens & Aiken, 1999). Consequently, nurses in leadership positions must be educationally prepared to develop and implement sound models for the effective delivery of client care. Although many health care organizations collect large sets of data and are beginning to use scientific methods to improve the services they render, these activities are typically fragmented, isolated from day-to-day nursing management, and lack alignment with any organizational strategy. The Canadian Nurses Association (CNA) concurs with the Canadian Adverse Events Study that errors occur as a result of system failure rather than human failure (Baker & Norton, 2001). Before criticizing the age of this article, recognize that this is one of a few seminal studies! This chapter will discuss the strategic planning process and the importance of aligning the organization's strategic vision with the mission, philosophy, and values of the organization and the communities served by the organization. In addition, unit or departmental goals and objectives need to align with those of the organization.

STRATEGIC PLANNING

As Lewis Carroll observed in *Alice's Adventures in Wonderland*, "If you don't know where you are going, any road will do." A health care organization needs to have a good idea of where it fits into its environment and the types of programs and services that are needed and demanded by its clients or stakeholders. This approach applies at both a broad organizational level and at a unit level.

A nurse manager in an ambulatory medicine clinic needs to have an understanding of which programs and services are valued by the client population that the clinic serves and how the unit's ongoing activities fit with the overall strategy of the larger organization. Staff should also consider clients' needs when developing new services.

STRATEGIC PLANNING DEFINITION

The scenario described in the interview with Dr. Carruthers (see the Real World Interview) is an example of factors that affect strategic planning. A **strategic plan** can be defined as the sum total or outcome of the processes by which an organization engages in environmental analysis, goal formulation, and strategy development with the purpose of organizational growth and renewal. Robbins et al. (2002) define strategic planning as "plans that apply to the entire organization, that establish the organization's overall objectives, and that seek to position the organization in terms of its environment" (p. 55). Strategic planning is ongoing and is especially needed whenever the organization is experiencing problems or internal or external review problems.

THE PURPOSE OF STRATEGIC PLANNING

The purpose of strategic planning is twofold. First, it means that everyone shares the same idea or vision for where the organization is headed; and second, a good plan can help to ensure that the needed resources are available to carry out the initiatives that have been identified as important to the unit or agency. In addition, a clear plan allows the manager to select among seemingly equal alternatives based on the alternatives' potential to move the organization toward the desired end goal. Senge (2006) states that people with a strong sense of personal direction can join together to create a powerful synergy toward what "we truly want" (p. 197). **Reengineering** is the fundamental rethinking and redesign of the process under review to bring about radical and dramatic improvements and increases in value. Often called business process reengineering, it implies an approach that will allow dramatic changes and yield dramatic improvements in the manner in which the business processes are carried out. Strategic planning is a major component of business process reengineering.

STEPS IN THE STRATEGIC PLANNING PROCESS

In any strategic planning process, steps need to be followed in a particular order. This process is similar to the nursing process, in which one assesses and plans before implementing an intervention. Similarly, when developing an organizational, unit, or program plan, it is important to progress in a systematic manner. The first step consists of an environmental assessment.

REAL WORLD INTERVIEW

Recent efforts to expand the range of ambulatory services available at St. Joseph's Hospital have centred on consolidating the orthopedic and rheumatology services. Clients with a myriad of conditions, such as sprains, dislocations, and fractures, and who require consultations or medication alteration would benefit from the consolidation of these services in one location. In addition, outpatient radiology and laboratory facilities would be in close proximity to the orthopedic and rheumatology clinics, creating a user-friendly environment for the clients. The majority of the clients are elderly, or have compromised mobility. Consolidation of services will result in increased satisfaction for clients, staff, and physicians.

Chris Carruthers, MD
Orthopedics

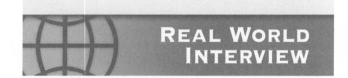

REAL WORLD INTERVIEW

The pivotal value of strategic planning is that it requires an organization to focus on its raison d'être, its mission, and to test how its operations are leading to accomplishment of that mission. Simply put, strategic planning determines where an organization is going over the next few years or more, how it's going to get there, and how it'll know if it got there or not.

Brian Williams, MScN
Health Care Consultant

ASSESSMENT OF EXTERNAL AND INTERNAL ENVIRONMENT

As outlined in Figure 13-1, **strategic planning** involves clarifying the organization's philosophical values; identifying its mission or why the organization exists; articulating a vision statement; and then conducting an environmental assessment, or **SWOT analysis**, which examines the strengths, weaknesses, opportunities, and threats of the organization. This information provides data that then drive the development of three- to five-year strategies for the organization. Tactics are then created and prioritized. Finally, goals and objectives are solidified into annual operating work plans for the organization. This same process is used for unit or departmental strategic planning. See Figure 13-2 for an example of a SWOT analysis.

COMMUNITY AND STAKEHOLDER ASSESSMENT

A frequently overlooked but highly important area for analysis is the stakeholder assessment. A **stakeholder** is any person, group, or organization with a vested interest in the program or project under review. A **stakeholder assessment** involves a systematic consideration of all potential stakeholders to ensure that the needs of each of these stakeholders are incorporated in the planning phase.

For a program to be successful, the involvement of those who will be affected is essential, whether the stakeholders are in the community or are the unit staff who will be affected by a proposed strategic plan. When stakeholders are not involved in the project planning, they do not gain a sense of ownership and may accept a program or strategic goals with only limited enthusiasm, or not at all.

OTHER METHODS OF ASSESSMENT

A number of methods can be used to support involvement in the strategic planning process. Thoughtful planning is required to determine which method to use when another method is appropriate.

SURVEYS AND QUESTIONNAIRES

Frequently, surveys or questionnaires are used when there is both a large number of stakeholders and a general idea of the options available. For example, staff might be polled to determine whether they would attend continuing education and which days and times would be most desirable.

FOCUS GROUPS AND INTERVIEWS

Focus groups are small groups of individuals selected because of a common characteristic, such as a recent diagnosis of diabetes. People are invited to meet as a group and respond to questions about a topic in which they have an interest or an expertise. An example of a focus group would be a group of clients who have recently had experiences with childbirth. They might be asked to come together to discuss their obstetric experiences at the institution in the hope that the discussion will lead to insights or information that could be used for improving care in the future. Focus groups are usually more time-consuming and expensive to conduct than questionnaires or surveys. They work best when the topic is broad and the options are not clear.

ADVISORY PANEL

Large projects often benefit from an advisory panel, selected from various constituencies affected by a proposed program. The advisory panel does not have formal authority over a program, but it is instrumental in reviewing the planned program and making recommendations and suggestions. Because the advisory panel is deliberately selected to reflect representation from

REAL WORLD INTERVIEW

At our academic health science centre, leaders in the organization, board members who represent the community, and customer stakeholders develop the strategic plan. Once the strategic plan is developed, it is published and reviewed at a centre-wide management meeting. It is then reviewed in divisional meetings and presented to staff through unit staff meetings, where the voice of the chief nursing officer has the most impact. I essentially interpret the rationale for the corporate strategic plan to my staff and glean their reactions. I then communicate the staff's feedback to the corporate level.

In our organizational newsletter for all staff, articles are published describing the plan and addressing points of clarification. Each division and department then undertakes the process of developing divisional and departmental plans that support the strategic plan. For example, a few years ago, the strategic plan articulated that our academic centre would become a major cardiac centre with a state-of-the-art cardiac catheterization laboratory. The department of cardiac services then included development of a state-of-the-art cardiac catheterization laboratory into its plan.

Anne L. Bernat, RN, MSN, CNAA
Chief Nursing Officer

Vancouver Coastal Health Strategic Framework

Lens	People First
Vision	We will be leaders in promoting wellness and ensuring care by focusing on quality and innovation.
Mission	We are committed to supporting healthy lives in healthy communities with our partners through care, education and research.
Values	Service	Integrity	Sustainability
Drivers	Patient/Community Focus	Engaged Team	Operational Excellence	Financial Sustainability

Goals

| Provide the best quality of care. | Promote better health for our communities. | Optimize our workforce and prepare for the future. | Use our resources efficiently to sustain a viable health care system. |

Objectives

1.1 Use a standardized, rigorous process to accelerate the creation and broad use of evidenced-based protocols in all clinical areas and programs.

1.2 Develop a regional program for Mental Health and Addiction and Cardiac Sciences to improve quality of care.

1.3 Build a regional medication reconciliation system across the continuum.

2.1 Reduce health inequities in the populations we serve through focused improvements in core public health programs.

2.2 Build on VCH integration strategies to support implementation of the MoHS directive to deliver integrated primary care, home and community care and community mental health services.

3.1 Enhance workforce utilization and match staffing to clinical volumes and patient acuity.

3.2 Recruit and retain the best people by fostering a culture of excellence, recognition and respect.

3.3 Build organizational capacity by strengthening leadership and management competencies.

4.1 Embed LEAN thinking at all levels to fulfill objectives and to deliver quality outcomes.

4.2 Develop and implement best practices in care management to reduce unnecessary days of stay.

4.3 Deliver administrative and support efficiencies through the shared services organization and consolidation.

4.4 Respond to provincial patient-centered funding model.

4.5 Develop service agreements with funders and service providers.

4.6 Develop and implement a strategy to secure increased capital funding.

4.7 Continue our commitment to "Green Care" alternatives by reducing waste and our carbon footprint.

Figure 13-1a Vancouver Coastal Health Strategic Framework

Source: Vancouver Coastal Health. Retrieved from http://www.vch.ca/media/Strategic%20Framework.pdf, May 28, 2011. Reprinted with Permission.

Saskatoon Health Region Strategic Directions, Goals and Objectives for 2011-2012
May 6, 2011

Vision: Healthiest People, Healthiest Communities, Exceptional Service

Mission: We improve health through excellence and innovation in service, education and research, building on the strengths of our people and partnerships.

Values: Respect, Compassion, Excellence, Stewardship, Collaboration

Promise: Every moment is an opportunity to create a positive experience in the way we treat and care for people, in how we work and interact with each other, and in how we deliver quality service. We promise to seize every opportunity.

TRANSFORM THE CARE AND SERVICE EXPERIENCE	PARTNER TO IMPROVE HEALTH OF THE COMMUNITY	TRANSFORM THE WORK EXPERIENCE	BUILD A SUSTAINABLE, INTEGRATED SYSTEM
Provide exceptional care and services that exceeds client expectations and is consistent with best practices	*Improve the overall health of the population and reduce health disparities*	*Create a workplace that optimizes capabilities, capacity, engagement and quality of worklife for providers and learners*	*Manage and align our resources to ensure sustainability of the health system*
Place clients and families first; and **Provide culturally safe and competent care with a focus on First Nations and Métis people:** • Develop and begin implementation of a 10 year plan for patient and family centred care **Achieve timely access to services:** • Establish spine clinic • Implement other SkSI strategies to meet surgical volume and wait time targets • Repatriate deceased donor kidney transplants to ensure full range of surgery and	**Identify health needs and priorities with community partners:** • Implement first steps of rural health strategy to support and partner with all communities ready to engage in joint health service planning, including but not limited to: Watson, Wakaw/Cudworth, Nokomis, Lanigan, and Watrous **Focus on health promotion, protection and disease prevention:** • Participate in priority projects of the Saskatchewan Population Health Council, with emphasis on Phase One implementation of SHR HIV strategy	**Work together to create safe and supportive work places:** • Continue implementation of the SHR Workplace Excellence plan, collaborating with employees to improve their health as well as our organization's workplace and financial health, resulting in reductions in sicktime and WCB time lost **Develop a highly skilled, workforce with a sufficient number and mix of service providers:** • Focusing on employee, workplace and financial health, continue	**Maximize efficiencies and reduce waste:** • Implement operational efficiencies to achieve SHR 2011/12 budget targets • Develop a multi-year SRHA-approved strategy to spread Lean across the care continuum • Implement Lean in redesign related to Emergency Optimization), Home Care, Lab and hospital discharge planning • Participate in provincial shared services and procurement **Strategically invest in facilities, equipment and information technology:** • Implement capital project plans for: ▪ RUH Pharmacy

(Continued)

Figure 13-1b Saskatoon Health Region 2011–2012 Strategic Directions, Goals, and Objectives

Source: Saskatoon Health Region, *2011–2012 Strategic Directions, Goals and Objectives.* Retrieved from http://www.saskatoonhealthregion.ca/about_us/strategic_home.htm, May 28, 2011. Reprinted with Permission.

Saskatoon Health Region Strategic Directions, Goals and Objectives for 2011-2012
May 6, 2011

- nephrology services available to patients in SHR
- Meet provincial target for numbers of assessed hospital patients awaiting LTC transfer
- Enhance capacity to respond to surges in demand for clinical care
- Implement priority projects related to SCH redevelopment

Eliminate harm and avoidable deaths:

- Enhance medication safety
- Implement *SHN!* Falls Prevention bundle in 100% of LTC facilities
- Continue implementation of surgical site infection bundle
- Improve communication among care providers and with patients and clients at all points of care provision transfer
- Implement IHI global trigger tool in acute care to inform focus for quality and safety improvements

Collaborate with communities and governments to reduce disparities in health status:

- Finalize the Health Care Equity Audit framework in the pilot areas of Public Health (immunization), Chronic Disease Management (diabetes care), and Psychiatry (suicide attempt)

Begin implementation of the Aboriginal Health strategy:

- Support the Provincial MOU on First Nations Health and Well-being process by ensuring alignment of our SHR initiatives with the intent of the MOU
- Establish and engage the Aboriginal Health Council in providing guidance on building a representative workforce, planning the Children's Hospital and developing a culturally safe and competent environment

implementing SHR plan to reduce overtime

Promote teamwork and interprofessional practice:

- Complete rollout of Releasing Time to Care on all medical and surgical wards
- Begin to introduce The Productive Operating Theatre (TPOT) in at least one operating theatres Develop and begin implementation of strategy and program for physician engagement and physician and dyad leadership development

Develop a diverse workforce, ensuring enhanced representation from First Nations and Métis populations:

- Implement the Awaken the Power of Change: 2010-14 Representative Workforce Action Plan

- Watrous/Manitou Lodge redevelopment
- Parkridge remediation
- Major VFA improvements
- SPH Surgery renovation)
- Plan for Children's Hospital
- Plan for new MRI and service delivery/research PET
- Further develop electronic health record Implement voice recognition for dictation
- Implement bed management system

Foster research, learning and innovation:

- Implement Saskatoon Centre for Patient-oriented Research
- Develop capacity in health systems research and program evaluation

Measure and report performance, benchmarking with high performing health systems and other industries:

- Develop and communicate portfolio-specific annual plans and balanced scorecards

Figure 13-1b Continued

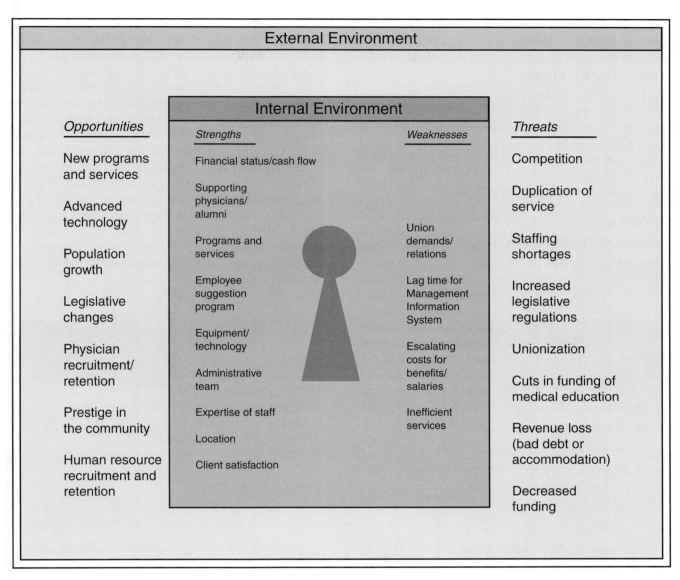

Figure 13-2 Key to Success in Strategic Planning: SWOT Analysis

various stakeholders and areas of expertise, the panel is expected to be able to identify potential concerns and provide sound guidance for the program.

REVIEW OF LITERATURE RELATED TO IDENTIFIED PROGRAMS

A review of the literature should be completed prior to strategic planning or beginning any new project or program. This review will allow the project team to identify similar programs, their structures and organization, potential problems and pitfalls, and successes. Referring to the case described in the Johnson interview, it was helpful, prior to designing the program, to have an understanding of the methods and strategies identified in the literature as effective when working with children and educators. Reviewing the literature is an ongoing process. As programs are tentatively identified, the

literature is searched for best practices and best evidence on how to conduct a program; then the program ideas are refined.

RELATIONSHIP OF STRATEGIC PLANNING TO THE ORGANIZATION'S MISSION

All strategic planning and goals and objectives must be examined with an eye to the purpose or mission of the organization. Organizations can get into trouble when they move too far from their core mission. Consequently, each new project needs to be evaluated in light of its congruence with the main mission that has been identified. It is fine for an organization to move to another project, but only if the new project is in line with the mission.

Otherwise, the new programs risk draining energy from the main focus of the mission.

PLANNING GOALS AND OBJECTIVES

After all strategic goals and objectives have been identified, they need to be prioritized according to strategic importance, resources required, and time and effort involved. A timeline should be set to allow a thoughtful evaluation of each goal and objective and the degree to which each can be implemented in the specified time frame and with the available resources. To avoid misunderstandings and unmet expectations, this timeline and its goals and objectives should be communicated to all stakeholders.

DEVELOPING A MARKETING PLAN

When the strategic planning process involves new programming for external audiences, and even if only an internal redesign or restructuring is involved, the strategic plan and the goals and objectives will need to be communicated to all involved constituencies. Such communication will be needed, for example, when an institution is planning to implement a new information system to ensure that it meets provincial government expectations for reporting data. Designing, implementing, training, and evaluating this new system will require substantive changes in both work flow and in the way that employees carry out their day-to-day work. If adequate thought has not been given to communication across the organization about the project, the chance of success is less and the risk of poor cooperation is greater. See Table 13-1 for a summary of the steps involved in strategic planning. See Table 13-2 for an illustration of aligning the balanced scorecard with typical strategic directions.

TABLE 13-1	SUMMARY OF STEPS IN STRATEGIC PLANNING

1. Perform an environmental assessment.
2. Conduct a stakeholder analysis.
3. Review the literature for evidence and best practices.
4. Determine congruence with the organizational mission.
5. Identify planning goals and objectives.
6. Estimate resources required for the plan.
7. Prioritize according to available resources.
8. Identify timelines and responsibilities.
9. Develop a communication plan.
10. Write and communicate the business or strategic plan.
11. Evaluate.

TABLE 13-2	ALIGNING THE BALANCED SCORECARD WITH TYPICAL STRATEGIC DIRECTIONS

Balanced Scorecard	Typical Strategic Directions
Clinical Utilization and Outcomes	Quality Patient Care/Improvement
Financial Performance and Condition	Organizational Effectiveness
Patient Satisfaction	Patient and Family Focused Care
System Integration and Change	Partnerships, Collaboration and Integration

Source: Brun, L. (2003). The Dos and Don'ts of Strategic Planning. *Healthcare Management Forum,* 16(4): 37–38. Reprinted with Permission.

LITERATURE APPLICATION

Citation: Young, J., Bell, R., Khalfan, A., & Lindquist, E. (2008). Evaluating the balanced scorecard at the University Health Network: An impact assessment. *Healthcare Quarterly*, 11(2): 52–56.

Discussion: The University Health Network implemented a new Balanced Scorecard approximately one year prior to its evaluation. The development, rollout and management methodology was based on the principles of Kaplan and Norton's strategy-focused organization principles. The purpose of the study was to determine the extent to which the scorecard had focused and aligned the various organizational units and departments around shared goals and objections. It was also planned to assess the scorecard's impact on frontline staff, and how it should be modified in the next stage. A survey, interviews and focus groups were used to evaluate the results.

Implications for Practice: Although UHN was found to be on the right track, it needed to provide frontline management with the tools and expertise they need to feel comfortable discussing scorecard issues with their staff. Many staff with UHN believe there has been insufficient dialogue. Eighteen recommendations, developed from the four evaluation methods, were grouped according to four themes: education, communication, process, and balanced scorecard revisions. They were designed to increase staff engagement, understanding, and buy-in.

ORGANIZATIONAL PURPOSE, MISSION, PHILOSOPHY, VALUES

Every organization has a purpose and a guiding philosophy. Most often, the purpose and philosophy are explicitly stated and detailed in a formal mission statement. Typically, this mission statement reflects the organization's values and indicates the behaviour and strategic actions that can be expected from that organization. The mission statements of most health care organizations relate to providing high quality or excellence in client care. Some mission statements focus exclusively on providing care, whereas others assume a broader view and

consider the education of health care professionals and the promotion of research as contributing to a broader mission. The mission of other organizations may be community-based, and these organizations consequently will focus on providing community outreach and population-based services to a specific community or population within a community.

MISSION STATEMENT

The **mission statement** is a formal expression of the purpose or reason for the existence of the organization or a department within it. It declares the organization's primary driving force, or its vision of the manner in which it believes care should be delivered. (For examples of actual mission statements, refer to Exploring the Web, p. 288–289)

Covey (1990) states, "An organizational mission statement—one that truly reflects the shared vision and values of everyone within that organization—creates a unity and tremendous commitment" (p. 139). For the unit mission statement to have the greatest effect, all members of the unit work team should participate in its development.

Questions to be answered by the group charged with development of the unit mission include the following:

- What do we stand for?
- What principles or values are we willing to defend?
- Whom are we here to help?

There are three criteria for a unit mission statement:

- A mission statement is no longer than a couple of sentences.
- It states the unit's purpose using action words.
- It should be simple and from the heart. (Jones, 1996)

Mission statements are so broad that units often adopt the organization's mission statement.

PHILOSOPHY

The **philosophy of an organization** is typically embedded in the mission statement. In essence, it contains a value statement of the principles and beliefs that direct the organization's behaviour. A careful reading of the mission statement will usually provide a good understanding of the institutional philosophy or value system. Mission statements with phrases such as *with respect for the dignity of each elderly resident, a brighter future for all children,* or *vigorous rehabilitation to maximize each individual's utmost potential* provide clues to the type of service that one can expect from that organization. In the best of worlds, the behaviours of the organization are consistent with its stated mission, philosophy, and values.

From a unit perspective, the core beliefs may be complex, such as those expressed in Table 13-3, or they can be short statements developed from a staff

TABLE 13-3	CORE BELIEFS

- Quality exists where shared purpose, vision, values, and partnerships are lived.
- Each person has the right to health care, which promotes wholeness in body, mind, and spirit.
- Each person is accountable to communicate and integrate his/her contribution to health care.
- Partnerships are essential to plan, coordinate, integrate, and deliver health care across the continuum.
- Continuing to learn and think in different ways is essential to improve health.
- A healthy culture begins with each person and is enhanced through self-work, partnerships, and systems supports.

Source: From B. Wesorick, December 2000. *CPM Resource Center Mission and Core Beliefs.* Copyright © 2000, CPM Resource Center, an Elsevier Inc. business. All rights reserved. Used with permission.

brainstorming session, such as "client centred," "partnering," and "healing environment." A unit's core beliefs or values are then incorporated into the unit's mission and vision statements.

VISION

The **vision** of an organization provides a clear picture of what the future will look like for that organization. It usually defines the key results achieved and the goals that are still to be accomplished. It also describes the key behaviours that the organization needs to demonstrate to be successful. The boundaries of the organization will be clearly described.

The unit vision statement reflects the organization's vision. A unit vision statement exemplifies how the mission and vision of the unit will be actualized within the organization's mission and vision.

Following are four criteria of a vision:

1. It is written down.
2. It is written in present tense, using action words, as though it were already accomplished.

3. It covers a variety of activities and spans broad time frames.
4. It balances the needs of providers, clients, and the environment. This balance anchors the vision to reality. (Wesorick et al., 1997)

The surgical unit vision statement in Table 13-4 exemplifies the core values of the unit: client centred, partnering, healing environment, and knowledge. The written statement tells the reader the work of the unit, why it is done, how, and for what reasons. In short, it delineates how the unit fulfills its mission.

VALUES

Values describe the boundaries the organization will have while pursuing its vision. Both core values (i.e., those values that will not be compromised) and aspirational values (i.e., those values that are wished for) will be described.

In order to be meaningful, values must be described in clear behavioural terms and must be measurable.

TABLE 13-4	SURGICAL UNIT VISION STATEMENT

The work we do: Affects the outcomes that clients desire in their pursuit of wellness.

Why we do it: To provide a healing environment in which an individual's physical, mental, emotional, and spiritual well-being will be nurtured.

Who we are: Practising within partnering relationships that communicate respect while recognizing and valuing diversity.

How we do it: By committing to continued learning. Our knowledge fosters our growth; our mentoring nurtures our practice. (Roesch, 2000)

CRITICAL THINKING

Examine these two mission statements and then respond to the questions that follow.

Hospital A: "Our mission is to improve the health and well-being of our community and provide quality health care, through cooperation with our partners—the community, providers, educators, and researchers. We will create a supportive team environment for clients, employees, and clinical staff. We will create and maintain an integrated, accessible, and affordable health system, with excellence as our constant goal."

Hospital B: "We are a Catholic health care community that respects the sacredness of all aspects of life. Inspired by the healing ministry of Jesus Christ, our staff, physicians, and volunteers are dedicated to service and to the support of one another. In this environment of service, support, and respect, we meet the physical, emotional, social, and spiritual needs of those served through compassionate care, teaching, and research."

Which of these institutions do you think would be more likely to organize a client lecture series on living with diabetes? Value the contributions of nursing? Provide experimental therapy for cancer? Be open to scheduling routine, client care visits for preadmission orientation?

LITERATURE APPLICATION

Citation: Iron, K. (2006). ICES Report: Health Data in Ontario: Taking Stock and Moving Ahead. *Healthcare Quarterly*, 9(3): 24–26.

Discussion: Policymakers, planners, administrators, and the public are able to see how well the health care system is performing by evaluating the information provided to them in balanced scorecards. Many system characteristics and data sources must be used to present a complete picture. Ontario has been a leader in reporting in many clinical areas, such as surgical procedures, cardiac care, and the use of drugs for the elderly. However, other key areas, such as chronic disease management and preventive care, cannot be fully evaluated because the relevant data are either of poor quality or unavailable. This article describes how health information could be improved in Ontario, and the types of data that are required. One of the primary recommendations is to create a centralized and dedicated health information agency in order to have a real-time health service and clinical information system, vital for improving the health of Ontarians.

Implications for Practice: The importance of accurate collection, interpretation, and dissemination of data cannot be overemphasized. Although great strides have been made, the ability to measure how the health system works is necessary to understand and improve client outcomes and system efficiency.

Sometimes an organization's values are formally stated and explicit, as in a mission statement. At other times the values are implicit and become part of the organizational culture. It is always important to assess an organization's values, as depicted in its mission statement, prior to considering employment; when important individual and organizational values collide, the result will likely be a constant source of frustration for both the employee and employer.

ORGANIZATIONAL STRUCTURE

Organizations are structured or organized to facilitate the execution of their mission, strategic plans, reporting lines, and communication within the organization. This need for structure applies to both entire organizations as well as individual nursing units. Organizational structures can be described in a number of ways by identifying their selected characteristics, which tend to exist on a continuum. For example, under the category of type or level of authority in an organizational structure, a highly bureaucratic, highly authoritarian structure is at one end of the continuum and a highly democratic, participative structure is at the other end. The highly authoritarian model is well suited for the purposes of the military, where it is seen most often. When decisions need to be made quickly, with clarity and not with challenges or discussion, as in a battle situation, a highly authoritarian organizational structure works well.

An example at the other end of the continuum would be a multidisciplinary group of professionals meeting to determine the care management of a client or client population. This group might be a hospice team task force made up of nurses, social workers, physicians, home care personal support workers, bereavement specialists, and chaplains, all meeting to discuss the care planning for a dying client. In this situation, team members of each discipline need to be able to freely contribute according to their particular area of knowledge and expertise. This type of organizational structure can function successfully only in a participative, democratic manner.

TYPES OF ORGANIZATIONAL STRUCTURES

Although a poor structure makes a high performance impossible, the best structure in the world will not ensure good performance (Drucker, 1973).

Most often, the existing organizational structures are communicated by means of an organizational chart. Figure 13-3 is an example of an organizational chart for a large acute care general hospital system. This organization has a tall bureaucratic structure with many layers in the hierarchy, or chain of command, and a centralized formal authority in the board of trustees. It represents a formal, top-down reporting structure.

MATRIX STRUCTURE

Because of the greater complexity of today's health care system, more organizations are using matrix structures. Figure 13-4 shows a matrix design (Shortell & Kaluzny, 2000).

FLAT VERSUS TALL STRUCTURE

Organizations are considered flat when there are few layers in the reporting structure. A tall organization would have many layers in the chain of command. An example of a flat organizational structure is a school of nursing that has no departments and many faculty members report to one dean of nursing.

DECENTRALIZED VERSUS CENTRALIZED STRUCTURE

The terms *centralized* and *decentralized* refer to the degree to which an organization has spread its lines of authority, power, and communication. A tall, bureaucratic design like the one depicted in Figure 13-3 would be considered highly centralized. A matrix design like the one in Figure 13-4 would be on the decentralized end of the continuum. As can be seen in Figure 13-4, the nursing manager can interface with the Alzheimer's disease program manager without going through a central, hierarchical core, as would happen in a bureaucratic structure like that in Figure 13-3.

Other characteristics or attributes can be used to assess organizations. Many typologies exist that may be used for this purpose. For example, Shortell and Kaluzny (2000)

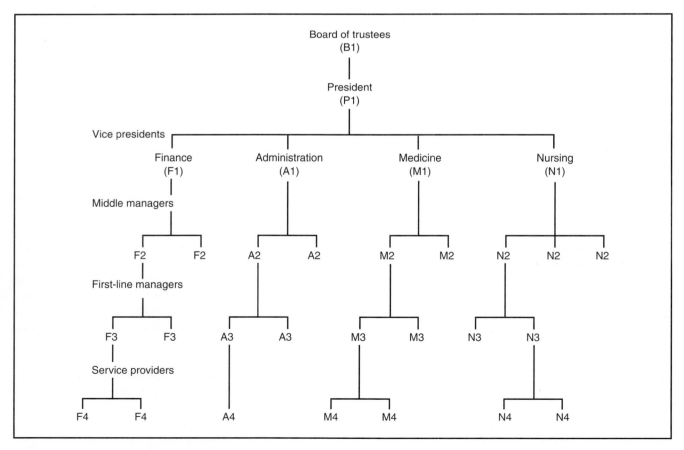

Figure 13-3 Organizational Chart, Formal Authority Structure: Acute Care General Hospital

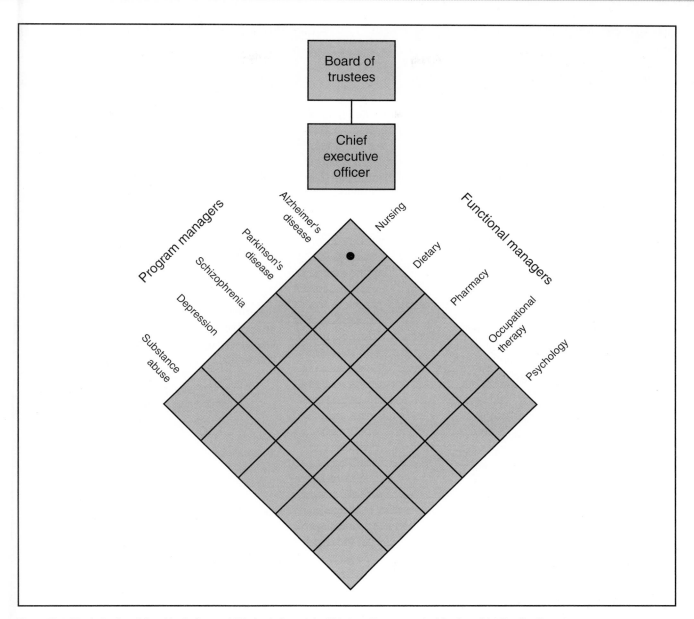

Figure 13-4 Matrix Design: A Psychiatric Centre. A Worker is Part of the Alzheimer Program and a Member of the Nursing Department

suggest using external environment, mission and goals, work groups and work design, organizational design, inter-organizational relationships, change and innovation, and strategic issues. Refer to Table 13-4 for an example of how these attributes can be assessed in four different health service organizations (Shortell & Kaluzny, 2000).

DIVISION OF LABOUR

The way the labour force is divided or organized has an effect on how the mission is accomplished. The functional organizational chart in Figure 13-5 graphically depicts how the formal authority in this organization is structured (Shortell & Kaluzny, 2000). At the highest level, the board of trustees delegates authority to the

chief executive officer, who delegates to the vice presidents, and so on. At the vice presidential level, there are five department directors for each branch. The department directors each report to their respective vice president. The nurse managers report to their department director of nursing. The charge nurse reports to the nurse manager of her unit. The treatment nurse and the medication nurse report to the charge nurse. In this functional design, the division of labour is efficient and specialized. A danger with a functional division of labour is that individuals may be so focused on their own specific area that they have little perspective on the overall picture. For example, a treatment nurse may focus on treatments and have little information about the total client.

TABLE 13-5		TYPOLOGY OF FOUR HEALTH SERVICES ORGANIZATIONS		

Attribute	Regional Health Authorities	Home Health Care Agencies	Hospitals	Pharmaceutical Companies
External environment	Complex High change Highly integrated	Relatively simple Moderate change Increasingly competitive	Complex High change	Moderate complexity Moderate change Highly competitive
Mission and goals	Acute and primary care emphasis; keep people well	Quality of life Maintaining functional status	Acute care emphasis; curing illness	Research and development (R&D) emphasis; new product development
Work group and work design	Program and cross-program teams; high need for coordination Coordination of care across continuum	Simple design; primarily one-on-one client contact	Departmental and cross-departmental teams; high need for coordination	Separation of functions possible; R&D versus sales; relatively low need for coordination
Organization design	Functional, divisional, and matrix, integrating primary care physicians, specialists, and all professions	Functional	Divisional and matrix	Divisional and strategic business units
Inter-organizational relationships	Vertically and horizontally integrated health system	Expand client base and gain economies of scale	Key to becoming part of vertically integrated health systems	Important for global expansion
Change and innovation	Respond to and create new client-focused and organization-focused care management approaches	Respond to demographic and social changes	Respond to the new paradigm; implement new roles within vertically integrated systems	Respond to new product development demands
Strategic issues	Fit into an expanded and changing health care delivery system	Demonstrate continuing value and, therefore, reimbursement for services	Fit into an expanded and changing delivery system	Decrease time to develop new drugs

In the matrix structure shown in Figure 13-4, the structure was less important; and the workforce roles and reporting relationships were based on the project or task to be accomplished, rather than on a rigid hierarchy. An example of a matrix structure is the planning involved in the preparation for an Accreditation Canada review. The organization teams could be composed of various individuals at varying levels of responsibility and from programs across the organization, but they could interact with staff at all levels and report

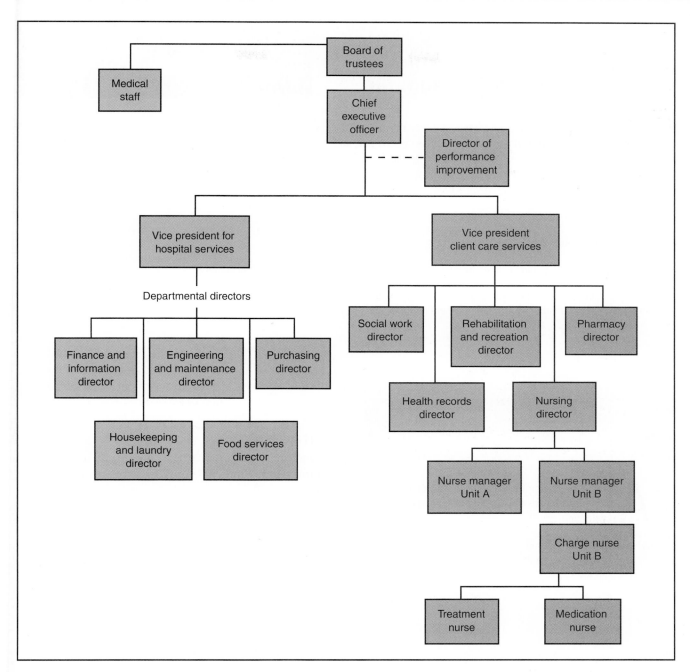

Figure 13-5 A Functional Design: Nursing Home

as a task force for the purposes of the accreditation survey.

ROLES AND RESPONSIBILITIES

Note that exact roles and responsibilities within each level and division are not defined on the organizational charts beyond specifying the given division, for example, nursing. The scope of responsibilities, specific duties, and specific job requirements are provided in documents such as individual job or position descriptions.

REPORTING RELATIONSHIPS

An organizational chart, such as the one in Figure 13-5, shows the formal reporting relationships, depicted with a solid line. Sometimes dotted lines are used in an organizational chart to indicate dual or secondary reporting relationships. An example of such a relationship might be the role of the director of quality improvement, who not only reports directly to the chief executive officer but also has position accountabilities to the board of trustees. The formal reporting relationships may or may not reflect the actual communications that occur within the institution.

CASE STUDY 13-1

A client presented to the emergency department with complaints of nausea, vomiting, and diarrhea over three hours. The triage nurse determined that the client was of low-risk, and referred him to the "fast track," an area that was completely staffed by licensed practical nurses. When a licensed practical nurse assumed the care of the client, she noticed that his vomitus was becoming blood tinged, and she contacted the physician. The client's condition progressively worsened, and he was eventually admitted to the intensive care unit.

What could have been done differently?

Was anyone at fault? Who?

Why is good communication especially important when there is a functional division of labour?

What types of problems could you expect if staff members focused on their own tasks and failed to communicate with each other about the client's emotional, psychosocial, educational, and discharge needs?

CRITICAL THINKING

A number of studies have demonstrated that primary nursing leads to improved client and nurse satisfaction.

Why do you think this might be? Can you think of any disadvantages to a primary nursing care model for organizing care?

DIVISION OF LABOUR BY GEOGRAPHIC AREA

Care delivery can be efficiently divided according to geography or location. Such a division of labour might consist of the hospital and ambulatory care or, at smaller unit levels, the north team and the west team. Frequently, care provided by home health agencies is divided by geographic district for travel efficiencies. At the health care system level, geographical division could mean that each major area, such as the hospital and the supporting ambulatory clinics (located two blocks away), would have separate supporting services, such as two pharmacies, one in the ambulatory clinic and one in the hospital. Both ambulatory clinic and inpatient areas could, and often do, have separate health records departments. An

obvious concern in such arrangements is lack of coordination and duplication of services.

DIVISION OF LABOUR BY PROGRAM

Sometimes, care delivery is organized around programs. A division of labour by program is a type of functional division of work, but is based on a client's diagnosis or the specialty care required by a client. For example, care delivery might be divided into a cardiology program, a woman's health program, and an oncology program. Division of labour by program can lead to improved quality of care and decreased confusion for the client because the information and protocols used in the outpatient area would be consistent with the information and protocols used in the hospital and across the entire health care system. Figure 13-6 demonstrates a program design (Shortell & Kaluzny, 2000).

PRIMARY NURSING

Primary nursing care describes a model of care in which one nurse is primarily responsible for all aspects of client care for a given client or clients. The client is assigned a primary nurse upon admission, and, when possible, that nurse will be the client's primary caregiver throughout the hospitalization. In this model, an associate nurse is usually assigned to assume care responsibilities when the primary nurse is not available.

Many factors affect strategic planning, such as highlighted by the SWOT analysis discussed in this chapter (page 267). Nurses need to prepare to address these many factors.

Figure 13-6 Program Design

CRITICAL THINKING

You have been asked to take a leadership role in identifying potential concurrent disorder programs that could be implemented in the community-based mental health centre where you work as a community health nurse. You normally report to the mental health manager, but for this project you are designated as the coordinator of concurrent disorder programs. As you begin your assessment of potential programs, you will need to interact with a number of functional departments across the organization, such as dietary, pharmacy, occupational therapy, and psychology. In addition, you will have to examine the other mental health programs to ensure you are not duplicating services.

Given this situation, what would be some advantages of working in an institution that had a matrix design such as the one depicted in Figure 13-4? What might be the disadvantages?

THE STRUCTURE OF PROFESSIONAL PRACTICE

In an organization that values professional nursing practice, strategic initiatives are most effectively developed and implemented through a structure of shared governance and shared decision making between management and clinicians.

SHARED GOVERNANCE

Shared governance is an organizational framework grounded in a philosophy of decentralized leadership that fosters autonomous decision making and professional nursing practice (Porter-O'Grady, 1992). Shared governance, by its name, implies the allocation of control, power, or authority (i.e., governance) among mutually (i.e., shared) interested vested parties (Stichler, 1992). In most health care settings, the vested parties in nursing fall into two distinct categories: (1) nurses practising direct client care, such as staff nurses; and (2) nurses managing or administering the provision of that care, such as managers. In shared governance, a nursing organization's management assumes the responsibility for organizational structure and resources. Management relinquishes control over issues related to clinical practice. In return, staff nurses accept the responsibility and accountability for their professional practice.

The most successful unit-based shared governance occurs when an organization-wide structure of shared governance is in place and unit-based functions can articulate with this structure. Organizational shared governance structures are usually council models that have evolved from pre-existing nursing or institutional committees. In a council structure, clearly defined accountabilities for specific elements of professional practice have been delegated to five main arenas: clinical practice, quality, education, research, and management of resources (Porter-O'Grady, 1992). Figure 13-7 illustrates a shared governance model.

CLINICAL PRACTICE COUNCIL

The purpose of the clinical practice council is to establish the practice standards for the work group. Often, this council or committee is a unit-level committee that works in conjunction with the organizational committee that is accountable for determining policy and procedures related to clinical practice. Initiatives that foster an evidence-based practice based on research ensure the development of practice standards based on current science of clinical practice, not merely tradition.

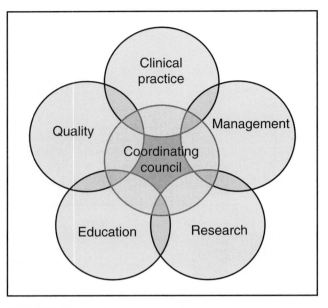

Figure 13-7 A Shared Governance Model

QUALITY COUNCIL

The purpose of the quality council is twofold: (1) to credential staff and (2) to oversee the unit's quality management initiatives. In the role of credentialing staff, this committee is responsible for interviewing potential staff and reviewing their qualifications, or credentials. It then makes recommendations regarding hiring. The quality committee also serves as the body that reviews staff credentials on an ongoing basis and makes recommendations regarding promotion. Quality management initiatives for which the council is responsible can include review of indicators of the unit's overall clinical performance, such as medication errors, client falls, family satisfaction, and response time in answering call lights. At times, a unit will also participate in an organizational disease management study by looking at the care of a specific client population, such as clients with diabetes.

EDUCATION COUNCIL

The purpose of the education council is to assess the learning needs of the unit staff and develop and implement programs to meet these needs. This council usually works closely with organizational education and training departments. Unit orientation programs and training programs related to new clinical techniques and new equipment are examples of programs sponsored by the education council.

RESEARCH COUNCIL

At the unit level, the research council advances the use of research for the purpose of incorporating research-based findings into the clinical standards of unit practice. In the process of research utilization, staff critique available

REAL WORLD INTERVIEW

As an administrator, it is imperative that I consider the needs of the staff when planning for the Nursing Practice Council. Although I have a vision of the roles and responsibilities of this council, it is important that the staff share this vision, or create one of their own that is congruent with the mission of the organization. Staff represented on the Nursing Practice Council include those providing direct client care, nurse educators and clinical nurse specialists, nursing managers, and directors of nursing. To provide this opportunity to the staff, we held a two-day facilitated retreat offsite to formulate and, subsequently, articulate the mission, vision, and values of the Nursing Division within the Health Sciences Centre, and to articulate goals and objectives for the next two years.

Dorothy Johnson, PhD, MSN
Chief Nursing Officer, Health Sciences Centre

REAL WORLD INTERVIEW

We plan every year, but I'd say we look at our unit philosophy based on our core values and re-evaluate the strategic plan every two to three years. We had three core values that guided us, and then this year, with all the external pressures, we added a fourth. We keep these core values in the forefront when we do our annual planning. The process we used to develop and re-evaluate the core values was really very powerful and staff driven.

SPAN—Staff Planning Action Network—is our unit-based shared governance organization. SPAN met and developed draft mission and vision statements from our philosophy, which is based on our current core values—a client-centred, partnering, and healing environment. They then transcribed these draft statements onto three flip charts and for 15 minutes per shift circulated these terms throughout the unit and got staff's reaction and feedback to the statements. Revisions were made from the feedback received. These revisions were then presented at a staff meeting. What was emerging from the feedback was a focus on the need for continuing education and training related to the rapidly changing environment. So we added a fourth value—knowledge.

Our unit philosophy, stemming from our core values, is what we believe in. We've expanded these core values into a vision statement that demonstrates what it is to practice on this unit.

Pat Roesch, BSN, RN
First-Line Unit Manager

research literature and then make recommendations to the practice council. In this way clinical policies and procedures can be based on evidence-based research findings. The research council may also coordinate research projects if advanced practice nurses are employed at the institution.

MANAGEMENT COUNCIL

The purpose of the management council is to ensure that the standards of practice and governance agreed upon by unit staff are upheld and that adequate resources are

available to deliver client care. The first-line unit manager is a standing member of this council. Other members include the assistant nurse managers and the charge or resource nurses from each shift.

COORDINATING COUNCIL

Shared governance structures also include a coordinating council, whose purpose is to facilitate and integrate the activities of the other councils. This council is usually composed of the first-line unit manager and the chairpersons of the other councils. This council usually

LITERATURE APPLICATION

Citation: Jeffs, L., Merkley, J., Jeffrey, J., Ferris, E., Dusek, J., & Hunter, C. (2006). Case study: Reconciling the quality and safety gap through strategic planning. *Canadian Journal of Nursing Leadership*, 19(2): 32–40.

Discussion: An essential outcome of professional practice environments is the provision of high-quality, safe nursing care. To mitigate the gap between quality and safety, nursing leadership at St. Michael's Hospital in Toronto undertook a strategic plan to enhance the environment of nursing professional practice. This case study outlines the development of the strategic planning process.

Implications for Practice: The nursing strategic plan is an essential step towards the transformational change required to support any organization's vision that provides for safe, quality health care. Leadership is required at all levels of the nursing division, and a change-management approach is necessary. The aim is to transform practice settings.

facilitates the annual review of the unit mission and vision and develops the annual operational plan (Sellers, 1996).

Unit-based shared governance structures may be less diverse. Often, some of the councils are combined into one council, for example, education and research. Or a council may contain subcommittees whose purposes are to perform very specific tasks, for example, to credential and promote staff or to recruit and retain staff. Unit-based structures are varied, with the primary purpose being to empower staff by fostering professional practice while meeting the needs of the work unit.

ENSURING COMPETENCY AND PROFESSIONAL STAFF DEVELOPMENT

Professional practice through the vehicle of shared governance requires competent staff. Competency is defined as possession of the required skill, knowledge, qualification, or capacity (Webster's Encyclopedic Unabridged Dictionary, 1996) and is best determined in practice by a group of one's peers. Alspach (1984) defines competency as a determination of an individual's capability to perform to defined expectations (p. 656). Competency of professional staff can be

ensured through credentialing processes developed around a clinical or career ladder staff promotion framework. A **clinical ladder** acknowledges that staff members have varying skill sets based on their education and experience. As such, depending on skills and experience, staff members may be rewarded differently and carry differing responsibilities for client care and the governance and professional practice of the work unit.

CRITICAL THINKING

As a nurse practising in a shared governance organization, you remember a decade ago when the organization decentralized, made a commitment to nursing professional practice, and implemented shared governance. Everywhere you went, people were talking about it and displaying posters and other signs of nursing's importance to the organization. That was years ago, before managed care and all its changes and before this latest nursing shortage. Now you do not hear people talking about it so much. You wonder, Does professional practice still exist? How can you tell? How does your organization compare with other organizations that do not have shared governance? Is it possible that professional practice has become the culture and so there is no need to talk about it anymore?

BENNER'S NOVICE TO EXPERT

Benner's (1984) model of novice to expert provides a framework that, when developed into a clinical or career promotion ladder, facilitates professional staff development by building on the skill sets and experience of each practitioner. Benner's model acknowledges that practitioners can be expected to have acquired tasks, competencies, and outcomes that are based on five levels of experience.

Benner's model of novice to expert is based on the Dreyfus and Dreyfus (1980) model of skill acquisition applied to nursing. Benner's model has five stages: novice, advanced beginner, competent, proficient, and expert. Novice nurses are recognized as being task-oriented and focused. After they have mastered most tasks required to perform their ascribed roles, they move on to the phase of advanced beginner. The nurse who can demonstrate marginally acceptable independent performance illustrates the advanced beginner.

CASE STUDY 13-2

You are a competent nurse who is a member of the credentialing committee of the quality council. A fellow peer has presented his credentials for review in hopes of being promoted to the next level on the clinical ladder. You review the packet and make the recommendation that he be promoted. However, at the credentialing committee meeting, you learn that the first-line unit manager and the individual's preceptor, another member of the committee, have not recommended promotion.

You wonder whether your colleague is aware of concerns about his performance.

Are there guidelines and standards that you are not aware of that have not been met?

What is the next course of action for the committee?

What should your response be at this meeting?

REAL WORLD INTERVIEW

There are five levels to our clinical ladder, which is similar to Benner's novice to expert model. The RN Is, or novices, are the new graduates and people in orientation. The experts are the clinical specialists. A lot of them have also become nurse practitioners so that the organization can receive some reimbursement for their client care services. This is a good thing because, otherwise, I'm afraid we wouldn't have these expert nurses anymore. They are the true mentors for nursing staff, especially when you are working with a very complex or difficult client situation.

Staff nurses also mentor each other. During orientation, your preceptor guides you along the path from RN I to RN II. When you decide you'd like to advance to RN III, you can choose another mentor. RN IIIs provide much more clinical leadership for staff and for the overall unit. I decided I was ready to be promoted to that level when other staff consistently were coming to me for clinical guidance and with client care questions. Now, as an RN III, I am the chairperson of our unit-credentialing committee, which is part of the quality council of our shared governance model.

Our clinical ladder uses a portfolio as the main tool to evaluate the nurse's readiness to advance. When you are an RN I in orientation, you are first introduced to the idea of a portfolio and how to put it together. It is difficult at first, because people do not know what is expected. However, after that first time when you are promoted from an RN I to an RN II, it becomes easier. You just build on what is already in the portfolio.

A portfolio should include the following:

Registrations

Your résumé

Letters of reference

Evaluations

Examples of participation in development of the team plan of care

Exemplars

CEU certificates

(Continued)

Clinical documentation of client care	Presentations
Validations for competencies related to technical skills (medication administration, IV therapy)	Publications

The portfolio tells the story of your practice. When a group of people are ready for promotion, the members of the credentialing committee meet. We review the portfolios and make recommendations related to advancement. The nurse manager is a member of this committee. She always reviews the portfolio and gives us her feedback even if she is unable to attend the credentialing meeting. I enjoy reading the exemplars the best. Exemplars are mini-stories that paint the pictures of each nurse's practice, and they are all so different.

Stacey Conley, RN, BS
Staff Nurse

A competent nurse is one who has been in the same role for two to three years. These nurses have developed the ability to see their actions as part of the long-range goals set for their clients. The conscious, deliberative planning that is characteristic of this skill level helps achieve efficiency and organization.

Proficient nurses characteristically perceive situations as wholes rather than as series of tasks. They develop a plan of care and then guide the client from point A to point B. They draw on their past experiences and know that in a typical situation, a client must exhibit specific behaviours to meet specific goals. They realize that if those behaviours are not demonstrated within a certain time frame, then the plan needs to be changed.

The experts are those nurses who intuitively know what is going on with their clients. Their expertise is so embedded in their practice that they have been heard to say, "Something's wrong with this client. I'm not sure what's going on, but you had better come and evaluate this." Not heeding the call derived from the intuitive sense of an expert nurse has resulted in a client's cardiac arrest. These expert nurses often seek advanced education and become clinical specialists.

Although nurses don't participate in "credentialing" per se in Canada, the notion of career laddering exists. Perhaps learning can take place by examining some of the career laddering models in the United States. Exploration of one such model follows.

The Colorado Differentiated Nursing Practice Model (see Figure 13-8) builds on the work of Benner (1984) regarding career ladder stages. Stage I is characterized as the entry or learning stage. Stage II is characterized by

the individual who competently demonstrates acceptable performance while adapting to time and resource constraints. Stage III is characterized by the individual who is proficient. And stage IV is characterized by the individual who is an expert. The stages in this model are specifically defined by behaviours that are consistently exhibited or practised over a defined period of time.

THE PROCESS OF PROFESSIONAL PRACTICE

Ongoing professional staff development is part of the regular performance feedback that staff can expect from the first-line unit manager. The first-line unit manager also provides ongoing professional development of staff in their daily interactions on the unit, and identifies projects and activities that meet a staff member's readiness for leadership development and advancement.

SITUATIONAL LEADERSHIP

The leadership framework developed by Hersey and Blanchard (1993) can be combined with an individual's position on a clinical/career ladder to assist the first-line unit manager in discerning the best approach for developing the potential of staff members. **Situational leadership** maintains that there is no one best leadership style, but rather that effective leadership lies in matching the appropriate leadership style to the individual's or the group's level of task-relevant readiness. Readiness refers

Colorado Differentiated Practice Model

The Colorado Differentiated Practice Model for Nursing has a separate clinical ladder for the six preparatory backgrounds depicted on the conceptual model (Diagram 1). A nurse selects the education clinical ladder according to the nursing credential s/he has attained.

The framework for each educational ladder has four distinct stages. These stages allow nurses to self-pace their advancement. A nurse is placed in a stage according to his or her own competency and experience.

Each nursing ladder has four weighted components as follows:
- Competency Statements 60%
- Institutional Goals 15%
- Skills 10%
- Professional Activities 15%

Conceptual model

Sample ladder

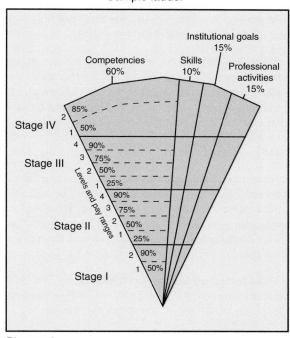

Diagram 1

Diagram 2

Figure 13-8 Colorado Differentiated Nursing Practice Model

Source: Courtesy of Marie E. Miller, Colorado Nursing Task Force.

to how able and motivated an individual is to perform a particular task. A basic assumption of situational leadership is that a leader should help followers grow in their readiness to perform new tasks as far as they are able and willing to go. This development of followers is accomplished by adjusting leadership behaviour through four styles along the leadership curve.

According to Hersey and Blanchard's (1993) model, individual followers with low task readiness, such as novice nurses, require a telling style on the part of the leader. They need to be told what to do and to be given strong direction if they are to be successful and productive. As these followers grow in readiness, the leader should shift to a selling style, with more positive reinforcement and socio-emotional support. Once individuals reach higher levels of readiness, as a proficient or expert nurse, the

leader should respond by decreasing control. The leader moves first to a participatory style characterized by a high degree of relationship with staff and a lower need to give task direction. Then, with expert staff, the leader moves to a style of delegating that involves communicating a sense of confidence and trust, because highly competent individuals respond best to greater freedom.

An individual's readiness to learn and accept new tasks may change for a variety of reasons. When first-line managers discern a change, they must readjust their style of interaction with the nurse—moving forward or backward through the leadership curve—to provide the appropriate level of support and direction to facilitate that individual's continued development, productivity, and success as a member of the client care team. The development of staff based on their innate readiness

REAL WORLD INTERVIEW

I have a particularly touching story to tell you. D.T. was a 44-year-old man who was admitted from our ear, nose, and throat clinic with a large mass at the base of his tongue. Upon arrival on the unit, the client appeared very anxious, not knowing what he would face in the next few days. The client and his wife had been told that he would have a tracheostomy placed, which was quite a shock to them. They were both feeling overwhelmed with the situation.

As it happened, I was present for every major event that occurred with this family during that admission. I can recall the day when the client was told that the mass was cancerous. He and his family were devastated. I went to talk with the family and proceeded to tell them I could not begin to imagine what they must be going through, but that if they needed to talk, I was a good listener. I could tell that they very much appreciated that.

During the next few days, the family began to accept what was going on, and we began working together to teach them all they needed to know about tracheostomies and how to care for them. D.T. and his wife learned quickly how to be independent with tracheostomy care. In the coming days, the client underwent a feeding tube placement so that he could get some nutrition. I taught him and his wife how to care for the feeding tube and how to hang tube feedings. They learned so quickly that toward the end of the hospital stay, they were doing all his care independently. The client was informed that he would need to undergo radiation and chemotherapy. In preparation for the treatment, the client needed to have a complete dental extraction. Considering all that D.T. and his wife went through in such a short time, they both responded quite well to the situation.

Upon discharge, I set the client up with Lifeline (an emergency response service), nursing services, and equipment for the tracheostomy and tube feedings. This was no easy task because they did not have much money and their insurance company was quite difficult to deal with. As their primary nurse, I spent days on the phone in preparation for their discharge. It was quite challenging but rewarding when all was accomplished. It was both a happy and a sad day when the client and his wife were discharged. Since the client has left, I have kept in touch through writing, and I've talked to him in person when he has been readmitted to the medical floor for his chemotherapy treatment. I am glad to report that thus far D.T. is doing well.

This was a particularly touching experience for me. This family was very special to me, and I am glad for the opportunity I had to get to know them and be a special part of their lives. As an unknown author has said, in the end, we will not remember the years we spent nursing, we will only remember the moments.

Stacey Conley, RN, BS
Staff Nurse

---

to accept new tasks and responsibilities facilitates their promotion along a continuum of novice to expert and ensures that a professional client care team is able to consistently deliver accountability-based client care.

ACCOUNTABILITY-BASED CARE DELIVERY

Accountability-based care is essential in today's value-driven workplace. Individuals who are accountable are, by definition, able to report, explain, or justify their actions (Webster's Encyclopedic Unabridged Dictionary, 1996). Accountability is about achieving outcomes and is the foundation for evaluation (Porter-O'Grady, 1995). The following care delivery systems are built on the tenet of accountability to the clients who are the receivers of nursing care. As such, they provide systems or processes of care that are congruent with professional practice.

MEASURABLE QUALITY OUTCOMES

An important component of management is regular evaluation of a unit's performance to ensure that the outcomes of care delivery are meeting the objectives of professional practice as outlined in the unit's annual operational plan. The development of process improvement measures in today's health care organizations is driven by the multiple domains of quality required by the Accreditation Canada (AC).

UNIT-BASED PERFORMANCE IMPROVEMENT

To develop a comprehensive unit-based continuous quality improvement program to meet the requirements

Y ou are a primary nurse working as part of the interprofessional orthopedic team. You notice that an increasing number of diabetic clients are being admitted for elective total hip surgery. Because the length of stay is so short and your team has such a surgical focus in caring for clients, the clients' underlying chronic diseases have not been a focus on the unit. However, you are aware that the larger organization is beginning to evaluate how different populations of clients, such as diabetics, are cared for across the continuum of care.

What should you do to improve care for your clients?

of today's health care system, the manager should track outcomes from four domains: access, service, cost, and clinical quality (G. Vasile, Cooperstown, NY, Bassett Healthcare, personal communication, August 16, 2000). See Figure 13-9 for the performance improvement plan.

Outcomes of unit continuous quality improvement programs can be succinctly displayed using the Quality Compass (Nelson, Mohr, Batalden, & Plume, 1996). The Bassett Quality Compass in Figure 13-10 measures quality from four domains: functional status, clinical outcomes, cost and utilization, and client (patient) satisfaction. This Quality Compass depicts the outcomes of an organization-wide disease management asthma study prior to an asthma disease management intervention. The Quality Compass tells us that functionally 30 percent of the population has moderately severe asthma and that the majority of asthmatics have had little documented teaching on the use of a peak flow metre or metred-dose inhalers (MDIs),

which is the current standard of care. More than 30 percent of the client visits for asthma are urgent visits. This indicates that a large portion of the asthma population would benefit from a disease management intervention that increases client teaching and develops individual, specific, asthma care plans. The Quality Compass provides a framework to guide the development of a unit-based quality improvement program, and it provides a tool with which to present the quality improvement outcomes in the succinct, visual format of an executive summary.

The manager is the fundamental operations person in the health care system. Successful orchestration of a client care unit in today's health care system is achieved through vision-driven professional practice. Implementing this vision is achieved through a unit governance structure of shared decision making, an accountability-based client care delivery system, and regular evaluation of performance based on the tenets of performance improvement.

INPATIENT SURGICAL UNIT

2000 PERFORMANCE IMPROVEMENT PLAN

As part of Bassett's commitment to quality, the Surgical Unit will strive to improve performance through a cycle of planning, process design, performance measurement, assessment and improvement. There will be ongoing assessment of important aspects of care and service and correction of identified problems. Problem identification and solution will be carried out using a systematic intra- and interdepartmental approach organized around patient flow or other key functions, and in concert with the approved visions and strategies of the organization. Priorities for improvement will include high risk, high volume and problem-prone procedures.

The Surgical Unit will:

• promote the Plan-Do-Check-Act methodology for all performance improvement activities
• provide staff education and training on integrated quality and cost improvement
• collect data to support objective assessment of processes and contribute to problem resolution

In identifying important aspects of care and service, the Surgical Unit will select performance measures in the following operational categories:

A. Clinical Quality
1. Patient safety

• Patient falls
• Indicator: # of patient falls per month/# of patient days with upper control limits set by the research department based on statistical deviation

• Medication and IV errors
• Indicator: # of patient IV/medication errors per month/# of patient days with upper control limits set by the research department based on statistical deviation

• Restraint use
• Indicator: % of compliance with policy for use of restraints and overall rate of restraint use

2. Pressure ulcer prevention
• Indicator: Rates of occurrence-quarterly tracking report

3. Surveillance, prevention, and control of infection
• Indicator: Infection control statistical report of wound and catheter associated infections
• Indicator: Quarterly monitoring of compliance with standards for Acid Fast Bacilli (AFB) room use; evidence of staff validation in AFB practice

4. Employee safety
• Injuries resulting from
• Back and lifting-related injuries
• Morbidly obese patients
• Orthopedic patients
• Indicators: # of injuries sustained by employees and any resultant workmen's compensation (Human Resources quarterly report)
• 100% competency validation in lifting techniques and back injury prevention
• Respiratory fit testing
• Indicator: competency record of each employee

5. Documentation by exception
Indicators:
• 100% validation of RN/LPN staff
• Monthly chart audit (10% average daily census or 20 charts) meeting compliance with established standards

B. Access:
• Maintenance of the 30 minute standard for bed assignment of ED admissions
• Indicator: Quarterly review of ED tracking record

C. Service:
Patient Satisfaction
Indicator: Patient Satisfaction Survey: 90% or above response to, "Would return," and "Would recommend"

D. Cost:
• Nursing staff productivity will remain at 110% of target of 8.5 worked hours per adjusted patient day within a maximum variance range of 10%

For each of the above performance measures, this performance improvement plan will:

• address the highest priority improvement issues
• require data collection according to the structure, procedure and frequency defined
• document a baseline for performance
• demonstrate internal comparisons trended over time
• demonstrate external benchmark comparisons trended over time
• document areas identified for improvement
• demonstrate that changes have been made to address improvement
• demonstrate evaluation of these changes; document that improvement has occurred or, if not, that a different approach has been taken to address the issue

The Inpatient Surgical Unit will submit biannual status reports to the Bassett Improvement Council (BIC) through the Medical Surgical Quality Improvement Council (MSQIC).

Approved by:_____Date:_____

(Chief or Vice President)

Figure 13-9 Performance Improvement Plan

Source: Courtesy of Patricia Roesch, BS, RN, Bassett Healthcare.

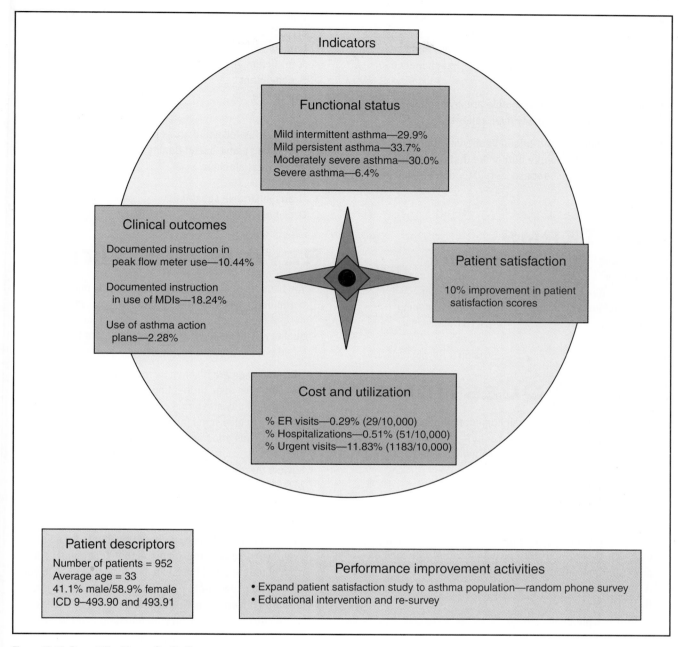

Figure 13-10 Bassett Healthcare Quality Compass

Source: Courtesy of Kathleen F. Sellers, PhD, RN, Bassett Healthcare.

KEY CONCEPTS

- Successful orchestration of a client care unit in today's health care environment is achieved through vision-driven professional practice.

- Strategic planning is a process designed to achieve goals in dynamic, competitive environments through the allocation of resources (Andrews, 1990).

- Shared governance is an organizational framework grounded in a philosophy of decentralized leadership that fosters autonomous decision making and professional nursing practice.

- A clinical or career promotional ladder provides a framework that facilitates professional staff development by building on the skill sets and experience of each practitioner.

- Situational leadership maintains that there is no one best leadership style, but rather that effective leadership lies in matching the appropriate leadership style to the level of task-relevant readiness of each individual or group.

- Individuals who are accountable are, by definition, able to report, explain, or justify their actions.

- A comprehensive unit-based quality improvement program should include outcomes that are tracked from four domains: access, service, cost, and clinical quality.

KEY TERMS

clinical ladder	stakeholder
focus groups	stakeholder assessment
mission statement	strategic plan
philosophy of an organization	strategic planning
reengineering	SWOT analysis
shared governance	values
situational leadership	vision

REVIEW QUESTIONS

1. Which of the following is a document that describes the institution's purpose and philosophy?
   A. the organizational chain of command
   B. the organizational chart
   C. the mission statement
   D. the strategic plan

2. Which of the following is the outcome of the processes by which an organization engages in environmental analysis, goal formulation, and strategy development with the purpose of organizational growth and renewal?
   A. stakeholder assessment
   B. SWOT analysis
   C. strategic planning
   D. mission development

3. Which of the following is contained in an organizational chart for the most formal and hierarchical organizational structure?
   A. a matrix design
   B. many layers of command
   C. a program design
   D. a number of dotted lines representing reporting relationships

4. Which of the following describes shared governance?
   A. an accountability-based care delivery system
   B. a tested framework of organizational development
   C. a competency-based career promotion system
   D. the allocation of control, power, or authority (i.e., governance) among interested parties

5. Which of the following is *not* one of the five levels of a clinical promotion ladder built on Benner's theoretical framework?
   A. proficient
   B. competent
   C. orientee
   D. expert

6. Which of the following areas is *not* considered when developing a unit-based Quality Compass?
   A. client satisfaction
   B. cost
   C. administrative satisfaction
   D. clinical outcomes

REVIEW ACTIVITIES

1. You have been asked by your first-line unit manager to participate in a performance improvement team looking at care of the diabetic client. What areas other than clinical quality will you evaluate? Identify indicators for each area to measure. What are you seeking to improve?

2. You have been practising now for three years. This summer you have been precepting a new graduate who is having difficulty mastering changing a sterile dressing. You need to give some feedback, but you are uncertain how to do this effectively and wonder whether you are part of the reason this new graduate is having difficulty. Review the section on situational leadership (pages 282–283). At what level of readiness is this new graduate? Has your leadership style been appropriate for that level of experience and motivation?

3. You have been practising as a new graduate for a little over a year. You are feeling more confident about your clinical practice and think you might want to expand your leadership experience. Your unit governance framework is shared governance. Review the common councils of shared governance. Given your education and experience, which council would you like to join?

EXPLORING THE WEB

- Upon completion of your nursing degree, you are planning to interview for a position at an area hospital. In preparation for your interview, you want to understand the hospital's mission and other information, all of which is readily available on the web. For example, if you are planning to apply at Alberta Health Services (*http://www.albertahealthservices.ca/*), go to *http://www.albertahealthservices.ca/careers.asp*. The exact address of the mission statement of the health system is available at *http://www.albertahealthservices.ca/190.asp*.

- Another example is the Hospital for Sick Children in Toronto at *http://www.sickkids.ca/*. The exact web address of the mission statement is *http://www.sickkids.ca/AboutSickKids/who-we-are/Vision-Mission-Values/index.html*.

- Look at these web pages, paying particular attention to the descriptions they provide of the organizations' missions. What impressions do you form about these organizations and their missions? Does the stated mission seem to fit with the general impression you get from the website? Could you easily find information about positions available? About the institution? Try this exercise with your local hospital or medical centre.

- Look at the following websites for examples of strategic plans and the approach used to create the plan.

- *http://www.saskatoonhealthregion.ca/about_us/strategic_home.htm*

- *http://www.rohcg.on.ca/about/strategic-e.cfm*

- Go to *http://www.nursingsociety.org*. This site provides weekly literature updates from Sigma Theta Tau International, the nursing profession's honour society. What new books and periodicals are available that may be helpful to you in your practice?

REFERENCES

Baker, G. R., & Norton, P. (2001). Making patients safer! Reducing error in Canadian healthcare. *Healthcare Papers,* 2(1), 10–31.

Baker, G. R., & Norton, P. (2004). Next steps for patient safety in Canadian healthcare. *Healthcare Papers,* 5(3), 75–80.

Baker, G. R., Norton, P. G., Flintoft, V., Blais, R., Brown, A., Cox, J., et al. (2004). The Canadian Adverse Events Study: The incidence of adverse events among hospital patients in Canada. *Canadian Medical Association Journal,* 170(11), 1678–1686.

Benner, P. (1984). *From novice to expert.* Menlo Park, CA: Addison-Wesley.

Brun, L. (2003). The dos and don'ts of strategic planning. *Healthcare Management Forum,* 16(4), 37–38.

Clifford, J., & Horvath, K. J. (1990). *Advancing professional nursing practice: Innovations at Boston's Beth Israel Hospital.* New York: Springer.

Covey, S. R. (1990). *The seven habits of highly effective people.* New York: Fireside.

Devitt, R., Klassen, W., & Martalog, J. (2005). Strategic management system in a healthcare setting – moving from strategy to results. *Healthcare Quarterly,* 8(4), 58–65.

Dreyfus, S. E., & Dreyfus, H. L. (1980). *A five stage model of the mental activities involved in directed skill acquisition.* Unpublished report supported by the Air Force Office of Scientific Research, USAF (Contract F49620-79-C-0063), University of California, Berkeley, CA.

Hall, S., Thabet, R., & Dummet, M. (2009). Building a sustainable system: The making of the WTIS. *Healthcare Quarterly,* 12(Special issue), 43–51.

Havens, D. S., & Aiken, L. H. (1999). Shaping systems to promote desired outcomes: The magnet hospital model. *Journal of Nursing Administration,* 29(2), 14–20.

Hersey, R. E., & Blanchard, T. (1993). *Management of organizational behavior.* Edgewood Cliffs, NJ: Prentice-Hall.

Iron, K. (2006). ICES report: Health data in Ontario: Taking stock and moving ahead. *Healthcare Quarterly,* 9(3), 24–26.

Jeffs, L., Merkley, J., Jeffrey, J., Ferris, E., Dusek, J., & Hunter, C. (2006). Case study: Reconciling the quality and safety gap through strategic planning. *Nursing Leadership,* 19(2), 32–40.

Jones, L. B. (1996). *The path: Creating your mission statement for work and for life.* New York: Hyperion.

LaPorta, J. A., King, G., Cathers, T., Havens, L., Young, C., & Aylward, S. (2003). A test of a centre's vision. *Healthcare Management Forum,* 16(1), 34–36.

Ludemann, R. S., & Brown, C. (1989). Staff perceptions of shared governance. *Nursing Administration Quarterly,* 13(4), 49–56.

MacGregor-Burns, J. (1979). *Leadership.* New York: Harper & Row.

Marquis, B. L., & Huston, C. J. (2012). *Leadership roles and management functions in nursing theory and application* (7th ed.). Philadelphia: Lippincott, Williams, & Wilkins.

Marr, J., Tam, R., Simms, S., & Bacchus, F. (2011). Implementing a comprehensive support service solution at a major community hospital in Ontario, Canada: Lessons learned. *White Papers.* Retrieved from http://www.longwoods.com/content/22091/print

Nelson, E., Mohr, J. J., Batalden, P. B., & Plume, S. K. (1996). Improving health care, part 1: The clinical value compass. *Journal of Quality Improvement,* 22(4), 243–258.

Porter-O'Grady, T. (1992). *Implementing shared governance: Creating a professional organization.* St. Louis, MO: Mosby-Year Book.

Porter-O'Grady, T. (1995). *The leadership revolution in health care.* Gaithersburg, MD: Aspen.

Reisdorfer, J. T. (1996). Building a patient-focused care unit. *Nursing Management,* 27(10), 38, 40, 42, 44.

Robbins, S. P., DeCenzo, D. A., & Stuart-Kotze, R. (2002). Fundamentals of management: *Essential concepts and applications* (3rd Canadian ed.). Toronto: Prentice-Hall.

Roesch, P. (2000). Surgical unit practice. *Nursing Matters,* 7(3), 1.

Seaman, A., Elias, M., O'Neill, B., & Yatabe, K. (2010). Strategic implementation and accountability: The case of the long-term care alliance. *Healthcare Quarterly,* 13(2), 44–48.

Sellers, K. F. (1996). *The meaning of autonomous nursing practice to staff nurses in a shared governance organization: A hermeneutical analysis.* Unpublished doctoral dissertation, Adelphi University, Garden City, NY.

Senge, P. M. (2006). *The fifth discipline: The art & practice of the learning organization.* New York: Doubleday.

Shortell, S., & Kaluzny, A. (2000). *Health care management: Organization design and behavior* (4th ed.). Clifton Park, NY: Delmar Learning.

Stichler, J. F. (1992). A conceptual basis for shared governance. In N. D. Como & B. Pocta (Eds.), *Implementing shared governance: Creating a professional organization* (pp. 1–24). St. Louis, MO: Mosby.

Webster's encyclopedic unabridged dictionary of the English language (2nd ed.). (1996). New York: Random House.

Wesorick, B. (2000). Mission and Core Beliefs. *CPMRC Connections ... for Continuous Learning,* 3, 3.

Yoder-Wise, P. S. (1999). *Leading and managing in nursing* (2nd ed.). St. Louis, MO: Mosby.

Young, J., Bell, R., Khalfan, A., & Lindquist, E. (2008). Evaluating the balanced scorecare at the University Health Network: An impact assessment. *Healthcare Quarterly*, 11(2), 52–56.

SUGGESTED READINGS

Aiken, L. H., Havens, D. S., & Sloane, D. M. (2000). The magnet nursing services recognition program. *American Journal of Nursing*, 100(3), 26–35.

Alspach, J. (1984). Designing a competency-based orientation for critical care nurses. *Heart and Lung*, 13, 655–662.

Andrews, M. (1990). Strategic planning: Preparing for the 21st century. *Journal of Professional Nursing*, 6(2), 103–112.

Bell, C. (1996). *Managers as mentors*. San Francisco: Berrett-Koehler.

Bridges, W. (2000). *Managing transitions: Making the most of change*. New York: Perseus Books Group.

Cormak, M., Brady, J., & Porter-O'Grady, T. (1997). Professional practice: A framework for transition to a new culture. *Journal of Nursing Administration*, 27(12), 32–41.

Drucker, P. (1973). *Management tasks, responsibilities, and practices*. New York: Harper & Row.

Duckett, L., Henly, S., Avery, M., Potter, S., Hills-Bonczyk, S., Hulden, R., et al. (1998). A theory of planned behavior-based structural model for breast-feeding. *Nursing Research*, 47(6), 325–336.

Fraser, B., & Hollett, R. G. (2003). Use of a program logic model to guide the development of a strategic plan for Wellington County Hospitals Network. *Healthcare Management Forum*, 16(3), 12–17.

Institute of Medicine. (1999). *To err is human*. Washington, DC: National Academy Press.

Jones, K. R., DeBaca, V., & Yarbrough, M. (1997). Organizational culture assessment before and after implementing patient-focused care. *Nursing Economics*, 15(2), 73–80.

Kaplan, R. S., & Norton, D. P. (2001). *The strategy focused organization*. Boston: Harvard Business School.

Korabek, B., Slauenwhite, C., Rosenau, P., & Ross, L. (2004). Innovations in seniors care: Home care/physician partnership. *Canadian Journal of Nursing Leadership*, 17(3), 65–78.

Kouzes, J. M., & Posner, B. Z. (2002). *The leadership challenge* (3rd ed.). San Francisco: Jossey-Bass, A Wiley.

Myers, I. B. (1993). *Introduction to type*. Palo Alto, CA: Consulting Psychologists Press.

Sellers, K. F., Hargrove, B., & Jenkins, P. (2000). Asthma disease management programs improve clinical and economic outcomes. *MEDSURG Nursing*, 9(4), 201–203, 207.

Senge, P. (1990). *The fifth discipline*. New York: Doubleday.

Senge, P. (1994). *The fifth discipline fieldbook* (p. 49). New York: Doubleday.

Silvetti, C., Rudan, V., Frederickson, K., and Sulivan, B. (2000). Where will tomorrow's nurse managers come from? *Journal of Nursing Administration*, 30(4) 157–159.

Wesorick, B. (1998). *The way of respect in the workplace* (p. 15). Grand Rapids, MI: Practice Field.

Zemke, R., Raines, C., & Filipczak, B. (2000). *Generations at work: Managing the clash of veterans, boomers, xers and nexters in your workplace*. New York: AMACOM.

CHAPTER 14

Change and Conflict Resolution

Margaret M. Anderson, EdD, RN-C, CNAA
Adapted by Heather Crawford, BScN, MEd, CHE

It is not the strongest of the species that survives, nor the most intelligent, but rather the one most responsive to change.

(Charles Darwin)

OBJECTIVES

The purpose of this chapter is to enable the reader to

- define change from personal, professional, and organizational perspectives;
- identify the change theorists;
- discuss the concept of the learning organization;
- identify the driving and restraining forces of change within a structured setting;
- discuss change strategies;
- discuss the role and characteristics of a change agent in the change process;
- use the change process to plan, implement, and evaluate a change project;
- identify conflict situations; and
- identify steps in the conflict resolution process.

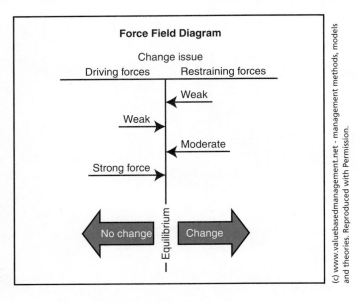

Force Field Diagram

Change issue

Driving forces   Restraining forces

Weak

Weak

Moderate

Strong force

Equilibrium

No change   Change

JoAnne has been a nurse manager for five years. During that time, she has had no fewer than five directors. In addition, she has had two different medical directors for her unit, two different methods of care delivery, and the amalgamation of two nursing units, resulting in a change of culture and mission. JoAnne has just started her master of science in nursing (MScN) degree, and wonders whether she can make it through another change. She shuts her desk drawer, looks in the mirror, and says to her reflection, "You can do it. You know you love a challenge. The only thing that is constant is change, and this will give you an opportunity to apply your education to the current exciting change initiatives!" JoAnne immediately straightened her shoulders, put her head up, and walked out of her office. She smiled at her staff and said, "Hello."

What do you think JoAnne is feeling?

How should JoAnne go about introducing yet another change to her staff?

In health care, is change inevitable, pervasive, and exciting?

This chapter is designed to introduce the concepts of change and conflict resolution. Change is an inevitable and frequent occurrence in health care and in life. Technology, biomedical discoveries, and advances in disease treatment and medications cause revolutions in the treatment and course of illness. These advances also make changes in wellness and health promotion rapid and sweeping. Along with change, conflict is also inevitable. The resolution of that conflict is necessary for the good of the client and the organization. Although conflict in itself is not a bad thing, unresolved conflict can thwart the efforts of the best-intentioned change agent and cause stagnation and tension in a work team.

This chapter will help to alleviate the anxiety surrounding change and conflict as well as teach the importance of embracing change and confronting conflict. Change is frightening only when you are not a part of it or you have no input into it. The staff nurse has a responsibility

to provide input, even if it is not invited, and to become involved in the planning and implementation of change. Equally important is the evaluation of change. Evaluating honestly and making necessary modifications are as important to the success of a change project as the planning and orderly implementation. If nothing else is learned, learn to embrace change as an opportunity to improve client care and to advance the profession of nursing. Look at conflict resolution as an opportunity to learn something new or as the opportunity to persuade others.

CHANGE

There are many definitions of change, and there are many types of change. For simplicity, **change** can be defined as "the act, process, or result of altering or modifying" (Nelson Canadian Dictionary, 1997, p. 233). The outcome may be the same, but the actions performed to reach the outcome may be different. For instance, because of road closures, how you get to work might be different. Although the goal of getting to work remains the same, you might try a different method: for example, driving a different route or taking the bus rather than driving. In the professional nursing setting, new client admission forms may require a different method of assessing the client or may change the number of people involved in the admission process. Rather than one registered nurse conducting the entire admission process, the process may be broken down so that individuals with different skill levels conduct different parts of the process. The goal is still the admission of the client to a unit; how it is done may be different. Most change is implemented for a good or reasonable purpose. Most organizational change is planned. The change is intentional and goal-oriented, with activities that are proactive and purposeful (Robbins & Langton, 2002). If employees do not understand the reason behind change, they should ask.

For purposes of discussion, **personal change** is a change made voluntarily for one's own reasons, usually for self-improvement. Personal change may include altering your diet for health reasons, taking classes for self-improvement, or removing yourself from a destructive or unhealthy environment or situation. **Professional change** may be a change in position or job, such as obtaining education or credentials that will benefit your current position or allow you to be prepared for a future position. Professional change is often planned and can involve extensive change in both your personal and professional lives. Both personal and professional change may be stressful. However, if the change is voluntary and carries intrinsic or extrinsic rewards, it is often considered important and worth the stress.

Organizational change is the type of change that often causes the most stress or concern. **Organizational**

CRITICAL THINKING

Think about a time you were determined to make a personal change in your life. What emotions did you experience? Did you have support for this change? Did you set a realistic goal for yourself?

LITERATURE APPLICATION

Citation: Edgar, L., Herbert, R., Lambert, S., MacDonald, U., Dubois, S., & Latimer, M. (2006). The joint venture model of knowledge utilization: A guide for change in nursing. *Canadian Journal of Nursing Leadership,* 19(2): 41–55.

Discussion: This research article discusses knowledge utilization (KU) as an essential component of today's nursing practice and health care system. Although much knowledge has been generated, the gap between practice and research continues. Knowledge utilization models have moved from factors affecting individual nurses to include a broader perspective related to practice environments and the socio-political context. This paper proposes the Joint Venture Model of Knowledge Utilization (JVMKU). It describes its development and suggested uses at both local and organizational levels.

Implications for Practice: The Joint Venture Model of Knowledge Utilization includes a global analysis of the factors influencing KU and provides a guide for knowledge use at the nursing unit level as well as at the organizational level. It supports the position that people who use their skills and knowledge are effective change agents within work settings that are motivating. The JVMKU proposes that KU and its subsequent outcomes be determined by the following: interaction among leaders, emotional intelligence, individuals and organizations, knowledge within the practice environment or workplace, and the broad socio-political environment. This model is generic and broad enough that users can fill in the details with information pertinent to their situation. For example, a nurse leader at any level of an organization who wants to introduce a change can examine the model's concepts for areas of strength and areas for improvement. Then the nurse leader can make improvements, focus on the most favourable conditions, or defer change until a more suitable time.

LITERATURE APPLICATION

Citation: Ducharme, J., Buckley, J., Adler, R., & Pelletier, C. (2009). The application of change management principles to facilitate the introduction of nurse practitioners and physician assistants into six Ontario emergency departments. *Healthcare Quarterly,* 12(2): 70–77.

Discussion: This article describes a project that was funded by the Ontario Ministry of Health and Long-Term Care. MedEmerg facilitated the introduction of three new providers into six emergency departments. A managed change process is described, and the project emphasized the importance of a managed process in the implementation of the change.

Implications for Practice: The results of the change indicated that there was a need for better understanding of the cultural environment, more consistent communication with stakeholders, better engagement of physicians, more resources to support staff involvement, and the management of expectations. Key strengths included the benefit of using a team-building process to motivate and support change, the applicability of the Participatory, Evidence-Based, Patient-Focused Process for Advanced Practice Nursing (PEPPA) framework and the values of advanced environmental scanning. These lessons learned will benefit others who want to make changes within their health care settings.

change can be defined as "an alteration of an organization's environment, structure, technology or people" (Robbins, DeCenzo, & Stuart-Kotze, 2002, p. 183). Sometimes a lot of preparation and discussion precedes organizational change. Sometimes it comes as a surprise to the employees and causes a great deal of consternation and stress. Organizational change can affect five different aspects of an organization: its culture, structure, technology, physical setting, and human resources. Changing an organization's culture may be one of the most difficult changes and challenges because the underlying values and goals of the organization need to change. Changing structure involves altering authority relations, job design, or similar variables. Changing technology includes modification in the way work is processed, or in the methods and equipment used. Changing the physical setting involves altering the space and layout arrangements. Changing human resources refers to changes in employee skills, expectations, or behaviour (Robbins & Langton, 2002).

TRADITIONAL CHANGE THEORIES

The change theories discussed here are Lewin's Force-Field Model (1951), Lippitt's Phases of Change (1958), Havelock's Six-Step Change Model (1973), and Rogers' Diffusion of Innovations Theory (1983). These are classic change theories and are based on Lewin's original model.

Lewin's model has three simple steps. The steps are unfreezing, movement, and refreezing. Unfreezing refers to a thawing of the current or old way of doing things. Individuals begin to be aware of the need for doing things differently, that change is needed for a specific reason. In the next step, the intervention or change is introduced and explained. The benefits and disadvantages are discussed, and the change—the move to a new level—is implemented. In the third step, refreezing occurs, meaning that the new way of doing is incorporated into the routines or habits of the affected people. Although these steps sound simple, the process of change is, of course, more complicated (Flower & Guillaume, 2002).

Lippitt's Phases of Change are built on Lewin's model. Lippitt defined seven stages in the change process: (1) diagnosis of the problem, (2) assessment of the motivation and capacity for change, (3) assessment of the change agent's motivation and resources, (4) the selection of progressive change objectives, (5) choosing an appropriate role for the change agent, (6) maintenance of the change once it has been started, and (7) termination of the helping relationship. Lippitt emphasized the participation of key personnel and the change agent in designing and planning the intended change project. Lippitt also emphasized communication during all phases of the process (Sullivan & Decker, 2001).

Havelock designed a six-step model of the change process. This model is based on Lewin's model, but Havelock included more steps in each stage. The planning stage includes (1) building a relationship, (2) diagnosing the problem, and (3) acquiring resources. This planning stage is followed by the moving stage, which includes (4) choosing the solution and (5) gaining acceptance. The last stage, the refreezing stage, includes (6) stabilization and self-renewal. Havelock emphasized the planning stage. He believed that resistance to change can be overcome with careful planning and inclusion of the affected staff. Havelock also believed that the change agent, the person responsible for planning and implementing the change, should encourage participation of the affected employees. The more the people affected by the change participate in the change, the more they are likely to make the change successful and to support the necessity for the change (Sullivan & Decker, 2001; Tappen, Weiss, & Whitehead, 2004).

In 1983 Rogers published his Diffusion of Innovations Theory. Although based on Lewin's model, this theory is much broader in scope and approach. He developed a five-step innovation and decision-making process. Rogers believed that change can be rejected initially and then adopted at a later time. He believed that change is a reversible process and that initial rejection does not necessarily mean the change will never be adopted. This theory also works in reverse—the change may initially be adopted and then rejected at a later time. Rogers' approach emphasized the capriciousness of change. In his theory, timing and format take on new meaning and importance—as the time involved in change implementation grows longer, the more the change process takes on a life of its own and the original change and reasons for it may be lost. The change process must be carefully managed and planned to ensure that it survives mostly intact. Table 14-1 is a comparison chart of these change models.

The theories described in Table 14-1 are linear in nature, meaning they more or less proceed in an orderly manner from one step to the next. This linearity and the fact that they are all based on Lewin's theory make them similar in complexity and in use. These theories work well for low-level, uncomplicated change. They do not work well in highly complex and nonlinear situations. Health care organizations are very complex and require more sophisticated theories of change.

EMERGING THEORIES OF CHANGE

Much more complex in breadth and depth than the theories previously discussed are two often-used and emerging theories of change: the chaos theory and the learning organization theory. According to Wagner and Huber (2003), "organizations can no longer rely on rules, policies, and hierarchies, or afford to be inflexible; and small changes in the initial conditions of a system can drastically affect the long-term behaviour of that system." Chaos theory hypothesizes that chaos actually has an order. That is, although the potential for chaos appears, at first glance, to be random, further investigation reveals some order to the chaos.

Health care organizations have experienced chaos in the past 10 to 15 years, which, according to chaos theory, is normal. Most organizations go through periods of rapid change and innovation and then stabilize before chaos erupts again. Even though each chaotic occurrence is similar to the one that occurred before, each is different. The political, scientific, and behavioural components of the organization are different from before, so the chaos looks different. Order emerges through fluctuation and chaos. Thus, the potential for chaos means that the organization must be able to organize and implement change quickly and forcefully. Little time is available for orderly linear change. Leaders in these organizations are expected to act quickly and be flexible to meet the

TABLE 14-1	**COMPARISON CHART OF CHANGE THEORIES AND THEIR USES**			
Theorist and Year	Lewin (1951)	Lippitt (1958)	Havelock (1973)	Rogers (1983)
Title of Model	Force-Field Model	Phases of Change	Six-Step Change Model	Diffusion of Innovations Theory
Steps in Model (The steps in the models are spaced to indicate their correlation to Lewin's model.)	1. Unfreeze 2. Move 3. Refreeze	1. Diagnose problem 2. Assess motivation and capacity for change 3. Assess change agent's motivation and resources 4. Select progressive change objective 5. Choose appropriate role of change agent 6. Maintain change 7. Terminate helping relationship	1. Build relationship 2. Diagnose problem 3. Acquire resources 4. Choose solution 5. Gain acceptance 6. Stabilization and self-renewal	1. Awareness 2. Interest 3. Evaluation 4. Trial 5. Adoption

Source: Adapted from *Introductory Management and Leadership for Nurses* (2nd ed., p. 327) by R.C. Swansburg and R.J. Swansburg (1998). Boston: Jones & Bartlett Publishers.

challenge of the potentially chaotic forces. Organizations today are required to deal with highly unstable environmental conditions, and they are compelled to change in a manner that allows for constant fluidity and continuous renewal (Ayers, 2002).

Peter Senge (2006) first described learning organization theory. Learning organizations demonstrate responsiveness and flexibility. Senge believed that because organizations are open systems, they can best respond to unpredictable changes in the environment by using a learning approach in their interactions and interdisciplinary workings with one another. The whole cannot function well without a part regardless of how small that part may seem. For example, a well-equipped stove cannot work without a source of either electricity or gas. It does not matter how new, innovative, or energy efficient the stove is; it cannot function without an energy source. An example in health care is that the laboratory department cannot complete an accurate test and assessment without the cooperation of the physician, nurse, nurse assistant, or unit clerk. If the physician does not order the appro-

priate test, and the nurse does not adequately prepare the client for the test, then the laboratory cannot prepare an accurate report. Without the proper requisition, the laboratory cannot perform the appropriate test on the specimen. The learning organization understands these interrelationships and responds quickly to improve relationships. This response may be through dialogue or team problem solving, but all parties must understand what is at stake for cooperation to occur.

Senge developed five disciplines that he believed are necessary for organizations to achieve the "learning organization status" to deal effectively with chaos: systems thinking, personal mastery, mental models, building shared vision, and team learning. Senge defined a discipline as "a body of theory and technique that must be studied and mastered to be put into practice" (Senge, 2006, p. 10). In the learning organization, each individual has something to offer that melds with what others have to offer to determine the right steps to take in sorting out the causes of chaos and responding positively to it. The goals of the organization and individual are mutually related so that quick response to chaos occurs, with positive results for both the organization and the individual. The key to development of Senge's five disciplines is two-way communication or open discussion, dialogue, and being a lifelong learner (Senge, 2006). Most experts agree that few, if any, health care organizations have evolved to the learning organization status. Although this is a goal to work toward, health care itself has not evolved to the point of quick reaction to chaos and a rapidly changing environment.

THE CHANGE PROCESS

Planned change in the work organization is not much different from planned change on a personal level. The major difference is that more people are involved, the scale is larger, and more opinions must be considered. There are three basic reasons to introduce a change: (1) to solve a problem, (2) to improve efficiency, or (3) to reduce unnecessary workload for some group (Marquis & Huston, 2012). To plan change, one must know what has to be changed. Change for the sake of change is unnecessary and stressful (Bennis, Benne, & Chin, 1969).

STEPS IN THE CHANGE PROCESS

The change process can be related to the nursing process. Using the nursing process as a model, the first step in the change process is assessment.

ASSESSMENT

In assessment, one identifies the problem or the opportunity for improvement through change, by collecting and analyzing data. The data collection and analysis should be from several perspectives: structural, technological, and people.

A structural perspective is one of physical space or the configuration of physical space. For instance, a medical-surgical unit in a hospital may plan to move to the space vacated by the obstetrics unit. The space is large enough but is not configured to be conducive to the care of medical-surgical clients. Assessment of the structural components may include examination of the location of elevators, supply stations, client charts, telephones, call lights, and other physical or structural components. Structural components often mandate how the work is done or the process of doing the work. Poor structural configuration may require the work team to perform extra steps to accomplish its goals.

A technological perspective may address a lack of wall outlets for necessary equipment, poorly situated computer locations, and lack of computer system interface ability. Sometimes, technology lags behind the goals of a work team and therefore slows down the team. The team spends more time troubleshooting technology than in providing care.

A perspective on people may bring to light personnel with inadequate training to accomplish the goals, an unwillingness to meet the goals, a lack of commitment to the organization, or a lack of understanding for the need for change.

Assessment data are collected from internal and external sources. Lewin identified forces that were supportive of change as well as forces that were barriers to change. He called these driving and restraining forces. If the restraining forces outweigh the driving forces, then the change must be abandoned because it cannot succeed. Driving and restraining forces include political issues, technology issues, cost and structural issues, and people issues. The political issues include the power groups in favour of or in opposition to the proposed change, and may include physicians, administrators, civic and community groups, or provincial and federal restrictions. The technology issues include whether to update old equipment, computer systems, or methods for accounting for supply use. Cost and structural issues include the costs, desirability, and feasibility of remodelling or building new construction for the change project. People issues include the commitment of the staff, their level of education and training, and their interest in the project. The most common people issue is fear of job loss or fear of not being valued. It bears repeating that if the restraining forces outweigh the driving forces, the change will not succeed, and it should be abandoned or rethought.

During data analysis, potential solutions may be identified, sources of resistance may come to light, determination of strategies may become apparent, and some areas of consensus may become evident. Statistical analysis is an important component of analysis, which should be conducted whenever possible to provide persuasive information in favour of the change, especially when the issue is either meeting the cost objectives or the mission objectives. The goal of data analysis is to support the need to change and to offer data to support the potential solution selected. The people who are potentially most affected by the change need to be involved in the assessment, data collection, and data analysis. They have a vested interest in the change and must not only support the change but also be willing to implement change (Bennis et al., 1969).

PLANNING

The next step is to plan. This step determines who will be affected by the change and when change will occur. All the potential solutions are examined. The driving and resisting forces are again examined and strategies determined for implementing the change. The target date for implementation and also the outcomes or goals are clearly delineated and stated in measurable terms. Again, the most successful plan for change is one in which the individuals who will be most affected are involved, satisfied, and committed.

The plan should also address how the change will be implemented, although it may require modification as the implementation begins. For instance, how many work groups or units will implement the change at once? Will the change implementation be staggered from month to month or week to week? Will the supports that are necessary to manage the change be implemented first? Just how will this change be implemented? Finally, the overall plan includes strategies for evaluation. It is crucial that evaluation be built in. Expected outcomes must be identified in measurable terms, and the plan to evaluate those outcomes and a timetable for evaluation must be evident. Unevaluated change will not succeed.

IMPLEMENTATION OF CHANGE STRATEGIES

Bennis et al., (1969) identified three strategies to promote change in groups or organizations: the power-coercive strategy, the normative-reeducative strategy, and the rational-empirical strategy. Different strategies work in different situations. The power or authority of the change agent influences the strategy selected. Most change agents use a variety of strategies to promote successful change.

The power-coercive strategy is very simple—"do it or get out." This strategy is based on the application of power by a legitimate authority, economic sanctions, or the political clout of the change agent (Marquis & Huston, 2012). Little effort is required to encourage participation of employees, and little concern surrounds their acceptance or resistance to the proposed change. An example of this strategy would include implementation of the Canadian government's privacy legislation across the nation. This group of strategies is generally reserved for situations in which resistance is expected but not important to the power group.

The second group-change strategy is normative-reeducative. This strategy is based on the assumption that group norms are used to socialize individuals. This strategy focuses on using the individual's need for satisfying social relationships in the workplace. Very few individuals can withstand social isolation or rejection by the work group. Compliance and support for a change are garnered by focusing on the perceived loss of social relationships in the workplace. Although some resistance to change may be expected, this strategy assumes people are interested in preserving relationships and will go along with the majority. The change agent does not necessarily require a legitimate power base, but gains power by skill in interpersonal relationships (Marquis & Huston, 2012).

The third group of strategies is rational-empirical. This group assumes that humans are rational people and will use knowledge to embrace change. It is assumed that once the self-interests of a group are evident, the group will see the merit in a change and embrace it. Knowledge and training are the components used to encourage compliance with change. This strategy is very successful when little resistance is anticipated. Table 14-2 summarizes the three strategies for change.

EVALUATION OF CHANGE

In the evaluation step, the effectiveness of the change is evaluated according to the outcomes identified during the planning phase. Evaluation is the most overlooked component, although it is considered by some experts to be the most important aspect of change. Usually, not enough time is allowed for the change to become effective or stable, which is a grave error. The time intervals for evaluation should be identified and allowed to elapse before modifications are made and declarations of failure are asserted. A certain period of confusion and turmoil accompanies all changes, whether large or small. If the outcomes are achieved, then the change was a success. If not, then some revision or modification may be necessary to achieve the outcomes that were anticipated.

STABILIZATION OF CHANGE

After effectiveness has been determined, stabilization of the change is complete. The project is no longer a pilot or experiment but is a part of the culture and function of the organization. Although there is no magical time frame for stabilization to occur, it should be encouraged as soon as possible to make the change project complete. Often, re-evaluation is planned after the first six months or year of implementation to ensure that stabilization of the change has occurred.

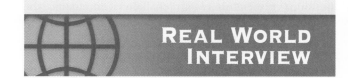

REAL WORLD INTERVIEW

"Beyond changes specific to client care, nurses have to be adept at dealing with other sorts of changes, such as changes in policies, functions, regulations, technology and their workplace."

Lori Adler, RN
Manager, Practice Standards,
College of Nurses of Ontario

Source: College of Nurses of Ontario. (2011). Be a change leader: How to thrive in a changing healthcare environment. *The Standard,* 36(1): 10–12.

TABLE 14-2	STRATEGIES FOR CHANGE
Strategy	**Description**
Power-coercive approach	Uses authority and the threat of job loss to gain compliance with change.
Normative-reeducative approach	Uses social orientation and the need to have satisfactory relationships in the workplace as a method of inducing support for change. Focuses on the relationship needs of workers.
Rational-empirical approach	Uses knowledge as a power base. Once workers understand the organizational need for change or understand the meaning of the change to them as individuals and the organization as a whole, they will change.

CRITICAL THINKING

Consider one of the changes you have experienced in a personal or work setting. Was there any plan for evaluation of the change? Was any thought given to making some modification in the change when it was obvious the change could not be implemented as designed? What could have been done differently?

RESPONSES TO CHANGE

People do respond to change. The most typical response to change is resistance. Humans like order and familiarity; they enjoy routine and the status quo. The more the relationships or social mores are challenged to change, the more resistance there is to change. Marquis and Huston (2012) point out that nurses are more likely to accept a change in an intravenous pump rather than a change in who can administer the intravenous fluid. This finding suggests that the social mores of a group are more important than technology in a change. The social mores dictate the roles and responsibilities of groups of workers, such as registered nurses, licensed practical nurses, unregulated care providers, and so on. Registered nurses are often less concerned with technology and more concerned with maintaining traditional roles and responsibilities.

Several factors affect resistance to change. The first is trust. The employee and employer must trust that each is doing the right thing and that each is capable of producing successful change. In addition to capability, predictability

is important. The employee wants a predictable work environment and security. When change is introduced, then that predictable environment—and, therefore, the employee's comfort zone—begins to come into question (Lapp, 2002). Another factor is the individual's ability to cope with change. Silber (1993) points out four factors that affect an individual's ability to cope with change[*]:

1. Flexibility for change, that is, the ability to adapt to change
2. Evaluation of the immediate situation, that is, if the current situation is unacceptable, then change will be more welcome
3. Anticipated consequences of change, that is, the impact change will have on one's current job
4. Individual's stake or what the individual has to win or lose as an effect of the change, that is, the more individuals perceive they have to lose, the more resistance they will offer

Change is a scary prospect for those who have not had much experience with change or who have had only negative experiences with change. It is important to help people remember that change is inevitable and ever present. Developing an attitude of embracing and accepting change is desirable.

Bushy (1993) has identified six behavioural responses to planned change. These behavioural responses are usually apparent in every health care facility and every nursing unit[†].

1. Innovators: Change embracers. They enjoy the challenge of change and often lead change.
2. Early adopters: Open to change. They are receptive to but not obsessed with change.

[*] Silber, M. B. (1993). The "C"s in excellence: Choice and change. *Nursing Management, 24*(9): 60–62.

[†] Bushy, A. (1993). Managing change: Strategies for continuing education. *The Journal of Continuing Education in Nursing, 23:* 197–200.

3. Early majority: Enjoy and prefer the status quo. They do not want to be left behind, and they adopt change before the average person.

4. Late majority: Often known as the followers. They adopt change after expressing negative feelings and are often skeptical.

5. Laggards: Last group to adopt a change. They prefer tradition and stability to innovation and are suspicious of change.

6. Rejecters: Openly oppose and reject change. They may be surreptitious or covert in their opposition, and may hinder the change process to the point of sabotage.

Other responses to change have been identified, including grief, denial, anger, depression, and bargaining (Marquis & Huston, 2012). Regardless of the importance and necessity of change, the human response is very important and cannot be dismissed. So often, in one's zeal to respond to a need, the change agent forgets that the human side of change must be dealt with. People have a right to their feelings and a right to express them. The important point is the change agent helps people respond and then move on to the goal of implementing the change. Gently but firmly, people must be guided toward acceptance.

Many people are dissatisfied with their situation in either their personal or professional lives, but don't know how to change. Maybe by understanding some principles of change, one can become more willing to participate in change and eagerly engage in effecting change. See Table 14-3 for some principles of change.

THE CHANGE AGENT

Throughout this discussion of change, the term **change agent** has been used instead of manager, leader, or administrator. The change agent is the person responsible for implementing a change project. This person may be from within or outside an organization. Often the change agent is a leader or manager because people in these roles are usually innovators and likely enjoy change. A change agent is ultimately responsible for the success of the change project, large or small. The role of the change agent is to manage the dynamics of the change process, which requires knowledge of the organization, knowledge of the change process, knowledge of the participants in the change process, and understanding of the feelings of the group undergoing change. Probably the most important role of the change agent is to maintain communication, momentum, and enthusiasm for the project while still managing the process. Table 14-4 summarizes the roles and characteristics of the change agent.

The recipients of change must trust the change agent's interpersonal skills to provide information and manage change but also the agent's personal integrity and honour as an honest, principled individual. The executives in the organization must trust that the change agent will accomplish the established goals, given the proper support. The change agent also needs to recognize that

TABLE 14-3	PRINCIPLES OF CHANGE

A change in one part affects other parts and other systems.

People affected by the change should participate in making the change.

People should be informed of the reasons for the change.

Concrete and specific feedback about the process of change will enhance its acceptance.

People need assistance in dealing with the effects of the change.

People's suggestions and contributions about the implementation of change should be sought and incorporated.

A change must be reinforced or the system will revert to its old practices.

Conflict may occur at any step during the change process.

The more compatible the new ideas are with one's values and needs, the more easily a change will be adopted.

The more trust one has in the initiator of change, the more likely one is to support the change.

One's past experience with change can profoundly affect one's willingness to support a new idea.

Source: Grossman, S.C., & Valiga, T.M. (2009). *The New Leadership Challenge: Creating the Future of Nursing,* 3rd edition. FA Davis Company, Philadelphia, PA with permission.

TABLE 14-4	**ROLES AND CHARACTERISTICS OF THE CHANGE AGENT**

- Lead the change process by example
- Manage process and group dynamics and show others how to adapt to change
- Demonstrate that the change is critical and inspire response from others
- Understand feelings of the group experiencing the change and engage them in the process
- Maintain momentum and enthusiasm
- Maintain vision of change
- Communicate change, progress, and feelings
- Knowledgeable about the organization
- Honest and direct
- Respected
- Intuitive

REAL WORLD INTERVIEW

I have always enjoyed trying new things and developing to my potential. However, I have no patience for a manager who is not truthful. Once she pretends to have the answers, and makes up her plan as she goes, I lose all respect, and trust is destroyed. It's okay to say, "I don't know," *but* you need to find the answer, and report back to me. Don't lie to me.

Margaret Mary Chester, RN
Staff Nurse

those who develop the project need to have some definite inclusion concepts folded into the vision for success. Inclusion concepts are those ideas or concepts that the affected parties believe are absolutely necessary for their peace of mind or moral value. When these concepts are included, people feel ownership and value—a piece of them or their idea is in the plan.

Finally, the change agent must use some intuition during the evaluation steps to be able to bow out of the change and to allow those affected to accept ownership. This decision is a matter of timing and insight into when the staff is ready to accept and incorporate the change as its own. Bennis (1989) warns that not stepping away from the project and cutting the ownership bonds means that

it is the change agent's project for many years to come, even after that person leaves the organization. During evaluation, the change agent must support modifications and revisions that help transfer project ownership.

CHANGE AGENT STRATEGIES

Following are some strategies the change agent can use in managing the process:

1. Begin by articulating the vision clearly and concisely. Use the same words over and over. Constantly remind people of the goals and vision.
2. Map out a tentative timeline and sketch out the steps of the project. Have a good idea of how the project should go.
3. Plant seeds or mention some ideas or thoughts to key individuals from the first step through the evaluation step; then an idea of what is expected can be under consideration.
4. Select the change project team carefully. Make sure it is heavily loaded with those who will be affected and other experts as needed. Select a variety of people. For example, an innovator, someone from the late majority group, a laggard, and a rejecter are probably good to include. These people provide insight into what others are thinking.
5. Set up consistent meeting dates and keep them. Have an agenda and constantly check the timeline for target activities.
6. For those not on the team but affected by the project, give constant and consistent updates on progress. If the change agent does not update staff, someone on the project team will, and the change agent wants to control the messages.

7. Give regular updates and progress reports both verbally and in writing to the executives of the organization and those affected by the change.

8. Check out rumours and confront any conflict head on. Do not look for conflict, but do not back away from it or ignore it.

9. Maintain a positive attitude and do not get discouraged.

10. Stay alert to political forces both for and against the project. Reach consensus on important issues as the project goes along, especially if policy, money, or philosophy issues are involved. Obtain consensus quickly on major issues or potential barriers to the project from both executives and staff.

11. Know the internal formal and informal leaders. Create a relationship with them. Consult them often.

12. Having self-confidence and trust in oneself and one's team will overcome a lot of obstacles. (Lancaster, 1999)

Leaders and managers must act as role models during the change process. It is important that change is presented in a positive light, particularly because change frightens most people. Remember the phrase "fear of the unknown." Does it apply to change? One can never over communicate when it comes to change, particularly to those affected by the change. The only thing really constant about change is change itself! Porter-O'Grady and Malloch (2003) suggest that "change is ... a never-ending journey" (p. 12). Every point of arrival is also a point of departure. As a result, leaders must carefully balance periods of effort and action with periods of rest and celebration so that the stakeholders will be regularly refreshed and re-energized to meet future challenges.

CONFLICT

An important part of the change process is the ability to resolve conflict. Conflict resolution skills are leadership and management tools that all registered nurses should have in their repertoire. Conflict itself is not bad. Conflict is healthy. Like change, conflict allows for creativity, innovation, new ideas, and new ways of doing things. It allows for the healthy discussion of different views and values and adds an important dimension to the provision of quality client care. Conflict can occur in almost any situation about almost anything. Conflict can arise over a matter as trivial as the size of an earring allowed in the dress code or as serious as who has the final authority on client care policy. Without some conflict, groups or work teams tend to become stagnant and routinized. Nothing new is allowed to penetrate the "way we have always done it" mentality. The change agent and the nurse manager

quickly become targets if they introduce new ideas or new systems of operating.

There are a variety of definitions of conflict. Conflict can be defined as two or more parties holding differing views about a situation (Tappen, 2001), or as the dynamic content of diversity, with human conflict as the diversity being worked out in the human community (Porter-O'Grady & Malloch, 2003). As can be surmised from these definitions, **conflict** can be defined as a disagreement about something of importance to each person involved. Not all disagreements become conflicts, but all disagreements have the potential for becoming a conflict, and all conflicts involve some level of disagreement. The astute manager can determine which disagreements might become conflicts and which ones will not. This discussion of conflict resolution does not include professional communication skills, which are discussed in Chapter 6.

SOURCES OF CONFLICT

Whenever there is an opportunity for disagreement, there is a potential source of conflict. The common sources of conflict in the professional setting include disputes over resource allocation or availability, personality differences, differences in values, threats from inside or outside an organization, cultural differences, and competition. In recent years organizational, professional, and unit goals have served as major sources of conflict. Nurses frequently see financial goals and client care goals as being in direct conflict. In many organizations, this issue is the most frequently mentioned source of emotionally charged conflict (Sullivan & Decker, 2001).

Sources of conflict in personal arenas include differences in values, threats to security or well-being, financial problems, and cultural problems. Family relationships are often sources of conflict because of the complexity of these relationships.

TYPES OF CONFLICT

There are three broad types of conflict: intrapersonal, interpersonal, and organizational. Intrapersonal conflict occurs within the individual. For example, if Marilyn is not granted her requested day off, she may have an internal conflict about whether to call in sick, or to take the day off without pay, or to go to work. Or Marilyn may have conflict about priorities: should she attend her daughter's softball game or write her paper for school?

An interpersonal conflict occurs between two people or between groups or work teams. A disagreement may arise in philosophy or values, or policy or procedure. It may be a personality conflict; for example, two people just irritate each other. This type of conflict is not unusual in work situations. People new to a team may have ideas that are not totally acceptable to the team members already in place. Individuals who transfer from one unit to another

TABLE 14-5	SOURCES OF CONFLICT

Environmental Sources	Individual Sources
Cultural	Ego
Nationality	Personality
Religion	Identity
Class	Intimate relationships
Economics	Beliefs
Politics	Perceptions
Society	Perspectives
Resources	Education
Race	Position and role

Source: T. Porter-O'Grady & K. Malloch, *Quantum Leadership A Textbook of New Leadership,* p. 81. Copyright (c) 2003: Jones and Bartlett Learning, Sudbury, MA. www.jblearning.com. Reprinted with permission.

often create a certain amount of conflict over processes and procedures. For example, the nurse transferring from the intensive care unit (ICU) to the coronary care unit (CCU) may be comfortable with one way of making assignments, but then try to encourage the new peers to adopt that methodology without sharing the rationale for why the new way is better.

Organizational conflict can be a healthy way of introducing new ideas and encouraging creativity. Competition for resources, organizational cultural differences, and other sources of conflict help organizations identify areas for improvement. Conflict helps organizations identify legitimate differences among departments or work teams based on corporate need or responsibility. When organizational conflict is highlighted, corporate values and differences are aired and resolved.

THE CONFLICT PROCESS

Before attempting to intervene in a conflict situation, the conflict's five stages should be accurately assessed. The five stages are "latent conflict, which implies the existence of antecedent conditions; perceived conflict, which often involves issues and roles; felt conflict, which occurs when the conflict is emotionalized; manifest or overt conflict, when action is taken; and conflict aftermath" (Marquis & Huston, 2012). Conflict always has consequences, whether they are positive or negative. If the

conflict is managed effectively, the people involved will believe their issues were heard and the situation was dealt with appropriately. If the conflict was handled poorly, the conflict issues are unresolved and are almost guaranteed to resurface at a later date and then cause further conflict (Marquis & Huston, 2012).

CONFLICT RESOLUTION

The ideal goal when attempting to resolve conflict is to create a win-win solution. Such a solution is not always possible, but the manager is·responsible for controlling the conflict so that individual differences are minimized. There are essentially seven methods of conflict resolution that dictate the outcomes of the conflict process.

Although some methods are more desirable or produce more successful outcomes than others, all the methods have a place in conflict resolution, depending on the nature of the conflict and the desired outcomes. Table 14-6 is a summary of these methods and highlights some of their advantages and disadvantages.

Avoiding is a very common technique. The parties involved in the conflict ignore it, either consciously or subconsciously.

Accommodating is often called cooperating. In this technique, one side of the disagreement decides or is encouraged to adjust or adapt to the other side by ignoring or sidestepping their own feelings about the

CRITICAL THINKING

Recall a time of conflict in your life. Looking at it with a different perspective, what antecedent conditions led to the conflict? What was the core of the conflict? Were personal goals or values at stake? How would you look at the same conflict now?

issue. People often accommodate when the stakes are not that high and the need to move on is pressing. Frequent use of this method, however, can lead to feelings of frustration or being used—one person is "used" to get the cooperation of another. Sullivan (2004) suggests that losing this conflict is advisable, if the payoff assists you to win in the long-term.

Competing is a conflict resolution technique that produces a winner and loser. The concept is that there is an all-out effort to win at all costs. This technique may be used when time is too short to allow other techniques to work or when a critical, though unpopular, decision has to be made quickly. This technique is often called forcing because the winner forces the loser to accept the winner's stance on the conflict.

TABLE 14-6	**SUMMARY OF CONFLICT RESOLUTION TECHNIQUES**	
Conflict Resolution Technique	**Advantages**	**Disadvantages**
Avoiding—ignoring the conflict	Does not make a big deal out of nothing; conflict may be minor in comparison to other priorities	Conflict can become bigger than anticipated; the source of conflict might be more important to one person or group than others
Accommodating—smoothing or cooperating; one side gives in to the other side	One side is more concerned with an issue than the other side; stakes are not high enough for one group and that side is willing to give in	One side holds more power and can force the other side to give in; the importance of the stakes is not as apparent to one side as the other; can lead to parties feeling used if they are always pressured to give in
Competing—forcing; the two or three sides are forced to compete for the goal	Produces a winner; good when time is short and stakes are high	Produces a loser; leaves anger and resentment on the losing side
Compromising—each side gives up something and gains something	No one should win or lose, but both should gain something; good for disagreements between individuals	May cause a return to the conflict if what is given up becomes more important than the original goal
Negotiating—high-level discussion that seeks agreement but not necessarily consensus	Stakes are very high and solution is permanent; often involves powerful groups	Agreements are permanent, even though each side has gains and losses
Collaborating—both sides work together to develop the optimal outcome	Best solution for the conflict and encompasses all important goals to each side	Takes a lot of time; requires a commitment to success
Confronting—immediate and obvious movement to stop conflict at the very start	Does not allow conflict to take root; very powerful	May leave the impression that conflict is not tolerated; may make something big out of nothing

Compromising is a method used to achieve conflict resolution in situations in which neither side can win and neither side should lose. Compromise is rampant in our society and is useful for goal achievement when the stakes are important but not necessarily critical. Compromise is often seen as appeasement—each side gives up something and each side gains something. Compromise is a good technique for minor conflicts or conflicts that cannot be resolved satisfactorily for both sides. Both parties win and lose.

Collaboration occurs in conflict resolution when both sides work together to develop a mutually acceptable outcome. It is an assertive and cooperative means of achieving important goals, which results in a win-win solution. This technique requires both sides to seek an acceptable solution to the conflict so that all parties feel their goals or objectives have been achieved.

Negotiating requires careful communication techniques and highly developed skills. The optimum solution for the conflict may not be reached, but each side has some wins and some losses. The term *negotiation* is often used in reference to collective bargaining or politics; however, it is a very useful technique for conflict resolution at all levels. Negotiating is used when the stakes are considerably higher or when return to the conflict cannot occur. Return to the conflict may not be possible for a variety of reasons, such as a union contract, a permanent change in policy or governance, or career or life changes. The idea of negotiation is that each party will gain something. Therefore, general agreement is reached, but consensus—that is, agreement in concept—is not necessarily the goal.

According to Lewicki, Hiam, and Olander (1996), there are five basic approaches to negotiating: collaborative (win-win), competitive (win at all costs), avoiding (lose-lose), accommodating (lose to win), and compromise (split the difference). These five approaches to negotiation are influenced by the importance of maintaining the relationship relative to the importance of achieving one's desired outcomes (see Figure 14-1).

Sometimes agreement cannot be met through negotiation. In these situations, alternative dispute resolution may be used to keep the dispute private and avoid expensive litigation. The College of Nurses of Ontario has an alternative dispute resolution called the Participative Resolution Program (PRP). This program is an alternative to the complaint investigation process. It allows the complainant, nurse, and the College to work together to create solutions that satisfy everyone involved. The PRP attempts to bring an effective solution to the complaint that will continue to protect the public interest. This process supports the College's efforts to encourage quality improvement in nursing practice and, at the same time, reflects the trend toward the use of non-adversarial ways of dealing with conflict.

REAL WORLD INTERVIEW

One of the biggest mistakes a leader can make is to assume all information provided to you is 100 percent accurate. The leader who doesn't question, who takes everything at face value, and believes that all is well, is not a leader, but an avoider and procrastinator. A problem will not be solved by ignoring the fact that there are two sides to every issue.

Marcy Ogilvie, MScN
Nurse Executive

Pawl (2009) suggests that "most disputes—if they are really disputes at all—can be resolved successfully in an informal fashion" (p. 42). However, parties cannot reach agreement through negotiation. In these circumstances, alternative dispute resolution (ADR) may be needed to keep some privacy in the dispute and to avoid expensive litigation. Types of ADR include medication, fact finding, arbitration, due process hearings, and the use of an advocate or ombudsperson (Marquis & Huston, 2012).

One other technique used in conflict resolution is *confronting*. This technique heads off conflict as soon as the first symptoms appear. Both parties are brought together, the issues are clarified, and some outcome is achieved.

Success of the techniques presented here depends on several factors. The importance of the issue in the conflict to the various sides has an enormous impact on the technique selected and the degree of success that will be achieved. Conflict resolution is never really permanent because new issues will always arise. The challenge for the leader or manager is to determine which conflicts require intervention and which techniques stand the best chance of success. If one technique does not work, try another. Conflicts should be suppressed or avoided only under special circumstances that are dependent on the issues involved and the importance of the issues to the parties. Keep in mind that little problems become big problems later if the stakes are high and the issue is important to someone.

STRATEGIES TO FACILITATE CONFLICT RESOLUTION

Open, honest, clear communication is the key to successful conflict resolution. The nurse manager and leader and all parties to the conflict must agree to communicate

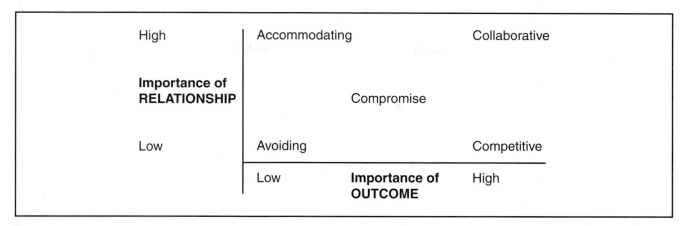

Figure 14-1 Negotiation Strategies

with one another openly and honestly. Courtesy in communicating is to be encouraged, which includes listening actively to the other side.

When you choose a setting for the conflict resolution discussions, find a place where people can be private, relaxed, and comfortable. It's best if external interruptions from phones, pagers, overhead speakers, and other personnel can be avoided or kept to a minimum. Establish a setting on neutral territory so that no one feels overpowered. At the outset agree to ground rules, such as not interrupting, who speaks first, and time limits. Ensure that the ground rules are respected and adhered.

One of the expectations for the conflict resolution process is that both sides in the conflict comply with the results. If one party cannot agree to comply with the decisions or outcomes, there is no point to engaging in the process. In such cases, if the employee is disrupting the team's function or interfering with goal achievement disciplinary action should be considered. In the rare cases of noncompliance or non-adherence to an agreed-upon conflict resolution, the leader or manager will need to seek expert legal counsel within the organization. In most conflicts, the parties are more than willing to comply with the results, and the outcomes prove to be positive. A tool for assessing conflict is identified in Figure 14-2. This tool can be used to determine whether interpersonal or inter-group conflict exists within an organization and whether a given conflict is functional or dysfunctional.

LEADERSHIP AND MANAGEMENT ROLES

Often, the roles of leader and manager are carried out by different people, but both these roles may also be the responsibility of one person. Marquis and Huston (2012) have identified the importance of integrating leadership skills and management functions in dealing with conflict. The manager must be able to discern constructive conflict from destructive conflict. Constructive conflict will result in creativity, innovation, and growth for the individuals concerned. When conflict is destructive, managers must deal appropriately with the conflict or risk follow-up activity that may be more destructive than the original conflict (Marquis & Huston, 2012). A leadership role includes the role modelling of conflict resolution methods as soon as a conflict is evident. Using this strategy, the leader demonstrates awareness, works to resolve intrapersonal or interpersonal conflict, and directs the conflict resolution process towards a goal that lets both parties win. The leader also works to reduce differences in perception about the conflict and tries to encourage each side to see the other's view. The nurse manager or leader assists the conflicting parties to identify techniques that may resolve the conflict and accepts differences between the parties without judgment or accusation. The leader fosters open and honest communication.

The manager role includes the creation of an environment conducive to conflict resolution. The manager uses authority to solve conflicts, which can include competition for immediate or unpopular decisions. When necessary, the manager can facilitate conflict resolution in a formal manner, compete and negotiate for available resources for the unit's needs, and compromise unit goals to achieve another more important unit goal. Ultimately, the manager negotiates consensus or compliance to conflict resolution outcomes or goals. Although the same person may have the roles of both leader and manager, during conflict resolution the leadership role is more important for resolution and compliance. The manager has formal power that can be used when necessary, but this is best reserved for important issues that are truly irresolvable.

Interpersonal or inter-group?

1. Who?
   - Who are the primary individuals or groups involved? What are their characteristics (values, feelings, needs, perceptions, goals, hostilities, strengths, past history of constructive conflict management, self-awareness)?
   - Who, if anyone, are the individuals or groups that have an indirect investment in the result of the conflict?
   - Who, if anyone, is assisting the parties to manage the conflict constructively?
   - What is the history of the individuals' or groups' involvement in the conflict?
   - What is the past and present interpersonal relationship between the parties involved in the conflict?
   - How is power distributed among the parties?
   - What are the major sources of power used?
   - Does the potential for coalition exist among the parties?
   - What is the nature of the current leadership affecting the conflicting parties?

2. What?
   - What is (are) the issue(s) in the conflict?
   - Are the issues based on facts? Based on values? Based on interests in resources?
   - Are the issues realistic?
   - What is the dominant issue in the conflict?
   - What are the goals of each conflicting party?
   - Is the current conflict functional? Dysfunctional?
   - What conflict management strategies, if any, have been used to manage the conflict to date?
   - What alternatives exist for managing the conflict?
   - What are you doing to maintain the conflict?
   - Is there a lack of stimulating work?

3. How?
   - What is the origin of the conflict? Its sources? Precipitating events?
   - What are the major events in the evolution of the conflict?
   - How have the issues emerged? Been transformed? Proliferated?
   - What polarizations and coalitions have occurred?
   - How have parties tried to damage each other? What stereotyping exists?

4. When and Where?
   - When did the conflict originate?
   - Where is the conflict taking place?
   - What are the characteristics of the setting within which the conflict is occurring?
   - What are the geographic boundaries? Political structures? Decision-making patterns? Communication networks? Subsystem boundaries?
   - What environmental factors exist that influence the development of functional versus dysfunctional conflict?
   - What resource persons are available to assist in constructive conflict management?

Functional or dysfunctional?	YES	NO
Does the conflict support the goals of the organization?	[ ]	[ ]
Does the conflict contribute to the overall goals of the organization?	[ ]	[ ]
Does the conflict stimulate improved job performance?	[ ]	[ ]
Does the conflict increase productivity among work group members?	[ ]	[ ]
Does the conflict stimulate creativity and innovation?	[ ]	[ ]
Does the conflict bring about constructive change?	[ ]	[ ]
Does the conflict contribute to the survival of the organization?	[ ]	[ ]

(Continued)

Figure 14-2 Guide for the Assessment of Conflict

	YES	NO
Does the conflict improve initiative?	[]	[]
Does job satisfaction remain high?	[]	[]
Does the conflict improve the morale of the work group?	[]	[]

A yes response to the majority of the questions indicates that the conflict is probably functional. If most of the responses are no, then the conflict is most likely a dysfunctional conflict.

Figure 14-2 (Continued)

CONFLICT MANAGEMENT AND CHANGE

Conflict management and resolution are important parts of the change process. Change can often threaten individuals and groups; thus, conflict is an inevitable part of the process. Keep in mind that some conflicts resolve themselves; the change agent should not be too quick to jump into an intervention mode. Figure 14-3 provides a guide for assessment of the level of conflict. If the level of conflict is too high, the nurse manager must apply conflict resolution strategies.

Is conflict too low?	YES	NO
Is the work group consistently satisfied with the status quo?	[]	[]
Are no or few opposing views expressed by work-group members?	[]	[]
Is little concern expressed about doing things better?	[]	[]
Is little or no concern expressed about improving inadequacies?	[]	[]
Are the decisions made by the work group generally of low quality?	[]	[]
Are no or few innovative solutions or ideas expressed?	[]	[]
Are many work-group members "yes-men"?	[]	[]
Are work-group members reluctant to express ignorance or uncertainties?	[]	[]
Does the nurse manager seek to maintain peace and group cooperation regardless of whether this is the correct intervention?	[]	[]
Do the work-group members demonstrate an extremely high level of resistance to change?	[]	[]
Does the nurse manager base the distribution of rewards on "popularity" as opposed to competence and high job performance?	[]	[]
Is the nurse manager excessively concerned about not hurting the feelings of the nursing staff?	[]	[]
Is the nurse manager excessively concerned with obtaining a consensus of opinion and reaching a compromise when decisions must be made?	[]	[]

A yes response to the majority of these questions can indicate a too-low conflict level in a work group.

Is conflict too high?	YES	NO
Is there an upward and onward spiralling escalation of the conflict?	[]	[]
Are the conflicting parties stimulating the escalation of conflict without considering the consequences?	[]	[]
Is there a shift away from conciliation, minimizing differences, and enhancing goodwill?	[]	[]
Are the issues involved in the conflict being increasingly elaborated and expanded?	[]	[]
Are false issues being generated	[]	[]
Are the issues vague or unclear?	[]	[]

(*Continued*)

Figure 14-3 Guide for the Assessment of Level of Conflict

Is job dissatisfaction increasing among work-group members?	[ ]	[ ]
Is the work-group productivity being adversely affected?	[ ]	[ ]
Is the energy being directed to activities that do not contribute to the achievement of organizational goals (e.g., destroying opposing party)?	[ ]	[ ]
Is the morale of the nursing staff being adversely affected?	[ ]	[ ]
Are extra parties getting dragged into the conflict?	[ ]	[ ]
Is a great deal of reliance on overt power manipulation noted (threats, coercion, deception)?	[ ]	[ ]
Is there a great deal of imbalance in power noted among the parties?	[ ]	[ ]
Are the individuals or groups involved in the conflict expressing dissatisfaction about the course of the conflict and feel that they are losing something?	[ ]	[ ]
Is absenteeism increasing among staff?	[ ]	[ ]
Is there a high rate of turnover among personnel?	[ ]	[ ]
Is communication dysfunctional, not open, mistrustful, and/or restrictive?	[ ]	[ ]
Is the focus being placed on non-conflict relevant to sensitive areas of the other party?	[ ]	[ ]

A yes response to the majority of these questions can be indicative of a conflict level in a work group that is too high.

Figure 14-3 (Continued)

CASE STUDY 14-1

Jane's supervisor has just appointed her to the role of coordinator. However, the current coordinator, Gwen, will remain working in the same department with Jane. Gwen tends to be negative about change and the organization, but she has excellent clinical knowledge.

What do you think Jane should do to help Gwen adjust to the change? Should Jane explore Gwen's feelings about the change? Which situation will be more stressful for Jane—being the coordinator or working with Gwen? Should Jane's supervisor have done something to prepare either Jane or Gwen for this change? What should have been done?

KEY CONCEPTS

- Change is inevitable, exciting, and anxiety provoking.

- Change is defined as making something different from what it was.

- Major change theorists include Lewin, Lippitt, Havelock, and Rogers.

- Senge's model of five disciplines describes the learning organization. This model describes organizations undergoing continuous and unrelenting change.

- The change process is similar to the nursing process.

- Strategies for change include the power-coercive approach, the normative-reeducative approach, and the rational-empirical approach.

- The change agent plays an important role in the change process. The change agent is responsible and accountable for the project.

- Conflict is a normal part of any change project.

- Conflict comes from many sources, including value differences, fear, and goal disagreement.

- The techniques for conflict resolution include avoiding, accommodating, compromising, competing, confronting, collaborating, negotiating, and alternative dispute resolution.

■ There are several strategies for conflict resolution. Clear, open communication is key.

■ Conflict can move the change process along if it is handled well. Conflict can stop the change process if it is handled poorly or allowed to get out of control.

KEY TERMS

change

change agent

conflict

organizational change

personal change

professional change

REVIEW QUESTIONS

1. What is the most desirable conflict resolution technique?
   A. avoiding
   B. competing
   C. negotiating
   D. collaborating

2. What is the most common source of conflict in today's health care organization?
   A. goals
   B. values
   C. resource allocation disputes
   D. competition

3. Which of the following characteristics describe both the change agent and the person responsible for conflict resolution?
   A. secretive and wilful
   B. trustworthy and a good communicator
   C. ambitious and avoiding
   D. powerful and dictatorial

REVIEW ACTIVITIES

1. Select a change project that you have either personally achieved or experienced in a clinical situation. Discuss with your classmates how you felt and how the change agent maintained momentum and enthusiasm for the project. If you chose a personal change, how did you maintain enthusiasm?

2. Recall a conflict you have been involved with in the clinical setting. Discuss each of the methods of conflict resolution identified in the chapter. Identify which methods would have helped. Did the conflict ever get resolved? How?

3. Discuss with a nurse manager how to determine whether a conflict is occurring. What steps does the nurse manager take to bring it out in the open? Share the information with your classmates.

4. Discuss with a nurse manager what it feels like on a personal level to have constant change? How did the nurse manager present an impending change to the staff? Did the nurse manager use any of the techniques discussed in this chapter? Was the change successful?

EXPLORING THE WEB

■ Look up this journal and describe its purpose. Would this journal be useful to the new nurse manager? A new nurse? Anyone else in health care?

■ Journal of Conflict Resolution: *http://jcr.sagepub.com/*

■ The College of Nurses of Ontario has an alternative dispute resolution called the Participative Resolution Program (PRP): *http://www.cno.org/en/search/?q= participative+resolution+process&p=1*. Describe the PRP's resolution process.

REFERENCES

Agnew Peckham Health Care Planning Consultants. (2010). *Forces of change in the health care environment*. Toronto: Author.

Ayers, D. F. (2002). Developing climates for renewal in the community college: A case study of dissipative self-organization. *Community College Journal of Research and Practice, 26*(2), 165–185.

Bennis, W. (1989). *On becoming a leader*. Reading, MA: Addison-Wesley.

Bennis, W., Benne, K., & Chin, R. (Eds.). (1969). *The planning of change* (2nd ed.). New York: Holt, Rinehart, Winston.

Bushy, A. (1993). Managing change: Strategies for continuing education. *The Journal of Continuing Education in Nursing, 23*, 197–200.

College of Nurses of Ontario. (2011). Be a change leader: How to thrive in a changing healthcare environment. *The Standard, 36*(1), 10–12.

Ducharme, J., Buckley, J., Adler, R., & Pelletier, C. (2009). The application of change management principles to facilitate the introduction of nurse practitioners and physician assistants into six Ontario emergency departments. *Healthcare Quarterly, 12*(2), 70–77.

Edgar, L., Herbert, R., Lambert, S., MacDonald, U., Dubois, S., & Latimer, M. (2006). The joint venture model of knowledge utilization: A guide for change in nursing. *Nursing Leadership, 19*(2), 41–55.

Flower, J., & Guillaume, P. (2002). Surfing the edge of chaos. *Health Forum Journal, March/April*, 17–20.

Grossman, S. C., & Valiga, T. M. (2009). *The new leadership challenge: Creating the future of nursing* (3rd ed.). Philadelphia: F. A. Davis.

Havelock, R. G. (1973). *The change agent's guide to innovation in education*. Englewood Cliffs, NJ: Educational Technology.

Heslin, K, & Marr, J. (2008). Building organizational capacity for change. *Healthcare Management Forum, 21*(4), 44–49.

Institute of Medicine. (2010). *The future of nursing leading change, advancing health: Report recommendations*. Retrieved from http://www.iom.edu/nursing

Lancaster, J. (1999). *Nursing issues in leading and managing change*. St. Louis, MO: Mosby.

Lapp, J. (2002). Thriving on change. *Caring Magazine*, 21(5), 40–43.

Lewicki, R. J., Hiam, A., & Olander, K. W. (1996). *Think before you speak*. New York: John Wiley & Sons.

Lewin, K. (1951). *Field theory in social science*. New York: Harper & Row.

Lippit, R., Watson, J., & Westley, B. (1958). *The dynamics of planned change*. New York: Harcourt, Brace.

Marquis, B. L., & Huston, C. J. (2012). *Leadership roles and management functions in nursing: Theory and application* (7th ed.). Philadelphia: Lippincott, Williams & Wilkins.

Nelson Canadian dictionary of the English language. (1997). Toronto: ITP Nelson.

Porter-O'Grady, T., & Malloch, K. (2003). *Quantum leadership: A textbook of new leadership*. Mississauga: Jones & Bartlett Publishers Canada.

Robbins, S., DeCenzo, D. A., & Stuart-Kotze, R. (2002). *Fundamentals of management: Essential concepts and applications* (3rd Canadian ed.). Toronto: Prentice-Hall.

Robbins, S., & Langton, N. (2002). *Organizational behaviour: Concepts, controversies, applications* (2nd Canadian ed.). Toronto: Prentice-Hall.

Rogers, E. M. (1983). *Diffusion of innovations* (3rd ed.). New York: Free Press.

Senge, P. M. (2006). *The fifth discipline: The art and practice of the learning organization*. New York: Doubleday.

Silber, M. B. (1993). The "C"s in excellence: Choice and change. *Nursing Management*, 24(9), 60–62.

Sullivan, E. J. (2004). *Becoming influential: A guide for nurses*. Upper Saddle River, NJ: Pearson/Prentice Hall.

Sullivan, E. J., & Decker, P. J. (2001). *Effective leadership & management in nursing* (5th ed.). Menlo Park, CA: Addison-Wesley.

Swansburg, R. C., & Swansburg, R. J. (1998). *Introductory management and leadership for nurses* (2nd ed., p. 327). Boston: Jones & Bartlett.

Tappen, R. M. (2001). *Nursing leadership and management: Concepts and practice* (4th ed.). Philadelphia: F. A. Davis.

Tappen, R. M., Weiss, S. A., & Whitehead, D. K. (2004). *Essentials of nursing leadership and management* (3rd ed.). Philadelphia: F. A. Davis.

Wagner, C. M., & Huber, D. L. (2003). Catastrophe and nursing turnover: Nonlinear models. *Journal of Nursing Administration*, 33(9), 486–492.

SUGGESTED READINGS

Bennis, W., & Biederman, P. W. (1997). *Organizing genius: The secrets of creative collaboration*. Reading, MA: Addison-Wesley.

Bennis, W., & Nanus, B. (1985). *Leaders: The strategies for taking charge*. New York: Harper & Row.

Duck, J. D. (1993). Managing change: The art of balancing. *Harvard Business Review, November/December,* 109–118.

Heifetz, R. A., & Linsky, M. (2002). A survival guide for leaders. *Harvard Business Review, June,* 65–74.

Heim, P. (1995). Getting beyond "she said, he said." *Nursing Administration Quarterly*, 19(2), 6–18.

Johnson, S. (1998). *Who moved my cheese?* New York: G.P. Putnam.

Jost, S. G. (2000). An assessment and intervention strategy for managing staff needs during change. *Journal of Nursing Administration*, 30(1), 34–40.

Kotter, J. P. (1996). *Leading change*. Boston: Harvard Business School Press.

Marriner-Tomey, A. (2000). *Guide to nursing management and leadership* (6th ed.). St. Louis, MO: Mosby.

McDaniel, R. R. (1997). Strategic leadership: A view from quantum and chaos theories. *Health Care Management Review,* 22(1), 21–37.

McFarland, G., Leonard, H., & Morris, M. (1984). *Nursing leadership and management*. New York: Wiley.

Rosswurm, M. A., & Larrabee, J. H. (1999). A model for change to evidence-based practice. *Image: Journal of Nursing Scholarship,* 31(4), 317–322.

Schweikhart, S. B., & Smith-Daniels, V. (1996). Reengineering the work of caregivers: Role redefinition, team structures, and organization redesign. *Hospital & Health Services Administration,* 41(1), 19–36.

Simms, L. M., Price, S. A., & Ervin, N. E. (2000). *The professional practice of nursing administration* (3rd ed.). Clifton Park, NY: Delmar Learning.

Thietart, R. A., & Forgues, B. (1995). Chaos theory and organizations. *Organization Science,* 6(1), 19–31.

Zukowski, B. (1995). Managing change—before it manages you. *Medical Surgical Nursing,* 4(4), 325–326.

CHAPTER 15

Power

Terry W. Miller, PhD, RN
Adapted by Sandra Trubyk, MSA, BN, BA

We absolutely need people who are skilled at operating and implementing the various systems that make for efficient and consistent delivery of services. Managers play a vital role in overseeing the allocation of resources and clarifying roles and responsibilities of team members. But management is not synonymous with leadership. Our health system needs the transformative power of nurse leaders who will innovate, drive change and inspire those around them to achieve their full potential. (Shamian, 2011)

OBJECTIVES

The purpose of this chapter is to enable the reader to

- define the concept of power;
- identify the various sources of power—coercion, reward, legitimacy, expertise, referent, information, and connection;
- recognize power at a personal level, a professional level, and an organizational level;
- describe how a nurse's perception of power affects client care;
- describe the association of connection power and relationships; and
- explain why nurses are faced with a paradox within the context of information power.

Dale Hogan/iStockphoto

The facility manager, Bryan, has been heard boasting about the authority he has over the nursing staff. Bryan's background is in social work. The hospital has several part-time facility managers with backgrounds in fields other than nursing. Bryan is demanding to make bed changes on the medical ward 2A. The unit nurse, Sara, looks over the charts for clients in 2A and feels that all her clients are appropriate for the ward's program and should not be moved to accommodate a surgical client from the day surgery area.

What would you do if you were Sara?

How would you approach the facility manager, Bryan?

Effective nurses are powerful. They show objectivity, creativity, and knowledge throughout their practice and regardless of their work setting. They have power and can exert it appropriately when they understand the concept of power from multiple perspectives. They use this understanding to motivate others, accomplish organizational goals, and provide safe and competent care. Yet the nursing profession has been criticized for not accepting that they have power and for not knowing enough about it.

Nurses have struggled with the concept of power throughout the profession's history. Many outside the profession continue to challenge the role of nurses in wielding power at any level, including at the bedside. "Globally, the majority of nurses are women. Nurses make up the largest part of the health workforce, but they are at the bottom of the medical hierarchy in terms of authority, remuneration and opportunities" (Canadian Nurses Association, 2010, p. 23). According to a Statistics Canada survey in 2005, women still dominated

the nursing occupation, and male nurses accounted for approximately 5.5 percent of all nurses.[1] Nurses do have great responsibility, and linked to that responsibility is power. In some countries, for example Turkey, women have low status in a patriarchal society and are largely invisible. Women are rarely referred to in official reports on the health care system, even though they make up the majority of health care professionals. Until 2007 men were legally constrained from being nurses. Turkish men and women could take the same nursing education and could have similar work roles, but women were known as nurses and men became health officers. Now in Turkey, the female nurses are fighting to bring more men into the nursing profession so they can gain some power (Herdman, 2008). Nursing has a rich history, and many of its leaders overcame the prejudicial challenges that confronted them. This chapter will discuss power and how nursing power affects client care.

DEFINITIONS OF POWER

Power has been defined in many ways, some of which are not so positive. Typically, **power** is described as the ability to create, acquire, and use resources to achieve one's goals. When a person seeks to achieve goals that are self-determined, this implies greater power than when goals are made either by others or with others. Power can be defined at various levels: personal, professional, or organizational. Power, regardless of level, comes from the ability to influence others or to affect others' thinking or behaviour.

Power at the personal level is closely linked to how an individual perceives power, how others perceive the individual, and the extent to which an individual can influence events. Nurses who feel empowered at a personal level are likely to manifest a high level of self-awareness. They also understand nursing as a profession because it represents the group to which they belong. They also understand the structure and operations of health care because it represents their work environment.

Those perceived as health care experts have significantly more authority and influence, and this makes them more effective in their work than those not perceived as experts. An expert's influence can be manifest in at least two ways: (1) having one's expertise validated by being introduced and promoted to a group as an expert, and (2) becoming an expert by consistently demonstrating one's knowledge, skills, and abilities in practice settings. Remarkably, nurses are often reluctant to be identified as experts in the eyes of clients, physicians, administrators, other nurses, other health care workers, and the public. If the nursing profession is to achieve the status and degree of empowerment it seeks, this lack of awareness must be addressed. Nurses need to realize they have power and expertise and demonstrate this with confidence. The personal power of nurses is evident in the decisions they make on a daily basis. This can be seen in the way they organize their lives and their work so they can accomplish what they want and obtain what they need for themselves and their clients. The more that nurses believe they can influence events through personal effort, the greater their sense of power.

Many accept the idea that if individuals believe they can make a difference and influence events in their lives, they are likely to participate actively in trying to achieve what they want. This kind of participation will make them feel more powerful, even if their efforts are not all that successful. Most of us will try to attain and maintain a

CRITICAL THINKING

The work and contributions of some nurses are so significant that they change the world. To be effective, these nurses define themselves as something far more powerful than what others may want them to be. When we ignore the relevance and significance of nursing history, we discount the contributions nurses have made to improve the lives of others. Our lack of historical awareness empowers others to discount the value of nursing. Ultimately, we limit our own future as nurses by hindering our potential for making even greater contributions to the future of health care.

Name two nurses who represent powerful figures in modern history. (If you need some help, see this chapter's Exploring the Web, page 322.) Why are their contributions so significant?

Can you identify some obstacles they experienced because they were nurses?

REAL WORLD INTERVIEW

In my years of clinical experience, I found the best nursing managers were the ones who gave away some of their power to the nursing staff. These were the managers that did not hover over you on the ward, but let you manage your workload and team. These managers knew when to delegate, to whom they could delegate, and they provided the right tools to perform the job. That is, I was recognized as a professional with sound nursing knowledge, organizational skills, and a caring attitude. This recognition enabled me to grow in my profession and heightened my self-esteem, which I conveyed to the clients I cared for. New graduates need a role model to assist them in improving their skills and knowledge. New graduates also need a leader who will guide but not take away their self-confidence. Managers who hold tightly onto the reins of managing are probably less confident in their own skills and knowledge, and that has an impact on the nurses they manage.

Sandra Martin, MS, RN

REAL WORLD INTERVIEW

We talked about the power of association. By definition, association means ... an organization of people with a common purpose and having a formal structure: it's a fairly simple and straightforward description. However, in my view, understates a critical dimension that is the power of association. Association membership is a commitment that allows each of us to accomplish in a group what we could not do alone. It allows us to pursue our individual passions or support others in the pursuit of their stated goals. In the case of RNAO, this occurs at the chapter, regional or interest group level.

David McNeil
President of RNAO

Source: RNAO Registered Nurse Journal, September/October 2010, p. 5.

power balance. If people feel powerless they may feel victimized. When people think their power is too strong, they can feel a great stress to perform flawlessly (Chilcote & Reece, 2009).

POWER AND ACCOUNTABILITY

Nurses have a professional obligation to view power not merely as a negative concept. Then they can avoid both power struggles and those who seem to savour power. Effective nurses view their ability to understand and use power as a significant part of their responsibilities to clients, their co-workers, the nursing profession, and themselves.

Traditionally, accountability has been considered one of the major hallmarks of the health care professions. Nursing is a profession and, as such, nurses have the primary responsibility for defining and providing nursing services. Yet some nurses appear to have a difficult time understanding the underlying accountability that comes with this powerful claim. Inherent in the role of the nurse are professional accountability and direct responsibility for decisions made and actions rendered.

SOURCES OF POWER

What **sources of power** do you use in your nursing? Chances are you use several types of power and, at times, may not even recognize you are using power. "Although the use of power in human interactions is often viewed negatively, it is a normal part of relationships, because people are frequently influencing and being influenced by one another" (Zastrow, 2009, p. 68). The terms *power* and *influence* can be used interchangeably and refer to having the ability to motivate others to follow through with actions or behaviour in a certain way. Power can be used to influence subordinates or peers or superiors. Power can also be obtained by having up-to-date knowledge on specific areas of health care. Effective nurses use sources of power known as expert, legitimate, referent, reward or coercion, connection, and information power. These are described below.

Expert power is derived from the knowledge and skills that nurses possess. However, special considerations should be kept in mind regarding expertise and power. The rapid explosion of knowledge has made expertise more valuable, and technological advances for accessing information have enabled more people to acquire expertise on any given subject. Someone who holds a legitimate position and also knows more about a subject than others has a decided advantage. However, when those with expertise are not acknowledged in a group, their expert power becomes less effective. When a reciprocal acknowl-

edgement of expertise is visible among group members power becomes balanced and productivity is enhanced. On the other hand, a lack of reciprocal acknowledgement has the opposite effect. The combination of expertise and a high position is most powerful, particularly if someone consistently demonstrates expertise.

Legitimate power is derived from the position a nurse holds in a group, which also indicates the nurse's degree of authority. Registered nurses have legitimate power based on receiving their registration from their regulatory body (Sullivan-Marx & Gray-Micell, 2008). The more comfortable nurses are with their legitimate power as nurses, the easier it is for them to fulfil their roles. Nurses in legitimate positions are expected to use their authority and may be punished for not doing so. Sometimes nurses are given responsibility for leading, but they have too little legitimacy or authority. People generally follow legitimate leaders with whom they agree. Although having legitimacy is a significant part of influence and control, legitimate power is not universally effective and is not sufficient as one's only source of power.

Referent power or charismatic power is derived from the degree to which others respect and like an individual, group, or organization. Nurses who are trusted and respected by others are most able to exert their influence. People want to agree with and follow those with referent leadership. Such leaders tend to be charismatic, and followers often rationalize or explain away any incongruent behaviour to maintain their high level of trust in the referent. It is erroneous to assume that only people who are less intelligent than the charismatic or referent leader will follow that leader. The referent leader who inspires trust and confidence also makes other people feel valuable.

Reward power and coercive power is the ability to reward or punish or create fear in others to influence them to change their behaviour. There are meaningful rewards other than money, such as formal recognition before one's nursing peers at an awards ceremony. The manner in which rewards are distributed is important. Rewards seldom motivate as effectively as a vision that unifies the members of the group. Therefore, reward power is an uncertain instrument for long-term change. Rewards are not likely to permanently change attitudes. Withholding rewards or achieving a goal by instilling fear in others often results in resentment.

People who have the ability to administer punishment or take disciplinary actions against others have coercive power. Wielding this type of power is often considered the least desirable tactic used by people in positions of authority. Typically, people do not enjoy being coerced into doing something and often perceive punishment as humiliating.

All types of power may be used to influence a peer or subordinate but attempting to influence superiors may meet with counter power and leave little choice other than to comply with their wants (Greenberg & Baron, 2000).

Connection power refers to the extent to which nurses are connected with others who have power. Teamwork, collaboration, networking, and mentoring are some of the ways in which nurses can become more connected and therefore more powerful. Leaders can dramatically increase their influence by understanding that people are attracted to those with power and their associates. As a new nurse, when you go to the office of the director of nursing services, or the chief nursing officer, or the president of the health care facility, do not forget that the clerical workers in the outside office have relationships with their boss—thus, they have connection power. If you try to go around them and take their power lightly, or insult or patronize them, you risk your own power base in relation to the director, or chief nursing officer, or president. Similarly, if a nurse bypasses a person who is directly responsible for a situation, the attempted circumvention reflects negatively on the nurse. Nurses should work to resolve issues at the appropriate level before they take their concerns to a higher level of authority. Nurses are expected to understand the structure and policies of the organizations in which they provide services.

Information power refers to peoples' ability to influence others by means of the information they provide to a group. Authoritarian leaders attempt to control information. Charismatic leaders provide information that is seductive for many people. Information leaders provide a sense of stability with the use and synthesis of information. If one knows how to get it and what to do with it, the greatest power may be in information.

Regardless of a nurse's leadership style, information plays an increasingly critical role. Legitimate power, reward power, and coercive power tend to be bestowed on individuals by their organizations. These forms of power tend to be effective for a short period of time only, unless accompanied by another form of power such as information power. Information power is especially important because, to be functional, health care teams and organizations require accurate and timely information that is shared. To be seen by others as having information power, nurses must share knowledge that is both accurate and useful. Information sharing can improve client care, increase collegiality, enhance organizational effectiveness, and strengthen one's professional connections. See Table 15-1 for a summary of the different types of power.

Nurse managers can have legitimate power due to their position in a health care facility and also other forms of power, such as expertise and charisma. They must decide what sources of power to use in each situation and with

TABLE 15-1	PRINCIPLES FOR UNDERSTANDING AND USING DIFFERENT TYPES OF POWER
Concept	**How It Works**
Expert power	—obtained based on knowledge and skills in a particular area of nursing
Legitimate power	—based on an individual's position within a group or organization; commonly associated with having a formal job authority or a position of influence on the unit
Referent power	—derived from desirable personal qualities, having vision, ability to inspire confidence, ability to influence actions of others based on charisma, and being liked and respected by peers and others
Reward and coercive power	—rewarding or punishing or creating fear in others to influence change in their behaviour
Connection power	—based on strong personal and professional relationships, having enhanced resources, capacity for learning and information sharing, and ability to increase one's overall sphere of influence
Information power	—possessions can be taken away, but one's internalized information, such as knowledge and wisdom, cannot be taken away. Information helps people exert their influence on others, regardless of whether the other has provided consent (Srinath, 2006).

TABLE 15-2	CHARACTERISTICS OF A POWERFUL PROFESSIONAL PRACTICE

1. Nurses with a powerful practice acknowledge their unique role in the provision of client-centred and family-centred care.

2. Nurses with a powerful practice commit to continuous learning through education, skill development, and evidence-based practice.

3. Nurses with a powerful practice demonstrate professional comportment and recognize the critical nature of presence.

4. Nurses with a powerful practice value collaboration, and they partner effectively with colleagues in nursing and other disciplines.

5. Nurses with a powerful practice strive to develop an impeccable character: to be inspirational, compassionate, and to have a credible, sought-after perspective.

6. Nurses with a powerful practice position themselves to influence decisions and resource allocation.

7. Nurses with a powerful practice recognize that the role of the nurse leader is to pave the way for nurses' voices to be heard and to help novice nurses develop into powerful professionals.

8. Nurses with a powerful practice evaluate the power of nursing and the nursing department in organizations they enter, by assessing the organization's mission and values and its commitment to enhancing the power of diverse perspectives.

Source: Adapted from Authors and Disclosures. (2010). The power of professional nursing practice: Discussion sessions about power with nurse leaders. *OJIN, The Online Journal of Issues in Nursing,* 12(1). Retrieved from http://www.medscape.com/viewarticle/553405_3

particular individuals in order to meet their goals. When they do so, they are using a power strategy, that is, a plan to use their sources of power in relation to key individuals and groups so there can be similar sources of power on both sides of an argument (Hibberd & Smith, 2006).

See Table 15-2 for a summary of the characteristics of a powerful professional practice.

PERSONAL ORIENTATION AND THE INTERNET

A person may desire power for impact, strength, or influence. In the simplest terms, the desire for power takes one of two forms: (1) an orientation toward achieving personal gain and self-glorification, or (2) an orientation toward achieving gain for others or the common good. The idea that power is corruptive or evil is reflected in the 19th-century quote attributed to Lord Acton: "All power corrupts, but absolute power corrupts absolutely" (Bothamley, 1993). According to this perspective, some believe that people who have power should not have power because they will potentially misuse it. They also

believe that people who desire power should not be trusted because their motivation is inherently wrong—their desire for power is for personal gain at any cost.

Many believe the Internet will level the playing field of power for everyone. The free flow of information will empower nurses and others—that is, all those who have access to the Internet and have the ability to use it effectively.

EMPOWERMENT AND DISEMPOWERMENT

Manojlovich (2007) suggests that there are compelling reasons to empower nurses. Powerless nurses are ineffective nurses. They are less satisfied with their jobs and more susceptible to burnout. Although information technology and the Internet have given us access to information worldwide, and allowed for quick response, they have also raised the standards for success and effectiveness. Consequently, leaders and managers must be able to see the wealth of talent in their staff. Empowered employees are engaged, involved, and they assist to a great extent in improving outcomes for both the organization and the client. In order to be empowered, individuals need to recognize the power that exists in their experience, knowledge, and internal motivation (Carlos, Randolph, & Blanchard, 2009).

In the late 1960s and early 1970s, and related to the self-help and political awareness movements, the concept of **empowerment** emerged (Ryles, 1999). Chandler (1986) was among the first to describe the process of empowerment in nursing. Chandler (1992) also distinguished between power and empowerment, noting that empowerment enables one to act, whereas power connotes having control, influence, or domination. Ongoing research on empowerment in nursing has demonstrated that highly motivated, empowered nurses share their sources of power in order to motivate and empower others (Laschinger & Havens, 1996). Empowered nurses experience less burnout (Laschinger, Finegan, Shamian, & Wilk, 2003) and less job strain (Laschinger, Finegan, & Shamian, 2001). Disempowerment creates feelings of frustration and failure in staff nurses.

By empowering others, the nursing manager passes on responsibility and, with it, authority. To effectively empower others to meet planned goals, the manager should share the appropriate information and knowledge with the staff nurse (Greenberg & Baron, 2000).

Nurses empower themselves and others in many ways. Basically, they empower others because they perceive them to be powerful. If an individual, a group, or an organization is perceived as being powerful, that perception can empower that individual, group, or organization. Some health care provider groups are viewed as more powerful than others because of the alliances they have formed with associations that are known to be powerful, such as the Canadian Medical Association (CMA). Similarly, nurses disempower themselves if they see nurses or nursing as powerless.

ROLE OF THE MEDIA

People who work in the media recognize the relationship between power and perception. Those who work in advertising, marketing, and public relations understand that public perceptions can be created or changed through advertising and marketing campaigns, damage control, timely press releases, and well-orchestrated media events.

The media can present nursing to the public in ways that can either empower or disempower nursing. Nurses have not consistently used the media as effectively as other more powerful occupational groups. To date the media have failed to recognize nursing as one of the largest groups in health care. It is hoped that the media's coverage of the rapidly growing nursing shortage over the next decade will improve public perception of nursing as a career and human service. The media need to show nurses as decision-makers, coordinators of care, and primary care providers, as well as those who follow orders in the health care field. Too often the media has presented a stereotypical, insignificant view of nurses,

and too often nurses fail to view nursing as the honourable profession it is.

One strategy for empowering nursing is to employ the media to create a stronger, more powerful image of nursing. For this strategy to succeed more nurses need to become active participants in a formal part of their profession: the Canadian Nurses Association (CNA); their provincial or territorial regulatory body and professional association; or one of the nursing specialty organizations, such as the Canadian Association of Critical Care Nurses (CACCN) or the Canadian Hospice Palliative Care Association (CHPCA).

A PLAN FOR PERSONAL EMPOWERMENT

A novice nurse who understands power can become more effective, make better decisions, and better help others. It is important for nurses both personally and professionally to understand power from a variety of perspectives. By doing so, nurses can gain more control of their work lives and their personal lives.

The future can be imagined in three ways: (1) what is possible, (2) what is probable, and (3) what is preferred. As a nurse who wants to experience a preferred future, think about what is happening to you as a person and as a nurse, what possibilities you have as a person and as a nurse, and what you are going to do about it.

POWER AND THE LIMITS OF INFORMATION

Even if nurses could fully trust the completeness and accuracy of information they have in their practice, they would have insufficient data. Things are always changing; therefore, information always needs to be updated. Nurses should never stop assessing and gathering information. To make good decisions, nurses must be able to gather enough data and realistically interpret its value, as well as share and apply information in a safe, competent manner. Effective nurses understand time constraints and set priorities to ensure that what is most important receives the most attention. These nurses are willing to take the inherent risk of making a decision, while understanding there will always be more information to gather and analyze. They recognize that choosing to make no decision is a decision in itself and that information is never complete. Table 15-3 presents a framework for becoming empowered using information.

TABLE 15-3	A FRAMEWORK FOR BECOMING EMPOWERED USING INFORMATION
Background	As an empowered nurse, you have the ability to discover important information and to use it to your advantage, as well as to the advantage of your clients.
Steps	■ Find and maintain good sources of information. ■ Get involved beyond direct client care. ■ Ask questions. ■ Listen to and analyze the answers. ■ Make a plan with the information acquired. ■ Evaluate the plan.
Information for providing care	■ Assess the client's condition using relevant, objective measurements. ■ Consult with other nurses, physicians, and other health care workers involved in the care of your clients. ■ Consult with the client's significant others, family members, and friends.
Information for becoming more effective in the work setting	■ Get involved beyond direct client care. ■ Volunteer for committee assignments that will challenge you to learn and experience more than what is expected of you in a staff nurse role. ■ Think about the following when involved with committees: 1. What is the committee trying to do? 2. What specific information does the committee use to make decisions? 3. How does the committee's work apply to my practice, my colleagues, my clients, my organizational unit, and the organization as a whole? ■ Assess the strength of the information you have in relation to your clients, your colleagues, your organizational unit, the organization as a whole, and the profession of nursing. ■ Readily share information with others who will value it and use it to a good end.
Evaluation	Periodically, re-examine your plans. Did you achieve your expected outcomes? If not, why not? Were there staffing problems or client crises? Were the activities that were necessary for outcome achievement carried out? What have you learned from this evaluation that you can apply to the future?

CRITICAL THINKING

Are you interested in becoming the best nurse possible? Do you enjoy meeting and associating with people who are successful? Do you feel most comfortable when you are in control over personal situations? Do you feel uncomfortable when you have little or no influence over the actions of others? Responding yes to these questions suggests that you have motives for personal achievement, being affiliated with others, and having power. **Achievement** refers to accomplishment of goals through effort. **Affiliation** refers to associations and relationships with others. From a behavioural perspective achievement, affiliation and power are interrelated and can be positive attributes of one's personality. Or, they can lead to highly destructive behaviour. A person's need for affiliation and power are predominantly interpersonal. The need for achievement is predominantly intrapersonal, that is, motivated by a personal conviction to be capable and competent. People with high achievement needs tend to rely on themselves to get things done. They activate their intrapersonal motivation. Consequently, they expend a high degree of energy and focus on improving their personal skills and learning new things. Depending on their past experiences and current interests, nurses engage in a variety of behaviours that reflect their needs for achievement, affiliation, or power Can you think of two nurses who are highly motivated in terms of their achievements, position, and power? Would these two nurses be role models for you? Why, or why not?

REAL WORLD INTERVIEW

Ms Cox is 38 years old and has been hospitalized four times. She underwent surgery this past spring and has encountered nursing care and nurses in various roles throughout the health care system. Ms Cox is articulate and reflective. She earned a degree in English and currently holds a position at a selective liberal arts university as an admissions counsellor. She states, "I don't think nurses know they are powerful.... Nurses can take on more than they think they can. They have the power to change the system in which they work. Yet I see nurses as the most overworked, underpaid, and underachieving professions also. There is so much more they could be doing if they didn't spend so much time railing against the machine. They are telling the wrong people—each other—that they are frustrated. They should be telling the ones with real power, or better yet, more of them should become the ones in power. Instead, they suffer with each other and stay angry. It appears almost passive-aggressive how nurses deal with power. My concern is that it can affect client care in such a negative way. Believe me when I say clients value nurses, but the people writing the paycheque for nurses must value nurses. Clients need nursing far more than they need anything else. The better nurses who have cared for me have been instrumental in my healing. Beyond knowing when I need medication or doing some procedure, it is the smile, the touch, and the well-placed word of encouragement that has gotten me through. This is where nurses have power because no one but a real nurse can provide it. It comes from the heart."

Audrey Cox (Client)

MACHIAVELLI ON POWER

Machiavelli wrote in his political treatise, *The Prince*, "There is nothing more difficult to try, nor more doubtful of success, nor more dangerous to deal with, than to take it upon oneself to introduce new institutions, because the introducer makes enemies out of all those who benefit from the old institutions and is feebly defended by all those who might benefit from the new ones" (Machiavelli, 1532/1996, p. 51).

CASE STUDY 15-1

Maria and Haley work on the same nursing unit in a large, metropolitan hospital. Both predominantly work the evening shift and have less than one year's experience since graduating from nursing school. Maria has been offered increasingly difficult client assignments, been entrusted with charge duties and, recently, was selected for a two-week leadership training program.

Haley has not adapted as well and has withdrawn from what was once a close friendship with Maria. Haley seeks consolation with the nurses she and Maria claimed they would never emulate. Haley takes her breaks and eats dinner with two nurses who complain that the best nurses are undervalued in the organization, yet these same nurses were not supportive of Maria or Haley or any other new nurses oriented to their unit.

Maria seeks out others she perceives to be knowledgeable and more satisfied in their professional roles. She strives to participate in non-mandatory meetings as well as clinical rounds, using them as an opportunity to ask questions. Thus, she is beginning to increase her personal level of power by connecting with the other staff and gathering information.

One night after a difficult shift, Haley accuses Maria of abandoning her and playing up to administration, and says that Maria is being used by the unit's nurse manager. Haley tells Maria that the other nurses are planning to file a complaint against the unit supervisor for selecting Maria to attend the leadership training program over the nurses that have been on the unit longer.

How should Maria respond to Haley?

LITERATURE APPLICATION

Citation: Manojlovich, M. (2007). Power and empowerment in nursing: Looking backward to inform the future. *OJIN: The Online Journal of Issues in Nursing,* Vol. 12(1), Manuscript 1.

Discussion: This article begins with an examination of the concept of power and provides an historical review of nurses' power over nursing practice. It describes what kinds of power over nursing care are required for nurses to make the best possible contributions to practice. The current state of nursing empowerment related to nursing care is the final area of review. The author suggests that three components need to be present for nurses to be empowered: (1) a workplace that has the requisite structures to promote empowerment, (2) a psychological belief in one's ability to be empowered, and (3) acknowledgement that there is power in the relationships and caring that nurses provide.

Implications for Practice: Nursing research has demonstrated the relationship between the first two components and empowerment. However, further research is needed to examine the power that exists in relationships. A more thorough understanding of these three components may help nurses to become empowered, and use their power for their practice and for better client care.

REAL WORLD INTERVIEW

Power is the ultimate responsibility one has in caring for the client. Our assessment and subsequent actions can determine whether a client will live or die. I feel confident in my abilities for the future, but as a new nurse, it is difficult to feel powerful because there is so much to learn. I believe that nurses tend to perceive power as being able to stand up to those above or higher up in the work setting. I think nursing is changing for the better because of the power gained with nurses having more autonomy. There is more trust put into the nurse's judgment because women's roles in society have changed and more men are entering the profession. Equal opportunity programs have created the structure to protect women and others who have been vulnerable to those in positions of greater power. I have learned that you do not have to be afraid to advocate for your client. If you need to call the attending physician during the night, then you do it. I have come to realize that power is not abusing the people working under you. Also, to understand power, it is important to understand people's roles and where they are coming from.

Julie Bergman
New Nursing Graduate

KEY CONCEPTS

- Effective nurses are powerful. They show objectivity, creativity, and knowledge throughout their practice and regardless of their work setting.

- Effective nurses have power and exert it appropriately by understanding the concept of power from multiple perspectives. They then use this understanding to motivate others, accomplish organizational goals, and provide safe, competent care.

- Power has been described as the ability to create, acquire, and use resources to achieve one's goals.

- Power can be defined at a personal level, a professional level, and an organizational level.

- The personal and information power of nurses is evident in the decisions they make.

- Hibberd and Smith (2006) help the nurse to understand how different people perceive power by describing sources of power as expert, legitimate, referent, reward and coercive, connection, and information.

KEY TERMS

achievement	legitimate power
affiliation	power
connection power	referent power
empowerment	reward power and coercive power
expert power	sources of power
information power	

REVIEW QUESTIONS

1. Which of the following describes how the most effective nurses use power?
   A. in one primary way
   B. to influence others or affect others' thinking or behaviour
   C. predominantly at an organizational level
   D. only to gain the necessary resources to be a better nurse

2. How has power been described in the literature?
   A. consistently as a negative concept
   B. most often as a manifestation of personal ambition
   C. as maintained through one's position in society, a work setting, or family
   D. in multiple ways, some not so positive

3. People sometime fear another person enough to act or behave differently from how they would otherwise. Which of the following is the name for the source of the other person's power?
   A. coercive power
   B. reward power
   C. expert power
   D. connection power

4. What source of power has become increasingly important because of technological innovation in the past decade?
   A. expert power
   B. information power
   C. connection power
   D. legitimate power

5. In which of the following ways do nurses disempower themselves?
   A. by facilitating the participation of others in decision making
   B. by taking action within an environment where there is an equitable distribution of power
   C. by believing they are empowered
   D. by discounting the role the media plays in the public's perception of nursing

6. In which of the following ways can a nurse's personal power be enhanced?
   A. by collaborating with colleagues on special projects outside the work setting
   B. by developing skills that do not apply directly to client care
   C. by volunteering to serve on organizational committees led by people who are not nurses
   D. all of the above

REVIEW ACTIVITIES

1. Identify a nursing leader. Observe this person and note the type of power this leader uses to meet objectives.

2. Watch a television show that portrays nurses. Note how nurses use or do not use the different types of power available to them. What do you observe?

3. Observe our national leaders. What examples of the use of power do you see? Is power used in helpful or unhelpful ways? Explain.

EXPLORING THE WEB

Visit the following sites for information on nursing leaders and nursing history:

- *http://www.cna-aiic.ca/cna/search/default_e.aspx?cx=0 17995081769602664776%3Amo7p1eqo4vc&cof=FORID %3A11&ie=UTF-8&q=nursing+leaders+and+nursing+ history'#1042*

- *http://www.chsrf.ca/browsebytopic/results. aspx?tag=Leadership*

- *http://www.longwoods.com/home.php?cat=252*

- *http://www.chsrf.ca/browsebytopic/results. aspx?tag=Research+capacity*

Visit the following sites for information on power, leadership, and women:

- *http://www.guide2womenleaders.com/*

- *http://feminine-leadership.com/*

- *http://ksgexecprogram.harvard.edu/Programs/wp/ overview.aspx*

Visit the following sites for information on political power for clients:

- *http://www.nursingworld.org/MainMenuCategories/ ANAMarketplace/ANAPeriodicals/OJIN/TableofCon- tents/Volume122007/No1Jan07/tpc32_216091.aspx*

- *http://www.nursingworld.org/MainMenuCategories/ ANAMarketplace/ANAPeriodicals/OJIN/TableofCon- tents/Volume112006/No1Jan06/ArticlePreviousTopic/ KibbutzNursing.aspx*

- *http://www.i2i.org/main/article.php?article_id=1112*

- *http://www.healthcarereform.net*

The following sites discuss a variety of nursing resources and issues, including collective power:

- *http://www.cna-nurses.ca/cna/default_e.aspx*

- *http://www.nursingworld.org*

Go to the site for the Ontario Training Centre for Health Services and Policy

- *http://www.otc-hsr.ca/.* Note the onsite and online courses offered to nurses interested in health policy.

Here are some other sites related to health policy:

- *http://www.cihr-irsc.gc.ca/e/13733.html*

- *http://chspr.queensu.ca/*

- *http://www.chspr.ubc.ca/*

REFERENCES

Aiken, L. H., Clarke, S. P., Sloane, D. M., Sochalski, J., & Silber, J. H. (2002). Hospital nurse staffing and patient mortality, nurse burnout, and job dissatisfaction. *JAMA*, 288(16), 1987–1993.

Authors and Disclosures. (2010). The power of professional nursing practice: Discussion sessions about power with nurse leaders. *OJIN, The Online Journal of Issues in Nursing*, 12(1). Retrieved from http://www.medscape.com/viewarticle/553405_3

Bothamley, J. (1993). *Dictionary of theories*. London: Gale Research International.

Bower, F. L. (2000). *Nurses taking the lead: Personal qualities of effective leadership*. Philadelphia: Saunders.

Canadian Nurses Association. (2010). Access – Taking action on gender equity. *Canadian Nurse*, 106(9), 23.

Carlos, J. P., Randolph, A. & Blanchard, K. (2009). *Empowerment takes more than a minute; engage people and watch your organization soar* (2nd ed.). San Francisco: Berrett-Koehlar.

Chandler, G. E. (1986). *The relationship of nursing work environment to empowerment and powerlessness*. Unpublished doctoral dissertation, University of Utah, Salt Lake City, UT.

Chandler, G. E. (1992). The source and process of empowerment. *Nursing Administration Quarterly*, 16(3), 65–71.

Chilcote, A., & Reece, S. (2009). Power Paradox. *Leadership Excellence*, 12(6), 8–9.

Greenberg, J., & Baron, R. (2000). *Behavior in organizations* (7th ed.). Upper Saddle River, NJ: Prentice Hall.

Herdman, E. (2008). Gender equality or patriarchal dividend: Structural change in Turkish nursing. *Nursing and Health Sciences*, 10(2), 159–163.

Hibberd, J. M., & Smith, D. L. (2006). *Nursing leadership and management in Canada* (3rd ed.). Toronto: Elsevier Canada.

Kelly, L. Y., & Joel, L. A. (1996). *The nursing experience: Trends, challenges, and transitions* (3rd ed.). New York: McGraw-Hill.

Laschinger, H. K. S., Finegan, J., & Shamian, J. (2001). Promoting nurses' health: Effect of empowerment on job strain and work satisfaction. *Nurses Economics*, 19(2), 42–52.

Laschinger, H. K. S., Finegan, J., Shamian, J., & Wilk, P. (2003). Workplace empowerment as a predictor of nurse burnout in restructured healthcare settings. *Hospital Quarterly*, 6(4), 2–11.

Laschinger, H. K. S., & Havens, D.S. (1996) Staff nurse work empowerment and perceived control over nursing practice: Conditions for work effectiveness. *JONA*, 26(9), 27–35.

Laschinger, H. K. S., & Wong, C. (1999). Staff nurse empowerment and collective accountability: Effect on perceived productivity and self-rated work effectiveness. *Nursing Economics*, 17(6), 308–316.

Machiavelli, N. (1996). *The prince* (P. Sonnino, Trans.). Atlantic Highlands, NJ: Humanities Press International. (Original work published 1532)

Manojlovich, M. (2007). Power and empowerment in nursing: Looking backward to inform the future. *OJIN, The Online Journal of Issues in Nursing*, 12 (1), Manuscript 1. Retrieved from http://www.nursingworld.org/MainMenuCategories/ANAMarketplace/ANA...ents/Volume122007/No1Jan07/LookingBackwardtoInformtheFuture.aspx

Marquis, B. L., & Huston, C. J. (2009). *Leadership roles and management functions in nursing: theory and application* (6th ed.). Philadelphia: Lippincott, Williams, & Wilkins.

Matthews, S., Laschinger, H. K. S., & Johnstone, L. (2006). Staff nurse empowerment in line and staff organizational structures for chief nurse executives. *Journal of Nursing Administration*, 36(11), 526–533.

McNeil, D. (2010). President's view: Power in association. *RNAO Registered Nurse Journal, September/October,* 5.

Nasrabadi, A. N., Lipsion, J. G., & Emami, A. (2004). Professional nursing in Iran: An overview of its historical and sociocultural framework. *Professional Nurse*, 20(6), 396–402.

Rowland, H. S., & Rowland, B. L. (1997). *Nursing administration handbook*. Rockville, MD: Aspen.

Ryles, S. M. (1999). A concept analysis of empowerment: Its relationship to mental health nursing. *Journal of Advanced Nursing*, 29(3), 600–607.

Shamian, J. (2011). President's Message. *Canadian Nurse*, 107(3), 4. Retrieved from http://www.canadian-nurse.com/index.php?option=com_content&view=article7id=357%

Srinath, S. (2006). *The power law of information: Life in a connected world*. Thousand Oaks, CA: Sage Publications.

Sullivan-Marx, E. M., & Gray-Micell, D. (2008). *Leadership and management skills for long-term care*. New York: Springer.

Zastrow, C. J. (2009). *Social work with groups: A comprehensive workbook* (7th ed.). Belmont, CA: Thomson Brooks/Cole, Cengage Learning.

SUGGESTED READINGS

Anderson, M. A. (2001). *Nursing leadership, management, and professional practice for the LPN/LVN* (2nd ed.). Philadelphia: F. A. Davis.

Apker, J., Ford, W. S. Z., & Fox, D. H. (2003). Predicting nurses' organizational and professional identification: The effect of nursing roles, professional autonomy, and supportive communication. *Nursing Economics,* 21(5), 226–232.

Belle, F. (2002). Women managers and organizational power. *Women in Management Review,* 17(3/4), 151–156.

Benner, P. E. (2000). *From novice to expert: Excellence and power in clinical nursing practice* (commemorative ed.). Upper Saddle River, NJ: Prentice Hall.

Denis, J. L., Lamoth, L., & Langley, A. (2001). The dynamics of collective leadership and strategic change in pluralistic organizations. *Academy of Management Journal,* 44(4), 809–837.

Fairhurst, G. T. (2010). *The power of framing: Creating the language of leadership*. San Francisco: John Wiley and Sons.

Hanna, L. A. (1999). Lead the way. *Nursing Management,* 30(11), 36–39.

Haslam, S. A., Reicher, S. D. and Turner, J. C. (2010). *The new psychology of leadership: Identity, influence and power*. New York: Psychology Press.

Kellerman, B. (2010). *Leadership: Essential selections on power, authority and influence*. New York: McGraw-Hill.

Kuokkanen, L., & Katajisto, J. (2003). Promoting or impeding empowerment? Nurses' assessments of their work environment. *JONA,* 33(4), 209–15.

Leddy, S., & Pepper, J. M. (1998). *Conceptual bases of professional nursing* (4th ed.). Philadelphia: Lippincott.

Leiter, M. P., & Laschinger, H. K. S. (2006). Relationships of work and practice environment to professional burnout. *Nursing Research,* 55(2), 137–146.

Short, P. M. (1998). Empowering leadership. *Contemporary Education,* 69(2), 70–72.

Spitzer, K. L., Eisenbery, M. B., & Lowe, C. A. (1998). *Information literacy essential skills for the information age*. Syracuse, NY: ERIC Clearinghouse on Information & Technology.

Stelter, N. (2002). Gender differences in leadership: Current social issues and future organizational implications. *Journal of Leadership and Organizational Studies,* 8(4), 88–99.

CHAPTER ENDNOTE

1. Health Canada, Health Care System, "Findings from the 2005 National Survey of the Work and Health of Nurses." Retrieved from http://www.hc-sc.gc.ca/hcs-sss/pubs/nurs-infirm/2005-nurse-infirm/index-eng.php

CHAPTER 16

Managing Performance and Outcomes Using an Organizational Quality Improvement Model

Mary McLaughlin, RN, MBA
Karen Houston, RN, MS
Adapted by Heather Crawford, BScN, MEd, CHE

*Opportunity is missed by most
people because it is dressed in
overalls and looks like work.*
(Thomas Edison)

OBJECTIVES

The purpose of this chapter is to enable the reader to

- articulate the major principles of quality and continuous quality improvement (CQI), including customer identification, participation at all levels, and process improvement rather than criticism of individual performance;

- describe how quality improvement affects the client and the organization;

- identify how data are used for continuous quality improvement (CQI);

- describe the difference between enterprise risk management and CQI; and

- describe how the principles of CQI are implemented in an organization.

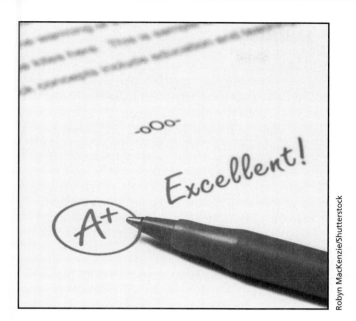

Robyn MacKenzie/Shutterstock

Saskatchewan's Health Quality Council (HQC) was launched in 2003 with a mandate to not only measure and report on healthcare but also work with a range of partners to improve the province's health system. In late 2007, HQC's board decided it was time for Saskatchewan to reinvent its healthcare system, using the highest performing systems in the world as its model. And in 2008, HQC launched Accelerating Excellence, a multi-level program to rethink, redesign, and renew healthcare.

To help maintain momentum and show other provinces whether high-performing healthcare can be achieved in Canada, HQC is documenting its journey.

Like instant gratification? Don't look for a job in quality improvement.

"It's hard. It's one of those jobs where you never go home and think, 'I have done everything I could today. My desk is clear,'" admits Felecia Watson, director of quality improvement and strategic planning for Sun Country Health Region in Southeastern Saskatchewan. Instead, Watson finds herself struggling daily to choose among dozens of Sun Country activities that would benefit from a systematic quality improvement exercise.

Continuous quality improvement has been shown to be a powerful tool to help make health care organizations more effective. Rondeau and Wagar (2002) report that it is generally believed that the failure of most total quality management (TQM) and continuous quality improvement programs is not the result of flaws in either the philosophy or the principles of quality improvement but the result of ineffective implementation systems. These sources of failure include

---

Source: Coutts, J. (2011). Small Steps ... Improving Quality One Team at a Time in Saskatchewan. *Healthcare Quarterly,* 14(1): 25.

a lack of commitment and understanding on the part of organizational leaders and ineffective management of the change process. The improvement philosophies of quality experts, such as Deming (1986) and Crosby (1989), also emphasize the commitment of management.

Quality improvement is described as both a science and an art. The science of improvement is the development of new ideas, the testing of those ideas, and the implementation of change. As Langley, Nolan, Norman, Provost, and Nolan (1996) described, W. Edwards Deming has provided an important contribution to the science of improvement. Deming's components of appreciating a system, understanding variation, and applying knowledge and psychology are fundamental improvement principles. Quality improvement is also described as an art that taps into creative, out-of-the-box ideas. It is about systematically testing new ideas to improve customer care. Health care customers include clients, families, staff, community, and agencies. If the change is planned, measured, and does not negatively affect the quality of customer care, the possibilities for what can be achieved are limitless.

Adapting the concepts of science and art in improving health care can create an enthusiasm for change and a passion for results. This chapter will discuss and provide examples of the application and implementation of quality improvement principles in a health care setting.

HISTORY OF QUALITY ASSURANCE

Berwick Blanton Godfrey, and Roessner (1991) suggested that process complexity results in a tremendous amount of waste and rework. Some studies suggest the amount of waste and rework can amount to 25 to 30 percent of total costs of production. Consider Berwick and Plsek's red bead example (1992): In a group of beads in a bag, there are 90 blue beads and 10 red beads. There are four workers whose job it is to take blue beads out of a bag. They cannot see what colour bead they are taking. The supervisor watches to see how many red beads are pulled out of the bag. The first day, worker A has 1 red bead, worker B has 4 red beads, worker C has 3 red beads, and worker D has 2 red beads. The supervisor states that worker A has done a great job and worker B has done a terrible job. He tells them they have to improve. The beads go back in the bag and they start over the next day. This day, worker A has 4 red beads, worker B has 0 red beads, worker C has 2 red beads, and worker D has 4 red beads. The supervisor praises worker B for the improvement and yells at workers A and D for not doing a good

CRITICAL THINKING

Children with cancer, who present to an Emergency Department (ED), with a fever and who have a low white blood cell count (Febrile Neutropenia) require timely assessment and administration of antibiotics. In December, 2003, a Child Health Standards audit indicated the average time from triage to antibiotic administration was 5 hours. Opportunities for improvement were identified.

A working group, established in June 2004, developed a physicians' standard order sheet that was implemented in the Children's Hospital ED in December 2004. During the next year, twenty-four children were admitted from the ED to the inpatient oncology unit with Febrile Neutropenia. An analysis of the charts has shown that the average time from triage to antibiotic administration has decreased to 1.46 hours—a significant improvement in providing safe and timely care (see Figure 16-1).

Congratulations to the ED staff for all their support of and interest in this initiative. Thank you to the members of the Febrile Neutropenia Working Group.

What would you have done to improve the quality of care? How could you bring your ideas to other staff members without making them feel that the quality of their care was being criticized? What measures would you use to ensure that while you were improving some aspects of care, you were not decreasing other critical outcome measures?

Source: Galloway, L. (2006). "Improving Timeliness of Care." *Quality for Kids Newsletter,* 5(1): 2. Reprinted with permission of Winnipeg Regional Health Authority.

job. The truth is these workers do not have any ability to change the number of red beads that they pull out of the bag.

This example demonstrates random variation. Using reward or punishment in the face of random variation results in tampering with the system rather than quality improvement. The tampering encourages staff to look for someone to blame rather than changing the process to improve outcomes. So the question is, How much variability can reasonably be expected? Variability can be calculated on a time series chart, discussed in detail later in this chapter.

Quality assurance (QA) emerged in health care in the 1950s. It began as a method of inspection to ensure that health care institutions—mainly hospitals—maintained minimum standards of care. Quality assurance's methods consisted primarily of chart audits of various client diagnoses and procedures. For example, nurses completed chart audits to determine whether or not bowel movements had been documented on the graphic vital signs sheet! The use of Quality assurance grew over time. QA departments became the organizational mechanism for measuring performance against standards and reporting incidents and errors, such as mortality and morbidity rates. This approach was reactive and fixed the errors after a problem was noted. The method was thought to be punitive, with its emphasis on "doing it right," and did little to sustain change or proactively identify prob-

lems before they occurred. The culture was one of blame rather than learning. It did, however, accomplish the task of monitoring minimum standards of performance.

TOTAL QUALITY MANAGEMENT

Total quality management (TQM), also referred to as continuous quality improvement (CQI) and **performance improvement (PI),** began in the manufacturing industry with W. Edwards Deming and Joseph Juran in the 1950s. The total quality management approach revolutionized the industrial world with the search for manufacturing excellence through higher productivity, lower cost, and a competitive edge. Deming is credited with being the main generating force in Japan's post–World War II rise to manufacturing excellence as a world industrial leader. The lessons learned from Deming's strategy for quality are applicable to the achievement of excellence and quality in health care management.[1]

Seeman and Brown (2006) reviewed Peter Drucker's most significant writings, including his prediction in the 1940s of the rise of the knowledge worker. They conducted an empirical review of his impact on contemporary quality improvement principles in health care by examining academic citations to his work and ideas. In their article, Seeman and Brown cited Drucker's 1988 article, "The Coming of the New Organization" published in the

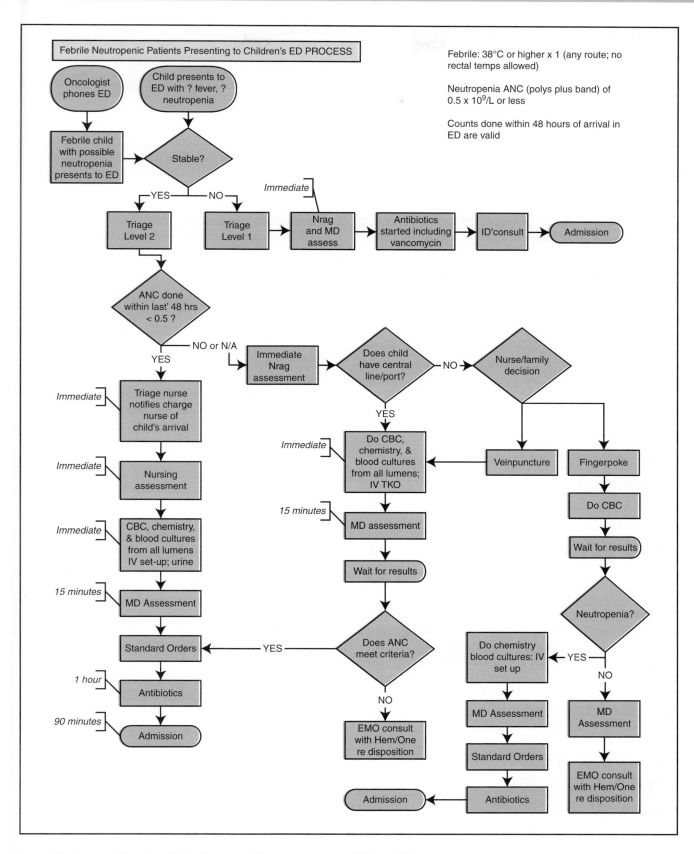

Figure 16-1 Example of Flow Chart Febrile Neutropenic Patients Presenting to Children's ED Process

Source: Galloway, L. (2006). Improving timeliness of care, Child Health Quality Team, *Quality for Kids Newsletter,* 5 (1): 2. Reprinted with permission of Winnipeg Regional Health Authority.

TABLE 16-1	DIFFERENCE IN FOCUS BETWEEN QUALITY ASSURANCE AND CONTINUOUS QUALITY IMPROVEMENT

Focus of Quality Assurance (doing it right)

1. Assessing or measuring performance
2. Determining whether performance conforms to standards
3. Improving performance when standards are not met

Focus of Continuous Quality Improvement (doing the right thing)

1. Meeting the needs of the customer
2. Building quality performance into the work process
3. Assessing the work process to identify opportunities for improved performance
4. Employing a scientific approach to assessment and problem solving
5. Improving performance continuously as a management strategy, not just when standards are not met

Harvard Business Review (Drucker, 1988). According to Drucker, efficiencies could be achieved through formalizing communication and information-sharing across the organizations, and he identified hospitals specifically as knowledge-based organizations.

TQM, CQI, and PI are terms that are frequently interchanged. For the purposes of this chapter, **continuous quality improvement (CQI)** will be referred to as a systematic process used to improve outcomes based on customers' needs. This proactive approach emphasizes "doing the right thing" for customers, and the end result of this method is to satisfy customers. The goal of CQI is to consistently meet or exceed the needs of clients, families, staff, health professionals, and community. This approach was integrated into the health care industry in the 1980s when cost and quality of care pressures were steadily increasing. Movement into QI is thought to be more an overall management approach than a single program. Integrating concepts of quality into daily organizational operations are key to successful outcomes. Table 16-1 notes the difference in focus between quality assurance and quality improvement.

GENERAL PRINCIPLES OF QUALITY IMPROVEMENT

Quality improvement is a structured system for creating organization-wide participation and partnership in planning and implementing continuous improvement methods; the aim is to understand and meet or exceed customer needs and expectations. Quality improvement principles include the following:

- The priority is to benefit clients and all other internal and external customers.
- Quality is achieved through the participation of everyone in the organization.
- Improvement opportunities are developed by focusing on the work process.
- Decisions to change or improve a system or process are made based on data.
- Improvement of the quality of service is a continuous process.
- Committed leadership is necessary to make it happen.
- Both education and long-term commitment are required.

Early quality assurance (QA) literature focused on fixing problems, "doing it right," and having zero defects. Over time, a gap was found between theory and practice, and it was determined that quality is not about being perfect. Three significant aspects of quality improvement have been identified. First, it is about being better, doing things right the first time. This approach increases an organization's chances of survival during highly turbulent and competitive times.

Second, quality improvement is about health care professionals seeing themselves as having customers or clients. For the health care professional, the notions of "customer" or "client" require a major shift in mind-set. These terms are frequently used in business and, initially, referring to a patient as a customer or a client was thought to undermine the professional care provided to patients. Designing health care processes from the customer's point of view as opposed to the professional's point of view is a challenge and requires changes in thinking and the redesign of health care processes. Health care involves work processes in which one step leads to the next. Improving these steps is an important part of improving care and customer satisfaction. Customer satisfaction is rooted in the way health professionals treat their clients/customers and in the quality of their outcomes. Having the goal of astounding clients with quality in every interaction is key to achieving satisfaction and loyalty.

Third, quality improvement directs health professionals to give their customers more than the basics. By doing so, their customers will recommend and demand these services. This goal is achieved by being proactive and seizing opportunities to perform better, driving for quality consistently and continuously, and not waiting for problems to be pointed out or pressure from external stakeholders before making improvements. When interprofessional teams collaborate and decisions about change are supported by data, improvements can be sustained over time.

The primary benefits of adopting quality concepts and principles include the following: (1) being able to discover performance issues more quickly and efficiently by looking at every problem as an opportunity for improvement, (2) improving staff satisfaction by involving staff in how the work process is designed and carried out, and (3) empowering staff to identify and implement change. Two additional quality concepts relate to increasing the customer's perception that you care by designing work processes to meet the customer's needs—rather than the health care provider's needs—and decreasing unnecessary costs from waste and rework, lost time, and not meeting provincial requirements. These quality concepts should be emphasized until they become work habits and part of an organization's daily operations.

CUSTOMERS IN HEALTH CARE

A customer is anyone who receives the output of your efforts. There are internal and external customers. An internal customer is anyone who works within the organization and receives the output of another employee. Internal customers include health care staff, such as physicians, nurses, pharmacists, physical therapists, respiratory therapists, occupational therapists, pastoral caregivers, recreation therapists, and lab technicians. An external customer is anyone who is outside the organization and receives the output of the organization. Clients are external customers, but they are not the only external customers. Other external customers include private physicians; insurance companies, such as Blue Cross; government departments, such as Health Canada; Accreditation Canada (AC); and the community you serve.

PARTICIPATION OF EVERYONE IN THE ORGANIZATION

Continuous quality improvement (CQI) is achieved through the participation of everyone in the organization at all levels. A participation and empowerment initiative must be built by first offering employees the opportunity for appropriate involvement. An organization that encourages empowerment promotes a culture of employee ownership. Such a culture is characterized by employees who do the following:

■ take responsibility for the success or failure of an organization
■ take an active part in developing new ways of doing things
■ trust that their efforts are valued

A new staff member can participate on an individual, unit, or organizational level in designing and improving daily work practices and processes. For example, as an individual, a nurse could change the organization of her day to spend more time with clients' families. On a unit level, a nurse could work with others on the unit to make the client report more time efficient. On an organizational level, a nurse could suggest that the process for notifying the pharmacy about a missing medication could be improved, and the nurse could participate on a team to find a solution.

All members of the staff are encouraged to participate in quality improvement processes, including physicians, registered nurses, physical therapists, occupational therapists, speech language technologists, pharmacists, community case management workers, social workers, medical technologists, and any member of the health care team who cares for clients or contributes to the care of clients. The goal of CQI efforts, as well as the process being worked on, determines who participates on the team.

For example, if you were trying to decrease the time a client waits outside the diagnostic imaging department for a test, your CQI efforts would need to include the client transportation staff, unit clerks, unit registered nurses, and diagnostic imaging staff. If you were trying to ensure that clients with congestive heart failure are discharged understanding the importance of weighing themselves daily, you would need the participation of the cardiac unit's registered nurse, the clinical dietician, home care association staff, the primary care physician, the cardiologist, the pharmacist, and the client and the client's family.

The key to determine who participates in CQI is to include the point-of-care staff: the frontline workers who do the direct care involved in the work process that you are trying to change. Because these people have the most

REAL WORLD INTERVIEW

I am more excited every day as I see nurses, physicians, and others embrace the concept of quality improvement. Initially, the process was tedious, because there was skepticism, but as ideas were introduced, implemented, and were successful, the enthusiasm rose exponentially. Our decisions are based on clinically relevant data. It is important to gain support from key players who have to deal with the implementation of any change.

Sharon Townsend, BScN
Quality Officer

CRITICAL THINKING

The emergency department team has successfully completed an accreditation review. Although commendations were made, some areas for improvement were noted. One of the areas for improvement was to strengthen the medication reconciliation process for both admitted and discharge clients from the department.

What suggestions would you make to the team? What processes would be involved? How could the processes be improved? Who would participate with you to identify ways to strengthen the medication reconciliation process?

knowledge of the work process, they can look for potential areas of improvement. It is important for staff to have a clearly identified way to suggest opportunities for improvement in things they see in their day-to-day work. For example, an X-ray technologist may note steps in the process of scheduling and transporting clients that create a long wait time for X-ray testing. A mechanism for suggesting improvement in the diagnostic imaging department would encourage the technologist to suggest and test ideas for change.

FOCUS ON IMPROVEMENT OF THE HEALTH CARE WORK PROCESS

Improvement opportunities are focused on the process of work that the health care team delivers. The dictionary defines a **process** as a series of actions, changes, or functions that bring about a result. All work processes have inputs, steps, and outputs. An example of a work process is a client attending a preoperative clinic. All the steps of the preoperative visit can be measured. These steps are then reviewed, applying evidence-based principles, as appropriate, to improve client care. Steps may be eliminated or changed and then standardized so that all staff uses the improved work process.

IMPROVEMENT OF THE SYSTEM

A **system** is an interdependent group of items, people, or processes with a common purpose (Langley et al., 1996). In a system, the processes as well as the relationships among the processes lead to the outcome. You can improve the outcome by examining the processes and relationships. In a system, every step of a process affects the following step. For example, if the X-ray staff

members place the client who has had a chest X-ray in the hall and call transportation to take the client back to his room but do not consider the transportation process, they may decrease the total time a client is in diagnostic imaging but increase the client's time in the hall waiting for transportation. You cannot improve care unless you review all the steps in the system's process.

A CONTINUOUS PROCESS

Improvement of service quality is a continuous process. Walter Shewhart, the director of Bell Laboratories in the mid-1920s, is credited for the concept of the cycle of continuous improvement. This concept suggests that products or services are designed and made based on knowledge about the customer. Those products or services are marketed to and judged by the customer. As the customer makes judgments, changes are made to improve the product or service (Al-Assaf & Schmele, 1997). Hence, the process of QI is continuous because it is linked to changing customer needs and judgments.

IMPROVEMENT BASED ON DATA

Decisions to change or improve a system or process are made based on data. When someone tells you that the clients are waiting too long to return from diagnostic imaging, it is time to look at the data. Review the wait time data to see whether wait times are increasing. The data will clarify these claims.

Using data correctly is important. Data should be used for learning, not for judging. It is critical to look at work processes rather than people for improvement opportunities. In the diagnostic imaging example, if you jumped to the conclusion that someone was not doing his job correctly, you might criticize the transportation staff person who returned the client from diagnostic imaging. This approach would not foster improvement ideas. Health care professionals could miss finding opportunities for real improvement if they do not analyze the process—for example, the client has a chest X-ray, is put in hall, a clerk calls transportation, and the transportation clerk pages transportation aide—and the relationships among the processes— for example, waiting times between calls, transportation phone process, page system. Perhaps it has nothing to do with the transportation person who returned the client to the room. The actual root cause may be a long delay in the paging system. Reviewing the wait time data is an example of examining the process, not the people carrying out the process.

IMPLICATIONS FOR CLIENT CARE

The implications of quality improvement for client care can be measured by the overall value of care. Value is a function of both quality outcomes and cost.

Outcomes can be a client's clinical or functional outcomes. For example, did the client live, can the client go back to work? Outcomes can also be measured by client satisfaction. For example, would the client recommend this health care facility to someone else?

Cost is the cost of both direct and indirect client care needs. Direct cost is the cost of the care of the client: for example, cost of medications, operating room equipment, and direct client caregiver salaries. **Indirect costs** are the costs of other care activities, including utility costs, such as electricity, and salaries of those who are not involved in direct client care, such as secretaries, unit clerks, and human resource staff.

$$\text{Value} = \frac{\text{Quality of outcomes}}{\text{Cost}}$$

In most QI efforts, as quality is improved by standardizing care delivery processes and applying evidence-based principles, the cost of care decreases.

METHODOLOGIES FOR QUALITY IMPROVEMENT

Several models outline methods for quality improvement. One is reviewed here: the FOCUS-PDSA quality improvement model (Plan-Do-Study-Act [PDSA] Cycle and the FOCUS methodology). Improvement comes from the application of knowledge (Langley et al., 1996). Thus, any approach to improvement must be based on building and applying knowledge. (This acronym is also known as

FOCUS-PDCA—Plan-Do-Check-Act (PDCA) Cycle and the FOCUS methodology.)

THE PLAN-DO-STUDY-ACT CYCLE

The PDSA Cycle starts with three questions:

1. What are we trying to accomplish?
2. How will we know that a change is an improvement?
3. What changes can we make that will result in improvement?

Then testing needs to be done to evaluate the effect of a proposed change and to learn about different alternatives (see Figure 16-2). The goal is to increase the ability to predict the effect that one or more changes would have if they were implemented (Langley et al., 1996). The plan for testing should cover who will do what, when they will do it, and where they will do it. Using the PDSA cycle encourages ongoing quality improvement.

THE FOCUS METHODOLOGY

The FOCUS methodology describes a stepwise process for how to move through the improvement process (see Figure 16-3).

F: Focus on an improvement idea. This step asks the question, Is there a problem? During this phase, an improvement opportunity is articulated and data are obtained to support the hypothesis that an opportunity for improvement exists.

O: Organize a team that understands the process. Identify a group of staff members (i.e., key players) who are direct participants in the process to be examined: the point-of-care staff. A team leader is identified who will appoint team members.

C: Clarify what is happening in the current process. A flow diagram (see Figure 16-4) is very helpful for identifying and understanding the current flow of events, and for determining where standardization might be possible. A detailed flowchart can be analyzed in two ways to uncover possible problems—at a macro level and at a micro level.

At the macro level scan the flowchart for any indication that the process is broken. Red flags include the following:

■ Many steps that represent quality checks or inspections for errors. Too many boxes in your flow diagram that describe similar steps could indicate rework or a lack of clarity in roles.

■ Areas in the process that are not well understood or cannot be defined. If the process cannot be defined well, you can be certain it is not being

CRITICAL THINKING

Winnipeg Children's Hospital has joined a Canadian Collaborative on Medication Reconciliation. The Collaborative was a joint initiative of the Canadian Association of Pediatric Health Centres and the Canadian Patient Safety Institute's Safer Healthcare Now! campaign. Medication reconciliation is a formal process of obtaining a complete and current list of each client's current home medications, including name, dosage, frequency, and route, and comparing it to the physician's admission, transfer and/or discharge orders. Discrepancies are brought to the attention of the prescriber, and if appropriate, changes are made and documented. There are three types of discrepancies: (1) intentional discrepancy, where the physician makes an intentional change and the choice is clearly documented; (2) undocumented intentional discrepancy, where the physician makes an intentional choice to change, but it is not clearly documented; and (3) unintentional discrepancy, where the physician unintentionally changed, added, or omitted a medication that the client was taking prior to admission. The second and third choices put the clients at risk of a medication error.

What kind of process can you envision implementing to determine the rate of discrepancy? What potential recommendations can you make regarding the care provided to the clients?

Source: Adapted from Galloway, L., Caligiuri, C., & Epp, G. (2006). Medication reconciliation. *Child Health Quality Team, Quality for Kids Newsletter,* 5(1), 3.

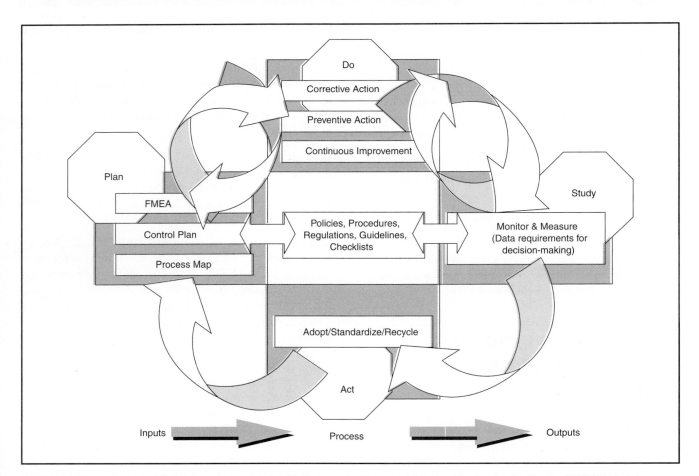

Figure 16-2 Plan-Do-Study-Act (PDSA) Example: Interrelationship Between the Elements of Advanced Product Quality Planning (APQP) Methodology

Source: Keeler, C., Johnson, A., & Lee, A. (2009). Understanding failure: Taking and maintaining control. *Healthcare Management Forum,* 22(2): 46. Reprinted with Permission.

LITERATURE APPLICATION

Citation: Lees, M., Chapman, P., & Dickson, S. (2011). A process improvement strategy for patient safety. *Healthcare Management Forum,* 24(1), Supplement: 25–28. Reprinted with Permission.

Discussion: This article describes an Executive Training for Research Application (EXTRA) project. The authors sought to establish an effective approach to implementing and sustaining a process improvement program for patient safety practices in response to a government policy decision to publicly report hospital standardized mortality ratio. The intervention focused on sustaining compliance with two safety initiatives of Safer Healthcare Now! Bundles—Medication Reconciliation (Med Rec) and Acute Myocardial Infarction (AMI). This article presents the results of the process improvement project on the two safety programs as well as the key lesson learned.

Implications for Practice: The lessons learned include the importance of teamwork, training, leadership, frontline champions, and the courage to create the conditions for change. Managing change and improvement projects is difficult, but it can be done successfully if there is strong and consistent leadership support. The support should occur within the setting of a proven framework for quality improvement and guided by clear aims and goals that are measurable and pursued by a team that is enabled for success.

	Table 1 FOCUS-PDCA model for AMI project
F	Find a process for improvement opportunity (purpose, determine if there is a problem)
O	Organize a team who understands the process (key players)
C	Clarify the current knowledge of the process (process mapping)
U	Uncover the root cause of variation and poor quality (root cause analysis) Use data analysis
S	Select the process improvement and clarify the aim of goal
P	Plan the process improvement and data collection
D	Do the improvement data collection and analysis
C	Check/study the result of improvement and lessons learned
A	Act to hold the gain by adopting, adjusting or abandoning the change

Figure 16-3 FOCUS-PDCA Model for AMI (Acute Myocardial Infarction) Project

Source: Aldarrab, A. (2006). "Application of Lean Six Sigma for Patients Presenting with ST-Elevation Myocardial Infarction: The Hamilton Health Sciences Experience." *Healthcare Quarterly,* 9(1): 56–61. Reprinted with Permission.

performed efficiently and with maximized outcomes.

- Many wait times between processes. Wait times should always be minimized to improve efficiency of the process.
- Multiple paths that show lots of people involved in the activity or delivering the service to the customer. The involvement of too many staff is wasteful and confusing to the client.

If the process seems reasonable, with one or two areas needing improvement, then undertake a micro-level analysis of your flow diagram.

- Examine decision symbols (i.e., diamonds) that represent quality inspection activities. Can these activities be eliminated? Do some errors go undetected? Is the check redundant? This examination will ensure limited rework and maximum clarity.

Figure 16-4 Application of Lean Six Sigma for Patients Presenting with ST-Elevation Myocardial Infarction

Source: Aldarrab, A. (2006). "Application of Lean Six Sigma for Patients Presenting with ST-Elevation Myocardial Infarction: The Hamilton Health Sciences Experience." *Healthcare Quarterly,* 9(1): 56–61. Reprinted with Permission.

- Examine each process in the diagram for redundancy and value. If a step is repeated or does not have any value for the customer, it should be eliminated.
- Examine processes for waiting time areas. The process should be changed to eliminate these wait times.
- Examine all processes for rework loops. A step should not be repeated. Resources are always limited, especially in hospitals today.
- Check that handoffs are smooth and necessary. Handoffs are times when a process is passed from one staff person or department to another. Handoffs always leave room for error. They are also common times for wait areas. During this phase, cause-and-effect diagrams and Pareto charts can be helpful. These tools are discussed on pages 339–340.

U: Understand the degree of change needed. In this stage, the team reviews what it knows and enhances its knowledge by reviewing the literature, available data, and competitive benchmarks. How are other health care organizations doing the process?

S: Solution: Select a solution for improvement. The team can brainstorm and then choose the best solution. It can then use the PDCA Cycle to test this solution. An implementation plan should be used to track progress and the steps required. This implementation plan can be in the form of a work plan or Gantt chart. A Gantt chart is a chart in the form of a table that identifies what activity is to be completed, who is responsible for it, and when it is going to be completed (see Figure 16-5). It outlines the steps needed to implement the change.

Improvement strategies identified at the organizational level involve benchmarking, meeting government requirements, identifying opportunities for system changes following sentinel event review, using a balanced scorecard, and using a storyboard.

OTHER IMPROVEMENT STRATEGIES

BENCHMARKING

Benchmarking is the continual and collaborative discipline of measuring and comparing the results of key work processes with those of the best performers. Learning how to adapt these best practices can help to achieve breakthrough process improvement and build healthier communities (Gift & Mosel, 1994). Benchmarking focuses on key services or processes: for example, length of time in the operating room for a total hip replacement or length of stay in hospital post-procedure. A benchmark study will identify gaps in performance and provide options for selecting work processes to improve, ideas for redesign

of care delivery, and ideas for better ways of meeting customer expectations (Youngberg, 1998).

REGULATORY REQUIREMENTS

Accreditation Canada (AC) assists health organizations across the country to examine and improve the quality of care and the service they provide to their clients. Accreditation Canada introduced a new accreditation program in 2008 called Qmentum, which emphasizes health system performance, risk prevention planning, client safety, performance measurement, and governance.[2] See Chapter 1, pages 21–23, for further discussion on Qmentum and Accreditation Canada's accreditation process.

Accreditation is an ongoing cycle. It starts when a health care organization first applies to become accredited. Subsequently, the organization prepares for an accreditation visit and review by setting objectives and building teams. The purpose of establishing the teams is not only to prepare for the accreditation survey but also to assist with ongoing processes related to quality improvement and operations. The organization then assesses whether it complies with the national standards and required organizational practices, submits its self-assessment, and is evaluated by an external team of independent peer reviewers when the AC survey team visits. Following the conclusion of the site visit, the facility receives a brief verbal summary of the findings. A formal written report, highlighting strengths and offering suggestions for improvement, is received within a few weeks. The survey results provide ideas for future CQI strategies.

SENTINEL EVENTS

A **sentinel event** is an unexpected incident related to system or process deficiencies, and which leads to death or major and enduring loss of function for a recipient of health care services. The major and enduring loss of function refers to sensory, motor, or psychological impairment that was not present at the time services were sought or begun. The impairment is not related to the natural course of the client's illness or to an underlying condition.[3] Events are called sentinel because they require immediate investigation. During analysis of these sentinel events, opportunities for improving the system will arise and should be taken advantage of. Linkage of the sentinel event review to the organization's performance improvement system will identify strategies for the prevention of future sentinel events. An example of a sentinel event is surgery performed on the wrong side of a client. Reviewing the surgical process and developing an effective system to mark the appropriate site exemplifies a change in process to prevent such future harmful occurrences.

BALANCED SCORECARD

To ensure value in care, measurement of progress has to be balanced. Effective measurement must be an integral part of the management process. The balanced

TABLE 16-2	CAUSES AND BRAINSTORMED SOLUTIONS OF DELAY FROM DOOR TO ECG TIME

Causes

- Level of skill of new nurses

- Availability of primary nurse

- Availability of bed

- ECG machines/supplies

- Triage assessment

Brainstormed Solutions

- Budding with experienced nurses and education

- ECG technician to do all ECGs
- To look at nurse: patient ratio
- Retention of staff
- Healthy work environment

- Designated bed for ECGs
- To always have one bed ready for the next patient arriving in the ED (12)
- ECG technician to do all ECGs
- EMS to do prehospital 12 lead ECG

- Need for new/more machines with 15 lead capability
- Use medical diagnosis unit machines during night time hours to add resources
- Synchronization of clocks and ECG machines (digitalized clocks)

- Standard scales to ensure consistent triage
- Triage nurses not to be pulled to regular nurse relief duties
- Clarification of triage/charge nurse roles
- Central bed manager on days
- Use more experienced nurses in the triage role
- Feedback loop to the ED nurses and MDs regarding meeting the timeline goals
- Continuous education

Source: Aldarrab, A. (2006). "Application of Lean Six Sigma for Patients Presenting with ST-Elevation Myocardial Infarction: The Hamilton Health Sciences Experience." *Healthcare Quarterly,* 9(1): 56–61. Reprinted with Permission.

Activity	Responsible	July	Aug	Sept	Oct	Nov
Discuss move with staff	Manager	X				
Form an ad hoc planning group	Team Leader	X				
Receive report from group re: order of move	Team Leader and Manager		X			
Discuss report with staff	Manager, Team Leader, and Staff		X			
Notify other departments			X	X		
Prepare offices in new building	Staff		X	X		
Pack office contents	Staff			X		
Move into new space and unpack	Staff				X	
Evaluate the moving process	Staff, Manager, and Team Leader				X	
Make recommendations re: future moves	Staff, Manager, and Team Leader					X

Figure 16-5 Example of a GANTT Chart: Preparation for an Office Move

REAL WORLD INTERVIEW

I felt benchmarking was useful because it helped us to identify best performance and provide a method to set targets for improvement for ourselves. It allowed us to see where we operate in comparison to other organizations. In addition, we were able to more appropriately determine our staff requirements.

Grant Fairfield, RN, MScN
Clinical Nurse Specialist, Rehabilitation

scorecard provides individuals with a framework that translates an organization's objectives into a set of linked performance measures (Kaplan & Norton, 1993). It provides answers to four basic questions: (1) how do customers see us? (i.e., customer perspective); (2) what must we excel at? (i.e., internal perspective); (3) can we continue to improve and create value? (i.e., innovation and learning perspective); and (4) how do we look to funders? (i.e., financial perspective). Generally, four cardinal domains of outcomes are measured: functional status of client, clinical outcomes, satisfaction, and costs (Caldwell, 1998).

Such an approach allows those reviewing data to examine all aspects of care. For example, client outcomes are reflected in a client's functional status and clinical status, which are balanced by client satisfaction and cost to ensure value. Data can be arranged to create a balanced scorecard; this approach uses the organization's priorities as categories for indicators. For example, three priorities might be customer service, cost-effectiveness, and positive clinical outcomes. These priorities help determine which indicators should be measured to give a balanced view of whether a strategy is working.

Indicators are selected based on what they have in common. If a change occurs in the cost-effectiveness category it will affect the data in another category. For example, if the number of client referrals to home care is increased, is the client's satisfaction affected positively or negatively? If the length of stay for these clients is decreased, are complication rates increased or decreased? After indicators are selected, data are tracked over time at regular intervals (e.g., every month or every quarter). See Figure 10-1 to see a balanced scorecard for the patient care team of a neonatal intensive care unit.

STORYBOARD: HOW TO SHARE YOUR STORY

Process improvement teams share their work with others through a storyboard. The storyboard usually takes the major steps in the improvement methodology and visually outlines the progress in each step. Displaying the storyboard in a high-traffic area of the organization will inform other staff of the QI efforts under way. Storyboarding can be done when a process is complete, or it can be used during the process to communicate information.

CLIENT SATISFACTION DATA

Client satisfaction data can be obtained in several ways. Most health care facilities have clients complete a questionnaire that asks how they felt about their health care encounter. It is most helpful if this data can be compared or benchmarked with other organizations' data. However, this requires that several organizations use the same data collection tools. All client responses are entered into a database so that results can be compared. Another method to obtain client satisfaction information is via a focus group or a post-care interview, which requires meeting with one or more clients after their discharge and asking for feedback on their perceptions of their stay.

LITERATURE APPLICATION

Citation: Fallah, S., Chen, X., Lefebvre, D., Kurji, J., Hader, J., & Leeb, K. (2011). Babies admitted to NICU/ICU: Province of birth and mode of delivery matter. *Healthcare Quarterly*, 14(2): 16–20.

Discussion: Neonatal intensive care units are specialized units that provide high levels of intensive care for premature babies and those with medical or surgical problems. Rates of admission to these units vary across Canada. Because of the highly specialized care that babies receive in these units, the costs are higher than for normal newborn lengths of stay. This study explored the variation in NICU/ICU admissions and the characteristics of mothers and newborns associated with an increased likelihood of NICU/ICU admission.

Implications for Practice: After excluding multiple births, preterm births, small-for-gestational-age births, and those babies delivered by women with select complications, the authors found an increased risk for NICU/ICU admission for babies born by Caesarian Section as their only indication.

Why is Jason in the hospital? Because he has a bad infection in his leg.

But why does he have an infection? Because he has a cut on his leg and it got infected.

But why does he have a cut on his leg? Because he was playing in the junkyard next to his apartment building and there was some sharp, jagged steel there that he fell on.

But why was he playing in a junkyard? Because his neighbourhood is run down. A lot of kids play there and there is no one to supervise them.

But why does he live in that neighbourhood? Because his parents can't afford a nicer place to live.

But why can't his parents afford a nicer place to live? Because his Dad is unemployed and his Mom is sick.

But why is his Dad unemployed? Because he doesn't have much education and he can't find a job.

But why......?

Source: Toward a Healthy Future: Second Report on the Health of Canadians. Health Canada, 1999. Reproduced with the permission of the Minister of Health, 2011.

As this story suggests, health, illness and early death depend on a variety of factors or "determinants" that surround individuals, families and nations. Getting to the root cause of Jason's illness and the other major health problems we face in Canada today requires action on the broader determinants of health. It also requires that we continue to provide high-quality health services that will help Jason heal.

USING DATA

Several different types of charts can be used to examine data during QI efforts: time series charts, Pareto charts, histograms, flowcharts, fishbone diagrams, pie charts, and check sheets.

TIME SERIES DATA

Time series data (see Figure 16-6) allow individuals to see changes in data over time. A time series chart allows the user to view a number of observations for a particular subject at regular intervals over time. An example of a time series chart is the weekly volume of clients waiting for more than 24 hours in the emergency department.

Tracking data over time allows you to see how a process is behaving, and a time series graph is able to illustrate this. Graphs or charts—rather than tables of numbers—are used to display data, because graphs are faster to interpret. The time series chart is used to look for trends, shifts, and unusual data.

CHARTS: PARETO, HISTOGRAM, FLOWCHARTS, FISHBONE DIAGRAMS, PIE CHARTS, AND CHECK SHEETS

In addition to time series data graphs, information can be displayed in several different ways to enhance decision making: Pareto diagrams, pie charts, flowcharts, and histograms. Figure 16-7 is an example of a fishbone diagram. (Fishbone diagrams are also referred to as root cause diagrams, cause-and-effect diagrams, or Ishikawa diagrams.) Note that many factors contribute to a problem. The review of a cause-and-effect chart encourages staff to look for all the causes of a problem, not just one cause. Figure 16-8 shows a check sheet, a Pareto chart, and a control chart. A full discussion of these tools is outside the scope of this chapter.

PRINCIPLES IN ACTION AN ORGANIZATION

How are these principles and tools of quality management actually used on a day-to-day basis in a health care facility? The organization sets up an appropriate structure and uses a process for quality and monitoring outcomes.

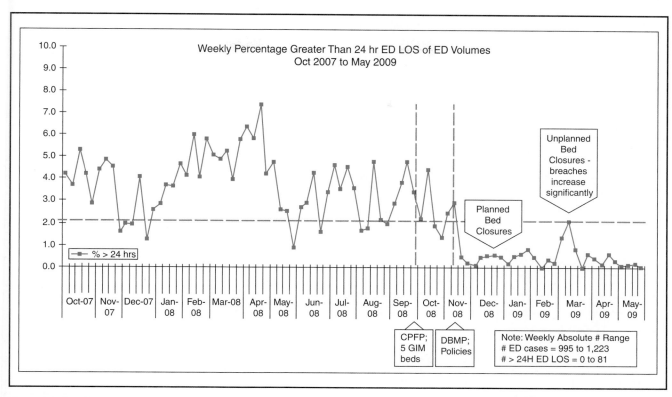

Figure 16-6 Time Series

Source: Alikan, L.M., Howard, R.J., & Bowry, R. (2009). From a project to transformation: How "going against the flow" led to improved access and patient flow in an academic hospital. *Healthcare Management Forum,* 22(3): 23.

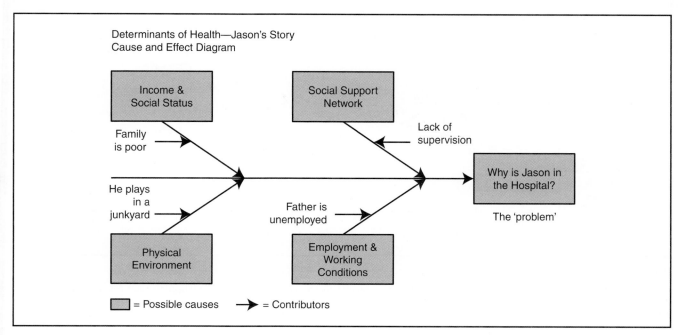

Figure 16-7 Root Cause/Fishbone Diagram/Cause and Effect Diagram/Ishikawa Diagram

Source: Child Health Team. *Quality for Kids Newsletter.* Reprinted with permission of Winnipeg Regional Health Authority.

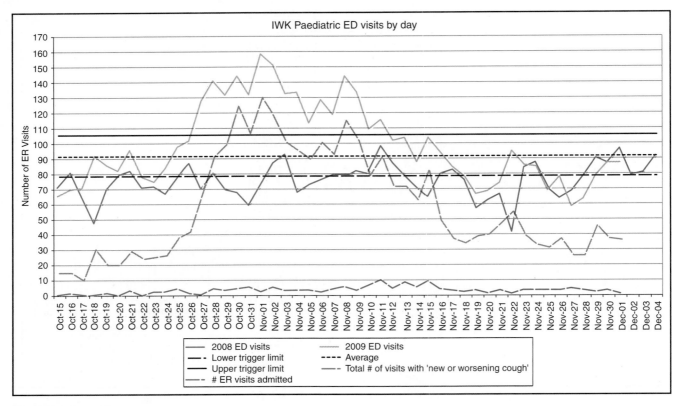

Figure 16-8a Pareto Chart

Source: Mahon, K., Blackmore, N., Thibeault, M., Belliveau, B., & Burgess, S. (2011). When ordinary days become extraordinary: The response to H1N1 at the Izaak Walton Killam Health Centre. *Healthcare Management Forum,* 24(1): 16.

Figure 16-8b Control Chart

Source: Jugenburg, M. (2006). "Children's Hospital's Newest Unit is Taking Off." *Quality for Kids Newsletter,* 5(2):1. Reprinted with permission of Winnipeg Regional Health Authority.

Quality Issues Identified and Improved Through Simulation*

Quality Issues identified	Hospital						Solutions
	A	B	C	D	E	F	
Environment /Room							■ Designated stocking person and stocking routine/schedule
Stocking and Storage							
Room stocking (e.g., vacuum, respiratory therapy, IV equipment) inconsistent or did not have designated individual to stock room	−	+	−	+	+	+	■ Ensured placement of equipment in room conducive to emergencies
Stool in bathroom farthest from patient and often blocked	−	−	+	−	−	−	
Tracking Time							■ Repeated simulations to test
Unaware of ability of fetal monitor to mark time	+	−	−	−	−	−	■ Modified equipment storage based on use and easy access
Inconsistently marked time	−	+	−	−	−	−	
Clock out of nurse's line of vision	−	−	−	+	−	−	■ Removal of out-of-date materials
Clinical Information							
Posters In room illustrate improper techniques (e.g., McRoberts technique)	−	−	−	−	−	−	
Medications, Devices, and Equipment							■ Created emergency kits (e.g.. post-partum hemorrhage kit) containing all related medications, syringes, and needles and taped card to kit with doses, route, and contraindications
Medications							
Inconsistent or inaccurate information listed on medications	+	+	+	+	+	+	
Inconsistent knowledge of where all medications stored	+	−	−	−	−		
Difficulty obtaining medications because of multiple storage locations	−	−	−	+	+	−	
Unlabeled IV lines when several present	−	+	−	−	−	−	
Electronic Health Record							■ Established alternative methods to obtain medication information (call the pharmacy, reference books, consul-tants)
Delayed documentation of key medical Information until after emergency	−	+	−	−	−	−	
Balloon Tamponade							
No/inconsistent awareness of balloon tamponade device	−	+	+	+	+	+	■ Conducted periodic in-service on emergency equipment and medica-tions and their storage locations and discussed expectations of stocking. including checking infrequently used emergency equipment
Inconsistent knowledge of where balloon stored	−	+	−	−	−	−	
No balloon available	−	−	+	−	+	+	
Miscellaneous Equipment							
Battery in emergency cordless phone did not work	−	−	−	−	+		■ Ensured consistent labeling of IV lines
							■ Standardized and communicated expectations regarding equipment and documentation of information
Staffing and Staff Roles							
Inconsistent expectations regarding identification and roles of helpers	+	−	+	−	−	+	■ Standardized roles and expectations of helpers, including family
Communication							
Hesitant to use transparent thinking (thinking out loud)	+	−	+	−	−	+	■ Developed examples of statements to use and practiced in simulations
Knowledge of Protocols/Documentation							
Inconsistent knowledge of emergency protocols (e.g., massive transfusion)	−	−	+	−	−	−	■ Conducted in-services on protocol locations and how to use. practice in simulations

* +, quality issue identified; −, quality or issue not identified: IV, intravenous.

Figure 16-8c Check Sheet

Source: Guise, J.M., Lowe, N.L., Deering, S., Lewis, P.O., O'Haire, C., Irwin, L.K., Blaser, M., Wood, L.S., & Kanki, B.G. (2010). Mobile in situ obstetric emergency simulation and teamwork training to improve maternal-fetal safety in hospitals. *The Joint Commission Journal on Quality and Patient Safety,* 36(10): 450. Reprinted with permission.

CASE STUDY 16-1

Y ou work in a busy emergency department, where you have a good working relationship with your nursing colleagues and with the emergency physicians. You believe that the care delivery in the department could improve, thereby increasing client satisfaction and reducing the length of time clients wait to be seen. How would you proceed? Whose support would you enlist first? Who should be involved? What quality indicators could be measured?

ORGANIZATIONAL STRUCTURE

Most organizations today are structured to maximize QI efforts, which allow it to be flexible and nimble in a very turbulent health care environment. This organizational structure encourages accountability and communication by focusing all staff on the priorities of the organization.

Figure 16-9 is an a framework that shows a structure for quality and enterprise risk management. Note that it includes a range of people, from board members to staff on individual quality improvement teams (QITs). Communicating priorities at all levels in the organization is key. Staff members must realize how their day-to-day work influences the accomplishment of strategic goals. Mission, vision, and value statements help accomplish this clarity of focus (see Chapter 13, pp. 269–270.)

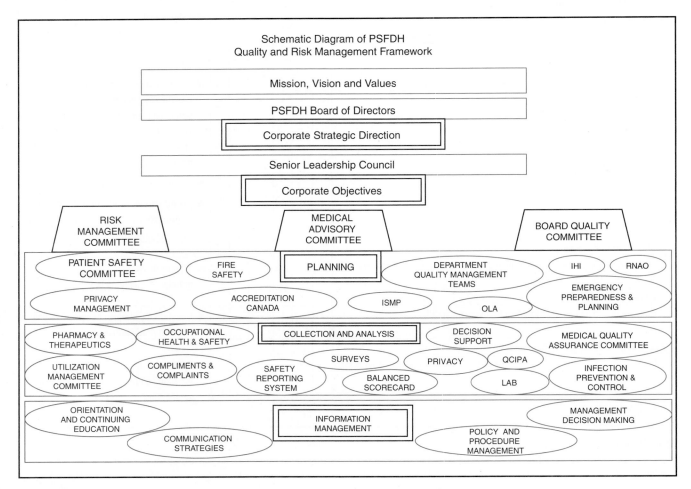

Figure 16-9 Schematic Diagram of PSFDH (Perth Smiths Falls District Hospital) Quality and Risk Management Framework

Source: Cassidy-Gifford, C., & Stepanuik, T. (2010). *Quality and Risk Management Plan.* Perth and Smiths Falls District Hospital.

CRITICAL THINKING

At times, some care providers, particularly physicians, see clinical pathways and other standardized guidelines as cookie-cutter medicine. All health care providers like to think they give their clients the best care possible. Standardization and evidence-based clinical guidelines are intended to communicate the latest evidence as to the best practice for a given client problem. Using these guidelines allows care providers to focus on specific individual client needs rather than spending their energy on determining the best evidence-based strategy according to the current research.

In developing a clinical pathway or other standardized guideline, evidence-based practice guidelines should be incorporated. In the absence of evidence-based practices, team consensus should be used to develop the clinical pathway. In the absence of consensus, the client's health care provider should make an independent decision, even though this is not included in the clinical guideline.

A group that was developing a clinical pathway for the care of clients with acute myocardial infarction noted evidence showing that these clients should receive acetylsalicylic acid (ASA) on admission. The research in this area was very clear, and most providers believed this practice was being followed. When a chart audit was performed to determine whether it was, in fact, the practice on the unit, it was discovered that only 48 percent of clients were receiving ASA within eight hours of admission. The team added this practice to the clinical pathway. After this change was implemented, 85 percent of clients received ASA within the first eight hours of admission.

What practices on your unit are based on an evidence-based clinical pathway? How can you participate in improving the care of more clients using evidence-based clinical pathways? Do you use clinical practice guidelines?

OUTCOMES MONITORING

Outcomes are a measurement of the client response to structure and process. Outcomes measure actual clinical progress. The development of process improvement measures in today's health care organizations is driven by the multiple domains of quality that Accreditation Canada and legislation require. Outcomes can be short term, such as the average length of stay (ALOS) for a client population, or long term, such as a measure of clients' progress over time—for example, survival rate for a transplant client at one, two, and three years after treatment. Outcomes can be studied to identify potential areas of concern, which may lead to an investigation of structure and process to determine any root causes. For example, when a postoperative infection rate was used as an outcome measure, an increase in the number of infections per month was noted. This finding led the team to review the client care process being used. The team discovered that preoperative prophylactic antibiotics were not given to the client because the order was not written. The team added this order to the initial order set, and all clients received prophylactic antibiotics. The number of postoperative infections decreased.

Research supports and demonstrates that Quality and Risk Management Goals are enhanced and achieved when the active measurement and monitoring of indicators is supported by leadership, education, training, and accountability. Figure 16-10 illustrates the interdependence of quality and risk priorities. It is a delicate act to balance efficiency, effectiveness, safety, quality, client satisfaction and stakeholder accountability. To achieve sustainable system improvements health care professionals need to work together. All health care providers at all levels are responsible for fostering a culture of safety and quality to promote and support quality management, enterprise risk management, and client safety. See Figure 16-10 to see how the Perth Smiths Falls District Hospital Strategic Plan is integrated with the Quality and Risk Management Framework.

ENTERPRISE RISK MANAGEMENT

Enterprise Risk Management (ERM) is a comprehensive process used to evaluate all risk exposures confronting an organization. Its three concrete aspects—framework, tools, and solutions (Carroll, 2004)—are designed to do the following:

Figure 16-10 Integration of PSFDH Strategic Plan and the Quality and Risk Management Framework

Source: Cassidy-Gifford, C., & Stepanuik, T. (2010). *Quality and Risk Management Plan.* Perth and Smiths Falls District Hospital.

■ Lessen the exposure to, frequency of and severity of risk, and assess the frequency, cost, and probability of risk

■ Assist the board in discharging corporate governance obligations

■ Formalize accountability by program or service

■ Standardize risk-assessment and analysis processes

■ Ensure transparency through effective reporting

■ Develop management awareness

■ Create an environment where risk management forms part of the overall decision-making process and is integrated into the daily business of the organization[4]

Enterprise Risk Management (ERM) at St. Joseph's Hospital incorporates the Health Insurance Reciprocal of Canada (HIROC, 2006b) Risk Management Self-Appraisal Module and corresponding action plans and aligns with Accreditation Canada's new Qmentum process.[5]

KEY CONCEPTS

■ Quality improvement is a continuous process focused on improving client care processes and outcomes.

■ Focus on client care needs to drive improvement opportunities.

■ Use data to drive decisions.

■ Link improvement initiatives to the organization's mission, vision, and values.

■ Communicate Organizational goals and objectives up and down within an organization.

■ Establish a balance in improvement goals that are focused on client clinical and functional status, cost, and client satisfaction outcomes.

■ Enterprise risk management is an integral part of an organization's quality management program.

KEY TERMS

benchmarking
continuous quality
  improvement (CQI)
enterprise risk management (ERM)
indirect costs

performance
  improvement (PI)
quality assurance (QA)
sentinel event
system

REVIEW QUESTIONS

1. Which of the following describes the benchmarking process?
   A. reviewing your own unit's data for opportunities
   B. collecting data on an individual client
   C. reviewing data in the literature
   D. comparing your data to that of other organizations to identify opportunities

2. Identifying opportunities in the health care arena is the responsibility of which of the following groups?
   A. administration
   B. physicians
   C. clients
   D. everyone

3. Following a sentinel event, which step would be initiated first?
   A. no action
   B. corrective action of personnel
   C. reporting to health department and doing root cause analysis
   D. immediate investigation

4. What document defines the purpose of an organization?
   A. mission statement
   B. fishbone diagram
   C. balanced scorecard
   D. process flowchart

5. What tool could be used to track a change in a process over time?
   A. flowchart
   B. histogram
   C. time series chart
   D. pie chart

REVIEW ACTIVITIES

1. Risk management, infection-control practitioners, and a benchmark study have revealed that your unit's use of Foley catheters is above average. Brainstorm reasons why the use is so high. Create a fishbone (root cause) diagram to help determine all the possible causes.

2. After you have identified the root causes for the above-average use of Foley catheters, use the PDCA Cycle to identify improvement strategies.

3. Think about your last clinical rotation. Identify one process that you believe could be improved. How would you begin improving the process? Use the FOCUS methodology in your analysis.

EXPLORING THE WEB

- Use these sites for potential benchmark data:

  Cochrane Collaboration:
  http://www.cochrane.org/

  Canadian Institute for Health Information:
  http://www.cihi.ca/CIHI-ext-portal/internet/EN/Home/home/cihi000001

- The following sites are recommended when looking for evidence-based guidelines or research studies for a particular diagnosis:

  Institute for Clinical Evaluative Sciences:
  http://www.ices.on.ca

  Health Information Research Unit:
  http://hiru.mcmaster.ca/

  Canadian Medical Association Clinical Practice Guidelines:
  http://mdm.ca/cpgsnew/cpgs/index.asp

  International Health Data Linkage Network:
  http://www.ihdln.org/member/

REFERENCES

Al-Assaf, A. F., & Schmele, J. (1997). *Total quality in healthcare.* Boca Raton, FL: St. Lucie Press.

Aldarrab, A. (2006). Application of Lean Six Sigma for patients presenting with ST-elevation myocardial infarction: The Hamilton Health Sciences experience. *Healthcare Quarterly, 9*(1), 56–61.

Alikhan, L. M., Howard, R. J., & Bowry, R. (2009). From a project to transformation: How "going against the flow" led to improved access and patient flow in an academic hospital. *Healthcare Management Forum, 22*(3), 20–26.

Behamdouni, G., & Millar, K. (2010). Implementation of an enterprise risk-management program in a community teaching hospital. *Healthcare Quarterly, 13*(1), 72–78.

Berwick, D., & Plsek, P. (1992). *Managing medical quality videotape series.* Woodbridge, NJ: Quality Visions.

Berwick, D. M., Blanton Godfrey, A., & Roessner, J. (1991). *Curing health care: New strategies for quality improvement.* San Francisco: Jossey-Bass.

Caldwell, C. (1998). *Handbook for managing change in health care.* Milwaukee, WI: ASQ Quality Press.

Cassidy-Gifford, C., & Stepanuik, T. (2010). Quality and Risk Management Plan. Perth and Smiths Falls District Hospital.

Child Health Quality Team. (2006). Children's Hospital's newest unit is taking off! *Quality for Kids Newsletter, 5*(2), 1.

Coutts, J. (2011). Small steps … Improving quality one team at a time in Saskatchewan. *Healthcare Quarterly*, 14(1), 25–27.

Crosby, P. B. (1989). *Let's talk quality*. New York: McGraw-Hill.

Deming, W. E. (1986). *Out of the crisis*. Cambridge, MA: Center for Advanced Engineering Study.

Dobrown, M. J., Sullivan, T., & Sawka, C. (2008). Shifting clinical accountability and the pursuit of quality: Aligning clinical and administrative approaches. *Healthcare Management Forum*, 21(3), 6–12.

Drucker, P. F. (1988). The coming of the new organization. *Harvard Business Review*, 66(1), 45–53.

Fallah, S., Chen, X., Lefebvre, D., Kurji, J., Hader, J., & Leeb, K. (2011). Babies admitted to NICU/ICU: Province of birth and mode of delivery matter. *Healthcare Quarterly*, 14(2), 16–20.

Federal, Provincial and Territorial Advisory Committee on Population Health. (1999). *Toward a healthy future: Second report on the health of Canadians*. Ottawa: Minister of Public Works and Government Services Canada. Retrieved from http://www.phac-aspc.gc.ca/ph-sp/report-rapport/toward/report-eng.php

Galloway, L. (2006). Improving timeliness of care. *Child Health Quality Team, Quality for Kids Newsletter*, 5(1), 2.

Galloway, L., Caligiuri, C., & Epp, G. (2006). Medication reconciliation. *Child Health Quality Team, Quality for Kids Newsletter*, 5(1), 3.

Gift, R. G., & Mosel, D. (1994). *Benchmarking in health care: A collaborative approach*. Chicago: American Hospital Publishing.

Guise, J. M., Lowe, N. L., Deering, S., Lewis, P. O., O'Haire, C., Irwin, L. K., et al. (2010). Mobile in situ obstetric emergency simulation and teamwork training to improve maternal-fetal safety in hospitals. *The Joint Commission Journal on Quality and Patient Safety*, 36(10), 443–453.

Kaplan, R., & Norton, D. (1993). Putting the balanced scorecard to work. *Harvard Business Review, September/October*, 134–147.

Keeler, C., Johnson, A., & Lee, A. (2009). Understanding failure: Taking and maintaining control. *Healthcare Management Forum*, 22(2), 44–48.

Langley, G. J., Nolan, K. M., Norman, C. L., Provost, L. P., & Nolan, T. W. (1996). *The improvement guide*. San Francisco: Jossey-Bass.

Lees, M., Chapman, P., & Dickson, S. (2011). A process improvement strategy for patient safety. *Healthcare Management Forum*, 24(Suppl. 1), 25–28.

Lesar, T., Briceland, I., & Stein, D. (1997). Factors related to errors in medication prescribing. *Journal of the American Medical Association*, 277(4), 312–317.

Mahon, K., Blackmore, N., Thibeault, M., Belliveau, B., & Burgess, S. (2011). When ordinary days become extraordinary: The response to H1N1 at the Izaak Walton Killam Health Centre. *Healthcare Management Forum*, 24(1), 14–19.

Rondeau, K. V., & Wagar, T. H. (2002). Implementing CQI while reducing the work force: How does it influence hospital performance? *Healthcare Management Forum*, 17(2), 22–29.

Seeman, N. & Brown, A. D. (2006). Remembering Peter Drucker: Inspiring the quality revolution in healthcare. *Healthcare Quarterly*, 9(1), 50–52.

Youngberg, B. (1998). *The risk manager's desk reference*. Gaithersburg, MD: Aspen.

SUGGESTED READINGS

Caro, D. (2011). Towards sustainable traumatic brain injury care systems: Healthcare leadership imperatives in Canada. *Healthcare Management Forum*, 24(1), 25–30.

Duffy, J. R. (2000). Cardiovascular outcomes initiative: Case studies in performance improvement. *Outcomes Management in Nursing Practice*, 4(3), 110–116.

Harrigan, M. L. (2000) *Quest for quality in Canadian health care: Continuous quality improvement* (2nd ed.). Ottawa: Health Canada. Retrieved from http://www.hc-sc.gc.ca/hcs-sss/pubs/care-soins/2000-qual/index_e.html

Henry, S. B. (1995). Informatics: Essential infrastructure for quality assessment and improvement in nursing. *Journal of the American Medical Information Association*, 2(3), 169–182.

Kaplan, R., & Norton, D. (1996). *The balanced scorecard: Translating strategy into action*. Boston: Harvard Business School Press.

Kelly-Heidenthal, P., & Heidenthal, P. R. (1995). Benchmarking. *Nursing Quality Connections*, 4(5), 4.

King, K. M., & Teo, K. K. (2000). Integrating clinical quality improvement strategies with nursing research. *Western Journal of Nursing Research*, 22(5), 596–608.

Kipp, J., McKim, B., Zieber, C., & Neumann, I. (2006). What motivates managers to coordinate the learning experience of interprofessional student teams in service delivery settings? *Healthcare Management Forum*, 19(2), 42–48.

Kitson, A. (2000). Towards evidence-based quality improvement: Perspectives from nursing practice. *International Journal of Quality in Health Care*, 12(6), 459–464.

Koivula, M., Paunonen, M., & Laippala, P. (1998). Prerequisites for quality improvement in nursing. *Journal of Nursing Management*, 6(6), 333–342.

Maleyeff, J., Kaminsky, F. C., Jubinville, A., & Fenn, C. (2001). A guide to using performance measurement systems for continuous improvement. *Journal of Healthcare Quality*, 23(4), 33–37.

McGowan, J., Straus, S. E., & Tugwell, P. (2006). Canada urgently needs a national network of libraries to access evidence. *Healthcare Quarterly*, 9(1), 72–74.

Meisenheimer, C. G. (1997). *Improving quality: A guide to effective programs* (2nd ed.). Gaithersburg, MD: Aspen.

Mor, V., Morris, J., Lipsitz, L., & Fogel, B. (1998) Benchmarking quality in nursing homes: the Q-Metrics system. *Canadian Journal of Quality in Health Care*, 14(2), 12–17.

Patrick, L. (2004). Building an effective risk management program in a healthcare setting. *Healthcare Management Forum*, 17(3), 27–29.

Pink, G. H., Brown, A. D., Daniel, I., Hamlette, M. L., Markel, F., McGillis Hall, L., et al. (2006). Financial benchmarks for Ontario hospitals. *Healthcare Quarterly*, 9(1), 40–45.

Plsek, P. E. (1993). Tutorial: Quality improvement project models. *Quality Management in Health Care*, 1(2), 69–81.

Rantz, M. J., Petroski, G. F., Madsen, R. W., Scott, J., Mehr, D. R., Popejoy, L., et al. (1997). Setting thresholds for MDS (Minimum Data Set) quality indicators for nursing home quality improvement reports. *Joint Committee Journal on Quality Improvement*, 23(11), 602–611.

CHAPTER ENDNOTES

1. Health Canada, "Quest for Quality in Canadian Health-care: Continuous Quality Improvement, the Focus of CQI (background)." Retrieved from http://www.hc-sc.gc.ca/hcs-sss/pubs/qual/2000-qual/intro-eng.php#a4

2. "Accreditation Canada." Retrieved from http://www.accreditation.ca/accrediation-programs/qmentum/

3. The Joint Commission. "Facts about the sentinel event policy." Retrieved from http://www.jointcommission.org/facts_about_the_sentinel_event_policy/

4. Behamdouni, G., & Millar, K. (2010). Implementation of an enterprise risk-management program in a community teaching hospital. *Healthcare Quarterly,* 13(1), 73.

5. Ibid.

CHAPTER 17

Decision Making

Sharon Little-Stoetzel, RN, MS
Adapted by John P. Angkaw, MBA (c), MEd, BScN

Nurses have known that their decisions have important implications for client outcomes. Today, they are being increasingly called to be active decision makers in healthcare. The frequency and types of decisions faced by nurses will be influenced by their work environment, perceptions of their clinical role, operational autonomy, and the degree to which they see themselves as active and influential decision makers. (Thompson, Cullu, McCaughan, Sheldon, & Raynor, 2004)

OBJECTIVES

The purpose of this chapter is to enable the reader to

- apply effective decision making to clinical situations, incorporating critical thinking and problem solving;
- facilitate group decision making by using various techniques;
- apply technology, as appropriate, to decision making;
- examine the nurse's role in client decision making;
- examine strategies to improve decision making and to build self-confidence;
- describe the nature of decision making and the resulting cascades;
- identify their personal style in decision making;
- identify a minimum of three intrinsic factors that influence decision making in a health care environment; and
- articulate the link between climate, culture, and locus of control.

mmm/Shutterstock

You are a staff nurse on the medical cardiology unit, and you have just come from a unit meeting, where your nurse manager reported the results of the most recent client care score card. The incidence of client falls has increased by 75 percent. In addition, 35 percent of the clients have had repeat falls within 48 hours of their initial fall. Second and subsequent falls have a high correlation to the rate of injury, and they result in increased diagnostic testing and extended lengths of stay. The manager has selected a task force to investigate potential solutions to this problem, and you have been appointed chairperson. The unit action council has been trending falls for the past year and has identified some reasons for the undesirable fall rate: inconsistent admission assessments, client demographics inconsistent with the cardiac population, and a lack of a fall risk assessment tool.

What is your emotional connection to the problem?

Is there enough information known?

Which is the focus: problem solving the situation to iden-tify the root cause or making a decision about the use of a fall predictive tool?

Are you excited about the opportunity to assume a leader-ship role?

What should be the first step of the task force?

Can the decision-making process help the group solve the situation?

This chapter explores the decision-making process and factors that promote or impede clinical and professional practice decision making. Strategies to facilitate both the frequency and quality of decision making are explored. Decision making is presented as an associated process within the problem-solving cycle. Critical thinking is essential when making decisions and solving problems. Application of decision-making models

to clinical and management decisions are presented. The chapter examines the advantages and the limitations of group decision making, as well as the use of technology in decision making. Finally, it discusses the nurse's role in client decision making and strategies for improving the decision-making process.

CRITICAL THINKING

A buzzword or a concept? The words **critical thinking** have found their way into the mainstream of nursing language among nurses and across organizations. How-ever, too many nurses use the term as a buzzword with little understanding of what critical thinking entails, how their own thinking differs from someone else's, and how to think critically in various situations (Alfaro-LeFevre, 2006). Critical thinking is essential when making deci-sions and solving problems. The Pew Health Professions Commission asserted that nurses must "demonstrate critical thinking, reflection, and problem-solving skills" to thrive as effective practitioners in the 21st century (Bellack & O'Neil, 2000, p. 16).

What does it mean to be a critical thinker? Scriven and Paul (2004), in a statement on critical thinking prepared for the National Council for Excellence in Critical Thinking Instruction, define critical thinking as "a mode of thinking—about any subject, content, or problem—in which the thinker improves the quality of their thinking by skilfully taking charge of the structures inherent in thinking and imposing intellectual standards upon them." Scriven and Paul also suggest that critical thinking can be seen as having two components: (1) a set of information and beliefs generating and processing skills; and (2) the habit, based on intellectual commit-ment, of using those skills to guide behaviour. Alfaro-LeFevre (2006) adds that critical thinking is contextual in that it changes depending on circumstances. Conse-quently, critical thinking needs to be viewed from three perspectives, namely: (1) thinking ahead, (2) thinking in action, and (3) thinking back.

Thinking ahead is the ability to be proactive and anticipate what might happen. Novice nurses or novice nurse managers, as a result of their limited experience, may have to tap into the expertise of others, or refer to procedure manuals or texts to enhance their skills in order to be proactive. Nurses caring for clients in a pediatric setting might anticipate that separation anxiety will alter the sleeping pattern of a child and might plan with the parents a schedule that includes frequent visits. A nurse manager might anticipate the need for a critical incident debriefing session following a sentinel event on the unit (e.g., a client death via suicide).

Alfaro-LeFevre describes thinking in action as the ability to think on your feet. It "represents rapid, dynamic reasoning that considers several cues and priorities at once." She cautions that this type of critical thinking is more prone to "knee-jerk" responses and decisions than the other types of thinking. For example, in cardiac arrest situations, the nurse makes the following decisions: (1) call for help; (2) access Airway, Breathing, Circulation; (3) initiate CPR; and (4) once the cardiac arrest team arrives, ensure an IV is initiated. Another example of thinking on your feet, as a manager, would be responding to a situation of a witnessed threatened client assault of a nurse. Thinking back, the process of reflective thinking, is described by Alfaro-LeFevre as the ability to recall and analyze one's reasoning process to look for flaws or omissions, gain increased understanding, and correct and improve thinking.

Paul (1992) is quick to point out the many accurate definitions of critical thinking, most of which are consistent with each other. A good critical thinker is able to examine decisions from all sides and take into account varying points of view. A good critical thinker does not say, "We've always done it this way," and refuse to consider alternate ways. The critical thinker generates new ideas and alternatives when making decisions. The critical thinker asks "why" questions about a situation to arrive at the best decision. Four basic skills—critical reading, critical listening, critical writing, and critical speaking— are necessary for the development of critical thinking

skills. These skills are part of the process of developing and using thinking for decision making. Ability in these four areas can be measured by the extent to which one achieves the universal intellectual standards illustrated in Table 17-1.

As you begin to apply critical thinking to nursing, use these universal intellectual standards when you are reading material from a textbook, listening to an oral presentation, writing a paper, answering test questions, or presenting ideas in oral form. Ask yourself whether the ideas are clear or unclear, precise or imprecise, specific or vague, accurate or inaccurate, and so forth. You will improve your critical thinking skills over time. Scriven and Paul (2004) conclude that "no one is a critical thinker through-and-through, and for this reason the development of critical thinking skills and dispositions is a life-long endeavour."

REFLECTIVE THINKING

John Dewey, as cited in Teekman (2000), was possibly one of the first and most influential educational theorists to initiate the process of reflective thinking. Dewey believed that reflective thinking occurred due to doubt, uncertainty, or mental obscurity that encouraged the person to inquire and find the material that would help overcome

TABLE 17-1	**THE SPECTRUM OF UNIVERSAL INTELLECTUAL STANDARDS**
Clear	Unclear
Precise	Imprecise
Specific	Vague
Accurate	Inaccurate
Relevant	Irrelevant
Consistent	Inconsistent
Logical	Illogical
Deep	Superficial
Complete	Incomplete
Significant	Insignificant
Adequate	Inadequate
Fair	Unfair

Source: Adapted from the Foundation for Critical Thinking, Dillon, CA. http://criticalthinking.org/university/unistan.html

doubt and uncertainty. He recognized the importance of past experiences for reflection and argued that results and recommendations are dependent on one's past experiences because they do not arise out of nothing.

Pesut and Herman (1999) describe **reflective thinking** as watching or observing ourselves as we perform a task or make a decision about a particular situation, followed by thinking about what we have done, and how we could have done it better. We have two selves: the active self and the reflective self. The reflective self watches the active self as it engages in activities. The reflective self acts as observer and offers suggestions about the activities. To be a good critical thinker, one must practise reflective thinking. Reflection upon a situation or problem after a decision is made allows the individual to evaluate the decision. Nurse educators assist students to become better reflective thinkers through the use of clinical journals. Using journals helps students reflect on clinical activities and improve their clinical decision-making abilities.

Reflective thinking is based on the fundamental assumption that learning from one's experience is critical in developing and maintaining competence because what was learned from a particular situation may be used as a guide for future situations, or be incorporated into one's existing knowledge (Mann, Gordon, & MacLeod, 2009).

Reflection and reflective practice has been identified as a method to increase the competency of today's health care professional.

Donaghy and Morss (2000) describe a process of guided reflection as a structured approach within the context of a reflective practice framework; it facilitates the individual's reflection because it is linked more closely with systematic critical enquiry, problem solving,

and clinical reasoning. In Canada the regulatory colleges for nurses have implemented continuing competence programs, which are designed to ensure ongoing competence and overall practice quality across the profession. Reflective thinking is becoming mainstream in all domains of practice (e.g., direct practice, administration, education, and research).

PROBLEM SOLVING

Problem solving is an active process that starts with a problem and ends with a solution. LeStorti et al. (1999) define a problem as the difference between the actual state and the desired state. The problem-solving process consists of five steps: identify the problem, gather and analyze data, generate alternatives and select an action, implement the selected action, and evaluate the action. Note the similarities to the nursing process steps of assessment, diagnosis, outcome identification, planning, implementation, and evaluation. The nursing process is applied to client situations or problems, whereas the problem-solving process may be applied to a problem of any type.

DECISION MAKING
AN INTRODUCTION

The mythology and legends of many different cultures include mythological creatures of human appearance but of extraordinary size and strength. *Giant* is the English word commonly used for such beings. The term *sleeping giant* has been coined to describe a calm, yet powerful force that is not to be disturbed for fear of the negative, unknown, or uncontrollable consequences that the force (i.e., the giant) can unleash.

REAL WORLD INTERVIEW

I believe that all nurses in all domains of practice should incorporate reflective thinking into their practice. It is required by my college in order to maintain my registration. However, it has also afforded me the opportunity to better myself both professionally and personally. It has forced me to revisit situations and evaluate the decisions I have made. Nursing is a constant learning experience and one must take it upon oneself to continually improve.

Catherine Terry, RN, MHA
Administrative Director,
Medicine and Ambulatory Care

REAL WORLD INTERVIEW

Thoughts lead on to purpose, purpose goes into action, actions form habits, habits decide character and character fixes our destiny.

Tyron Edwards
American Theologian (1809–1894)

Nursing in Canada is much like the sleeping giant, yet to be truly awakened. Described as the backbone of the health care system (Canadian Nursing Advisory Committee [CNAC], 2002), nursing comprises the largest number of health care professionals in Canada, with the number of registered nurses at 284,690, in 2009 (CNA, 2011). The active ingredient needed to awaken the giant is consistent and effective decision making. This process will provide individual nurses and the profession as a whole with a trajectory that is focused on nursing as a leader in the delivery of health care.

Imagine the health care system in Canada if nursing's voice was more influential than it currently is perceived. The impacts on current issues in nursing practice would be phenomenal, especially in the areas of defining and measuring workload, scope of practice and non-nursing tasks, the quality of the practice environment, autonomy and respect, as well as leadership and education. Empowerment, competence, and self-confidence are enhanced through effective decision making. And success in decision making builds further success and awakens the sleeping giant to achieve greatness.

Rapid changes in the health care environment (e.g., the contracting of resources, changes in the skill mix, staffing challenges, and more informed consumers) provide opportunities for expanded decision making for nurses at all levels. Government requirements for accountability for positive client outcomes and fiscal responsibility have led to an increase in decision making by nurses, which is pivotal to an agency's strategic and operational success. Shrinking budgets and other constraining factors require that nurse managers and direct practice nurses be more innovative and creative than ever before. As a result, decision making has rapidly become a core competency for all nurses. It is generally understood that client care is more complex today, given co-morbidities and the number of social and cultural factors. Client acuity (i.e., severity of illness) is generally perceived to be higher than in the previous decades. Because clients are being discharged from acute care institutions earlier, and with higher acuity, effective decisions regarding treatment must be made in a timely manner.

So what, then, is **decision making?** Decision making is the cognitive process leading to the selection of a course of action among alternatives. Every decision-making process results in a final outcome that can take the form of an opinion or an action. Decision making is a process of reasoning that begins when there is a perceived need to do something but we are not sure of what to do.

Clinical decision making occurs within the context of a health care environment and a therapeutic practitioner relationship or professional relationship. On a daily basis health care personnel apply their foundational knowledge to the information about clients through their history, an examination and integration of diagnostic test results, and dialogue with them in making important decisions about effective treatment. Despite the fact decision making seems so commonplace, Stanford School of Medicine's Centre for Immersive Simulation-Based Learning asserts "decision making is very complicated and hard to learn."[1] Further, Stanford suggests that decision making is more difficult to learn in situations in which decisions are complex and involve substantial discussion with clients or in settings, such as critical care units or the operating room, where time is a major factor.[2]

NATURE OF DECISION MAKING IN NURSING

Decision making can either be daunting or exciting to the new graduate nurse or to the nurse who has achieved expert status in practice. That response can be influenced by a number of individual and environmental factors (O'Reilly, 1993), which will be explored later in this chapter. Peter Block, author of *The Empowered Manager: Positive Political Skills at Work,* (1990) claims that we "walk the tightrope between advocating our own position and yet not increasing resistance against us by our actions (p. 7). In many cases, this tightrope is the juxtaposition that nurses in direct practice experience in often autocratic, hierarchical, practice environments. Block claims that the decision path we take in our organizational situations is essentially influenced by one of two factors. Namely, we are influenced by our individual choices, which are focused on adaptation, and secondly, by the norms and values of the organizations we find ourselves embedded within.

Nurses begin their careers making essentially two types of decisions. Nurses are involved in making clinical decisions within the context of a therapeutic relationship with a client. They also make decisions that relate to the context and system of care delivery. Finally, decisions are made about their own professional development and the career path they choose to follow. In each of these areas, nurses have the opportunity to choose maintenance versus greatness, caution versus courage, or dependency versus autonomy. Block (1990) describes these opportunities as the fundamental choices we make. Interestingly enough, these same fundamental choices are made by individual nurses, nursing managers, nursing executives within an organization, and by nursing as a discipline.

How does maintenance differ from greatness? Maintenance choices typically are those that permit us to hold on to what we have created or inherited—in other words, the status quo. This choice, repeated over time, although safe, does not result in forward direction. This type of decision making is characteristic in bureaucratic organizational cultures (Block, 1990). Personal safety is a strong driver in this key decision. Based on learned behaviour, staff in bureaucratic situations may have learned that their achievements are rewarded less and that their errors in decision result in personal repercussion or punishment.

Block states that the choice for maintenance is the choice to be led by others. Reflect for a moment on the current state of professional nursing within your clinical setting. Is nursing leading or being led by others outside of the discipline?

The alternative to maintenance is greatness. Block asserts that we tend to think of greatness as being something beyond our personal abilities because greatness is reserved for the Albert Schweitzers, the Bishop Tutus, or the Nelson Mandelas of the world. Yet these great people are ordinary individuals doing extraordinary things, all of which involved decision making at critical moments that were focused on greatness. Block defines greatness as giving up pessimism and the need for the insulation that comes with corporate structure and predictability. Choosing greatness requires knowledge, courage, and energy. All nurses have an opportunity to choose the status quo (i.e., maintenance) or positive change (i.e., greatness) in their daily practice and over the course of their careers. Choosing to accept the problem of ongoing staffing shortages is an example of accepting the status quo. Moving forward with a decision to explore a different skill mix, a change in staffing patterns, or to promote a full scope of practice would constitute making a decision of greatness.

What distinguishes caution from courage? Caution is a reflection of organizational values around risk-taking, autonomous decision making at the point of care, and organizational management style. Cautious decisions are often apparent in organizations in which staff feel a strong presence of supervision and management control. Language often heard is couched in caution, such as, "Be careful of so and so, who can be fatal if you get on his/ her wrong side" or "You have to be politically astute to survive in this organization." The opposite of caution is to choose courage. "In our culture, moving forward and creating an organization we believe in always requires an act of courage," (Block, 1990, p. 15).

To act courageously is to take an unpopular position or chart an unpopular path. The most solid example of courageous decision making by the nursing profession in Canada is illustrated in the fundamental change to degree education as an entry-to-practice requirement for all registered nurses. In the example above, the courage decision is to choose an unpopular path and examine staffing pattern changes or entertain revised skill mix. As the experienced decision maker has learned, often through trial and error, the hard part of choosing courage over caution is learning to avoid suicide.

The importance of professional nurse autonomy has been extensively addressed in the nursing literature over the past two decades. Nurse autonomy is a key indicator of quality work environments, yet definition, measurement, and interpretation of research findings have complicated the effective integration and promotion of this key indicator into nursing work environments (Tranmer, 2004).

Block claims the third type of choice we make as individuals is to choose between dependency and autonomy. He suggests that in many organizations a gap exists between articulating the value of autonomy and living it. In the nursing context, autonomy is a complex, multidimensional phenomenon—an interactive, relational process that occurs within the context of one's being and work. Wade (1999) differentiated among three types of autonomy: (1) structural and work autonomy as the worker's freedom to make decisions based upon job requirements; (2) attitudinal autonomy as the belief in one's freedom to exercise judgement in decision making; and (3) aggregate autonomy, which encompasses attitudinal and structural dimensions, the socially and legally granted freedom of self-governance, and control of the profession without influence from external sources.

Keenan (1999) and Scott, Sochalski, and Aiken (1999) identified two dimensions of nurses' work autonomy: organizational and clinical practice. The capacity of nurses to be involved as participants in the decision-making process provides direction and stewardship of work at the unit and organizational level. Macdonald (2002) described professional autonomy as the right to exercise clinical and organizational judgement within the context of an interdependent health care team in accordance with the socially and legally granted freedom of the discipline. Choosing autonomous decision making over dependency puts nurses in charge of what is happening at the moment, which is a very useful concept given the nature of nursing care and the frequency of decision making.

Block indicates that autonomous decision making helps us understand that we are the cause and not the effect. He also asserts that the fundamental vulnerability in the way most large organizations are managed is the pervasive feeling of dependency that is engendered. Language that might suggest a dependency environment may include "I was waiting for approval to do that" or "I'm counting on direction from above, or when top management gets its act together." This type of language is very much upward looking and is reflective of dependency. Is there a cost to individual nurses, managers, nurse executives, and to the discipline as a whole for choosing the dependency approach? Absolutely, and it gets paid in the form of a sense of helplessness in which we wait for clear instructions before acting— despite our inherent intuition that courage, greatness, and autonomy are required to change the trajectory of nursing leadership.

FACTORS INFLUENCING DECISION MAKING

As nurses, we need to have working knowledge of what drives individuals (i.e., our peers and our clients) to make choices that set up the cascade of courage, greatness, and autonomy as opposed to caution, maintenance, and dependency.

The research literature reports numerous factors that influence decision making (Pardue, 1987). These factors include individual variables, such as experience and knowledge (Benner, 1984; Benner & Tanner, 1987), creative thinking ability, education (Pardue, 1987), and self-concept (Joseph, 1985), as well as environmental and situational stressors (Cleland, 1967, Evans, 1990). These factors, either intrinsic or extrinsic, may serve to enhance or impede decision making in the area of clinical practice or professional development.

An examination of the intrinsic factors provides nurses with insight into the factors that are considered "controllable"—to borrow the word from the Heart and Stroke Foundation. Being controllable infers that we can make a conscious choice to alter or modify our behaviour to have an impact on the factor. Intrinsic factors include personal perception and preference, knowledge and experience, competence, self-confidence, and stress. Extrinsic factors that influence decision making include organizational climate and culture, client rights and choice, and legal legislative frameworks.

PERSONAL PERCEPTION AND PREFERENCE

Understanding how we perceive problems in clinical practice or in our professional lives helps us to see how we can influence our personal preference in decision making. ChangingMinds.org suggests that we have either subjective or objective perceptions.[3]

Objective perception is characterized by seeing the problem or decision point from the perspective of standing outside of our body. This viewpoint does not suggest any level of dispassion or disengagement; rather it simply represents an objective viewpoint, which is a comfortable place to be for many nurses. In this space of comfort, nurses can see things from a more impersonal, rational, and unemotional viewpoint. Typically, people who perceive opportunities for decision making in the objective view also tend to make *thinking decisions*. Thinking decisions are based on logic, an exploration of black and white tangible facts, and the use of clear rules. In organizations these types of decision makers may be perceived as cold and heartless by people who perceive opportunities for decision making on a more emotional basis.

Feelers tend to make decisions by considering the social context, listening to their heart, and considering the feelings of others. Feelers value harmony and use tact in their interactions with others.[4] Feelers are usually relationship-oriented and use a values base for decision making. As a result, feelers see the opportunity for decision making through the subjective lens, which tends to make them more empathetic and intuitive. Typically, thinkers, who are also objective, tend to be left-brain dominant, whereas feelers, who are subjective, tend to be right-brain dominant. The good news is that evidence now exists that shows that neither right- nor left-brain thinking is better than the other. Murphy (1985) asserts that each side is important, but each side also lacks something. In practical terms, both in a clinical and professional sense, we would never contemplate making a decision using only one-half of our brain.

KNOWLEDGE AND EXPERIENCE

Tanner, Padrick, Westfall, and Putzier (1987) studied the diagnostic reasoning approaches of nurses and nursing students and reported that increased knowledge and experience yielded more systematic data acquisition and greater diagnostic accuracy. Benner and Tanner (1987) also found that the difference in diagnostic accuracy was attributed to the ability of the expert nurse to intuitively determine the correct region for the assessment, select relevant data, and recognize the changing relevance of cues as the situation evolves. By contrast, Aiken, Clarke, Sloane, Sochalski, and Silber (2002) first reported a critical nurse-sensitive indicator called "failure to rescue," which refers to the lack of ability to pick up on these cues and intervene before a negative sequence of events begins to cascade. Benner and Tanner (1987) define intuition as "understanding without rationale" (p. 23). This level of expertise represents the hallmark of expert nursing judgement derived from the synergy of knowledge and experience. Evans (1990) suggests that ability to use intuition to rapidly identify important facts, and thereby limit the number of alternatives to be evaluated, reduces decisional conflict and stress and, therefore, is seen as a factor that enhances decision making.

On the flip side, Correnti (1992) dismisses intuition as irrational guessing. Given the heavy and appropriate focus on evidence-based nursing in today's curriculum of undergraduate nursing programs, many nurses are reluctant to follow their so-called gut feelings, and they reject the use of intuition in decision making.

O'Reilly (1993) suggests the attitude of dismissing intuitive judgement as irrational guessing will generate decisional conflict and create a barrier to expert nursing judgement. Given the current escalation of the client safety agenda by the 36 required organizational practices defined by Accreditation Canada, it is critical that all nurses possess and maintain honed intuitive decision-making skills. Such skills will ensure that nurses are in a position to activate the decision-making threshold and act sooner rather than later, thereby minimizing client safety risks. Within the required organizational practices, there are six client safety areas: safety culture, communication, medication use, infection control, work life and workplace, and risk assessment.[5] Correnti (1992) also supports the strategy of nurse educators teaching the application of intuitive skills, cultivating intuitive knowledge, and promoting the development of creating thinking abilities for problem solving.

Knowledge and experience are also influenced by past experience that includes education and decision-making experience (Marquis & Huston, 2012). Life experience plays a significant role in decision making. Maturity helps individuals to see a problem from more perspectives, based on their life experiences, which can yield a rich bank of alternatives. Possessing knowledge of the theories that underpin decision making and the process and tools involved also influence the knowledge and experience factor. Dwyer, Schwartz, and Fox (1992) found that nurses' desire for autonomy varies widely across the profession, and they postulate that nurses seeking autonomy are more likely to have experience with decision making than those who fear autonomy.

COMPETENCE

The Canadian Nurses Association (CNA) provides the following definition of competencies: the specific knowledge, skills, judgement, and personal attributes required for a registered nurse to practise safely and ethically in a designated role and setting (Canadian Nurses Association, 2007, p. 11). Campbell and Mackay (2001) have a different interpretation of competence, and they identify three concepts: (1) the ability to practise in a specific role; (2) the influence of the practice setting on competence; and (3) the integration of knowledge, skills, judgements, and abilities. Despite these definitions, no single universal definition exists of nursing competence. Nurses practise individually, and in groups, in a wide array of clinical, non-clinical, and non-traditional settings. What is common to all nurses is the need to make clinical and professional decisions in their practice. To be effective decision makers, nurses must have a solid anchoring in the core competencies related to their entry to practice, and they must possess knowledge and abilities related to problem solving and decision making within their professional practice.

The American Nurses Association states that the assurance of competence is the shared responsibility of the profession, individual nurses, professional organizations, credentialing and certification entities, regulatory bodies, employers, and other key stakeholders. The Canadian Nurses Association has numerous position statements where competence is key, such as "Promoting cultural competence in nursing," "Cultural competence and cultural safety in First Nations, Inuit and Métis nursing education," and "Promoting culturally competent care."

Hagbaghery, Salsali, and Ahmadi (2004) reported that effective clinical decision making depends on one's ability to gather, understand, and integrate data that focuses on clients' needs and the clinical situation. The best way for nurses to develop competence in decision making is to make decisions.

SELF-CONFIDENCE

Joseph (1985) claims that people who perceive themselves as less intelligent, less educated, and less competent than others relinquish their authority to those they perceive as being better. This observation plays itself out within health care facilities on a daily basis on many units. In nursing, one has to "earn one's stripes" by gaining the confidence and the respect of one's peers. New graduates and new nurses joining an established team often feel they need to prove themselves in order to be accepted by the more senior staff. Joseph also reports that an individual's locus of control (i.e., the extent to which people believe they can control events and outcomes), plays an important role in an individual's perception of self-efficacy and self-concept. Individuals with an external locus of control, often the "upward lookers," believe that events and outcomes are dependent on the action of others (Lazarus & Folkman, 1984).

Self-confidence is a term used to describe how secure people are in their own decisions and actions. This definition can be applied either generally or to specific situations or tasks. Nurses who possess a high degree of confidence believe they have the competence (i.e., the knowledge, judgement, and skill) to perform an action correctly or achieve some specific goal. Confident and competent nurses usually have little difficulty making clinical decisions, such as starting an intravenous in urgent or emergency situations, referring a client to social work, or ordering a pressure-reduction overlay mattress. Self-confidence is learned through repeated successful application of the decision-making process. Decisions that require courage, autonomy, and greatness, and result in positive client outcomes become strong motivators that support decision making. Decisions that illustrate caution, dependency, and maintenance have less intrinsic reward for the nurse, and, therefore, such decisions have little ability to motivate continued decision making. The outcome can be a lack of self-confidence, which is reinforced with every missed opportunity for decision making.

A lack of self-confidence is created when an individual holds a belief that a specific action or decision will not generate the desired results. This belief is reinforced when the outcome is less than desirable or if it results in repercussion from peers or the immediate supervisor. Making staffing decisions in the absence of the manager is an example of a decision that may not generate the desired results. The nurse may decide that a sick staff nurse does not need to be replaced because client acuity and complexity is aligned with the staff available at the time. However, this decision can lead to negative feedback from peers. On the other hand, staff replacement, particularly when it incurs overtime costs, may not be welcomed by the manager and will require the nurse to justify the decision with endless rationale. A lack of self-confidence is often coupled with self-consciousness, especially when someone is performing an action while being observed by others. Any mistake, however small, can be amplified by this preoccupation that someone is watching, and this perception will create an erosion of self-confidence and a heightening of self-consciousness. New graduates launching their professional careers need to be cautious not to fall into this trap.

STRESS

Stress arises when individuals perceive the environment to be demanding, because it exceeds their resources and threatens their personal well-being (Lazarus & Folkman, 1984). Bailey, Steffen, and Grout (1980) and Wakefield (1992) suggest that situations can be anxiety-provoking for some and stimulating for others, depending on how people perceive the environment. Generally speaking, nurses with an internal locus of control in a clinical setting perceive opportunities to influence outcomes for their clients, other nurses, and the organization. This approach leads to a greater sense of personal job satisfaction and reduction of stress. Staff members who have an external locus of control believe that external events and people are in control, and that they have very little choice over deciding their future.

Cleland (1967) studied the effects of stress upon nurses' thinking and concluded that moderate amounts of stress are required for optimal thinking. However, she also concluded that the long-term effects of functioning within highly stressful environments, such as today's health care settings, include stereotypical, unimaginative thinking, overgeneralization, and loss of interest. Bailey et al. (1980) found that nurses identified the following factors as producing the greatest stress: interpersonal conflict, inadequate staffing, lack of support when dealing with death, and physical environment. Coomber and Barriball (2007) found that stress and leadership issues exert influence of job dissatisfaction and turnover for nurses. To reduce workplace turnover and improve job satisfaction, organizations need to focus on the work environment, particularly at the unit level.

A study by Healy and McKay (2000) reveals significant positive relationships between nursing stress and mood disturbance, and a negative relationship between nursing stress and job satisfaction. In their study, they found that the use of avoidance coping and the perception of work overload were significant predictors of mood disturbance. There was no evidence to suggest that the use of humour had any moderating effect on the stress-mood relationship, but there was support for the influence of job satisfaction related to humour.

In 2007 the nursing profession found that stress is a constant and results in higher rates of job strain, lack of job satisfaction, and higher illness rates among nurses (Aiken et al., 2002). These results do not bode well for the future of nursing. Consequently, nurses and employers need to collaborate to create and maintain practice environments that support effective decision making at the point of care, and thereby contribute to a high sense of job fulfilment and autonomy for nurses.

EXTRINSIC FACTORS

ORGANIZATIONAL CLIMATE AND CULTURE

Organizational climate and culture provide the context in which nursing practice occurs and can have a profound impact on the efficacious and effective application of that practice. Carman et al. (1996) and Doran et al. (2002) conclude that organizational climate and culture are increasingly recognized as important variables in the success or failure of change initiatives, including quality improvement. Affonso and Doran (2000) add patient safety to the areas affected by an organization's climate and culture.

Hofstede (1998) noted that "culture is a characteristic of the organization, *not of individuals*" (p. 469). This description suggests that the culture in any organization is illustrated and measured through the language being used—both verbal and nonverbal—and the behaviours being exhibited by individuals and groups at the organizational level. Organizational culture can be influenced by individuals, organizational features, and external factors. Shein (1991) reported that individuals can facilitate cultural change through leadership that clarifies values and develops a common organizational vision. Organizational structures, routines, command and control expectations, and operational norms influence the organization's culture (Langfield-Smith, 1995).

Cultural factors have an impact on decision making. For example, a conservative organization that is risk averse, with a top-down bureaucratic operational style, is not likely to embrace a decentralized decision-making model in which nurses, nursing leaders, and nurse managers are encouraged to make pivotal decisions at the point of care. Block (1990) states that "if we sit on top of the pyramid we can have a very broad impact [i.e., influential decision making] on structure, policy, strategy and procedures" (p. 189). The opposite is true if nurses find themselves at the bottom of the pyramid. In this situation nurses may only have impact on decisions that affect personal actions. Block asserts that regardless of the staff position, "the challenge is to pursue our vision with as much courage and intensity as we can generate" (p. 189).

CLIENT CHOICE AND RIGHTS

The Canadian Healthcare Association indicates that there is no national bill of client rights approved for use in Canada. However, various interest groups have adopted a bill of rights for the people they represent; for example, the Arthritis Society of Canada has a bill of rights for people with arthritis. Typically, a bill of rights is organizationally driven and reflects the following principles: the client's right to self-determination, respect, privacy, confidentiality, continuity in care delivery, and financial billing rights. In every interaction, nurses, nurse leaders, and nurse managers must respect the client's rights to self-determination, which might mean accepting the client's decision to refuse treatment or to live at risk. Nurses also must be aware that a client may reach a point of being unable to make treatment decisions. Consequently, nurses need to understand the role of advanced directives; powers of attorney for care and finance; and substitute decision making, by either a substitute decision maker of the client's choice or a court-appointed guardian. They also must understand the legislative frameworks in which these various client representatives gain their power to act on behalf of the client. Above all, the client's wishes, directives, choices, and needs must be considered in the clinical decision-making process.

Following significant consultation with the public, the Excellent Care for All Act was proclaimed by the Ontario government in June 2010. This act mandated that a declaration of client values be published on each hospital website. The declaration of values could be in the form of a code of conduct, a value statement, or a client bill of rights. Most organizations have held focus groups, web site surveys, and individual interviews to determine what should be articulated in the bill of rights.

LEGISLATION AND REGULATION   External influences can include government legislation (e.g., Ontario's Regulated Health Professions Act, 1991), professional standards (e.g., the CNA Code of Ethics, various provincial regulators' standards of practice, and best practice guidelines), and various provincial government accountability agreements that outline performance standards. A classic example of the legislative and regulatory impact on decision making is the transfer of a controlled act from one discipline to another. In all provinces, nursing regulators have specific frameworks outlining how this transfer must occur. A nurse implementing a medical directive approved for use in the organization needs to use professional judgement in deciding whether to implement the directive. The nurse's actions within the directive are influenced by provincial legislation and professional regulation. This type of decision making in clinical practice is intense because of the speed of the decision and the consequences of indecision (e.g., deciding on whether to implement a medical directive on the management of chest pain).

Consideration of regulatory legislation, professional standards, best practice guidelines, and organizational policies and procedures is fundamental to effective clinical decision making. Thus, nurses must have knowledge and understanding of the regulatory framework that

governs their practice, and they must understand other regulatory practice requirements as defined in other types of federal and provincial legislation (e.g., the Personal Information Protection and Electronic Documents Act [PIPEDA], the Narcotic Control Act, acts governing consent and substitute decision makers, and health information protection acts).

STEPS IN THE DECISION-MAKING PROCESS

In everyday practice, nurses make decisions about client care. As nurses gain experience in clinical practice, decision making becomes more automatic, but the complexity of many decisions remains. Huber (2000) defines **decision making** as a "behaviour exhibited in making a selection and implementing a course of action from alternatives. It may or may not be the result of an immediate problem" (p. 378). Both decision making and problem solving use critical thinking. Table 17-2 reviews decision making and critical thinking. Figure 17-1 highlights the use of critical thinking in both problem solving and decision making.

Although decisions are unique to different situations, the decision-making process can be applied to each situation. The decision-making process is similar to the steps in problem solving. In the decision-making process, there are also five steps:

TABLE 17-2	REVIEW OF DECISION MAKING AND CRITICAL THINKING
Decision making	Decision making means making a selection and implementing a course of action from a group of alternatives. It may or may not involve a problem.
Critical Thinking	Critical thinking means analyzing the way one thinks. It should be incorporated into all steps of problem solving and decision making.

Figure 17-1 Critical Thinking Is Used in Both Problem Solving and Decision Making

- Step 1: Identify the need for a decision.
- Step 2: Determine the goal or outcome.
- Step 3: Identify the alternatives or actions along with the benefits and consequences of each action.
- Step 4: Decide which action to implement.
- Step 5: Evaluate the action.

In the following clinical application, the decision-making process is applied to a clinical situation.

CLINICAL APPLICATION

Your client is on droplet precautions because he has been diagnosed with tuberculosis. As per hospital policy, only two visitors are allowed at a time to see the client. No children under 12 years of age are allowed. The client does not speak English, and his family speaks very little English. You have noticed on two occasions that his visitors were not wearing masks. You inform the family about the importance of infection control practices and remind them of the hospital's policy regarding visitors. The family indicates to you that their grandfather really wants to see his four-year-old grandson, who came to visit him from another province. Use your skills in decision making and problem solving to help you decide what to do.

- Step 1: Identify the need for a decision. Should you allow the grandson to visit? Consider all the information (e.g., the hospital policy, professional practice standards, the client's wishes, and the client's anxiety level).
- Step 2: Determine the outcome. What is the goal? Consider the following questions: Can an exception to hospital policy be made? Is the goal to allow the client to see his grandson? Will the client and his family be satisfied?
- Step 3: Identify all alternative actions and the benefits and consequences of each. If you enforce hospital policy, the benefits are that all clients are treated equally and the written policy supports the decision. The consequences are that the client and his family may not be satisfied, and the grandson and grandfather may be upset. In addition, the grandson's health may be at risk. The alternative is to allow the grandson to visit. The benefits are that the client's level of anxiety will decrease, and the client and his family will be satisfied. The consequence is that a precedent is set that may make it difficult to enforce the existing hospital policy.
- Step 4: Arrive at the decision. Consider the two alternatives and the benefits and consequences of each. Make the decision and implement it.
- Step 5: Evaluate the decision. Was the goal achieved?

From the beginning of their careers, new graduate nurses are faced with the responsibility of making decisions regarding client care. Beginning nurses commonly have more questions than answers. When nurses are faced with a difficult clinical decision, Marquis and Huston (2012) recommend consulting with others, such as other RNs on the unit or supervisors, as early as possible. Depending on the situation, recognize that you have knowledge and intuition that are valuable. With more experience comes greater trust in your decision making.

MANAGEMENT APPLICATION

Nurse managers sometimes face complex decisions. Decisions related to budget are common in our current health care environment with its emphasis on cost containment and quality maintenance. Disciplining an employee also creates a complex situation in which managers must make decisions regarding the employee's future. A decision-making grid may help to separate the multiple factors that surround a situation. Figure 17-2 illustrates use of a decision-making grid by managers who were told they had to reduce their workforce by two full-time equivalents (FTEs). This grid is useful to visually separate the factors of cost savings, effect on job satisfaction of remaining staff, and effect on client satisfaction. The manager needs to determine the priorities when developing a grid.

A decision-making grid is also useful when a nurse is trying to decide between two choices. Figure 17-3 is an example of a decision grid used by a nurse deciding between working at hospital A or hospital B.

The Program Evaluation and Review Technique (PERT) is useful in determining the timing of decisions. The flowchart provides a visual picture depicting the sequence of tasks that must take place to complete a project. Jones and Beck (1996) provide an example of a PERT flow diagram depicting a case management project (see Figure 17-4). The chart shows the amount of time taken to complete the project and the sequence of events to complete the project. An advantage of the PERT diagram is that participants can visualize a complete picture of the project, including the timing of decisions from beginning to end.

DECISION TREE

A decision tree is a decision support tool that uses a graphlike model to outline the possible decisions and their associated benefits and consequences. Using this

CRITICAL THINKING

You are the manager on call at your hospital and at 2230 h. you were paged by the charge nurse on the medicine unit to seek your assistance. She informed you that there are visitors on the unit that are refusing to leave, and that said they will be staying the night. As per hospital policy, visiting hours are from 1100 to 2100 hours. All visitors who wish to stay overnight must obtain permission in advance. The visitors state that they are from out-of-town and want to spend as much time with their mother as possible. Furthermore, they stated that they had received permission to stay from the physician earlier.

How would you handle this request?

Apply the decision making process to this scenario.

tool is particularly helpful when dealing with a multi-stage decision-making process. It can be useful in making the alternatives visible. Figure 17-5 is a decision tree for choosing whether to go back to school.

Figure 17-6 identifies a decision analysis tree for a client who smokes.

GANTT CHART

A Gantt chart can be useful for decision makers to illustrate a project from beginning to end. It also highlights any key milestones or decision points along the way. Typically, a Gantt chart will outline the different phases and activities of a particular project. A Gantt chart is developed by having the horizontal (x) axis representing the lifespan of the project, usually specified in increments (i.e. days, weeks, months), and the vertical (y) axis

Methods of Reduction	Cost Savings	Effect on Job Satisfaction	Effect on Client Satisfaction
Lay off the two most senior full-time employees	$110,000	Significant reduction	Significant reduction
Lay off the two most recently hired full-time employees	$92,000	Significant reduction	Moderate reduction
Reduce by staff attrition	$78,000	Minor reduction	Minor reduction

Figure 17-2 Sample Decision-Making Grid

Elements	Importance Score (out of 10)	Likelihood Score (out of 10)	Risk (multiply scores)
If I work at hospital A			
Learning experience	10	10	100
Good mentor support	8	8	64
Financial reward	6	6	36
Growth potential	8	8	64
Good location	10	10	100
Total			364
If I work at hospital B			
Learning experience	8	8	64
Good mentor support	7	7	49
Financial reward	8	8	64
Growth potential	9	9	81
Good location	6	6	36
Total			294

Figure 17-3 Sample Decision-Making Grid for Weighing Options

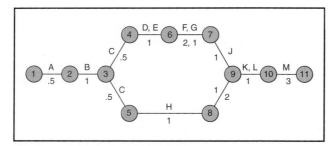

Figure 17-4 PERT Diagram with Critical Path for Implementation of Case Management

representing the task and activities that comprise the project. Figure 17-7 illustrates a Gantt chart used to show the progression of a nursing unit's pilot project.

GROUP DECISION MAKING

Certain situations call for group decision making. Vroom and Yetton (1973) identified certain questions that managers should ask themselves before making a decision alone. In some situations it is more appropriate for a group to make the decision rather than the individual manager.

REAL WORLD INTERVIEW

I often find decisions about disciplinary action the most difficult ones to make. But, when I use a decision-making model, it helps me make the best decision. My goal in the decision-making process is often twofold—to help the nurse to learn from the experience and to provide the nurse with appropriate tools to prevent similar mistakes happening in the future.

Erica
Nurse Manager Intensive Care Unit

Each situation is different, and an effective manager adopts the appropriate mode of decision making—group or individual. The eight questions in Table 17-3 may assist the manager in determining which mode to use.

According to today's leadership and management styles, the people who will be most affected by a decision are included in the decision-making process. Decisions

TABLE 17-3	INDIVIDUAL VERSUS GROUP DECISION-MAKING QUESTIONS

1. Does the manager have all the information needed?

2. Do the subordinates have supplementary information needed to make the best decision?

3. Does the manager have all the resources available to obtain sufficient information to make the best decision?

4. Is it absolutely critical that the team accept the decision prior to implementation?

5. Will the team accept the decision I make by myself?

6. Does the course of action chosen make a difference to the organization?

7. Does the team have the best interest of the organization foremost when considering the decision?

8. Will the decision cause undue conflict among the team?

Source: Material adapted from the chapter "Basic Consideration Underlying the Normative Model" from *Leadership and Decision-Making*, by Victor H. Vroom and Philip W. Yetton, (c) 1973. Reprinted by permission of the University of Pittsburgh Press.

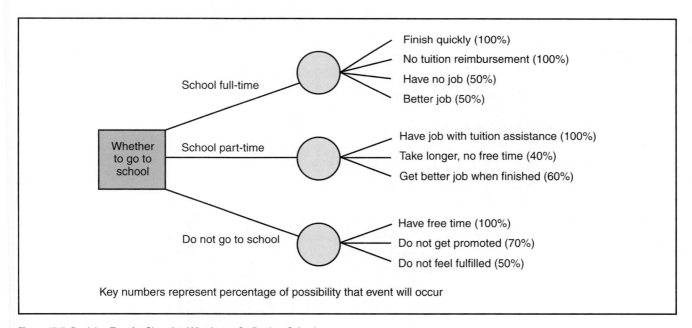

Figure 17-5 Decision Tree for Choosing Whether to Go Back to School

affecting client care should be made by those groups implementing the decisions.

The effectiveness of groups depends greatly on the group's members. The size of the group and the personalities of group members are important considerations when choosing participants. Because more ideas can be generated with groups, the group process allows for more choices, which increases the likelihood of higher quality outcomes. Another advantage of groups is that followers who participate in the decision-making process are more likely to accept the decision. Additionally, groups may be used as a medium for communicating the decision and its rationale.

A major disadvantage of group decision making is the time involved. Without effective leadership, groups can waste time and be non-productive. Group decision making can be more costly and can also lead to conflict. Groups can be dominated by one person or become the battleground for a power struggle among assertive members. See Table 17-4 for a list of the advantages and disadvantages of groups for decision making.

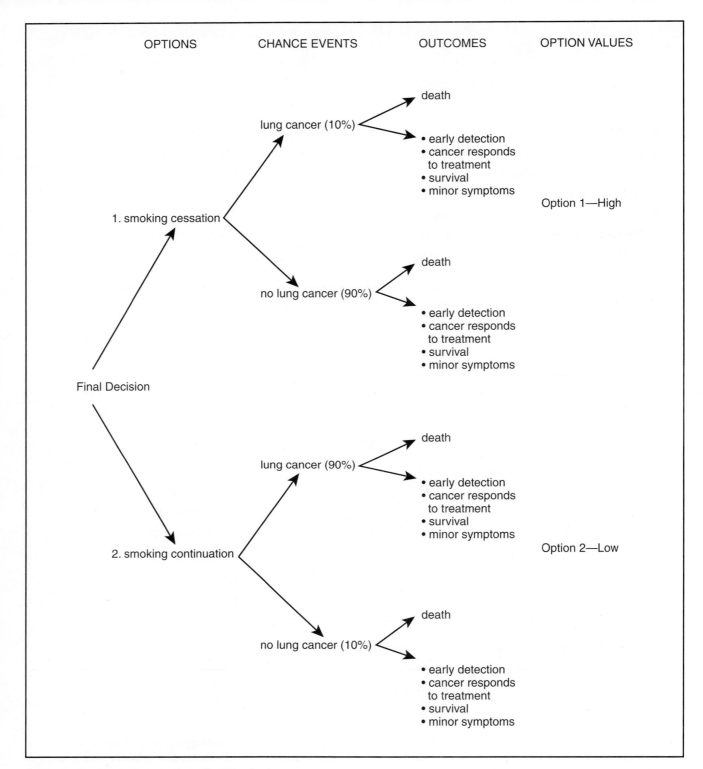

Figure 17-6 Decision Analysis Tree for a Client Who Smokes

TABLE 17-4	ADVANTAGES AND DISADVANTAGES OF GROUPS

Advantages

- Easy and inexpensive way to share information
- Opportunities for face-to-face communication
- Opportunity to become connected with a social unit
- Promotion of cohesiveness and loyalty
- Access to a larger resource base
- Forum for constructive problem solving
- Support group
- Facilitation of *esprit de corps*
- Promotion of ownership of problems and solutions

Disadvantages

- Individual opinions influenced by others
- Individual identity obscured
- Formal and informal role and status positions evolve—hierarchies
- Dependency fostered
- Time-consuming
- Inequity of time given to share individual information
- Existence of non-functional roles
- Personality conflicts

A nurse manager has agreed to have her unit pilot a new care delivery system within six months. The Gantt chart can be used to plan the progression of the project.

Activities	Sept	Oct	Nov	Dec	Jan	Feb	Mar	Apr	May
Discuss project with staff	------ X								
Form an ad hoc planning committee	------	—— X							
Receive report from committee			------ X						
Discuss report with staff			------ —— X						
Educate all staff to the plan				------	—— X				
Implement new system						------	——————		
Evaluate system and make changes							------	——	X

Key
------ Proposed Time
—— Actual Time
X Complete

Figure 17-7 Gantt Chart: Implementation of Care Delivery System

REAL WORLD INTERVIEW

Personally, I often have difficulty making decisions when there are conflicting opinions, because decisions can be very political in nature! I learned quickly that using a set of guiding principles really helped me make decisions affecting my daily practice. I prioritize my decision making by asking myself the following questions: What is best for the client? Is this aligned with the client goals? What is best for the clinicians? What is best for the organization? I find that by asking these questions, I am able to focus and consider the key factors to choose the best decision.

Tim McKinnon, RN, BScN
Staff Nurse, General Internal Medicine

CRITICAL THINKING

You are working for a home health agency that employs 17 registered nurses. As the agency's census has increased, concerns have arisen about the staffing and scheduling. The manager has said that until more staff can be hired, there will be an increased need for on-call and overtime scheduling. The manager has given the responsibility to the entire group to figure out the best way to cover the client assignments.

What would be the best group decision-making strategy to use? What should the group do first?

TECHNIQUES OF GROUP DECISION MAKING

Various techniques can be used in group decision making. Nominal group technique, Delphi technique, and consensus building are different methods to facilitate group decision making.

NOMINAL GROUP TECHNIQUE

The **nominal group technique** was developed by Delbecq Van de Ven and Gustafson in 1971. The word *nominal* refers to the nonverbal aspect of this approach (Cawthorpe & Harris, 1999). In the first step, no discussion occurs: group members write out their ideas or responses to the identified issue or question posed by the group leader. The second step involves presentation of the ideas of the group members along with the advantages and disadvantages of each. These ideas are presented on a flipchart or a whiteboard. The third phase may offer an opportunity for discussion to clarify and evaluate the ideas. The fourth phase includes private voting on the ideas. Those ideas receiving the highest rating are the solutions implemented.

DELPHI GROUP TECHNIQUE

Delphi technique differs from nominal technique in that group members are not meeting face to face. Questionnaires are distributed to group members for their opinions, and the responses are then summarized and disseminated to the group members. This process continues for as many times as necessary for the group members to reach consensus. An advantage of this technique is that it can involve a large number of participants and thus a greater number of ideas.

CONSENSUS BUILDING

Consensus is defined by the American Heritage Dictionary (2000) as "an opinion or position reached by a group as a whole; general agreement or accord" (p. 391). A common misconception is that consensus means everyone agrees with the decision 100 percent. Contrary to this misunderstanding, **consensus** means that all group members can live with and fully support the decision regardless of whether they totally agree. This strategy is useful with groups because all group members participate and can realize the contributions each member makes to the decision (Sullivan & Decker, 2001). A disadvantage to the consensus strategy is that decision making requires more time. This strategy should be reserved for important decisions that require strong support from the participants who will implement them. Consensus decision making works well when the decisions are made under the following conditions: all members of the team are affected by the decision; implementation of the solution requires coordination among team members; and the decision is critical, requiring full commitment by team members. Although consensus can be the most time-consuming strategy, it can also be the most gratifying.

GROUPTHINK

Groupthink and consensus building are different. In consensus, the group members work to support the final decision, and individual ideas and opinions are valued. In groupthink, the goal is for everyone to be in 100 percent agreement. Groupthink discourages questioning and divergent thinking. It hinders creativity and usually leads to inferior decisions (Jarvis, 1997). The potential for

LITERATURE APPLICATION

Citation: Hearns, G., Klein, M.C., Trousdale, W., Ulrich, C., Butcher, D., Miewald, C., Lindstrom, R., Eftekhary, S., Rosinski, J., Gomez-Ramirez, O., & Procyk, A. (2010). Development of a support tool for complex decision-making in the provision of rural maternity care. *Healthcare Policy,* 5(3): 82–96.

Discussion: The objective of this study was to develop a maternity care decision-making tool for the British Columbia Northern Health Authority (NH) for use in low birth volume settings. The authors wanted to clarify the influences affecting rural maternity care and develop a process to generate a set of value-focused objectives for NH in designing and evaluating rural maternity care alternatives. As a result of the study, a Decision Support Manual was developed to assist with assessing community needs and values, the context for decision making, and the capacity of the health authority or health care providers. It also assists in identifying key objectives for decision making, developing alternatives for care, and formulating a process for making trade-offs and balancing multiple objectives. The manual was effective.

Implications for Practice: The methodology provided a transparent communication tool to assist in making difficult decisions. While the manual was specifically intended to deal with rural maternity issues, the NH decision makers feel that the method can be easily adapted to assist decision making in other contexts where there are conflicting objectives, values, and opinions.

groupthink increases as the cohesiveness of the group increases.

An important responsibility of the group leader is to recognize symptoms of groupthink. Janis (as cited in Jarvis, 1997) described examples of these symptoms. One symptom is that group members develop an illusion of invulnerability, believing they can do no wrong. This problem has the greatest potential to develop when the group is powerful and group members view themselves as invincible. The second symptom of groupthink is the stereotyping of outsiders, which occurs when the group members rely on shared stereotypes—such as, all Conservatives are liberal or all Liberals are conservative—to justify their positions. The people who challenge or disagree with the decisions are also stereotyped. A third symptom is that group members reassure one another that their interpretation of data and their perspective on matters are correct regardless of the evidence showing otherwise. Old assumptions are never challenged, and members ignore what they do not know or what they do not want to know.

Strategies to avoid groupthink include appointing group members to roles that evaluate how group decision making occurs. Group leaders encourage all group members to think independently and verbalize their individual ideas. The leader allows the group some time to gather further data and reflect on data already collected. A primary responsibility of the managers or the group leader is to prevent groupthink from developing.

LIMITATIONS TO EFFECTIVE DECISION MAKING

Useem and Useem (2005) suggest that because our decision-making processes are sound we are not lemmings heading over a cliff However, in clinical practice or management decision making can be flawed when nurses encounter the classic pitfalls and are unable to recognize their impact.

What are the obstacles to effective decision making? Past experiences, values, personal biases, and preconceived ideas affect the way people view problems and situations. What helps prevent these factors from distorting the decision-making process is critical thinking. Hammond, Keeney, and Raiffa (1998) have identified pitfalls to effective decision making:

- making the decision based upon the first available information,
- being comfortable with the status quo or not wanting to rock the boat,
- making decisions to justify previous decisions even if those decisions are no longer satisfactory,
- pursuing supporting evidence that verifies the decision while ignoring evidence to the contrary,
- presenting the issue in a biased manner or with a leading question, and
- assigning inaccurate probabilities to alternatives.

LITERATURE APPLICATION

Citation: Woolf, S., et al. (2005). Promoting informed choice: Transforming healthcare to dispense knowledge for decision making. *Annals of Internal Medicine,* 143(4): 293–301.

Discussion: The public thrives at accessing information, but not necessarily when clients have to make a decision regarding their health. The roles and expectations associated with the health care provider and consumer have shifted through the years. Now consumers are active participants in their health care. Because clients are increasingly involved in their health care, it must be ensured that they receive the right information at the right time. In this way they can make the best possible decision about their care to obtain the desired outcome.

Implications for Practice: Although several approaches to enhance client decision making are proposed, each with their own strengths and weaknesses, the authors recommend a change to the entire health care infrastructure such that clients are delivered the relevant and timely information necessary to make an effective decision.

USE OF TECHNOLOGY IN DECISION MAKING

The best source of clinical decision making and judgement is still the professional practitioner. However, computer technology can be used to support information systems, including decision making, for managers (Tomey, 2000). Patient classification systems, inventory control, scheduling staff, documentation of client care, order entry for tests, appointments, and changes in policies and procedures are but a few examples of how computers can assist managers with tracking the information managers need. Computer software for the clinical practitioner is available for clinical decision making and should be carefully critiqued prior to use.

NURSES' ROLE IN CLIENT DECISION MAKING

In today's world, clients are taking a more active role in treatment decisions. Consumers of health care are more knowledgeable and have more options than in previous years. Nurses must be aware of clients' rights in making decisions about their treatments, and they must assist clients in their decision making. When clients are active participants, their compliance with prescribed treatments is more likely to follow. Empowering the client in this manner ultimately promotes a more positive outcome.

STRATEGIES TO IMPROVE DECISION MAKING

Comfort with decision making improves with experience. Early in their careers, nurses are usually indecisive or uncomfortable with making decisions. Alfaro-LeFevre (1995) has identified several strategies that help to improve critical thinking, which, in turn, will also help to improve decision making. Do you have all the information needed to make a decision? At times, delaying a decision until more information is obtained may be the best approach. Asking "why," "what else," and "what if" questions will help you arrive at the best decision. When more information becomes available, decisions can be revised. Very few decisions are set in stone. Another helpful strategy for improving decision making is to anticipate questions and outcomes. For example, when calling a physician to report a client's change in condition, the nurse will want to have pertinent information about the client's vital signs, lab values, and current medications readily available.

Nurses who practise strategies to promote their own critical thinking will, in turn, be good decision makers. A foundation for good decision making comes with experience and learning from those experiences. Table 17-5 shows some additional tips to consider when making decisions. By turning decisions with poor outcomes into learning experiences, nurses will enhance their decision-making ability in the future.

Nurses on a general surgery unit have identified several problems on their unit and want to take action to remedy them. The manager is accepting and supportive of their ideas and states that she will sponsor any initiatives that will help improve the unit. She suggests they should form a unit-based council. The manager identified the following issues from her perspective: shortage of staff, low staff satisfaction, lack of experienced nurses on the unit, high turnover, and low morale.

What are your initial thoughts?

What do you think the group should do? How will the group solve the problem?

TABLE 17-5	DOS AND DON'TS OF DECISION MAKING

Do	Don't
Make only those decisions that are yours to make.	Make snap decisions.
Write notes and keep ideas visible about decisions to utilize all relevant information.	Waste your time making decisions that do not have to be made.
Write down pros and cons of an issue to help clarify your thinking.	Consider decisions a choice between right and wrong but a choice among alternatives.
Make decisions as you go along rather than letting them accumulate.	Prolong deliberation about decisions.
Consider those affected by your decision.	Regret a decision; it was the right thing to do at the time.
Trust yourself.	Always base decisions on the "way things have always been done."

Source: Adapted from *The Small Business Knowledge Base,* 1999 <www.bizmove.com>

KEY CONCEPTS

- The changing health care landscape requires nurses to be active and effective decision makers. The ability of nurses to make appropriate decisions has a significant impact on both client and staff outcomes.

- A good critical thinker is able to examine decisions from all sides and take into account varying points of view. Use of the universal intellectual standards will improve a nurse's critical thinking.

- Practising reflective thinking helps individuals become better critical thinkers.

- Problem solving involves five steps: (1) identify the problem, (2) gather and analyze data, (3) generate alternatives and select action, (4) implement the selected action, and (5) evaluate the selected action.

- The decision-making process has five steps: Step 1—identify the need for a decision; Step 2—determine the goal or outcome; Step 3—identify alternatives or actions, along with their benefits and consequences; Step 4—decide on the action and implement it; Step 5—evaluate the action.

- Decision-making grids may be helpful to separate multiple factors during the decision-making process.

- The PERT model is useful for determining the timing of decisions.

- In some situations the nurse manager makes an individual decision. Other situations call for group decision making.

- Consensus is a strategy utilized when using group decision making.

- To be an effective decision maker, individuals must identify and avoid certain traps during the decision-making process.

- The decision tree is a tool used to visualize the alternatives.

- The Gantt chart is useful to outline the lifespan of a project.

- Groupthink occurs when individuals are not allowed to express creativity, question methods, or engage in divergent thinking. Managers must be able to identify the symptoms of groupthink.

- The nurse must recognize the importance of empowering clients in making their own treatment decisions. The nurse needs to provide the client with relevant and timely information and assist the client to explore all possible options to get the best outcome.

- Many strategies can be used to improve your decision making. Obtaining all the information, asking yourself "why" and "what if" questions, and developing good habits of inquiry are a few of the strategies that will help improve your decision-making skills.

KEY TERMS

consensus
critical thinking
decision making
Delphi technique

nominal group technique
problem solving
reflective thinking

REVIEW QUESTIONS

1. Which of the following best describes the uses of decision making?
   A. to solve a problem
   B. to choose between alternatives
   C. to reflect on a certain situation
   D. to generate ideas

2. Which of the following is the best description of consensus?
   A. Everyone in the group agrees with the decision 100 percent.
   B. All members of the group vote on the selected action.
   C. Every group member compromises.
   D. Every group member fully supports the decision, once it is made.

3. Which of the following is a symptom of groupthink?
   A. The group members continually disagree with one another.
   B. The group members cannot come to a decision.
   C. The group members stereotype outsiders.
   D. The group members share a common bond.

4. Occasionally, making a decision is difficult because of the multiple factors that surround certain situations. Which of the following will nurse managers use to separate these factors?
   A. decision grid
   B. nominal group technique
   C. Delphi group technique
   D. consensus strategy

REVIEW ACTIVITIES

1. You are the manager of a 12-bed surgical unit. Your supervisor informs you that 12 more beds will be opened for neurosurgical clients, and you are to be the manager. Draw a PERT diagram to depict the sequence of tasks necessary for the completion of the project.

2. The education forms are not being filled out correctly or in a timely manner on new admissions in your medical-surgical unit. Decide on your own the best action to take in this situation. Then, form a group and attempt to reach consensus on the best action to take. Compare the differences between individual and group decision making. What did you learn about developing consensus?

3. Identify a problem that you have been considering. Using the decision-making grid below, rate the alternative solutions to the problem that you have been considering—on a scale of 1 to 3—on the elements of cost, quality, importance, location, and any other elements that are important to you.

	Cost	Quality	Importance	Location	Other
Alternative A					
Alternative B					
Alternative C					

4. Did this exercise help you in thinking through your decision?

5. Identify a current problem in health care. Use the problem-solving process in a group to find a solution. Employ the nominal group technique and the Delphi technique.

EXPLORING THE WEB

- Identify the Canadian Nurses Association position statements. Check out the website *http://www.cna-aiic.ca/CNA/issues/position/default_e.aspx*

- Note the universal intellectual standards at the Foundation for Critical Thinking: *http://www.criticalthinking.org/articles/index.cfm*

- Note the following site for clinical decision making. This site includes software for clinical decision making: *http://groups.csail.mit.edu/medg/*

- Review this site on emotional intelligence: *http://eiconsortium.org/*

REFERENCES

Affonso, D., & Doran, D. M. (2002). Cultivating discoveries in patient safety research: A framework. *The Journal of Nursing Perspectives, 2*(1), 33–47.

Aiken, L. H., Clarke, S. P., Sloane, D. M., Sochalski, J., & Silber, J. H. (2002). Hospital nurse staffing and patient mortality, nurse burnout and job dissatisfaction. *Journal of the American Medical Association, 288*(10), 1987–1993.

Alfaro-LeFevre, R. (1995). *Critical thinking in nursing.* Philadelphia: Saunders.

Alfaro-LeFevre, R. (2006). *Critical Thinking Indicators™.* Stuart, FL: Author.

American heritage dictionary of the English language (4th ed.). (2000). Boston: Houghton Mifflin.

American Nurses Association website. (2011). *Education and competence. Knowledge from ANA.* Retrieved from http://www.nursingworld.org/MainMenuCategories/ThePracticeofProfessionalNursing/NursingEducation.aspx

Bailey, J. T., Steffen, S. M., & Grout, J. W. (1980). The stress audit: Identifying the stressors of ICU nursing. *Journal of Nursing Education, 19*(6), 15–25.

Bandura, A. (1986). *Social foundations of thought and action: A social cognitive theory.* Englewood Cliffs, NJ Prentice Hall.

Bellack, J. P., & O'Neil, E. H. (2000). Recreating nursing practice for a new century: Recommendations and implications of the Pew Health Professions Commission's final report. *Nursing and Health Care Perspectives, 21*(1), 14–21.

Benner, P. (1984). *From novice to expert.* Menlo Park, CA: Addison Wesley.

Benner, P., & Tanner, C. A. (1987). How expert nurses use intuition. *American Journal of Nursing, 87*(1), 23–31.

Block, P. (1990). *The empowered manager: Positive political skills at work.* San Francisco: Jossey-Bass.

Boblin, S., Baxter, P., Alvarado, K., Baumann, A., & Akhtar-Danesh, N. (2008). Registered nurses and licensed/registered practical nurses: A description and comparison of their decision-making process. *Nursing Leadership, 21*(4), 56–72.

Boud, D., Keogh, R., & Walker, D. (1985). *Reflection: Turning experience into learning.* London: Kogan Page.

Brooks, E. M., & Thomas, S. (1997). The perception and judgment of senior baccalaureate student nurses in clinical decision making. *Advances in Nursing Science, 19*(3), 50–69.

Campbell, B., & Mackay, G. P. (2001). Continuing competence: An Ontario nursing regulatory program that supports nurses and employers. *Nursing Administration Quarterly, 25*(2), 22–30.

Canadian Nurses Association. (2007). *Framework for the practice of registered nurses in Canada.* Ottawa: Author.

Canadian Nurses Association. (2011). *2009 Workforce Profile of registered nurses in Canada.* Ottawa: Author.

Canadian Nursing Advisory Committee (CNAC). (2002). *Our health, our future: Creating quality workplaces for Canadian nurses.* Ottawa: Author.

Carman, J. M., Shortell, S. M., Foster, R. W., Hughes, E. F., Boerstler, H., O'Brien, J. L., et al. (1996). Keys for successful implementation of total quality management in hospitals. *Health Care Management Review, 21*(1), 48–60.

Cawthorpe, D., & Harris, D. (1999). Nominal group technique: Assessing staff concerns. *Journal of Nursing Administration, 29*(7/8), 11, 18, 37, 42.

Cleland, V. (1967). Effects of stress on thinking. *The American Journal of Nursing, 67*(1), 108–111.

Coomber, B., & Barriball, K. L. (2007). Impact of job satisfaction components on intent to leave and turnover for hospital-based nurses: A review of the research literature. *International Journal of Nursing Studies, 44*(2), 297–314.

Correnti, D. (1992). Intuition and nursing practice implications for nurse educators: A review of the literature. *Journal of Continuing Nursing Education, 23*(2), 91–94.

Donaghy, M. E., & Morss, K. (2000). Guided reflection: A framework to facilitate and access reflective practice with the discipline of physiotherapy. *Physiotherapy and Practice, 16*(1), 3–14.

Doran, D. M., Baker, G. R., Murray, M., Bohnen, J., Zahn, C., Sidani, S., et al. (2002). Achieving clinical improvement: An interdisciplinary intervention. *Health Care Management Review, 27*(4), 42–56.

Dwyer, D. W., Schwartz, R. H., & Fox, M. L. (1992). Decision making autonomy in nursing. *Journal of Nursing Administration, 22*(2), 107–112.

Evans, D. (1990). Problems in the decision making process: A review. *Intensive Care Nursing, 6*(4), 179–184.

Fero, L., Witsberger, C., Wesmiller, S., Zullo, T., & Hoffman, L. (2009). Critical thinking ability of new graduate and experienced nurses. *Journal of Advanced Nursing, 65*(1), 139–148.

Giddens, J., & Gloeckner, G. (2005). The relationship of critical thinking to performance on the NCLEX-RN. *Journal of Nursing Education, 44*(2), 85–89.

Grinspun, D. (2007). Healthy workplaces: The case for shared clinical decision making and increased full-time employment. *Healthcare Papers, 7*(Special issue), 85–91.

Hagbaghery, M. A., Salsali, M., & Ahmadi, F. (2004). The factors facilitating and inhibiting effective decision-making in nursing: A qualitative study. *BMC Nursing*, 3(1), 2.

Hammond, J. S., Keeney, R. L., & Raiffa, H. (1998). The hidden traps in decision making. *Harvard Business Review*, 76(5), 47–58.

Healy, C. M., & McKay, M. F. (2000). Nursing stress: The effects of coping strategies and job satisfaction in a sample of Australian nurses. *Journal of Advanced Nursing*, 31(4), 989.

Hearns, G., Klein, M. C., Trousdale, W., Ulrich, C., Butcher, D., Miewald, C., et al. (2010). Development of a support tool for complex decision-making in the provision of rural maternity care. *Healthcare Policy*, 5(3), 82–96.

Hofstede, G. (1998). Attitudes, values and organizational culture: Disentangling the concepts. *Organization Studies*, 19(3), 477–492.

Huber, D. (2000). *Leadership and nursing care management*. Philadelphia: Saunders.

Marquis, B. L., & Huston, C. J. (2012). *Leadership roles and management functions in nursing: Theory and application* (7th ed.). Philadelphia: Wolters Kluwer, Lippincott, Williams and Wilkins.

International Council of Nurses. (2000). *Position statement: Participation of nurses in health services decision making and policy development*. Geneva: Author.

Jarvis, C. (1997). *Groupthink*. Retrieved from http://www.bola.biz/communications/groupthink.html

Jones, R. A. P., & Beck, S. E. (1996). *Decision making in nursing*. Clifton Park, NY: Delmar Learning.

Joseph, D. H. (1985). Sex-role stereotype, self-concept, education and experience: Do they influence decision making? *International Journal of Nursing Studies*, 22(1), 21–32.

Keenan, J. (1999). A concept analysis of autonomy. *Journal of Advanced Nursing*, 29(3), 556–562.

Langfield-Smith, K. (1995). Organizational culture and control. In A. Berry, J. Broadbent, & D. Otley (Eds.). *Management control theories, issues and practices* (pp. 179–202). London: Macmillan.

Lazarus, R. S., & Folkman, S. (1984). *Stress, appraisal and coping*. New York: Springer.

LeStorti, A., Cullen, P., Hanzlik, E., Michiels, J. M., Piano, L., Ryan, P. L., et al. (1999). Creative thinking in nursing education: Preparing for tomorrow's challenges. *Nursing Outlook*, 47(2), 62–66.

Luecke, R. (2006). *Decision making: 5 steps to better results*. Boston: Harvard Business School Press.

MacDonald, C. (2002). Nurse autonomy as relational. *Nursing Ethics*, 9(2), 194–201.

Mann, K., Gordon, J., & MacLeod, A. (2009). Reflection and reflective practice in health professions education: A systematic review. *Advancements in Health Sciences Education*, 14, 595–621.

Murphy, E. C. (1985). Whole brain management: Part 1. *Nursing Management*, 16(3), 66.

Ontario. (2010). Excellent Care for All Act S.O. 2010, c. 14.

Niadu, S., Oliver, M., & Koronious, A. (1999). Approaching clinical decision-making in nursing practice with interactive multimedia and case-based reasoning. *Interactive Multimedia Electronic Journal of Computer Enhanced Learning*, 1(2).

O'Reilly, P. (1993). Barriers to effective clinical decision making in nursing. In *St Vincent's nursing monograph: 1993 selected works* (pp. 34–43). Sydney: Author.

Pardue, S. (1987). Decision-making skills and critical thinking ability among associate degree, diploma, baccalaureate, and master's-prepared nurses. *Journal of Nursing Education*, 26(9), 354–361.

Paul, R. (1992). *Critical thinking: What every person needs to survive in a rapidly changing world*. Santa Rosa, CA: Foundation for Critical Thinking.

Paul, R., & Elder, L. (2005). *The nature and functions of critical and creative thinking*. Dillon Beach, CA: Foundation for Critical Thinking.

Pesut, D. J., & Herman, J. (1999). *Clinical reasoning: The art and science of critical and creative thinking*. Clifton Park, NY: Delmar Learning.

Scott, J. G., Sochalski, J., & Aiken, L. (1999). Review of magnet hospital research: Findings and implications for professional practice. *Journal of Nursing Administration*, 29(1), 9–19.

Scriven, M., and Paul R. (2004) Defining Critical Thinking. Santa Rosa, CA: Foundation for Critical Thinking. Retrieved from http://www.criticalthinking.org/aboutCT/define_critical_thinking.cfm

Shein, E. (1991). *Organizational culture and leadership*. San Francisco: Jossey-Bass.

Stone, P. W., Harrison, M. I., Feldman, P., Linzer, M., Peng, T., Roblin, D., et al. (2005). Organizational climate of staff working conditions and safety: An integrated model. *Advances in Patient Safety*, 2, 467–481.

Sullivan, E., & Decker, P. (2001). *Effective leadership and management in nursing*. Menlo Park, CA: Addison Wesley Longman.

Tanner, C. A., Padrick, K. P., Westfall, U. E., & Putzier, D. J. (1987). Diagnostic reasoning strategies of nurses and nursing students. *Nursing Research*, 36(6), 358–363.

Teekman, B, (2000). Exploring reflective thinking in nursing. *Journal of Advanced Nursing*, 31(5), 1125–1135.

Thompson, C., Cullu, N., McCaughan, D., Sheldon, T., & Raynor, P. (2004). Nurses, information use, and clinical decision making – the real world potential for evidence-based decisions in nursing. *Evidence Based Nursing*, 7, 68–72.

Tomey, A. (2000). Guide to nursing management and leadership. St. Louis, MO: Mosby.

Tranmer, J. (2004). Autonomy and decision making in nursing. In L. McGillis-Hall (Ed.), *Quality work environments: Nurse and patient safety*. Sudbury, MA: Jones and Bartlett.

Useem, M., & Useem, J. (2005). Great escapes: Nine decision-making pitfalls and nine simple devices to beat them. *Fortune*, 151(13), 97–100.

Vroom, V. H., & Yetton, P. W. (1973). *Leadership and decision-making*. Pittsburgh, PA: University of Pittsburgh Press.

Wade, G. H. (1999). Professional nurse autonomy: Concept analysis and application to nursing education. *Journal of Advanced Nursing*, 30(2), 310–318.

Wakefield, M. (1992). Stress control for nurses. *The Canadian Nurse*, 88(4), 24–25.

Woolf, S., Chan, E., Harris, R., Sheridan, S., Braddoc, C., Kaplan, R., et al. (2005). Promoting informed choice: Transforming healthcare to dispense knowledge for decision making. *American College of Physicians*, 143(4), 293–301.

SUGGESTED READINGS

Aiken, L. H., Clarke, S. P., & Sloane, D. M. (2002). Hospital staffing, organization, and quality of care: Cross-national findings. *International Journal for Quality in Health Care,* 14 (1), 5–13.

American Philosophical Association. (1990). *Critical thinking: A statement of expert consensus for purposes of educational assessment and instruction, recommendations prepared for the Committee on Pre-college Philosophy.* ERIC Doc. No. ED 315-423, p. 2.

Boblin-Cummings, S., Baumann, A., & Deber, R. (1999). Critical elements in the decision-making process: A nursing perspective. *Canadian Journal of Nursing Leadership,* 12(1), 6–13.

Bryons, A., & McIntosh, J. (1996). Decision making in community nursing: An analysis of the stages of decision making as they relate to community nursing assessment practice. *Journal of Advanced Nursing,* 24(1), 24–30.

Duchscher, J. (1999). Catching the wave: Understanding the concept of critical thinking. *Journal of Advanced Nursing,* 29(3), 577–583.

Girot, E. A. (2000). Graduate nurses: Critical thinkers or better decision makers? *Journal of Advanced Nursing,* 31(2), 288–297.

Godolphin, W. (2009). Shared decision-making. *Healthcare Quarterly,* 12(Special issue),186–190.

Golbasi, Z., Kelleci, M., & Dogan, S. (2008). Relationships between coping strategies, individual characteristics and job satisfaction in a sample of hospital nurses: Cross-sectional questionnaire survey. *International Journal of Nursing Studies,* 45(12), 1800–1806.

Goleman, D. (1998). What makes a leader? *Harvard Business Review, November/December,* 93–102.

Huston, C. J., & Marquis, B. L. (1995). Seven steps to successful decision-making. *Amercian Journal of Nursing,* 95(5), 65–68.

Kontryn, V. (1999). Strategic problem solving in the new millennium. *AORN Journal,* 70(6), 1035–1044.

Marquis, B. L., & Huston, C. J. (1998). *Management decision making for nurses: 124 case studies* (3rd ed.). Philadelphia: Lippincott.

Martinez de Castillo, S. L. (1999). *Strategies, techniques, and approaches to thinking: Case studies in clinical nursing.* Philadelphia: Saunders.

Parsons, L. (1999). Building RN confidence for delegation decision-making skills in practice. *Journal for Nurses in Staff Development,* 15(6), 263–269.

Radwin, L. (1995). Conceptualizations of decision making in nursing: Analytic models and "knowing the patient." *Nursing Diagnosis,* 6(1), 16–22.

Recker, D., Bess, C., & Wellens, H. (1996). A decision-making process in shared governance. *Nursing Management,* 27(5), 48A, 48B, 48D.

Schon, D. A. (1989). A symposium on Schon's concept of reflective practice: Critiques, commentaries, illustrations. *Journal of Curriculum and Supervision,* 5(1), 6–9.

Scordo, K. (1997). Reaching consensus through electronic brainstorming. *Computers in Nursing,* 15(2), 33–37.

Simms, L. M., Price, S. A., & Ervin, N. E. (2000). *Professional practice of nursing administration* (3rd ed.). Clifton Park, NY: Delmar Learning.

Swansburg, R. C., & Swansburg, R. J. (2002). *Introductory management and leadership for nurse managers* (3rd ed.). Boston: Jones and Bartlett.

CHAPTER ENDNOTES

1. Stanford University School of Medicine, "Decision-making." Retrieved from http://cisl.stanford.edu/what_is/learning_types/decision_mkng.html

2. Ibid.

3. ChangingMinds.org, "Subjective vs. Objectivity Preferences." Retrieved from http://changingminds.org/explanations/preferences/subjective_objective.htm

4. ChangingMinds.org, "Thinking vs. Feeling." Retrieved from http://changingminds.org/explanations/preferences/thinking_feeling.htm

5. Accreditation Canada. "Required organizational practices." Retrieved from http://www.accreditation.ca/knowledge-exchange/patient-safety/required-organizational-practices/

UNIT VI
Other Professional Considerations

CHAPTER 18

Legal Aspects of Client Care

Judith W. Martin, RN, JD
Sister Kathleen Cain, OSF, JD
Adapted by Heather Crawford, BScN, MEd, CHE

The Sinclair Report was the inquest report that told the story of 12 children who died and the health care providers who worked with them, during 1994, in the pediatric cardiac surgery program at the Winnipeg Health Sciences Centre. I chaired the Winnipeg Health Sciences committee that examined the recommendations and identified an implementation plan. The Sinclair Report raised many legal issues that continue to concern and affect nurses across Canada on a daily basis. (Heather Crawford)

OBJECTIVES

The purpose of this chapter is to enable the reader to
- discuss the effect of law on nursing practice;
- describe the importance of the Canadian Constitution and the Canadian Charter of Rights and Freedoms to health care;
- describe the requirements of informed consent;
- name the most common areas of nursing practice cited in malpractice actions and list actions a nurse can take to minimize these risks;
- describe the various forms of advanced directives and how these are commonly implemented;
- identify the lessons that can be learned from coroner's inquests;
- describe risk management and how it is used in the health care setting; and
- discuss the rights of the nurse as an employee.

You are working on a medical-surgical unit when you admit an 82-year-old female, Mrs. Perkins. She has a medical diagnosis of abdominal pain and is admitted for further investigation. She is accompanied by her daughter, who leaves the room while you complete your admission nursing assessment. During your assessment, you notice bruises and welts across Mrs. Perkins' back, approximately two centimetres wide and the same distance apart. You ask Mrs. Perkins about these marks, but she tells you that she doesn't know how she got them. When her daughter returns, you mention the marks to her. She tells you that her mother is very unsteady on her feet and had fallen down the stairs. You notice when the daughter is in the room, Mrs. Perkins no longer maintains eye contact and is reluctant to speak without looking at her daughter first. You are beginning to suspect that Mrs. Perkins has been physically mistreated.

Do you need any additional information to determine the validity of your suspicions?

If abuse has occurred, what action should you take?

Do client confidentiality concerns affect any actions you may take?

Historically, Canada was originally inhabited by explorers and settlers from France and the United Kingdom. What is now known as the province of Québec was governed exclusively under French civil law until the French colonies in North America were given to Great Britain from France in 1763. French civil law was based on the Roman law system. In Roman law, legal rules and principles that establish rights and responsibilities of individuals are formally written in a single document known as civil code.

With the exception of the province of Québec, Canada's legal system is derived from English common law. The majority of **common law** was not written down or codified as statute law. Many of the essential rules and principles that govern our everyday life have been developed through precedents, which are individual sets of judges' reasons for deciding individual cases. Precedents are usually published in volumes by category, such as jurisdiction (e.g., provincial, territorial, or federal), subject matter (e.g., criminal law, family law), or level of the court that provided the decision (e.g., Federal Court of Appeal, Supreme Court of Canada). Legal principles and rules are developed from these precedents and are then applied by judges to specific cases. This body of precedent is called case law (Keatings & Smith, 2010, p. 90).

This chapter reviews how laws are enacted and implemented, and how the various types of laws affect nursing practice.

SOURCES OF LAW

The authority to make, implement, and interpret laws is generally granted in a constitution. A **constitution** is a set of basic laws that specify the powers of the various segments of the government and how these segments relate to each other. Generally, it is the role of a legislative body, at the provincial, territorial, and federal levels, to enact laws. The government of Canada is made up of three branches: the judicial branch, which resolves disputes and creates common or case law; the executive branch—comprising the Queen's representative, the governor general; the federal ministers, including the prime minister; and the public servants who work with the federal ministers—which crafts, administers, and enforces laws; and the legislative branch, consisting of the federal Parliament and provincial or territorial legislatures, which make statutory law (MacIvor, 2006).

PUBLIC LAW

Public law consists of constitutional law and criminal law, and defines a citizen's relationship with government.

CONSTITUTIONAL LAW

The Canadian Constitution (1982), which includes the *Canadian Charter of Rights and Freedoms* (1982), is the highest law in Canada. The Constitution predominantly deals with the rights and powers of the provincial, territorial, and federal governments; whereas the Charter addresses basic legal and democratic rights of Canadians. Health care is predominantly a provincial or territorial responsibility, but the federal government maintains responsibility for approximately one million people in certain groups, such as First Nations people living on reserves, Inuit, serving members of the Canadian Forces and the Royal Canadian Mounted Police, eligible veterans, inmates in federal penitentiaries, and refugee protection claimants.[1]

Recently, many discussions have taken place among various provincial, territorial, and federal governments related to the future of health care. The report of the Commission on the Future of Health Care in Canada (2002), conducted by Roy Romanow, QC, is based on the five principles of the Canada Health Act (1984). In his report, Romanow recommended that the Health Council of Canada establish a national framework for measuring and assessing the quality and safety of Canada's health care system. This process would compare the outcomes with those of other countries and report regularly to Canadians (Commission on the Future of Health Care in Canada, 2002, p. 251).

Several categories of public law affect the practice of nursing. For example, nurses accommodate clients' constitutional rights to practise their religion every time they call a client's clergy upon request, follow a specific religious custom for the preparation of meals, or prepare a deceased person's remains for burial.

Controversial constitutional rights that may affect the nurse's practice include the recognized constitutional rights of a woman to have an abortion[2] and an individual's right to die.[3]

Nurses may not believe in either of these rights personally and may refuse to work in areas in which they would have to assist a client in exercising these rights. Nurses may not, however, interfere with another person's right to have an abortion or to forgo lifesaving measures.

CRIMINAL LAW

The *Criminal Code of Canada* (1985) defines criminal offences and identifies the procedures to be used in determining criminal conduct. Criminal law focuses on the actions of individuals that can intentionally do harm to others. Often the victims of such abusive actions are the very young or the very old; these two categories of people generally have a more difficult time defending themselves against physical or emotional abuse. Nurses may notice that a vulnerable client has unexplained bruises, fractures, or other injuries. Most provinces and territories have mandatory statutes that require nurses to report unexplained or suspicious injuries to the appropriate protective agency. Generally, health care institutions will have clear guidelines to follow in such a situation. Failure to report the problem as required by law can result in the nurse being fined for inaction.

Another aspect of criminal law that affects nursing practice is the provincial requirement for criminal background checks on specified categories of prospective employees who will work with the very young or the elderly in institutions such as schools and nursing homes. Again, this requirement is an attempt to protect the most vulnerable citizens from mistreatment or abuse. Failure to conduct the mandated background checks can result in the institution having to defend itself for

any harm done by an employee with a past criminal conviction. The third area in which criminal law concerns affect nursing practice is the prohibition against substance abuse. Federal, provincial, and territorial laws require health care agencies to keep a strict accounting of the use and distribution of regulated drugs. Nurses are expected to routinely keep narcotic records accurate and current.

Nurses' behaviour when off duty can also affect their employment status. Abusing alcohol or drugs on one's own time, if discovered, charged, and convicted, can result in both terminated employment and restriction or revocation of registration to practise as a nurse (College of Nurses of Ontario, 2005; College of Registered Nurses of British Columbia, 2009). Frequently, regulatory nursing bodies make recommendations related to programs for the nurse with a drug or substance abuse problem; completion of such a program may be required before the nurse can resume practising. Additionally, health care facilities may conduct random drug screens on their employees to identify those who may be using illegal substances.

STATUTORY LAW

The laws made by the provincial, territorial, and federal governments are called acts or statutes. After a bill has passed through the federal Parliament or the provincial or territorial legislature and received Royal Assent, it is proclaimed and published. It then becomes law.

A federal statute that affects health care is the Canada Health Act (1984). This act requires that each province and territory provide care that is publicly administered,

CRITICAL THINKING

One of the nurses who consistently works on your team seems to have a significant change in behaviour following her trips to the washroom. You notice that she becomes increasingly drowsy and her speech is slurred. When you used the staff washroom immediately after her, you noticed a needle and syringe discarded in the garbage. In addition, following the most recent coffee break, the nurse has returned to the unit with a fresh bandage applied to her arm.

Given this scenario what should you do as a nurse? Would you expect to find some guidance in your institution's policy and procedure manual?

universal, portable, accessible, and comprehensive. It also prohibits provinces and territories from charging user fees and extra billing by physicians. A penalty (i.e., a decrease in transfer payments) may be imposed by the federal government if this statute is violated.

Established in 1978, the Canadian Centre for Occupational Health and Safety (CCOHS) is a Canadian federal government agency based in Hamilton, Ontario. It reports to the Parliament of Canada through the federal minister of labour. Its vision is to eliminate all work-related illnesses and injuries. The CCOHS is governed by a council representing three key stakeholder groups: government (federal, provincial, and territorial), employers, and workers. This structure mandates the CCOHS's impartial approach to information dissemination.[4]

Most Canadian jurisdictions have, in their occupational health and safety legislation, a "general duty provision" that requires employers to take all reasonable precautions to protect the health and safety of their employees. This provision includes protecting employees from a known risk of workplace violence. British Columbia and Saskatchewan have specific workplace violence prevention regulations; Nova Scotia has guidelines on workplace violence prevention; and Alberta has an occupational health and safety code on the prevention of workplace violence. Québec has legislation regarding "psychological harassment," which may include forms of workplace violence. The Canada Labour Code (i.e., for federally regulated workplaces) specifies that supervisors and managers must take the prescribed steps to prevent and protect against violence in the workplace (the specific regulations are being developed). Many jurisdictions also have regulations regarding working alone, which may have implications for workplace violence prevention.[5] Ontario amended the Occupational Health and Safety Act on June 15, 2010, with Bill 168. Under Bill 168, Ontario is required to have the necessary policies, programs, measures, and procedures in place to prevent violence and harassment in the workplace.[6]

In addition, various organizations, such as St. Michael's Hospital in downtown Toronto, have taken steps to ensure their staff's safety. In April 2006, St. Michael's Hospital hosted a conference to look at protecting everyone in the emergency room. Posters now tell patients and visitors that violence will not be tolerated, and visitor access has been limited to some areas of the emergency room. Staff members are being more proactive in using the code white procedure, which calls on a team of trained individuals to respond to any dangerous situation before it escalates (Shaw, 2006).

The Registered Nurses Association of Ontario (RNAO) Healthy Work Environments Best Practice Guideline, published in November 2006, presented 21 recommendations to support the creation of healthy and safe work environments for nurses. An International Nursing Review editorial described nurses experiencing violence at a rate 16 times higher than other professions (Kingma, 2001). In addition, the International Council of Nurses revealed statistics in 2009 that found 72 percent of nurses don't feel adequately protected from assaults at work.[7]

Regulated professions, including nursing, are governed by provincial statutes and regulations. The primary mission of professional regulation is protection of the public. The regulatory bodies are given power by the provincial or territorial governments, through legislation, to set practice standards, registration requirements, entry-to-practice requirements, continuing competence requirements, quality assurance criteria, methods of handling complaints, discipline and disciplinary procedures, and development of codes of ethics. As a result, the public is assured that each professional is competent to practice. In Ontario nurses are affected by two pieces of legislation: the Regulated Health Professions Act (1991) and its amendment of 2009, which came into effect June 1, 2011; and the Nursing Act (1991), which was amended in December 2009.

CIVIL LAW

Keatings and Smith (2010) define **civil law** as a system of law based on Roman law, prevalent in most European countries and Québec. In this system, in which legal principles and rules are formally written (codified) in an organized fashion into a central statute or code.[8] These statutes govern relations, rights, and obligations among individuals, corporations, or other institutions.

CONTRACT LAW

Contract law regulates certain transactions between individuals and legal entities, such as businesses. It also governs transactions between businesses. An agreement between two or more parties must contain the following elements to be recognized as a legal contract:

- Agreement between two or more legally competent individuals or parties stating what each must or must not do
- Mutual understanding of the terms and obligations that the contract imposes on each party to the contract
- Payment or consideration given for actions taken or not taken pursuant to the agreement

The terms of the contract may be oral or written. However, a written contract may not be legally modified by an oral agreement, which is often expressed by the phrase *all of the terms of the contract are contained within the four corners of the document.* Therefore, if it is not written,

CRITICAL THINKING

You are assigned to a medical-surgical unit, working the night shift. Your supervisor calls and says that one of the registered nurses assigned to the critical care unit has called in sick and you must work that unit instead of your usual assignment. You have never worked in the critical care setting before and have received no orientation to this unit. You are now asked to work there when it is short of staff.

What should you do?

it is not part of the agreement or contract. A contract may be express or implied. In an express contract, the terms of the contract are specified, usually in writing. In an implied contract, a relationship between parties is recognized, although the terms of the agreement are not clearly defined, such as the expectations one has for services from the dry cleaner or the grocer.

The nurse is usually a party to an employment contract. The employed nurse agrees to do the following:

- adhere to the policies and procedures of the employing agency
- fulfill the agreed-upon duties of the employer
- respect the rights and responsibilities of other health care providers in the workplace

In return, the employer agrees to provide the nurse with the following:

- a specified amount of pay for services rendered
- adequate assistance in providing care
- the supplies and equipment needed to fulfill the nurse's responsibilities
- a safe environment in which to work
- reasonable treatment and behaviour from the other health care providers with whom the nurse must interact

This contract may be express or implied, depending on the practices of the employer. Sometimes, what is determined to be "reasonable" by the employer is not considered reasonable by the nurse. For instance, after 20 years of working as a nurse on the orthopedic unit, a nurse may not view it as reasonable to be assigned to the labour and delivery unit for duty. It would be prudent for the nurse to express any misgivings to the supervisor and to take assignments that are in keeping with the nurse's experience on an orthopedic unit.

TORT LAW

Keatings and Smith (2010) define **tort** as a civil wrong committed by one person against another, such that some injury or damage is caused to either person or property. A tort can be non-intentional, as occurs in negligence, or it can be intentional, as occurs in assault, when the infliction of harm is intended.

NON-INTENTIONAL TORTS

Negligence is the failure to provide the care a reasonable nurse would ordinarily provide in a similar situation. To win a negligence lawsuit, the person who is suing the nurse must demonstrate that all the following elements existed between the client and nurse:

1. A duty or obligation created by law, contract, or standard practice that is owed to the complainant by the professional
2. A breach of this duty, either by omission or commission (by failure to administer treatment or provide health care according to particular standards of care)
3. Harm, which can be physical, emotional, or financial, to the complainant (i.e., the client) as a direct result of the breach of the duty of care (Keatings & Smith, 2010).

When a nurse is listed as a party in a medical malpractice lawsuit, the nurse's liability is determined by provincial or federal laws, such as the Regulated Health Professions Act, the Public Hospitals Act, standards for the practice of nursing, and the institution's policies and procedures. Therefore, if provincial or territorial laws mandate that a nurse must have a doctor's order before taking an action, then a doctor's order must be present. Problems arise when the orders are verbal and later the doctor claims that the nurse misunderstood and acted in error. Another pitfall is illegible writing, which can be misinterpreted and result in causing harm to the client. Many nurses who have been in practice for a long time have encountered confused doctors who write orders that are contrary to accepted medical practice. In these situations, the nurse must exercise professional judgment and follow the policies and procedures of the institution. Usually these policies require the nurse to notify the physician involved to clarify the orders.

The institution's policies and procedures describe the performance expected of nurses in its employ, and a nurse deviating from these policies and procedures can be liable for negligence or malpractice. Occasionally, such failure to adhere to institutional protocol can result in the employer denying the nurse a defence in a lawsuit.

Practising nurses must also adhere to the standards of practice for the nursing profession in the community.

REAL WORLD INTERVIEW

The most common problem areas for nurses are the failure to properly document the care provided, failure to appropriately monitor the client's condition and document it, and failure to appropriately document when physicians are needed and fail to respond. To address these issues, all nurses are required to attend annual education sessions to reinforce the requirements of appropriate documentation. The main rule of thumb is, "if it's not documented, it's not done" (as far as the courts are concerned), so … DOCUMENT! DOCUMENT! DOCUMENT!

Jill Jefferies, BScN
Risk Manager

These standards include such things as checking "the five rights" in medication administration or repositioning the bed-bound client at regular intervals. It is not uncommon for the nurses to be conflicted between an employer's expectations and the nursing standards of care, which can result either in insufficient time or lack of staff to adhere to the standards as taught in nursing school, or poor evaluations for taking too long to render care. In these situations nurses must evaluate the standards to follow to preserve their practice and protect themselves from liability. In some cases such an evaluation will lead to a decision to change jobs.

INTENTIONAL TORTS

ASSAULT AND BATTERY **Assault** is a threat to touch another in an offensive manner without that person's permission. An example would be if someone lunges at you in a threatening manner, but doesn't actually hit you. However, you had reason to believe that you would be harmed and threat was imminent. The aggressor would still be liable to damages for assault (Keatings & Smith, 2010). **Battery** is the touching of another person without that person's consent. An example of battery is slapping a client (i.e., direct battery) or pulling away a chair, resulting in the person falling to the ground (i.e., indirect battery). In the health care arena, complaints of battery usually pertain to whether the individual consented to the treatment administered by the health care professional. Most provinces and territories have laws that require clients to make informed decisions about their treatment.

INFORMED CONSENT

Every nurse needs to know the elements required for consent to treatment and the elements that constitute *informed* consent. The Ontario Health Care Consent Act, 1996, S.O. 1996, c.2, Sch. A identifies the elements required for consent:

- Consent must relate to the treatment.
- Consent must be informed.
- Consent must be voluntary.
- Consent must not be obtained through misrepresentation or fraud.

In addition, the Act explains that consent to treatment is *informed* only if the person received all of the information pertaining to the treatment that a reasonable person in the same circumstances would need to make a decision about the treatment, and the person received responses to all requests for additional information about the treatment. All of the following details must be explained to the client: the nature of the treatment, the expected benefits, material risks, material side effects of the treatment, alternative courses of action, and the likely consequences of not having the treatment.

Fiesta (1999) explains that informed consent laws protect the client's right to practise self-determination. The client has the right to receive sufficient information to make an informed decision about whether to consent or to refuse a procedure. The individual performing the procedure has the responsibility of explaining to the client the nature of the procedure, benefits, alternatives, and the risks and complications. The signed consent form is used to document that this explanation was completed, and it creates a presumption that the client has been advised of the appropriate risks.

Often the nurse is asked to witness a client signing a consent form for treatment. When you witness a client's signature, you are vouching for two things: the client signed the paper and the client was aware of signing a consent form (Olsen-Chavarriaga, 2000). For a consent form to be legal, in most provinces, the client must be at least 16 years old, or old enough to understand the nature of the treatment; must be mentally competent; must have had the procedures, their risks, and their benefits explained in an understandable manner; must be aware of the available alternatives to the proposed treatment; and must consent voluntarily. The nurse must also be familiar with the other people who are allowed, by law, to consent to medical treatment for clients who cannot consent themselves. In Ontario a formal hierarchy of substitute decision makers is outlined in the *Substitute Decisions Act* (1992) (see Table 18-1). For related policy in Saskatchewan, see The Health Care Directives and Substitute Health Care Decision Makers Act. Other provinces and territories have their own acts governing consent and substitute decision making.

TABLE 18-1	**HIERARCHY FOR SUBSTITUTE DECISION MAKERS IN ONTARIO**

1. Guardian appointed by the court

2. Attorney for personal care

3. Representative appointed by the Consent and Capacity Board

4. Spouse, common-law spouse, or partner of client

5. Child (at least 16 years of age) of client, parent of client

6. Parent of client who only has a right of access

7. Brother or sister of client

8. Any other relative of client by blood, marriage or adoption

9. Public Guardian or Trustee

Source: Ontario Seniors Secretariat, (2011). "If you don't appoint a substitute decision-maker." Retrieved from http://www.seniors.gov.on.ca/en/advancedcare/dontappoint.php

If no expressed written consent has been found in the chart of a client who is having surgery, and the nurse notes that the client has been sedated, does a written consent still need to be obtained? Keatings and Smith (2010) state that the written consent form itself cannot stand alone. It is only evidence that consent has been provided, but a mentally competent client may withdraw consent at any time, regardless of whether there is a form that existed providing previous consent. The most important consideration is that an informed consent has been provided. If the physician has documented in the chart that the client has provided consent, and that there has been disclosure related to the risks, consequences, and benefits of the procedure then this will usually be sufficient, regardless of whether the client had signed a consent form.

A nurse may also face a charge of battery for failing to honour an advance directive, such as a power of attorney for personal care or living will. Organizations may require that a hospital ask clients, upon admission, whether they have a living will; if they do not, the hospital may ask clients whether they would like to enact one. A **living will** is a written advance directive voluntarily signed by clients that specifies the type of care they desire if and when they are in a terminal state and cannot sign a consent form or convey this information verbally. The living will can be a general statement such as "no life-sustaining measures" or specific, such as "no tube feedings or respirator."

Often, the client's family has difficulty allowing health care personnel to follow the wishes expressed in a living will, and conflicts arise. These situations should be communicated to the hospital ethics committee, the pastoral care department, the risk management department, or the hospital department responsible for handling such issues. If clients have verbalized their wishes regarding end-of-life care to the family, such difficult situations can sometimes be avoided. When possible, clients should be encouraged to discuss these issues with their family. The nurse should be familiar with the requirements for the implementation of a living will in the province or territory where the nurse practises. Figure 18-1 is an example of a living will.

DO NOT RESUSCITATE (DNR) ORDERS

There is a distinction between "no CPR" and "DNR." Keatings and Smith (2010) state that the latter is a concept that includes any treatment given to sustain life, up to and including blood transfusions, antibiotic therapy, and artificial ventilation. According to the authors, CPR is limited to the technique of compressing the client's chest without applying artificial ventilation. Therefore, it is important to document the precise wishes of the client or substitute decision maker with respect to the request. Molloy (1992) suggests using the term *personal health care directive* to articulate one's wishes.

The attending physician may write a do not resuscitate (DNR) order on an inpatient, which directs the staff not to perform the usual cardiopulmonary resuscitation (CPR) in the event of a sudden cardiopulmonary arrest. The doctor may write such an order without evidence of a living will on the medical record, and the nurse should be familiar with the institution's policies and provincial or territorial law regarding when and how a physician can write such an order in the absence of a living will.

Declaration made this _____ day of _____, 2011.

I,_____ being of sound mind, wilfully and voluntarily make known my desire that my dying shall not be artificially prolonged under the circumstances set forth below and do hereby declare:

If at any time I should either have a terminal and irreversible incurable injury, disease, or illness or be in a continual profound comatose state with no reasonable chance of recovery, certified by two physicians who have personally examined me, one of whom shall be my attending physician, and the physicians have determined that my death will occur whether or not life-sustaining procedures are utilized and where the application of life-sustaining procedures would serve only to prolong artificially the dying process, I direct that such procedures be withheld or withdrawn and that I be permitted to die naturally with only the administration of medication or the performance of any medical procedure deemed necessary to provide me with comfort care.

In the absence of my ability to give directions regarding the use of such life-sustaining procedures, it is my intention that this declaration shall be honoured by my family and physician(s) as the final expression of my legal right to refuse medical or surgical treatment and accept the consequences of such refusal.

I understand the full import of this declaration and I am emotionally and mentally competent to make this declaration.

Signed: _____

City, County, and Province/Territory of Residence

The declarant has been personally known to me and I believe him/her to be of sound mind.

Witness _____

Witness _____

Figure 18-1 Sample of a Living Will* Declaration
*See provincial or territorial law requirements.

Often a DNR order is considered a medical decision that the doctor can make, preferably in consultation with the family, even without a living will executed by the client.

If the nurse feels such a DNR order is contrary to the client's or family's wishes, the nurse should consult the policies and procedures of the institution, which may require going up the chain of command until the nurse is satisfied with the course of action. This process may entail notifying the nursing supervisor, the medical director, the institution's chief of staff, or the chief medical officer. Often an institution has an ethics committee that examines such issues and makes a determination of the appropriateness of the order.

FALSE IMPRISONMENT

False imprisonment is the intentional restraint of individuals who are incorrectly led to believe they cannot leave a place. False imprisonment often occurs because the nurse misinterprets the rights granted to others by legal documents, such as powers of attorney for personal care, and does not allow a client to leave a facility because the person with the power of attorney for personal care (i.e., the agent) says the client cannot leave.

A **power of attorney** for personal care is a legal document executed by an individual (the principal) granting another person (the agent) the right to perform certain activities in the principal's name. The power of attorney can be specific, such as "initiate tube feedings," or general, such as "make all health care decisions for me." In most provinces and territories, a power of attorney for personal care is voluntarily granted by individuals and does not take away clients' rights to exercise their own choices. Thus, if the principal (i.e., the client) disagrees with the agent's decisions, the client's wishes will prevail. If a situation occurs in which an agent, acting on a power of attorney for personal care, disagrees with your client regarding discharge plans, contact your supervisor for further assistance in deciding an action consistent with your client's wishes and best interests.

A claim of false imprisonment may be based on the inappropriate use of physical or chemical restraints. Provincial and territorial laws mandate that health care institutions employ the least restrictive method of ensuring client safety. Physical or chemical restraints are to be used only when necessary to protect the client from harm when all other methods have failed. If the nurse uses restraints on a competent person who is refusing to follow the doctor's orders, the nurse can be charged with false imprisonment or battery. If restraints are used in an emergency situation, the nurse must contact the doctor immediately after application to secure an order for the restraints. Also, the nurse must check the institution's policies regarding the type and frequency of assessments required for a client in restraints and how often it

Y ou are working the night shift. One of your client's physicians has ordered a dose of a medication that you know is too high for this client. You are unable to locate the doctor to check the order. What would you do to ensure safe care for your client?

is necessary to secure a reorder for the restraints. These policies ensure the client's safety and must be consistent with provincial or territorial law.

RIGHT TO PRIVACY

In Canada there are two federal privacy laws: the Privacy Act (1983) and the Personal Information Protection and Electronic Documents Act (2001). The Privacy Act is a code of ethics for the government handling of personal information of the citizens of Canada. The Personal Information Protection and Electronic Documents Act, which was fully implemented by 2004, addressed the collection, storage, and use of personal information by organizations in the private and public sector. In addition, the provinces and territories may have their own laws related to privacy, such as the Personal Information Protection Act (2003) in British Columbia, Alberta's Freedom of Information and Protection of Privacy Act (2000), Manitoba's Personal Health Information Act, Newfoundland and Labrador's Personal Health Information Act (2008), Saskatchewan's Health Information Protection Act (1999), Access to Information and Protection of Privacy Act in Yukon, and the Personal Health Information Protection Act (PHIPA) (2004) in Ontario.

The right to privacy goes hand in hand with the right to confidentiality. These two rights affect all types of interaction with clients: from ensuring the curtains are drawn around a client's bed when bathing the client, to keeping information confidential and private when clients have told you something they don't want their family to know.

The nurse is required to respect the privacy of all clients. As a health care practitioner, the nurse may be privy to very personal information and must make every effort to keep it confidential. The need for confidentiality often necessitates policing conversations with co-workers to ensure that no client information is accidentally overheard by others.

Sometimes the protection of a client's privacy conflicts with the provincial or territorial mandatory reporting laws for the occurrence of specified infectious diseases, such as syphilis or human immunodeficiency virus (HIV). The need to protect an individual's privacy may also conflict with the provincial or territorial mandatory reporting laws

on suspected client abuse, discussed previously. Provincial or territorial law may also require the reporting of a client's blood alcohol level, incidences of rape and gunshot wounds, and adverse reactions to certain drugs.

Failing to strictly follow reporting laws could lead to criminal, civil, or disciplinary action and termination of employment. Nurses must consult the institution's policies and confer with its risk management department to ascertain their responsibilities and course of action. The Canadian Nurses Association (CNA) Code of Ethics for nurses states that nurses must be accountable for their practice. As a result, protection of the client and the public is required when incompetence or unethical or illegal practice compromise health care and safety. All provinces and territories have adopted this concept in their nurse practice acts. Nurses who observe unethical behaviour in a hospital should report this behaviour as directed in the institution's policies and procedures manual or by the laws of the province or territory.

LEGAL PROTECTIONS IN NURSING PRACTICE

As discussed earlier in this chapter, nursing practice is guided by provincial and territorial nurse practice acts and agency policies and procedures. Other resources for nurses include government inquiries, Good Samaritan laws, skillful communication, and risk management programs.

GOVERNMENT INQUIRIES

Special commissions, fatality inquiries, and coroners' inquests can have immediate and direct impact on nursing and organizational practices (Hibberd & Smith, 2006, p. 275). This effect has been demonstrated time and again in inquest and coroners' recommendations. Nurses traditionally are not aware of the numbers of coroner's recommendations that are published on an annual basis, or their content. In addition, they are not aware that these published reports are sent to health care facilities across the provinces and territories for their action. Nurses need to request these documents to ensure that recommendations are acted upon in their facility. For example, the two inquests following deaths at The Hospital for Sick Children in Toronto resulted in recommendations, some of which affected nurses directly.

The Sinclair Inquiry in Winnipeg, Manitoba, found that of the 12 pediatric cardiac deaths that occurred in 1994, five were preventable, four were possibly preventable, two were uncertain, and one was likely non-preventable (Sinclair, 2000). The central finding of the inquest was the following: "the evidence suggests that, during 1994, the Pediatric Surgery Program at the Health Sciences Centre did not provide the standard of health care that

it was mandated to provide and which parents believed, and had a right to expect, that their children would receive" (Sinclair, 2000, p. 465).

Some of the problems that the program faced related to the abilities of some of the individuals; however, the other problems were systemic in nature. Some issues related to the structure of the Health Sciences Centre, and specifically to policies and procedures related to staffing, leadership, teamwork, quality, communication, and decision making. Recommendations that related to the nursing division can be found in Table 18-2. It is important for nurses to pay heed to recommendations from coroner's inquests so that the practice and the profession of nursing is strengthened.

TABLE 18-2	NURSING-RELATED RECOMMENDATIONS FROM THE SINCLAIR REPORT

1. It is recommended that the HSC [Winnipeg Health Sciences Centre] establish a medical staff recruitment process for senior or specialized positions within the hospital that has as its main priority the creations of a mechanism that results in the best possible candidate being hired or appointed. The process should include the components ... Personnel in related fields, such as nursing, anaesthesia and perfusion, should have input into the criteria developed for the position. ... The recruitment process ... should include nurses. ...

2. It is recommended that there should be clear written lines of authority and responsibility within the Pediatric Cardiac Surgery Program. Efforts should be made to ensure that members understand these lines of authority.

3. It is recommended that there should be orientation and support for all new staff and for staff moving into new positions. This should be done even if the appointment is an Acting position.

4. It is recommended that the entire team, including those responsible for post-operative care, be prepared before the program moves to new procedures or higher-risk cases.

5. It is recommended that HSC restructure its nursing council to allow nurses to select its membership and to give it responsibility for nursing issues within the hospital. The nursing council should have representation on the hospital's governing body and be responsible for monitoring, evaluating, and making recommendations pertaining to the nursing profession within the hospital and for nursing care. The council should also serve as a vehicle through which nurses could report incident, issues, and concerns without risk of professional reprisal.

6. It is recommended that a clear policy be established on how staff is to report concerns about risks for clients. ... The government of Manitoba consider passing "whistle-blowing" legislation to protect nurses and other professionals from reprisals stemming from their disclosure of information arising from a legitimately and reasonable held concern over the medical treatment of patients.

7. It is recommended that there be a patient right's handbook that would include a section on the issue of informed consent ... as part of the consent process, that the information about a surgeon's experience in performing a particular procedure, as well as the experience of the hospital or surgical team be disclosed.

8. It is recommended that the HSC establish a clear policy on how staff is to report concerns regarding risks for clients ... and that all staff members are made aware of their responsibility to use incident reports and fully chart problems with the process of delivery of care and any complications in the outcome of care.

Source: Adapted from Sinclair, C.M. (2000). *The Report of the Manitoba Pediatric Cardiac Surgery Inquest: An Inquiry into Twelve Deaths at the Winnipeg Health Science Centre in 1994.* Winnipeg Provincial Court of Manitoba, pp. 467–483.

GOOD SAMARITAN LAWS

Good Samaritan laws are laws that have been enacted to protect the health care professional from legal liability. The essential elements of commonly enacted Good Samaritan laws are as follows:

- The care is rendered in an emergency situation.
- The health care worker is rendering care without pay.
- The care provided did not recklessly or intentionally cause injury or harm to the injured party.

Note that these laws are intended to protect the volunteer who stops to render care at the scene of an accident. These laws would not protect an emergency medical technician (EMT) or other health care professionals rendering care at the scene of an accident as part of their assigned duties and for which they receive pay. In doing their duties, these paid emergency personnel would be evaluated according to the standards of their professions.

Some of Canada's provinces have passed Good Samaritan laws. Ontario has the Good Samaritan Act, 2001; Alberta has the Emergency Medical Aid Act; British Columbia has the Good Samaritan Act; and Nova Scotia has the Volunteer Services Act. Except in Québec, no laws oblige people to help someone in need. Québec is unique in Canada because it imposes a duty on everyone to help a person in peril. The duty to take action stems from the Québec Charter of Human Rights and Freedoms, enacted in 1975, and the Civil Code of Québec, which came into force in 1994.

The Québec Charter includes a provision that states that if assistance can be provided without serious risk to the Good Samaritan or a third person, then the Good Samaritan is obligated to provide assistance. Little precedent exists to assist in interpretation of these provisions. Under the Civil Code every person is obligated to act as a reasonably prudent person. Failure to do so would amount to fault and lead to legal wrong.[9] Little uniformity exists among Canadian laws to protect the Good Samaritan. Some provinces' laws protect the rescuer from liability, unless evidence can prove gross negligence, but these laws do not force a person to assist. Every province except Prince Edward Island has a criminal compensation scheme to compensate Good Samaritans injured because of a criminal act. However, no common law province has established a general compensation scheme. Only five provinces and two territories have general legislation relieving a Good Samaritan from liability for negligence.[10]

SKILLFUL COMMUNICATION

The nurse must communicate accurately and completely both verbally and in writing. Often a case involving client care takes several years to come to trial; by that time, the nurse may have no memory of the incident in question and must rely on the written record from the time of the incident. This record is frequently displayed in the courtroom, enlarged to billboard size for all to see. All errors are apparent and omissions stand out by their absence, especially when data should have been recorded according to institutional policy. The old adage "if it isn't written, it wasn't done" will be repeated to the jury numerous times. Thus, it is essential that the nurse chart accurately and completely. To protect themselves when charting, nurses should use the FLAT charting acronym: F—factual, L—legible, A—accurate, T—timely

F: Charting should be *factual*—what you see, not what you think happened; only your own actions

L: Charting should be *legible*, with no erasures. Corrections should be made as you have been taught, with a single line drawn through the error and initialled.

A: Charting should be *accurate* and complete, clear, and concise. What colour was the drainage and how much was present? How many times, and at what times, was the doctor notified of changes? Was the supervisor notified?

T: Charting should be *timely*, completed as soon after the occurrence as possible. "Late entries" should be avoided or kept to a minimum. Regular entries should be made in chronological order.

Many health care teams are now documenting their practice by utilizing the acronym SBAR. The Situation-Background-Assessment-Recommendation (SBAR) technique provides a framework for communication among members of the health care team about a client's condition. It is an easy-to-remember, concrete mechanism, useful for framing any conversation—especially critical ones—requiring a clinician's immediate attention and action. It allows for an easy and focused way to set expectations for what and how something will be communicated among members of the team, which is essential for developing teamwork and fostering a culture of client safety. See Figure 18-2 and Figure 18-3 for information related to Q-TIPs (Quality Tools in Practice) and a sample of how to use SBAR respectively, both from Capital Health in Nova Scotia.

FOLLOWING DOCTORS' ORDERS

In most provinces and territories, nurses are required to follow the doctor's orders when giving care to clients unless doing so would cause them client harm. To follow this mandate, nurses must ensure that the orders are clear and accurate. If necessary, the nurse may need to contact the physician for clarification. If the nurse is still uncomfortable following the order, the supervisor should be notified and the institution's policies followed regarding notification. Because of the opportunity for

Q-TIPs

Quality Tools In Practice

SBAR
For Improved Communication!

Q-Tip #2
September 2006

	What is it?	The SBAR (Situation-Background-Assessment-Recommendation) technique provides a framework for communication between members of the health care team about a patient's condition.
	Why Use it?	• The SBAR tool ensures completeness of information and reduces the likelihood of missed data. • It allows for an easy and focused way to set expectations for what will be communicated and how it will be communicated. • Standardizes communication between healthcare providers, doctor-nurse, nurse-nurse, doctor-doctor.
	How do I do it?	• **S** – Situation – what's going on (5–10 seconds) • **B** – background – brief pertinent history, relevant context • **A** – Assessment – what I think, conclusion • **R** – Recommendation – what I need and in what time frame
	What will the Result look like?	An example is shown on the reverse of this page.

Source: www.ihi.org

Developed by: Michael Leonard
Doug Bonacurth
Suzanne Graham
Kaiser Permanente of Colorado

Capital Health

Figure 18-2 Q-TIPs (Quality Tools in Practice)

Source: Michael Leonard, Doug Bonacurth, Suzanne Graham, Kaiser Permanente of Colorado. Retrieved from <http:www.paediatricchairs.ca/safety_curriculum/domain3_docs/SBAR-Tool.pdf> April 21, 2011. Permission courtesy of Institute for Healthcare Improvement, Cambridge, MA.

A Sample of How to Use **SBAR**

SBAR REPORT TO PHYSICIAN ABOUT A CRITICAL SITUATION

S	**Situation – identify self, unit** **I am calling about** \<patient name and location\> **The problem I am calling about is** _____ **I have just assessed the patient personally and these are the changes in the patient's status:**

Background:

	NEURO	CV	RESP	GI	GU	LABS	MEDS
B	☐ GSC ☐ Sedation ☐ ICP/CPP ☐ Pupils	☐ BP/MAP ☐ HR ☐ ECG ☐ Rhythm ☐ Chest pain ☐ Temp ☐ PA and cardiac calcs ☐ CVP ☐ Bleeding ☐ IV access	☐ RR ☐ Sp)2 ☐ Change in ventilation or oxygenation ☐ Breath sounds ☐ ABG	☐ N/V ☐ OG/drain output ☐ Nutrition ☐ High residuals ☐ IAP ☐ Abdo pain	☐ U/O ☐ I/O ☐ Fluid balance	☐ Recent results ☐ Date of last cultures ☐ Blood glucose	☐ Current infusions and rates ☐ Increasing Inotropes ☐ Med Error

A	**Assessment** This is what I think the problem is: \<say what you think is the problem\> The problem seems to be \< cardiac infection neurologic respiratory _____ \> I am not sure what the problem is but the patient is deteriorating The patient seems to be unstable and may get worse, we need to do something.

R	**Recommendation**
	
	I request that you \<say what you would like to see done\>
	  ☐ Transfer the patient to critical care
	  ☐ Come to see the patient at this time
	  ☐ Talk to the patient or family about code status
	  ☐ Ask the on-call family practice resident to see the patient now.
	  ☐ Ask for a consultant to see the patient now
	
	Are any tests needed:
	Do you need any tests like CXR, ABG, EKG, CBC, or BMP?
	Others
	
	If a change in treatment is ordered then ask:
	  ☐ How often do you want vital signs?
	  ☐ How long do you expect this problem will last?
	  ☐ If the patient does not get better when would you want us to call again?
	
	Confirm:
	  ☐ I understand that the treatment plan is: "\<intervention and time frame for anticipated outcomes\>"
	  ☐ What should I do before you get here to assess the patient?

Additional samples are available at: http://www.cdha.nshealth.ca/quality/ihiTools.html

Figure 18-3 SBAR Report to the Physician

Source: SBAR Report to the Physician" was originally developed by Kaiser Permante. Permission courtesy of Institute for Healthcare Improvement, Cambridge, MA.

REAL WORLD INTERVIEW

The role of enterprise risk management in the health care environment is that of recognition, evaluation, and treatment of risks inherent in the organization. The goal of enterprise risk management is improving the quality of care provided by the organization while at the same time protecting its financial integrity. Enterprise risk management, while coordinated at a certain level of the organization, is not simply a one-department responsibility, but rather is the responsibility of each employee of the organization.

New graduates in nursing need to understand that in today's health care environment, each practitioner must look for ways to reduce the risks inherent in the delivery of health care. At a time when hospitals are having difficulty balancing budgets, our clients and consumers are demanding higher and higher quality of care.

Health care is at a crossroads, similar to the one that faced private industry during the 1970s. Our customers are demanding that we provide a safe environment and that we consistently strive for continuous quality improvement.

An incident report or occurrence form is a commonly used form that documents a variance from normal protocol or hospital procedures. It is not meant to place blame on an individual practitioner or department. It is used strictly to document the facts surrounding an event so the health care processes can be improved. Thus, the nurse should complete an incident report when any variance from a policy or a procedure is noticed. This assists in providing a culture of learning instead of a culture of blame.

When enterprise risk management receives the incident reports, they are logged into our database, and monthly reports are forwarded to nurse managers for follow-up and education with their staff.

Incident reports and the subsequent enterprise risk management department actions are generally reactive but we also do pro-active/preventive interventions in the health care setting. These include the following:

1. Education of students completing their senior year of study in nursing

2. Participation on client safety, occupational health and safety, pharmacy, nursing, and other hospital committees, which work on proactive programs to reduce risks

3. Facilitation of the slips and falls task force to reduce our clients' fall risk

4. Education of new nurses and physicians on principles of enterprise risk management

Harriet Percy, RN
Enterprise Risk Manager

misinterpretation and misunderstanding, verbal orders are not encouraged.

ENTERPRISE RISK MANAGEMENT PROGRAMS

Enterprise risk management programs in health care organizations are designed to identify and correct system problems that contribute to errors in client care or to employee injury. The emphasis in risk management is on quality improvement and protection of the institution from financial liability. Institutions usually have reporting and tracking forms to record incidents that may lead to financial liability for the institution. Enterprise risk management will assist in identifying and correcting the underlying problem that may have led to an incident, such as faulty equipment, staffing concerns, or the need for better orientation for employees. Once a system problem has been identified, the enterprise risk management department can develop educational programs to address the problem.

The enterprise risk management department may also investigate and record information surrounding a client or employee incident that may result in a lawsuit. This investigation will help personnel remember critical factors if called to testify at a later time. The nurse should notify the enterprise risk management department of all reportable incidents and complete all enterprise risk management or incident report forms as

TABLE 18-3	ACTIONS TO DECREASE THE RISK OF LIABILITY

- Communicate with your clients by keeping them informed and listening to what they say.
- Acknowledge unfortunate incidents and express concern about these events without taking the blame, blaming others, or reacting defensively.
- Chart and time your observations immediately, while facts are still fresh in your mind.
- Take appropriate actions to meet the client's nursing needs.
- Follow the facility's policies and procedures for administering care and reporting incidents.
- Acknowledge and document the reason for any omission or deviation from agency policy, procedure, or standard.
- Maintain clinical competency and acknowledge your limitations. If you do not know how to do something, ask for help.
- Promptly report any concern regarding the quality of care, including the lack of resources with which to provide care, to a nursing administration representative.
- Use appropriate standards of care.
- Document the time of changes in conditions requiring notification of the physician and include the response of the physician.
- Delegate client care based on the documented skills of regulated and unregulated personnel.
- Treat all clients and their families with kindness and respect.

mandated by institutional policies and procedures. Note also that employee complaints of harassment or discrimination can expose the institution to significant liability and should promptly be reported to supervisors and the enterprise risk management department, human resources, or whichever department is specified in the institution's policies. See Table 18-3 for a checklist of actions to decrease the risk of nursing liability.

MALPRACTICE AND PROFESSIONAL LIABILITY INSURANCE

Nurses may need to carry their own malpractice insurance. **Malpractice** refers to a professional's careless conduct in the discharge of professional duties or failure to meet standards of care for the profession that results in harm to an individual entrusted to the professional's care (Keatings & Smith, 2010). Nurses often believe their actions are adequately covered by their employer's liability insurance, but this is not necessarily so. If, in giving care, the nurse fails to comply with the institution's policies and procedures, the institution may deny the nurse a defence, claiming that because of the nurse's failure to follow institutional policy, or because of the nurse working outside the scope of employment, the nurse was not acting as an employee at that time. Also, nurses are being named individually as defendants in malpractice

suits more frequently than in the past. Consequently, it is advantageous for the nurse to be assured of a defence independent of that of the employer. Professional liability insurance provides that assurance and pays for an attorney to defend the nurse in a malpractice lawsuit.

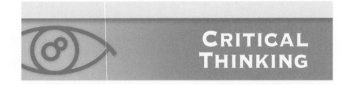

CRITICAL THINKING

You are the only registered nurse assigned to give 0900h medications on a 52-bed nursing home unit. To avoid being classified as a drug error according to the institution's policy and usual nursing practice, administration of the medications must occur within 45 minutes of the ordered time. Also, nursing practice mandates you verify the "five rights": the right drug, the right dose, the right client, the right time, and the right route.

What are the problems with this assignment? What would you do?

KEY CONCEPTS

- Nursing practice is governed by public and private laws.

- Nurses are responsible for providing a safe environment for clients entrusted to their care.

- Nurses need to be familiar with their institution's policies and procedures in giving care and in reporting variances, illegal activities, or unexpected events.

- Nurses must have good oral and written communication skills

- Common torts include negligence, assault and battery, and false imprisonment.

- Nurses need to be familiar with their provincial or territorial nurse practice act.

- Good Samaritan laws exist in many provinces or territories.

- Enterprise risk management programs improve the quality of care and protect the financial integrity of institutions.

KEY TERMS

assault	Good Samaritan laws
battery	living will
civil law	malpractice
common law	negligence
constitution	power of attorney
contract law	public law
false imprisonment	tort

REVIEW QUESTIONS

1. Which type of law authorizes nursing regulatory bodies to enact rules that govern the practice of nursing?
   A. provincial or territorial law
   B. federal law
   C. common law
   D. criminal law

2. If you make a threatening gesture to a client, with no contact having been made, you are liable for which of the following charges?
   A. assault
   B. defamation
   C. malpractice
   D. false imprisonment

3. Battery is an example of which of the following?
   A. intentional tort
   B. non-intentional tort
   C. assault
   D. negligence

4. Which of the following is a body of law that develops through precedents over time and has the force of law?
   A. contract law
   B. common law
   C. public law
   D. civil law

REVIEW ACTIVITIES

1. Talk to the enterprise risk manager at the hospital where you have your clinical assignments. How does the enterprise risk manager handle an incident report? Is it used for improving the hospital's care in the future? How?

2. Review the advance directive (i.e., living will) policy at the hospital where you have your clinical assignments. Notice the form that clients sign. How does it compare with the living will form on page 377?

3. Discuss how a nurse's off-duty behaviour can affect her practice as a nurse. Can the provincial or territorial regulatory body take action against the nurse's registration?

EXPLORING THE WEB

- Go to the following sites to find malpractice information for your province or territory: *http://www.cnps.ca/* and *http://www.cnps.ca/cnps_plus/index_e.html*

- Where can you find provincial and territorial laws regulating hospitals? *http://www.e-laws.gov.on.ca/index.html*

- You have a client who is to be transferred to a nursing home for recuperation. Where can you suggest the family look to evaluate the local nursing homes regarding their adherence to the provincial or territorial regulations for nursing homes? *http://app.infoaa.7700.gnb.ca/gnb/Pub/EServices/ListServiceDetails.asp?ServiceID1=9615&ReportType1=All*

- Where can you find a copy of the CNA Code of Ethics? *http://www.cna-aiic.ca/CNA/practice/ethics/code/default_e.aspx?pf=1*

REFERENCES

Capital Health website. *SBAR report to the physician (document)*. Retrieved from http://www.cdha.nshealth.ca/defaultnc.aspx?page=SearchResults&querySessionId=Query2548_86&siteId=1&siteFilter=1&xslpath=Resources%5csite_xsl%5csearchresults_anycontent_w_redirect.xsl

College of Nurses of Ontario. (2005). *How we protect the public*. Toronto: Author. Retrieved from http://www.cno.org/en/protect-public/

College of Registered Nurses of British Columbia. (2009). *Competencies in the context of entry-level registered nurse practice in British Columbia*. Vancouver: Author. Retrieved from http://crnbc.ca/registration/rnapplication/bcen/documents/375.pdf

Commission on the Future of Health Care in Canada. (2002). *Building on values: The future of health care in Canada*. Saskatoon: Author. Commissioner: Roy J. Romanow.

Fiesta, J. (1999). Informed consent: What health care professionals need to know, part 2. *Nursing Management,* 30(7), 6–7.

Hibberd, J. M., & Smith, D. L. (2006). *Nursing leadership and management in Canada* (3rd ed.). Toronto: W.B. Saunders.

Institute for Healthcare Improvement website. *SBAR technique for communication: A situational briefing model.* Retrieved from http://www.ihi.org/IHI/Topics/PatientSafety/SafetyGeneral/Tools/SBAR-TechniqueforCommunicationASituationalBriefingModel.htm

Keatings, M., & Smith, O. (2010). *Ethical and legal issues in Canadian nursing* (3rd ed.). Toronto: Mosby, Elsevier Canada Limited.

Kingma, M. (2001). Workplace violence in the health sector: A problem of epidemic proportion. *International Nursing Review,* 48(3), 129–130.

MacIvor, H. (2006). *Canadian politics and government in the Charter era.* Toronto: Nelson, a division of Thomson Canada Ltd.

Molloy, W., & Mepham, V. (1992). *Let me decide.* Toronto: Penguin Books.

Morris, J. (1991). *Canadian nurses and the law.* Toronto: Butterworths.

Olsen-Chavarriaga, D. (2000). Informed consent: Do you know your role? *Nursing,* 30(5), 60–61.

Ontario Seniors Secretariat. (2011). If you don't appoint a substitute decision-maker. Retrieved from http://www.seniors.gov.on.ca/en/advancedcare/dontappoint.php

Shaw, J. (2006). In harm's way. *Registered Nurse Journal,* 18(4), 12–16.

Sinclair, C. M. (2000). *The Report of the Manitoba pediatric cardiac surgery inquest: An inquiry into twelve deaths at the Winnipeg Health Sciences Centre in 1994.* Winnipeg: Provincial Court of Manitoba.

Zerwekh, J., & Claborn, J. C. (2000). *Nursing today: Transition and trends* (2nd ed.). Philadelphia: Saunders.

SUGGESTED READINGS

Brown, S. M. (1999). Good Samaritan laws: Protection and limits. *RN,* 62(11), 65–68.

Champion, J. B. (2001). When "enough" may not be enough: Informed consent and patient communication. *Risk Management in Canadian Health Care,* 2(8), 81–88.

DeLaune, S., & Ladner, P. K. (2002). *Fundamentals of nursing* (2nd ed.). Clifton Park, NY: Delmar Learning.

Fiesta, J. (1999a). Greater need for background checks. *Nursing Management,* 30(11), 26.

Fiesta, J. (1999b). Informed consent: What health care professionals need to know, part 1. *Nursing Management,* 30(6), 8–9.

Fiesta, J. (1999c). When sexual harassment hits home. *Nursing Management,* 30(5), 16–18.

LaDuke, S. (2000). What should you expect from your attorney? *Nursing Management,* 31(1), 10.

Mantel, D. L. (1999). Legally speaking: Off-duty doesn't mean off the hook. *RN,* 62(10), 71–74.

Martens, C. (2002). The Manitoba pediatric cardiac surgery inquest. *Risk Management in Canadian Health Care,* 3(7), 65–73.

McKee, R. (1999). Clarifying advance directives. *Nursing,* 29(5), 52–53.

Morris, M. R. (1998). Elder abuse: What the law requires. *RN,* 61(8), 52–53.

Perry, J. (2000). Legislating sharps safety. *Nursing,* 30(5), 50–51.

Provincial Court of Manitoba. (2001). *Report of the Review and Implementation Committee for the Report of the Manitoba Pediatric Cardiac Surgery Inquest.* Winnipeg: Review and Implementation Committee for the Report of the Manitoba Cardiac Surgery Inquest.

Sheehan, J. P. (2000). Protect your staff from workplace violence. *Nursing Management,* 31(3), 24–25.

Sloan, A. J. (1999). Legally speaking: Whistleblowing: There are risks! *RN,* 62(7), 65–68.

Spencer, P. C. (2002). Developing a hospital policy re: Disclosure of adverse medical events. *Risk Management in Canadian Health Care,* 4(6), 65–72.

Staten, P. A. (1999). How to cover all the bases on informed consent. *Nursing Management,* 30(9), 14.

Sullivan, G. H. (1999). Legally speaking: Minimizing your risk in patient falls. *RN,* 62(4), 69–70.

Sullivan, G. H. (2000). Legally speaking: Keep your charting on course. *RN,* 63(4), 75–79.

Ventura, M. J. (1999). Legally speaking: When information must be revealed. *RN,* 62(2), 61–62, 64.

Wilkinson, A. P. (1998). Nursing malpractice. *Nursing,* 28(6), 34–39.

CHAPTER ENDNOTES

1. Health Canada, "How Health Care Services Are Delivered." Retrieved from http://www.hc-sc.gc.ca/hcs-sss/pubs/system-regime/2005-hcs-sss/index-eng.php#a2

2. *R. v. Morgentaler,* [1993] 3 S.C.R. 463. Retrieved from http://www.canlii.org/en/ca/scc/doc/1993/1993canlii74/1993canlii74.pdf

3. *Rodriguez v. British Columbia (Attorney General),* [1993] 3 S.C.R. 519. Retrieved from http://www.canlii.org/eliisa/highlight.do?text=Rodriguez+v.+British+Columbia+%28Attorney+General%29%2C+%5B1993%5D+3+S.C.R.+519&language=en&searchTitle=Search+all+CanLII+Databases&path=/en/ca/scc/doc/1993/1993canlii75/1993canlii75.html

4. Canadian Centre for Occupational Health and Safety, "About CCOHS—Background." Retrieved from http://www.ccohs.ca/ccohs.html

5. Canadian Centre for Occupational Health and Safety, "Violence in the Workplace: Is there specific workplace violence prevention legislation?" Retrieved from http://www.ccohs.ca/oshanswers/psychosocial/violence.html

6. Industrial Accident Prevention Association (IAPA). "Resource articles. New legislation tackles workplace violence and harassment." Retrieved from http://www.iapa.ca/Main/Articles/2009_workplace_violence.aspx

7. International Council of Nurses, "Violence a worldwide epidemic." Retrieved from http://www.icn.ch/publications/violence/

8. Keatings, M., & Smith, O. (2010). *Ethical and Legal Issues in Canadian Nursing* (3rd ed., p. 421). Toronto: Mosby, Elsevier

9. Canadian Association of Food Banks, "Good Samaritan Law: Obligation to Help Someone in Trouble." Retrieved from http://foodbankscanada.ca/goodsamaritanlaw.htm

10. Search and Rescue Society of British Columbia, "Good Samaritan Legislation." Retrieved from http://www.island-net.com/sarbc/sarbc/legal-issues-in-sar.html

CHAPTER 19

Spirituality and the Profession of Nursing

Janet Stark, Certified Multifaith Chaplain

I held his hand while we talked, and we prayed together familiar words of comfort, the Our Father. Knowing I might not see him again, I gave him the Aaronic Blessing. At the end of our visit, I turned to leave. He said, "Thanks, Sister." I left feeling strangely blessed. I am not a nun, nor am I Roman Catholic. However, if he felt I acted as a nun toward him; if I acted for him as someone he trusted and respected in his faith tradition; then I was honoured to be filling that role. No corrections needed.[1]

OBJECTIVES

The purpose of this chapter is to enable the reader to

- define spiritual care, religious care, and culturally-appropriate care;
- describe how spiritual care is an integral part of holistic care;
- discuss the nurse's role and the leader's role in providing spiritual care;
- explain spiritual needs during illness;
- assess spiritual needs and spiritual distress;
- identify healthy spiritual practices;
- list effective tools to provide therapeutic spiritual intervention; and
- describe when and how to refer to chaplaincy or work with a spiritual care team.

Claudio Rossol/iStockphoto

You are the nurse manager on the medical-surgical floor of a busy hospital. You have a good understanding of holistic care and recognize the value that spiritual care brings to the ill client. Under your direction you have several nurses, all very capable of providing the best physical care. One of the most difficult areas of nursing proficiency, however, is the comfort level and standard of care when it comes to spiritual care. On your team you have

- *an older nurse who was trained by the Catholic nuns,*
- *a nurse with aboriginal roots who often feels that traditional medicine is at odds with his customs and practices,*
- *a young nurse who proudly claims to be an atheist,*
- *a middle-age nurse who is an evangelical Christian and attends every worship service held in the hospital,*
- *a nurse who is of Asian background and Buddhist in practice,*
- *a nurse who seems angry at the church and fights against any personal connection with organized religion, and*
- *a nurse who is very spiritual and finds strength in sports and nature.*

In reviewing their nursing backgrounds, you realize that there has been a vast range of educational experience when it comes to spiritual health. Some have had very little spiritual education, others have had the basics on chaplaincy services and religious care, and yet others have had a more current, broader focus on spirituality. How are you going to improve staff comfort level with the topic, educate all to reach the standard mandated by the Canadian Nurses Association (CNA), and ensure that clients are provided with the best practice spiritual care?

The topic of spiritual care is often misunderstood and poorly addressed in health organizations. We may profess to provide holistic care—body, mind, and spirit—but are we all "on the same page" when it comes to "spirit" care? If not all on the same page, how can we provide spirit care to a consistent standard? This chapter provides an opportunity for the reader to gain more understanding of the meaning of spiritual care as it applies to clients with many different diagnoses, ages, and stages of life.

SPIRITUALITY AND NURSING

Nurses may be aware that clients have spiritual needs, but many times are not able to respond to these needs. This may result from lack of education in nursing programs or because nurses see **spiritual care** as part of the psycho-social assessment completed by **pastoral care** workers. However, nurses are in the best position to provide spiritual care, particularly when they have established relationships with individuals at the end of life or with life-threatening illnesses. These clients are often more concerned about issues of a spiritual rather than a physical nature. The concept of providing spiritual care derives from an aspect of nursing theory that states humans are biological-psychological-spiritual beings.[2] Although nursing recognizes that clients have spiritual needs, the practice of spiritual care by nurses is often infrequent and is an underused aspect of client care. Narayanasamy (2006) states that recognition of the clients' spiritual needs is an integral part of holistic nursing because it forms part of the care of mind, body, and spirit. In a recent report, spiritual care was described as "an essential component of a holistic model of nursing" (Wordsworth, 2007). Spirituality is rarely discussed or debated, regardless of the fact that an awareness of spirituality is necessary for holistic care to be delivered (Petterson, 1998).

Recently, there has been much debate about a definition of spirituality. Jones (2004) suggests that an individual's perception of spirituality is unique. People who agree with this perspective believe that there can never be one universally accepted definition because spirituality means different things to different people. Guillory (2001) believes that spirituality is our inner consciousness, and that it is the source of inspiration, creativity, and wisdom. According to Guillory, "that which is spiritual comes from within—beyond our programmed beliefs and values" (p. 33) that have been taught but not tested by challenging life experiences. Increasingly, the concepts of spirituality and religion are being separated.[3] It is suggested that religion is more about systems: a social institution that is joined by individuals who share the same beliefs, traditions, and rituals.[4] It is characterized by boundaries, whereas spirituality cannot readily be defined by boundaries. Tanyi (2002) defines *spirituality* as "a personal search for meaning and purpose in life, which may or may not be related to religion" (p. 1). Regardless of its definition, a clear meaning of the term is important for not only enhancing communication, practice, education, and research but also reducing the gap between policy and expectations.[5]

The term spirituality is used not only in health care but also in society at large. Holistic health care includes the spiritual dimension. Society is both multicultural and ethnically diverse. As a result, for some individuals spirituality will be expressed and shaped by religious customs and practices that provide meaning to their existence. Nurses require the correct education and information about these customs and practices if they are to offer culturally sensitive religious and spiritual care and avoid stereotypical assumptions.[6]

Religion is an expression of spirituality reflected in the beliefs and practices that unite its adherents in the community. Religions are expressed through sacred writings, codes of behaviour, rituals, and ceremonies (Stark, 2008).

Spirituality is the *energy* within each person that looks for meaning and purpose in life. It is a unifying and integrating human factor. Spirituality is expressed through a vast array of means, both formal and informal (Stark, 2008).

Wright (2005) defines spirituality as "whatever or whoever gives ultimate meaning and purpose in one's life, that invites particular ways of being in the world in relation to others, oneself and the universe" (p. 4). Themes associated with the concept of spirituality include meaning, purpose, hope, faith, sense of peace, and connectedness.[7] The Canadian Nurses Association (CNA) (2009) believes that spirituality is an integral dimension of human health. See Table 19-1 for the CNA position statement on spirituality, health, and nursing practice.

LEADERSHIP: LEARNING AND GROWING

Nurses understand the need for continuing education and reflective practice—regulatory bodies require that nurses review their practice, identify areas requiring improvement and implement learning plans on a regular basis. In addition, continuing professional development is required related to professional standards of practice. Often the areas of focus are practical, such as how to use a new piece of equipment or a new treatment regime. Growing and learning in the spiritual realm is an area that is often neglected but can be fostered in a health care setting. Workshops on spiritual perspectives and issues can be offered. Opportunities for debriefing, and case reviews can help nurses to integrate spiritual practice into day-to-day nursing care. Three necessary components of positive learning include knowledge about the subject gained by study; skills taught or learned from experience; and attitude, which is possibly the hardest to change. Attitude, an inherent attribute, reflects the desire to stretch, grow, and self-reflect with respect to particular subject matter and skills.

TABLE 19-1	CNA POSITION—SPIRITUALITY, HEALTH, AND NURSING PRACTICE

- CNA recognizes that spiritual beliefs are diverse, reflecting both individual and cultural influences. To provide the best possible health outcomes, registered nurses are expected to respect this diversity in the same way they provide culturally competent care. Sensitivity to, and respect for, diversity in spiritual beliefs, support of spiritual preferences and attention to spiritual needs are recognized by CNA as required nurse competencies.

- CNA believes that being attentive to an individual's spirituality is a component of a holistic nursing assessment and nursing practice. When planning for and providing care, nurses have an ethical responsibility to be aware of and adjust for an individual's spiritual beliefs.

- CNA believes that through their practice, nurses are uniquely situated to ensure that an individual's spiritual values, beliefs and experiences are taken into account in the provision of ethically responsible health-care interventions.

- CNA supports the development, teaching and practice of communication strategies that create openness and skill in discussions with individuals about their spiritual beliefs. Continuing education, mentoring and workplace support can assist nurses in developing their abilities to be attentive to an individual's spiritual beliefs or values.

- CNA supports the interpretation and declaration – at national and international levels – of spirituality as an integral dimension of an individual's health, and believes such policy statements to be important to holistic health care and nursing practice.

Source: Canadian Nurses Association. (2009). *Position Statement, Spirituality, Health and Nursing* <http://www.cna-aiic.ca/CNA/documents/pdf/publications/PS111_Spirituality_2010_e.pdf>

LITERATURE APPLICATION

Citation #1: Penman, J., Oliver, M., & Harrington, A. (2009). Spirituality and spiritual engagement as perceived by palliative care clients and caregivers. *Australian Journal of Advanced Nursing,* Volume 26 Number 4: 29–35.

Discussion: Health professionals are inadequately prepared to provide spiritual care. Consequently, spiritual issues, more often than not, are overlooked and unresolved. This phenomenological inquiry set out to understand the lived experience of spirituality and engaging in spiritual matters for clients living with life-limiting conditions and their caregivers.

Implication for Practice: Evidence shows that clients would benefit from spiritual care, and may wish to discuss spiritual matters with health professionals; therefore, nurses would benefit from education toward increased comfort and competency providing such care.

Citation #2: Oldnall, A.S. (1996). A critical analysis of nursing: Meeting the spiritual needs of clients. *Journal of Advanced Nursing,* 23: 138–144.

Discussion: Nurses tend to equate spirituality with religion.

Implication for Practice: While nurses often feel it is inappropriate to get involved in religious matters, they often miss the bigger picture of helping with spiritual comforts.

Citation #3: Baldacchino, D. R. (2006). Nursing competencies for spiritual care. *Journal of Clinical Nursing,* 15(7): 885–896.

Discussion: Nursing assessment of clients' needs has been dominated by the medical model, which has been oriented primarily toward the physical needs. The author suggests that this is because the spiritual dimension was not considered as a relevant task in care. Renewal of the spiritual dimension in nursing care has been an area of focus during the past two decades, and researchers and practitioners have acknowledged its priority in care.

Implication for Practice: Spiritual care is a complex concept to understand. Nurses need to increase their awareness of the uniqueness of each individual client regarding the connection among mind, body, and spirit. The findings from this study will enable nurses to consider the importance of spiritual care. This may assist nurses to empower clients to find meaning and purpose during times of illness. Holistic care models teach that spiritual assessment should be integrated into the whole person assessment, not an optional add-on.

Citation #4: Edwards, A., Pang, N., Shiu, V., and Chan, C. (July 2010). The understanding of spirituality and the potential role of spiritual care in end-of-life and palliative care: A meta-study of qualitative research. *Palliative Medicine,* 24(8): 753–770. Retrieved from http://www.bmedreport.com/archives/15780, April 2, 2011.

Discussion: The aim of this study was to synthesize qualitative literature on spirituality and spiritual care at the end of life using a systematic review. Spiritual care is regarded as very important for many terminally ill clients, but professionals have difficulty defining what that care would include. This review examines articles from the perspectives of both the client and the health care provider. Quantitative studies have shown that 87 percent of clients consider spirituality to be important in their lives and between 51 percent and 77 percent of clients consider religion to be important.

Implication for Practice: It is evident that most people would benefit from spiritual care and that many would benefit from **religious care**. The articles cited a lack of training and suggested that to benefit and enhance care more training is needed in listening skills, awareness of individual needs, and different cultural beliefs.

(Continued)

LITERATURE APPLICATION (CONTINUED)

Citation #5: Belcher, A., & Griffiths, M. (2005). The spiritual care perspectives and practices of hospice nurses. *Journal of Hospice and Palliative Nursing, 7*(5): 271–279.

Discussion: Hospice nurses used traditional spiritual care interventions more frequently and held more positive perspectives regarding spiritual caregiving than did nurses in other practice settings.

Implication for Practice: It is noted that spiritual care is often reserved for those at the end of life and also that hospice or palliative care nurses are trained and comfortable providing psycho-social care. This type of care overlaps very easily with spiritual care.

Citation #6: Baldacchino, D. R. (2006). *Nursing competencies for spiritual care.* Journal compilation by the author, Blackwell Publishing Ltd.

Discussion: The outcome of spiritual care was found to enable clients to count their blessings in life, achieve inner peace, and explore coping strategies.

Implication for Practice: When nurses can see the results of positive spiritual intervention, they can feel profoundly rewarded.

HOLISTIC CARE

Different models describe holistic care. One model is a pie chart with physical, emotional, intellectual, and spiritual pieces. Another model shows the spirit on the outside of the circles, encompassing all of our collective parts. Figure 19-1 shows a model where the spirit is at the core of our individual being; it is what makes us personal and unique. The model also shows that the health of the body and mind are dependent on the health of the core self—the spirit.

MODELS OF SPIRITUALITY

All persons are spiritual in nature. However, not all persons are religious. Figure 19-2 describes the connection between religion and spirituality. Look at the small circle on the inside—imagine it in many different sizes. It could be very small for a person of Christian background who observes Christmas and Easter, but very little else of the Christian faith. Or it could be larger—for someone who

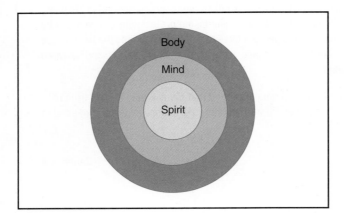

Figure 19-1 Holistic Self

Source: Stanford, M. (2008). *Grace for the afflicted.* Published by Paternoster (now BiblicaTM), Colorado Springs.

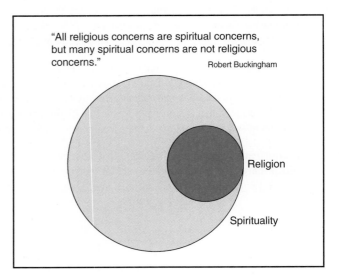

Figure 19-2 Our Spiritual and Religious Self

Source: Buckingham, Robert. School of Public Health & Social Policy, University of Victoria.

has a stronger faith practice. It could be a circle almost as big as the outer circle—for one where their religious faith is central to their very being (e.g., a faith leader, rabbi, or priest). The visual is of two circles where every person is fully spiritual in nature, with varying degrees of inner circles. It is quite reasonable to have a client who has no inner circle or religious nature; however, the outer circle depicts that spirituality is inseparable from the person.

HIERARCHY OF CARE

As in the circle model, Maslow's triangle includes all aspects of the person (see Figure 19-3). Spirituality touches each part from the most basic physiological needs through safety and upward to self-actualization. In health care, the focus is most often on the lower levels. When clients have acute illnesses, we can help them get well, and this means they move up the hierarchy, regaining their independence, and eventually they are discharged or empowered to manage chronic illness. When health care providers focus on basic needs, we are providing care. Helping people is a spiritual act, sharing part of oneself with another.

Maslow's model teaches that nurses must start to care for the ill person by providing for the basic needs first. Starting on the bottom level, we need to meet the physical needs such as food, water, sleep, and shelter. Next, the client must feel secure—that he will not fall out of bed or that he is safe in the nurse's care. When we move up toward love and belonging, we increase the opportunity for supportive care: companioning, affection, and spiritual care. The spiritual needs reside in the top three levels: belonging, confidence, comfort, hope, creativity, acceptance, and legacy. Maslow's model illustrates well the basic spiritual needs and shows that all aspects of care have a spiritual component.

HISTORY OF COMPASSIONATE CARE

Many nurses were originally motivated to serve others due to their religious and spiritual beliefs and practices. Florence Nightingale believed her work was "God's work." "The nurse was to acquire and apply knowledge about God's laws of health, and thus move mankind closer to perfection" (Dolamo, 2010). Nightingale's vision of nursing education by religious orders taught the morality of admission to health care by non-sectarian and non-class criteria. Kiley (2008) suggests that deans of Catholic nursing schools worry that a heightened emphasis on technical proficiency and scientific acumen has had the unintended consequence of de-emphasizing the spiritual essence of compassionate nursing care.

The following are examples of the religious roots of health care:

1. the parable of the Good Samaritan (Bible, Luke 10:25–37)
2. religious orders providing wayfare stations for travellers—the original hospice concept
3. the Order of Sisters of Charity of Montréal, commonly known as the Grey Nuns, founded in 1738 by Saint Marguerite d'Youville
4. early hospitals in South Africa were all mission hospitals, run by the church (Dolamo, 2010)

ASSESSMENT EDUCATION

Nurses need training in spiritual assessment, and they need a tool that is simple to use. This assessment is best incorporated into the basic nursing admission assessment and not simply perceived as an "extra" or "option." When nurses begin to understand that the spiritual assessment means discerning relationship needs, fears, worries, and

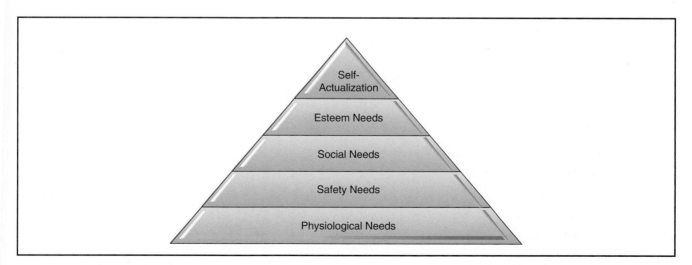

Figure 19-3 Maslow's Hierarchy of Needs

Source: Retrieved from http://www.abraham-maslow.com/m_motivation/Hierarchy_of_Needs.asp

important traditions, it may become less intimidating. Nurses who feel that it is too personal to ask religious questions must realize that, for many, this process brings information for accessing very helpful resources. Yes, spiritual care is personal, and so is bathing; yet bathing is recognized as essential and can be done with the utmost dignity! Consider carefully the questions outlined in Table 19-2, and you will see the value in collecting such information. Learn to internalize the questions. In this way you can ask them in your own words or in the cultural language of the client. The questions can be asked a few at a time, as a nurse develops a therapeutic relationship. But remember, these are not the kinds of questions one would ask and record on a clipboard, as with a dietary assessment.

Often a spiritual assessment is not done. Usually upon admission, clients are asked if they would like their religion recorded. Occasionally this question is met with hostility. However, it is a valuable question for most, and admission clerks interviewing the client need to find sensitive ways to ask this question. When a response is given, it is then recorded on the chart. Clients may give the name of their own clergy or faith leader. Also helpful is to ask the question: "Would you welcome a visit from the spiritual care team?" This implies that the invitation is given to all, and the question is too often perceived as "spiritual assessment."

Another paradigm that spiritual care services seek to change is an old idea that "If they ask me if I want to see a chaplain, then I must be dying." Belcher and Griffiths (2005) suggest that nurses may not complete a spiritual assessment with clients and their families for other reasons, including the following:

- not knowing what to ask or how to approach it
- no tool available

TABLE 19-2	SPIRITUAL AND CULTURAL ASSESSMENT

Patient/Client/Resident: _____

Faith Group/Religion/ Ethnic Background: _____

Spiritual Contact: _____ Phone # _____

Spiritual-Cultural History:
Do you have a faith practice or religion?
How would you describe your culture?
Do you have any rituals you wish to practice?
What spiritual practices gave you support in the past?
(Sometimes concrete examples need to be suggested: prayer, nature, reading, pets, art, music, worship services, visits from family, clergy)
Who gives you support?
Tell me about your family.
Is there anyone else who should be involved in making decisions about your care?

Goals of Care:
What is really important and meaningful to you right now?
Is there anything the care team needs to know about health practices or restrictions important to your culture/faith group?
What do you believe about your illness?

Spiritual Distress:
Is there anything bothering you right now?
Is there anything you are afraid of?
How are your loved ones coping right now?
What would help?
How can we include this in the hospital setting?
Are there any other concerns you would like to share with me?

Source: Stark, Janet. (2011). *Spiritual/Cultural Assessment.* Reprinted by permission of Janet Stark.

Self-awareness
What are my personal beliefs, values,
prejudices, assumptions, and feelings?
How may these influence the way in
which I nurse?

Spirituality
What does holistic care mean to me?
What other beliefs are there?
What do I know about different belief systems including
religious, humanist, and secularist?

Spiritual nursing (Reflection on personal client care—trigger questions)
Have I considered what things are important in this client's life?
Am I open to verbal and non-verbal cues?
How does the client relate to others? Who are the important people in the client's
life and how does she respond to them?
Is the client displaying possible signs of spiritual distress?
Is the client displaying any evidence of religious affiliation? (symbols,
religious texts, etc.)
Am I facilitating a trusting, open nurse-client relationship?
Am I providing the client with privacy as well as opportunity to talk and express feelings?
Am I able to provide holistic care or is a multi-disciplinary
approach needed? (e.g., chaplain, social worker, etc.)
Have I evaluated any spiritual intervention?

Figure 19-4 The ASSET Model

Source: Ellis, H.K., & Narayanasamy, A. (2009). An investigation into the role of spirituality in nursing. *British Journal of Nursing,* 18(14): 890.

- embarrassment and awkwardness
- reluctance to bring up a personal subject
- expectation that the social worker or chaplain will do it
- statement that "I don't believe in God"
- client unable to communicate
- short-term clients who are not in care long enough

Many authors believe that the use of formal assessment tools for spirituality is a move away from the simple caring ethos of nursing. Randall and Downie (2006) make the point that the assessment tool indicates that professional engineering is replacing quiet listening. They suggest that the use of these tools could constitute harassment and could act as a barrier to forming a therapeutic relationship with the client. They also believe that human relationships are at risk of being replaced by impersonal, ritualistic questionnaires.

On the other hand, Narayanasamy (2006) developed a cultural and spiritual assessment tool. Many nurses today do not have the skills to provide spiritual care without the use of definitions and assessment tools. In an ideal world, nurses could provide natural client-centred care without the use of assessment tools. However, if a trusting relationship is built between a nurse and a client, specific care plans and tools may encourage the nurse to consider the client's spirituality. If tools are used in this way, rather than as stencils, they can be effective guidelines for holistic care.[8] See Figure 19-4 for another example of an assessment tool. The ASSET model was created in response to a lack of education on spirituality in nursing education programs. It encourages those in education to become more self-aware and consider spirituality and the spiritual dimensions that are often excluded from common practice.

RELIGIOUS NEEDS

WHAT HEALTH PROFESSIONALS NEED TO KNOW

For many people, religious beliefs play a significant role in personal spiritual support. When one is ill, personal faith may be emphasized as one seeks to make meaning out of suffering. For others, it is a time of crisis of faith, when one cannot make sense of their situation. Some struggle to feel God's presence and to reconnect spiritually. A person may ask, "Why? Why me?" Real anguish is experienced by one who has a belief in a loving God but feels abandoned. Often this person can draw on his religious beliefs to bring him back to a place of acceptance.

Someone who has weak or broken ties to a faith community may wish to reconnect. Others may seek to form a new relationship with a spiritual power and may welcome support and direction. Nurses can identify this need and help make connections to the spiritual care team or community clergy.

To find inner peace, an ill person may need to identify, express, work through, and let go of spiritual anguish such as bitterness, guilt, or regret. Belief in a loving and forgiving spiritual power can help one let go and reach toward spiritual wellness. This can be a process, and for some it may be a struggle not completely settled at the time of death.

If prayer has been a part of the ill person's life, it can be a valuable resource. Prayer can acknowledge unspoken needs and desires and can be a tangible expression of suffering. Once articulated, that is "spoken out loud," a prayer can seek comfort, acceptance, and healing. Healing can be either physical or spiritual, or it can be both. Prayer happens in many ways—through the informally expressed word, meditation, touch, or more formal prayers and scripture passages. Other faith practices such as songs, readings, or rituals may often be a very comforting reminder.

The value of believing in life after death needs to be stressed, particularly because those from all religious backgrounds who believe in heaven or paradise or eternal life have a very strong asset in accepting impending death. Some may even welcome death as an end to suffering, an opportunity to be reunited with loved ones, seeing the face of God, or to have a new and healthy body. One may not be afraid to die but still be afraid to suffer or experience pain. One may also be afraid to be alone. Nurses can emphasize that the client will not be abandoned. Excellent **palliative care** should help ensure that an ill person will be as comfortable as possible in her final days. Nurses have shared many miracle moments—the signs and wonders a dying person has experienced. These are part of the profound experience of the mystery of spirituality.

WHAT ABOUT SHARING MY FAITH?

To provide spiritual care do your best to understand your clients and meet them on their own ground. Consider what to do when asked questions about your own religious beliefs. It is usually appropriate and even beneficial to share when two conditions are met: when the client and caregiver share the same faith and when the caregiver is asked.

When a member of staff or clergy seeks to convert clients to his or her own faith group, this is proselytizing and unethical. In most health facilities, community clergy are not allowed to make random hospital visits with the intent of converting clients.

Nurses tell many stories of unexplained occurrences, of miracles, and mysteries. Often they feel honoured to accompany a client who is having a deeply personal

CRITICAL THINKING

Last Call

An interesting story of a client who died *twice* was told to me by a retired nurse:

"It was over thirty years ago, and I remember it was a warm, sunny day. I was working in a small hospital, and caring for a lady who was near end-of-life. Suddenly the client stopped breathing, and I called for the doctor who was in another room. He came in, listened to her heart with his stethoscope, and pronounced her dead. At the time, I was thinking: *She doesn't look dead.* Usually, I pulled the sheet up to cover the face, but this time, I didn't. I also decided to wait awhile before I took her to the morgue. I left the room and a short time later, returned.

I found my dead client out of bed and fully ambulatory! I was dumbfounded! *She was actually on the phone, talking to a relative!* Again I left the room, and when I came back in the second time, she was back in bed, dead. The other nurses were just as stunned as I was! We didn't bother calling the doctor in, because he had already pronounced her dead!

I always will wonder, "Who did she call, and what did she tell them?"

What is your reaction to this story? Have you experienced a similar event? How does this make you feel?

Source: Stark, J. (2010). *Last call. Final scenes: Bedside tales at end of life.* Winnipeg: Word Alive Press.

REAL WORLD INTERVIEW

Dying is a very private and unique event for each senior and family. We should intrude as little as possible, and assist as much as we can.

Source: Dr. Elizabeth Latimer MD., CCFP., FCFP, Professor Emerita in the Department of Family Medicine, the Division of Palliative Care, McMaster University, Hamilton, Ontario.

spiritual experience. Whether one is religious or not, signs and wonders do take place. A collection of stories can be found in Maggie Callanan and Patricia Kelley's *Final Gifts* (1992). Sharing stories can be a means of learning and processing spiritual issues for clients, families, and staff.

CULTURAL CARE THEORIES

Culturally appropriate care extends the scope of spiritual and religious care. The term *cultural care* is a good one and a concept that Canadians are tolerant of. Culturally appropriate care includes the customs, traditions, and practices that are shared among a group of people. Sometimes by teaching this concept a way becomes open for discussing spiritual care.

CRITICAL THINKING

A beloved physician from our hospital died very suddenly. The staff members were visibly upset. Carrying on their duties in a professional manner that day was very difficult. The physician was a member of the Sikh faith. All had recognized his turban, his good looks, and affable manner. It was quite a loss for the hospital. His own community of faith organized a traditional Sikh service. It was in another city and many of the nursing staff could not attend. The Spiritual Care Department was asked to organize a memorial service for hospital staff as a tribute to his life and an opportunity for debriefing. The room was full, and the service was respectful of the Sikh traditions. Several staff members spoke about the beloved doctor. Some said the memorial service was an opportunity to process the loss and begin healing.

The memorial service could have been presented in the Christian tradition, as most of those present and also the clergy were of Christian background. Because the deceased was of the Sikh faith, it was decided to orient the service to be respectful of Sikh beliefs.

Do you think having a ceremony that represented Sikh beliefs was a good decision? Should the beliefs of the attendees paying respects affect the nature of the ceremony? Should the beliefs of the organizers? What kind of ceremony would you suggest in this scenario? What differences are there between a Sikh service and a traditional Christian one?

MULTICULTURALISM IN CANADA

Canada is known as a cultural mosaic, having people of many different ethnic backgrounds across the nation. Urban ethnic diversity in Canada gives us large areas of ethnic groups living together in cities. Local culture often manifests as a more homogenous group living in a local area. For example, in rural Québec, the local culture is francophone. In northern areas of each Canadian province, the local culture may be Aboriginal. In small towns and rural areas, there may be cultures almost entirely of English, Irish, and Scottish descent.

It is important for nurses to recognize that the Canadian population is transient, and staff travel far and wide as well. In a large city one can expect to care for ethnically diverse clients. Even in homogenous areas, accidents occur on major highways, bringing clients of all backgrounds into small-town emergency departments.

To be culturally sensitive, a care provider needs to be open and inquiring. A nurse does not need to know everything but, instead, know where to find information. A **multi-faith** manual could be a key resource. The spiritual care department should keep a current list of local practising clergy and leaders of all ethnic and faith groups. If copies of this list are kept in clinical areas and nurses are made aware of this list, they can be encouraged to contact the appropriate person without having to refer to the spiritual care department.

A culturally appropriate care plan is proactive, not reactive. A harm-reduction model suggests that we give a spiritual-cultural assessment early on, preferably on admission. The nurse needs to know right away who is going to speak for the client; always assume that clients speak for themselves unless they are incapable or they have made another directive. The nurse also needs to know if there are special considerations required in providing care, which also includes care upon death, handling of the body, and burial or cremation practices.

NEEDS

Spiritual

A spiritual need is anything a person needs to have: a sense of connectedness to others (relationship), a purpose in life (meaning), or a belief system in the transcendent (faith). Having spiritual needs met leads to wholeness, or holistic wellness.

Comfort

Good medical management seeks to control pain and other symptoms first, and then supportive care measures such as spiritual care can help.

Hope

Having hope is an optimistic approach—hope is a strong coping mechanism. We should not describe a client who has hope as being in denial, even though this is often seen as something negative. Instead, a client who shows a positive perspective is one who practises a belief in possibility to fuel spiritual strength. Sometimes denial is a temporary protection until one can process difficult feelings. Hope can help one to reserve the necessary energy for coping during illness.

Creativity

An ill person may find satisfaction in writing, drawing, or building. The creative instinct is strong, and many feel that creativity is an expression of spirituality. Using imagination and encouraging creativity can bring about a wealth of resources for the ill person. Music, art, pet therapy, care-clowning, and a host of other creative pursuits help to build spiritual wellness. Many health facilities incorporate creative and complementary practices in the care plan.

Legacy

Someone who is sick of being debilitated needs to be reminded of their value. If they are nearing the end of life, family need to let them know they will be remembered. The nurse can also provide validation: for example, by saying, "I can see your granddaughter is very pleased you taught her how to crochet," or "your son will always remember how much you appreciated those roses." *Legacy* means to remember one's value.

Reminiscence

Encourage story-telling because this often brings a person who is in physical or spiritual distress back to a happier, healthier time. Sharing stories, memories and old photos are great ways of diverting the focus from present suffering. This can be facilitated by sharing from photo albums or recording life stories orally or in written form.

SPIRITUAL DISTRESS

Spiritual distress can cause deep unrest and is often expressed emotionally. Sometimes clients are not sure why they feel distressed, or cannot articulate what the distress is, until a care provider or **chaplain** helps them work through issues and hears the client's story (refer to the questions on spiritual distress in the assessment Table 19-2). Sometimes it helps just to have the distressing emotion identified and articulated.

SPIRITUAL DISTRESSORS

Loss

From the time one hears bad news, there is often loss of hopes and dreams, which is called **anticipatory grief**. As illness progresses, a series of losses can be experienced by both the client and family. (See Critical Thinking—Five Stickies, and Experiences of Loss.)

Anger

Anger is a common grief reaction. A client may be angry at God—for not intervening, or for "punishing" them. Or they may be angry at themselves for not having had a healthier lifestyle. They may be angry at the physician or health system for failing them in some way.

Fear

A common fear relates to suffering or being in pain. Another fear is of being alone or isolated. Other fears are related to the unknown progression of illness, and fears about how loved ones are coping. When one can express concerns, fears often seem lighter.

Guilt

Remorse or regret about past behaviour, habits, and family relationships can weigh very heavily on an ill person. Some religions have histories of fostering guilt (see discussion on Spiritual Abuse). Sometimes it is helpful if a spiritual care provider can articulate forgiveness. This can help the client be positively motivated rather than paralyzed by the past.

Pain

Physical pain can be managed medically in most cases. The health care expertise related to physical pain is available, but not always assessed and handled well. **Total pain** is a type of pain often associated with serious illness. It is a combination of physical, emotional, and spiritual pain, which results in real hurt and must be addressed in all its aspects to be effective.

Loneliness

Feelings of abandonment or isolation are common. Even with many health providers coming to and going from the bedside, a client can feel lonely. They can be lonely to be heard, or lonely to be touched, or lonely to be accepted. Many residents of long-term care are truly lonely, having few or no family visits. In these circumstances, the staff often becomes their family.

EXPERIENCES OF LOSS

There are three expressions of loss: disappointment, demoralization, and depression. Generally speaking, disappointment is short term, demoralization may be long-term, and depression is a long-term clinical condition. For example disappointment, that is, when things are not as one had hoped, may be expressed a follows: "I can't go to my granddaughter's wedding because I fell and broke my leg." This person can, however, still find enjoyment in other things. This person needs support for a temporary loss. The term *demoralization* describes the undermining of a person's confidence or morale or

CRITICAL THINKING

Five Stickies

As we travel through life we grieve many losses. We grieve losing our first tooth, or our favourite primary school teacher. We grieve losing our ability to skip and jump as we grieve losing our youth. Some of us grieve losing our hair, and maybe again we grieve losing all of our teeth! At some point, we face the loss of our health. The normal life cycle consists of a series of losses.

To illustrate this point, take five small yellow sticky-notes, and on each one, write something you have in your life that is very meaningful to you. Put each of these five stickies on each finger of your left hand. With your right hand, take a sticky note from your neighbour and put it in front of you. Turn to your neighbour again, and take something else. Each of you now has only three stickies left. Once more, remove a sticky note from your neighbour. Stop when you only have one left.

You are eighty years old, and have been coping fairly well at home on your own, until one day you have a stroke. Your children try to take care of you for awhile, as best they can. One day they gather together and tell you how sorry they are, but you will need to move into a care home. You have arrived at the new nursing home, lonely and bewildered and suffering from limited movement from your stroke.

This is where the stickies come in: what things have you lost?

Now you can't get out to church and you miss it so, and all of your church friends too. No longer can you drive, as your licence has been taken away. You miss your old farmhouse where you spent many happy years, and your prize-winning flower garden. You miss your home-cooked meals because now you can't chew and swallow properly and are getting a minced diet. You are not over the loss of your husband, who died two years ago, and not only do you miss him, but you miss your cat, Spooky, also. Then the doctor comes in and tells you that the stroke has left permanent damage, and you will not walk again. The next week more test results come in and the doctor comes back in with more bad news. You also have a chronic illness, the beginnings of Parkinson's disease.

How do you feel now? What other perspectives do you need to consider when caring for a client? What last important thing in your life do you have left (sticky note)? What do you understand about the complex needs of a person with declining health? How would you foster a sense of hope?

Source: Stark, J. (2010). *Final scenes: Bedside tales at the end of life.* Word Alive Press. Winnipeg, MB. Reprinted by permission of Janet Stark.

being disheartened (Kissane, Wein, Love, Lee, & Clarke, 2004). It happens when one has lost one's spirit. It can be expressed in sadness due to a loss of health: "I'll never dance again after having my foot amputated"; "I had just retired and planned to tour Europe, when my heart gave way." The client, who may eventually accept the loss and adjust to a new reality, needs support and possibly counselling. Ignored, this condition may lead to depression. Depression is a condition that requires additional support and intervention to prevent prolonged or chronic depression. The client suffering depression may appear melancholy or flat. Things that might normally interest this person do not, and signs of depression point to a drop in general health. The term depression is often over used, when, in fact, the more accurate term for the person's condition is disappointment or demoralization.

SPIRITUAL ABUSE

Spiritual abuse can cause significant emotional damage to the vulnerable, especially to young children and those suffering from mental illness. According to Henke (1996),

Spiritual abuse is the misuse of a position of power, leadership or influence to further the selfish interests of someone other than the individual who needs help. Sometimes abuse arises out of a doctrinal position. At other times it occurs because of legitimate personal needs of a leader that are being met by illegitimate means. Spiritually abusive religious systems are sometimes described as legalistic, mind controlling, religiously addictive authoritarian.

Cases of spiritual abuse occur in cults, communal communities that deny individual rights and freedoms, abusive sexual relationships between clergy and children (pedophilia), sexual relationships between therapist and client. Common characteristics of abusive religious communities include an overemphasis on authority, secretiveness about doctrine, fundamental perfectionism, and suppression of criticism.

When a nurse or other health-care provider suspects a client has endured spiritual abuse, it is best to refer to chaplaincy and describe your observations. When privy to a story of spiritual abuse, the nurse should ask permission of the client to share this with the chaplain. Often these concerns are best handled by mental health practitioners and counselling. When a nurse suspects abuse from within the client's own faith group, it is not recommended to consult with their leader.

Some clients have been hurt by the church or by their past religious experiences and carry a deep resentment to any expression of organized religion. The church has helped many, but, historically, it has hurt many as well. Such experience also applies to nurses.

WORKING WITH A SPIRITUAL CARE TEAM

The team members involved in the spiritual care can be nurses, doctors, therapists, social workers, chaplains, or spiritual care coordinators, the client's own clergy or spiritual care advisor, and spiritual or hospice volunteers. Spiritual care can be provided by any member of this team. Clients who are ill and in need may not be able to differentiate between the exercises provided by a physiotherapist and the help provided by the nurse or support worker with toileting. The opportunity to be compassionate and sincere can accompany all activities of daily living.

Because nurses are in positions of trust and have mandates to provide holistic care, they are in a unique position to ensure that spiritual needs are assessed and addressed within the team. Often one team member will make a connection with a particular client, but professional practice demands that relationships with clients remain therapeutic. Even if a particular nurse makes a strong connection with a client, rather than taking over that client's spiritual care, she can chart well, report her experiences to the team members, and empower others to build strong connections to help in healing.

The nurse can consult with the chaplain and bring the chaplain to the bedside as a spiritual partner or resource, but without "turning things over to the expert."

Health care providers need to accept chaplaincy or the client's own spiritual care provider as members of the team. The client and family can identify and give permission for the appropriate person to be included early in the care plan.

LEADERSHIP ROLES FOR MODELLING SPIRITUAL AND CULTURAL CARE

A nurse manager should be prepared to mentor and lead staff toward best practice spiritual care by exhibiting the following behaviours:

- Understanding the concepts of spiritual, religious, and culturally appropriate care
- Understanding the scope of spiritual care within nursing standards of practice
- Modelling personal spiritual maturity and a comfort level with spiritual matters
- Encouraging staff to be open and share limitations and expertise within the team
- Providing and attending ongoing spiritual and cultural education for staff, and coordinating with the spiritual care department
- Developing a spiritual assessment tool and integrating it with routine nursing assessment
- Expecting that nurses will document spiritual care needs and interventions as they would physical ones
- Debriefing with staff when spiritual care has been particularly helpful, or difficult, or when there are incidences of staff grief
- Liaising with the spiritual care department and keeping open communication
- Encouraging staff to refer to and consult with the spiritual care department when necessary
- Keeping an up-to-date list of contact numbers for the area's clergy and multi-faith providers
- Encouraging staff to include the client's clergy in discussions as part of the team
- Developing better working relationships with volunteers and valuing the assistance they bring to spiritual care. Involving volunteers more effectively and inclusively as a helpful resource.
- Having resources available for nursing staff, such as a multicultural manual and spiritual care guidelines
- Having Bibles and other religious and scriptural books available for clients
- Having a quiet place available on the floor for family meetings, counselling, and grieving

NURSING LEADERSHIP

What can the nurse-manager do to encourage appropriate spiritual care? Nurse managers can model a level of comfort during discussions surrounding client spiritual needs which demonstrates confidence in the development of their own spiritual maturity. Nurses are in positions of trust and responsibility. As leaders in health care they need to pay attention to all aspects of learning and growth, including spiritual. If nurse leaders can share their own strengths and needs related to spirituality they will have more ability to empower nursing staff and students to provide evidence-based spiritual care. Table 19-3 shows the practices of a leader who heals.

SPIRITUAL PRACTICES EVERY NURSE CAN ADOPT

Show up! The presence of the nurse as one enters the room can lower the anxiety of the client. The client feels that "the nurse will take care of me." Studies have shown that a nurse with a confident, focused, and compassionate presence can have the effect of lowering the client's blood pressure.

Agapé love Have positive regard for all—the term means "love for all mankind."

REAL WORLD INTERVIEW

Active Listening for Spiritual Distress

Cardinal O'Connor described the importance of a caregiver's personal spirituality from the perspective of his extensive ministry to those with the human immunodeficiency virus:

"When I visited hundreds of persons with AIDS, I discovered something that has been infinitely more important to them than any physical or medical help we can give them—the opportunity to talk about their own spiritual state, the opportunity to talk about their fears and anxieties, their hope for the future. ... A doctor or nurse can do so much to relieve such anxieties by spiritual examples ... [and by] treating people with spiritual gentleness."

Source: O'Brien, M.E. (2001). *The nurse's calling – A Christian spirituality of caring for the sick.* Paulist Press. New Jersey.

Mercy and grace Show compassion and **empathy** while providing non-judgmental, non-preferential treatment. The nurse shows grace by allowing the client to be human: imperfections and all.

TABLE 19-3	SEVEN P'S OF LEADERSHIP: BLUEPRINT FOR A HEALING HOSPITAL

1. Personal Commitment: Are we giving ourselves fully to our work?
2. The Practice of Passion: We need to cultivate passion in our work—to love the people with whom we work and the place we work as well.
3. The Exploration of the Potential: We are so much stronger than we think we are.
4. The Practice of Presence: It is through true presence that we discover how to give our love to meet the needs of another.
5. The Practice of Positive Attitude: Positive attitudes are important because they create hope and energy.
6. Persistence: Persistence is the power that causes us to hang in there. ...
7. The Practice of Prayer and Meditation: The calming influence of reflection is an essential ingredient of self-healing.

Source: Chapman, E. (2003). *Radical loving care: Building the healing hospital in America.* Baptist Healing Hospital Trust, Nashville. Reproduced by permission of Rev. Eric Chapman, J.D.

Develop trust The therapeutic relationship between client and care provider can greatly assist healing. Sometimes a relationship is driven more by personality than by professional competence. A client who is experiencing vulnerability needs to feel safe.

Eye contact and smile These are your first "words" to your client, and they help the initial connection. A warm smile often paves the way for meaningful discussion.

Active listening It is so important to hear the stories of the clients. Perhaps this is more important than saying the right words. Listening, hearing, and accepting are very helpful, even when this doesn't always result in direct action (see Real World Interview).

Sincere words Communication skills are important, as are a few words chosen intuitively. Often fumbling words are accepted because of the tone and the intent. A reflection or acknowledgment of what you are hearing is often helpful.

Gentle touch A light touch of the hand or shoulder is often appropriate, and can convey what words alone cannot. Hand-holding can be a great comfort, but caregivers need to wash their hands frequently and carefully to prevent the risk of spreading infection.

Simple reflection/prayer/meditation A reflective statement, prayer, poem, or reading a card are ways to offer spiritual practice. There are many creative ways to help while, at the same time, meeting the comfort level of the nurse.

Be* rather than *do Just the opposite of what nurses are trained for! Nurses are taught "don't just stand there, do something!" Sometimes it is more appropriate to "Don't do something, just stand there."

SPIRITUAL CARE AT THE END OF LIFE

There are eight domains of issues in hospice palliative care, with the client and the family at the centre. They are disease management; physical, psychological, social, spiritual, practical, and end-of-life care; and loss and grief. A complete model to guide hospice palliative care has been developed by the Canadian Hospice Palliative Care Association (CHPCA) (2002) (see CHPCA website). Spiritual care assessment and intervention can be readily identified in the following domains: psychological, social, spiritual, end-of-life care, and loss and grief. However, spiritual practice can occur at some level in all of the domains of care—including disease management and responding to physical and practical needs. Spiritual care also applies to the physical and practical domains, because compassion can be extended when cleansing wounds, or feeding or washing someone's face. This confirms the concept of

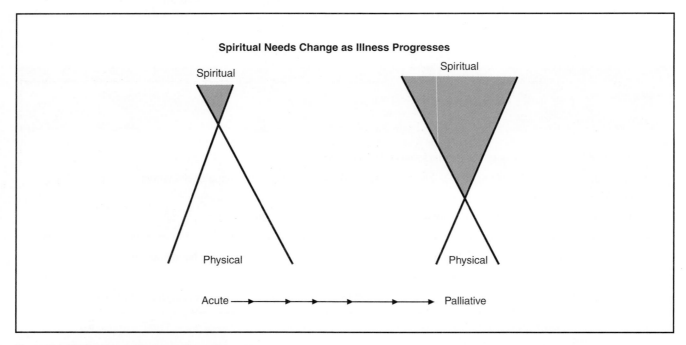

Figure 19-5 Spiritual Needs Change as Illness Progresses

Source: Lanark, Leeds & Grenville Palliative Care Education Manual (2008) compiled and edited by Janet Stark. Reprinted with permission.

providing spiritual care at all levels of Maslow's Hierarchy of Needs model. Opportunities for providing end-of-life spiritual care are the prevalent, which shows that it should not be treated as an additional or *add-on* therapy.

When illness is in the acute stage, the physical needs often outweigh all else (see Figure 19-6). The client requires treatment for pain and symptom control and active medical interventions. As an illness progresses toward palliative care, comfort measures increase. Then the spiritual needs are often manifest. When clients near the end of life, many turn to their spiritual or religious roots for grounding and support. This is the time when some clients make peace with (their) God.

The phrase, a dying client has "finished his business," may be about making relationships right and saying things that need to be said. There are several things that the dying client might want to say, one of which is "Good-bye". He may want to affirm his love and gratitude and provide a sense that any past wrongs are now forgotten. When people have made their relationships with loved ones right, they often die more peacefully. A nurse may not be able to heal broken relationships, but often acts as an enabler or conduit for bedside meetings to take place. It is indeed rewarding for nurses to know that they have played some small role in relieving the burden of guilt of a dying client.

ETHICAL CONCERNS

The concerns of privacy and confidentiality often come up in the area of spiritual care. As in any setting, nurses must maintain confidentiality if a client has "opened up" and shared deep secrets at a vulnerable time. Continuity of care can help to keep that confidentiality and trust in the therapeutic relationship. It is not always possible for the same nurse to continue working with the same client who has shared personal stories, as nurses often come and go from shift to shift.

Personal health information belongs to the client. However, the client can choose to include as an agent, whomever they wish in the circle of care. Consent to health information can be given verbally or in writing from the client or the substitute decision maker for a spiritual care provider to be consulted as part of the team. Information sharing will not be considered a breach of privacy when the client is aware of who is on the health team, and has given permission to discuss health matters related to her care plan.

Other ethical issues that might affect spiritual care include recent controversies about the definition of death, the right to refuse treatment, the role of parents in decision making for a pediatric client, and the withdrawal of treatment that may prolong life (see Chapter on ethics). These areas can cross over into spiritual or religious concerns, depending on the perspective of the client and family, and their beliefs and faith practices.

One of the best ways to determine the efficacy of providing spiritual care is in listening to the stories of clients and families. After a client has been discharged, or transferred, they often reflect on their care experience. Families who have had a loved one die in a health care setting often comment on their perception of their experience. Many times we hear positive comments about the quality of care related to compassion, presence, grief support, and other spiritual practices. This is qualitative evidence of the value of providing spiritual care and recognizing the importance of spirituality in a health setting.

May peace be with you
Calming your agitated heart,
Inviting you to be still
In your very being
May the blessing of peace be upon you.

Figure 19-6 A Universal Prayer

Source: Lanark, Leeds & Grenville Palliative Care Education Manual (2008) compiled and edited by Janet Stark. Reprinted with permission.

I am totally bedridden. I have extensive disease, unable to do anything for myself. I have total care provided by the community support worker and the home care nurse. I am not eating much, but I am mostly conscious and coherent, with periods of drowsiness and confusion. I am on several medications for pain and symptom control.

I know I am dying, and I have accepted this. I have spoken freely to all members of my family and they are in various stages of acceptance. All are supportive, but handling the news of my imminent death differently. My husband is great, and we talk about everything. He is very sad, but compassionate and provides much of my care when the nurses are not here. He will fall apart when I am gone.

I am in a hospital bed in my sunroom. I can see the back yards and fields beyond. I can hear the birds, and the neighbour's dog, and a plane flying overhead. Occasionally, I hear a car on the gravel lane and wonder who has come to see me today.

Even though there are pretty flowers on my bedside table, I can smell the taste of death all around me; the smell of sickness, stale air, and sweat. I smell the soaps and antiseptics and I can imagine I can even smell the medications. Maybe it is my imagination. I wonder if my family can smell it too; although they don't say anything. I bet even the dog smells death, but he also is too polite to protest, and he lies beside my bed on the mat. He misses our walks.

I try to enjoy bits of food, and sometimes I take in a bit, and sometimes it comes back up. Often even looking at food is hard. Everyone tries to encourage me to eat. At first I worried about hurting their feelings when they brought my favourite foods, so I would try. … But now, I think they get it: I just won't be eating much anymore. A few sips of water or ginger ale seem like a luxury.

I am thinking all kinds of things. I imagine all kinds of scenarios. My mind imagines my death in various ways, and the funeral. I can even imagine my loved ones sad and lonely after I am gone. Why can't my mind be still? I ask God for peace, and sometimes when I am alone I can feel peace, even taste it. Sometimes I feel so ready to let go, and at other times…I am scared.

I don't like a lot of fuss or noise, and ask that my house not turn into chaos. I can't stand chaos; it makes me feel like I'm not in charge. People come and go and I ask for my favourite music, not all the time, but a little each day. I have my photo albums beside me, and we take turns looking at them together. At first I did the commentaries myself, but now I am too tired and weak, and someone else must speak the stories. I can only manage ten minutes at a time.

My family asks nothing of me—I hope I have given them what they need. I have given them the blessing and they have given it back to me. I am fortunate in so many ways. I am ready now to be with the Lord. (Wow, I have heard that cliché before!) But it is so true. I am so tired…

Reflect on the holistic needs of this person.

What are the spiritual, physical, intellectual, emotional, and social needs of this person, and how well are they being met?

CRITICAL THINKING

A well-loved nurse died recently on the same floor where she had worked for many years. Staff members were recently upset during a murder trial because one of their colleagues had been killed. The staff was in crisis when they heard alarming news that one of their own had lost a child to suicide. Add to this, the normal incident of grieving for one's client who has died.

In providing a good spiritual care program for clients in hospital, we often overlook the needs of staff. Nurses need an opportunity to grieve and to express feelings and concerns. I recently learned that a nearby long term care home had more than eighty residents die last year. With all of this going on, nurses are expected to get up out of bed the next day, come to work with cheerful attitudes and be productive.

Spiritual Care services have to provide care for the staff as well as the clients. If the workers are well cared for, then it stands to reason that they in turn can provide better care. We have been called to do staff debriefings, last-minute prayer services, memorial services, and even funerals. A debrief is a time for reflection, meditation, prayer, and expression. The team gathers strength in knowing that they are united in their concerns or losses. It helps validate the stress level among the staff.

Another thing, of which we should all be aware, is that nurses bring their own family concerns with them. They may be experiencing difficulties, health problems in their families, and personal grief and loss. Even for a professional, it is hard to separate this personal weight when arriving at work to care for others. Let us remember to view the caregiver as a whole person, in the same way we do the client.

How do you ensure that staff are equally well looked after regarding their own grief? What does workplace wellness mean to you?

Source: Stark, J. (2010). *Final scenes: Bedside tales at the end of life.* Word Alive Press. Winnipeg, MB. Reprinted by permission of Janet Stark.

KEY CONCEPTS

- Spirituality
- Religion
- Culturally appropriate care
- Palliative care
- Spiritual assessment
- Spiritual history
- Spiritual distress

KEY TERMS

anticipatory grief
chaplain
empathy
multi-faith
palliative care

pastoral care
religious care
spiritual care
total pain

REVIEW ACTIVITIES

1. What does providing spiritual care mean to you?

2. Do you use a spiritual assessment? Can it be improved?

3. Have you experienced a *spiritually mystical* moment? How did you feel?

4. How do you respond to a nurse who is resistant to discussing spiritual care matters with clients?

5. Self-reflect on where you are on your spiritual journey.

6. As a nurse-manager, how would you mentor your nursing team?

7. Examine a case when you have provided spiritual care in the past. Would you have done anything differently?

8. What is your response when asked to pray with a client?

9. Prepare an outline for a thirty-minute on-unit in-service on spiritual care.

EXPLORING THE WEB

- A Guide to End-of-Life Care for Seniors: Chapter 7, Spirituality, and Chapter 8, Cultural Context, 2000, University of Toronto: http://www.chpca.net/uploads/files/english/resource_doc_library/a_guide_to_end_of_life_care_for_seniors_E.pdf

- Canadian Association for Spiritual Care: http://www.cappe.org

- Canadian Nurses Association: http://www.cna-aiic.ca

- Canadian Hospice Palliative Care Association: http://www.chpca.net/Home

- Ontario Multifaith Council: www.omc.ca

REFERENCES

Baldacchino, D. R. (2006). Nursing competencies for spiritual care. *Journal of Clinical Nursing*, 15, 885–896.

Belcher, A., & Griffiths, M. (2005). The spiritual care perspectives and practices of hospice nurses. *Journal of Hospice & Palliative Nursing*, 7(5), 271–279.

Canadian Hospice Palliative Care Association (CHPCA). (2002). A model to guide hospice palliative care: Based on national principles and norms of practice. Retrieved from http://www.chpca.net/model_to_guide_hpc

Canadian Hospice Palliative Care Association (CHPCA). (2004). *A caregiver's guide: A handbook about end-of-life care*. Ottawa: Author.

Canadian Nurses Association. (2009). Position Statement. Spirituality, Health and Nursing Practice. CNA Position. Retrieved from http://www.cna-aiic.ca/CNA/documents/pdf/.../PS111_Spirituality_2010_e.pdf

Chao, C. C., Chen, C. H., & Yen, M. (2002). The essence of spirituality of terminally ill patients. *Journal of Nursing Research*, 10(4), 237–244.

Chapman, E. (2003). *Radical loving care: Building the healing hospital in America*. Nashville, TN: Baptist Healing Hospital Trust.

Chung, L. Y. F., Wong, F. K. Y., & Chan, M. F. (2007). Relationship of nurses' spirituality to their understanding and practice of spiritual care. *Journal of Advanced Nursing*, 58(2), 158–170.

Davis, L. A., & Bishop, S. (2003). The Celtic knot project: A holistic nursing intervention teaching strategy. *International Journal of Human Caring*, 7(3), 8–12.

Dolamo, B. L. (2010). Spiritual nursing – Can one's religion make a nurse a better practitioner: A reflection on Florence Nightingale. *Nursing Update, May*, 22–24.

Edwards, A., Pang, N., Shiu, V., & Chan, C. (2010). The understanding of spirituality and the potential role of spiritual care in end-of-life and palliative care: A meta-study of qualitative research. *Palliative Medicine*, 24(8), 753–770.

Ellis, H. K., & Narayanasamy, A. (2009). An investigation into the role of spirituality in nursing. *British Journal of Nursing*, 18(14), 886–890.

Guillory, W. A. (2001). Spirituality in the workplace: A guide for adapting to the chaotically changing workplace. Salt Lake City, UT: Innovations International.

Henke, D. (1996). *Spiritual Abuse*. Retrieved from http://www.watchman.org/profile/abusepro.htm

Jones, C. (2004). Practicalities of spiritual assessment. *International Journal of Palliative Care*, 10, 372.

Kiley, G. (2008). Nursing school deans view spirituality as a core competency. *Catholic Health World*, 24(8). Catholic Health Association, United States. Retrieved from http://www.whausa.org/Nursing_school_deans_view_spirituality_as_a_core_competency/

Kissane, D. W., Wein, S., Love, A., Lee, X. Q., & Clarke, D. M. (2004). The demoralization scale: A report of its development and preliminary validation. *Journal of Palliative Care*, 20(4), 269–276.

Ledger, S. D. (2005). The duty of nurses to meet patients' spiritual and/or religious needs. *British Journal of Nursing*, 14(4): 220–225.

McClung, E., Grossoehme, D. H., & Jacobson, A. F. (2006). Collaborating with chaplains to meet spiritual needs. *MedSurg Nursing*, 15(3), 147–156.

Meraviglia, M., Sutter, R., & Gaskamp, C. D. (2008). Evidence-based guideline: Providing spiritual care to terminally ill older adults. *Journal of Gerontological Nursing*, 34(7), 8–14.

Mitchell, D. L., Bennett, M. J., & Manfrin-Ledet, L. (2006). Spiritual development of nursing students: Developing competence to provide spiritual care to patients at end of life. *Journal of Nursing Education*, 45(9), 365–370.

Narayanasamy, A. (2006a). *Spiritual care and transcultural care research*. London: Quay Books.

Narayanasamy, A. (2006b). The impact of empirical studies of spirituality and culture on nurse education. *Journal of Clinical Nursing*, 15(7), 840–851.

O'Brien, M. E. (2001). *The nurse's calling—A Christian spirituality of caring for the sick*. Mahwah, NJ: Paulist Press.

Oldnall, A. S. (1996) A critical analysis of nursing: Meeting the spiritual needs of clients. *Journal of Advanced Nursing*, 23,138–144.

Penman, J., Oliver, M., & Harrington, A. (2009). Spirituality and spiritual engagement as perceived by palliative care clients and caregivers. *Australian Journal of Advanced Nursing*, 26(4), 29–35.

Petterson, E. F. (1998). The philosophy and physics of holistic are: Spiritual healing as a workable interpretation. *Journal of Advanced Nursing*, 27, 287–293.

Stanford, M. (2008) *Grace for the Afflicted*. Colorado Springs, CO: Paternoster.

Stark, J. (2010). *Final Scenes: Bedside tales at end of life*. Winnipeg: Word Alive Press.

Stark, J. (Ed.). (2008). *Lanark, Leeds, & Grenville Palliative Care Education Manual Level 1*. Smiths Falls: Author.

Spear, H. J. (2004). I'll never forget...My first dying patient – Penny Jones. *Journal of Hospice and Palliative Nursing*, 6(2), 136–139.

Tanyi, R. A. (2002). Towards clarification of the meaning of spirituality. *Journal of Advanced Nursing*, 39, 500–509.

Tiew, L. H., & Creedy, D. K. (2010). Integration of spirituality in nursing practice: A literature review. *Singapore Nursing Journal*, 37(1), 15–22.

Wordsworth, H. (2007). Reclaim the spirit. *Nursing Standard*, 22(10), 22–25.

Wright, L. M. (2005). *Spirituality, suffering, and illness: Ideas for healing*. Philadelphia: F. A Davis.

Van Dover, L. J., & Bacon, J. M. (2001). Spiritual care in nursing practice: A close-up view. *Nursing Forum, 36*(3), 18–30.

VanLeeuwen, R., Tiesinga, L. J., Middel, B., Post, D., & Jochemsen, H. (2008). The effectiveness of an educational programme for nursing students on developing competence in the provision of spiritual care. *Journal of Clinical Nursing, 17*, 2768–2781.

SUGGESTED READINGS

Byock, I. (2004). *The four things that matter most; A book about living*. London: Free Press.

Cairns, M., Thompson, M., & Wainwright, W. (Victoria Hospice Society). (2003). *Transitions in Dying & Bereavement*. Winnipeg: Health Professions Press.

Callanan, M., & Kelley, P. (1992). *Final Gifts*. Toronto: Bantam Books.

Callanan, M. (2008). *Final Journeys*. Toronto: Bantam Books.

Jacobs, M. R. (2010). *A Clergy Guide to End-of-Life Issues*. Cleveland, OH: The Pilgrim Press.

Johnston Taylor, E. (2007). What do I say? Talking with patients about spirituality. Philadelphia: Templeton Foundation Press.

Ontario Multifaith Council on Spiritual and Religious Care. (2011). *Multifaith Information Manual* (5th ed.). Toronto: Author. Retrieved from http://www.omc.ca

Stark, J. (2010). *Final scenes: Bedside tales at end of life*. Winnipeg: Word Alive Press.

CHAPTER ENDNOTES

1. Stark, J. (2010). *Thanks Sister. Final scenes: Bedside tales at end of life* (p. 108). Winnipeg: Word Alive Press.

2. Wensley, M. (1995). Spirituality in nursing. Retrieved from http://www.ciap.health.nsw.gov.au/hospolic/stvincents/1995/a04.html

3. Tanyi, R. A. (2002). Towards clarification of the meaning of spirituality. *Journal of Advanced Nursing, 39,* 500–509.

4. Edwards, A., Pang, N., Shiu, V., & Chan, C. (2010). The understanding of spirituality and the potential role of spiritual care in end-of-life and palliative care: a meta-study of qualitative research. *Palliative Medicine, 24*(8), 753–770.

5. McSherry, W., Cash, K., & Ross, L. (2004). Meaning of spirituality: Implications for nursing practice. *Journal of Clinical Nursing, 13*, 934–941.

6. Gilliat-Ray, S. (2001). Sociological perspectives on the pastoral care of minority faiths in hospital. In H. Orchard (Ed.), *Spirituality in health care contexts* (Ch. 10). London: Jessica Kingsley.

7. World Health Organization Quality of Life Spirituality, Religiousness and Personal Beliefs Group (WHOQOL SRPB Group). (2005). A cross-cultural study of spirituality, religion, and personal beliefs as components of quality of life. *Social Science and Medicine, 62*, 1486–1497.

8. Ellis, H. K., & Narayanasamy, A. (2009). An investigation into the role of spirituality in nursing. *British Journal of Nursing, 18*(14), 889.

CHAPTER 20

Ethics and the Profession of Nursing

Nancy Walton, PhD

These virtues we acquire by first exercising them. ... Whatever we learn to do, we learn by actually doing it. ... By doing just acts, we come to be just ... by doing self-controlled acts, we come to be self-controlled; and by doing brave acts, we become brave.[1]

OBJECTIVES

The purpose of this chapter is to enable the reader to

- define ethics, morality, and ethical dilemma;
- differentiate between bioethics and nursing ethics;
- demonstrate an understanding of moral distress;
- apply ethical principles and theories to the examination of ethical dilemmas and challenging situations;
- describe the foundations of ethical health care in Canada;
- compare the codes of ethics used in professional nursing practice and appreciate their limitations;
- examine and analyze four ethical issues commonly encountered in nursing practice: consent and autonomy, resource allocation, end-of-life care, and truth telling;
- examine ethical challenges for nurse leaders;
- examine different roles in practical ethics and ethics in practice;
- demonstrate an understanding of the elements of an ethical environment in nursing; and
- examine two ethical decision-making models and evaluate their use in working through everyday ethical dilemmas found in practice.

beerkoff/Shutterstock

Fatima, a nurse manager of a busy regional dialysis unit, received a phone call from a frantic physician, who practised out of a small community hospital in a neighbouring town. The physician told Fatima that he had a 32-year-old client who was in dire need of urgent dialysis due to complications from bacterial endocarditis and septicemia. If she could receive dialysis, the client would have a good prognosis for a full recovery. Because the small community hospital did not have a dialysis unit, he was calling Fatima out of desperation. He had provided care for this client throughout the course of her complicated illness and had become friendly with her husband and small children. The client was an active community member and a dedicated, well-loved teacher at the local school. She had two small children, one with cerebral palsy, who required specialized care.

Fatima stated to the physician that the dialysis unit accepted clients on a first-come, first-served basis only. Frustrated and exhausted, the physician pleaded with Fatima to consider removing from dialysis a client who might be older with a poorer prognosis and offer his client a chance to return to her active life and small children. Adamantly, Fatima refused and reiterated that the unit treated all clients equally. Once again, the physician pleaded with Fatima to use common sense and stated that his client's age, family situation, and prognosis should be considered. He also objected to what he said was a completely arbitrary method of allocation. Fatima apologized and again refused, telling the physician that she would contact him if a space became available in the next few weeks. Quietly, the physician informed Fatima that the client would likely not survive the next few weeks without access to dialysis.

When Fatima hung up the phone, she felt terrible. On one hand, she had to abide by the unit policy of treating all clients equally, which, until now, she had felt was an effective and ethical way of allocating dialysis beds. On the other hand, she

wondered if the physician could be right—that allocating by a first-come, first-served method was somehow morally arbitrary. She had always felt that the current allocation method was fair, but if it meant that some clients were refused access altogether, then how could this method be fair?

Like many nurses, Fatima has been confronted with an ethical dilemma. Throughout history, nurses are faced with ethical challenges in all types of settings and, like Fatima, are forced to reflect upon and examine their practices, values, and beliefs, as well as those of the institutions in which they work. Fatima is confronted with a multidimensional dilemma. As a nurse manager, she occupies a "unique moral in-between position" (Storch, Rodney, & Starzomski, 2004, p. 2) because she must answer not only to the client of her unit and the larger community but to the nurses she supervises and the institution in which she practises.

As a manager, Fatima is compelled to abide by the policies of her unit, put in place by the institution. However, she had no involvement in setting these policies and, in practice, she finds herself unsure of their fairness. Also, as the enforcer of the admission policies on her unit, she feels she is required to act as a gatekeeper to care for individuals and the health care providers in the community. Within this role as ad hoc gatekeeper, Fatima feels she has little control over the decisions she must make and believes that some of these decisions are not what she would consider to be fair. Fatima has been confronted with an ethical dilemma that has arisen out of her everyday practice. For nurses, ethical dilemmas like Fatima's are a part of their daily lives in practice. These dilemmas require nurses to expend considerable energy and time devoted to serious reflection and meaningful inquiry.

ETHICS AND MORALITY

Ethics and morality are commonly used as interchangeable terms. Some agree that the two terms are very closely related, whereas others disagree, stating a difference in perception about what is understood to be *morality* and what is meant by *ethics*. **Ethics** can be defined as a way of understanding and reflecting upon social morality that encompasses moral issues, norms, and practices (Burkhardt & Nathaniel, 2002). Moral issues are those in which we find ourselves stating or reflecting that *something should happen, someone ought to act in a particular way, an action or intention is right or wrong, the consequences of an action are good or bad, there is a need to..., a person has a right to..., or we have a duty to a particular person or to act in a certain way.* Moral issues are matters that we find complicated, complex, dynamic, highly contextual, and difficult to resolve (Jameton, 1984). They are often the issues and situations that remain with nurses and other health professionals long after the clients have departed.

Morality can be defined as beliefs or traditions about what is determined to be right or wrong in terms of conduct towards ourselves and others (Beauchamp & Walters, 1999). Our ideas of morality are grounded in what we feel ought to happen, or what we believe people ought to do (Yeo, Moorhouse, Khan, & Rodney, 2010). Often these ideas are vague and may not provide clear guidance for approaching moral and ethical dilemmas. Additionally, many of our ideas about what is moral arise from our own values and beliefs and can differ significantly among rational, reasonable, and free-minded people. Although morality may provide some ideas or notions of what one ought to do, ethics is reflection and analysis upon the application of those ideas and notions (Yeo et al., 2010).

Within the field of ethical inquiry, **bioethics** is relatively new, having arisen in the mid-to-late 20th century in response to new technologies, choices, and concerns in matters of maintaining and intervening in the lives of human beings, such as health care, research, and the environment (Storch et al., 2004). Bioethics is sometimes referred to as health care ethics or biomedical ethics, although some suggest that these two terms are specific to the inquiry into issues of health care, health research, and interventions. The rise of bioethics has occurred alongside rapidly developing technological advances in health care, new frontiers in research and experimentation, and monumental advances in the dissemination of medical information via the media and the Internet. Furthermore, a noticeable change has occurred in the traditionally paternalistic model of the client–health care professional relationship, because clients and advocacy groups have challenged this model and have become empowered through knowledge of not only medicine and health care but of their rights and the rights of other individuals and groups.

One hundred years ago a common question in health care was likely, What can we do? Now, with increased choices, alternatives, and costly interventions, the question is, What should we do? (Boetzkes & Waluchow, 2000, p. 3). Such a question constitutes an **ethical dilemma**—a situation in which the best course of action is often not clear, and strong ethical reasons exist to support each position (Beauchamp & Walter, 1999). Often, in approaching an ethical dilemma, we feel forced to choose between two or more alternatives that each seem quite plausible or morally acceptable, depending on one's viewpoint and perspective. Alternatively, we may feel forced to choose between two or more alternatives, none of which is completely fitting or without seemingly negative consequences.

Strategies and models exist to help us in approaching ethical dilemmas but the reality is that such algorithms and frameworks can provide only guidance; they do not provide instant solutions to ethical dilemmas that are complex, multifaceted, and inherently human. Positive approaches to ethical dilemmas include gathering adequate information; sorting out facts from values; seeking the perspectives of all involved stakeholders; and problem solving and communicating with colleagues, clients, and their families.

An ethical dilemma can seem insurmountable because of lack of communication, confusion between facts and values, inadequate gathering of information, and problem solving in isolation, which can lead to moral distress. **Moral distress** results when ethical dilemmas are not acknowledged or effectively dealt with; when communication between team members, clients, and families is ineffective; or when professionals feel isolated or unsupported in their approach to solving such dilemmas. Simply put, it may be when the nurse knows the right thing to do but is unable to do it (Jameton, 1993). As the Canadian Nurses Association (CNA) states, moral distress can involve a compromise of the values and commitments of nurses (2008a). Moral distress involves and can lead to feelings of anxiety, frustration, and anger as well as guilt, emotional distress, and dissatisfaction with one's performance, action(s) or profession (Jameton, 1993; Keatings & Smith, 2010). Nurse leaders in the United States have created a document aimed at helping nurses recognize moral distress in practice (American Association of Critical Care Nurses, 2006). This document outlines "the 4 A's" for addressing moral distress (Ask, Affirm, Assess, and Act). The first step is to ask oneself about discomfort or unease with a situation to determine if moral distress is present. The second step is to affirm distress and a commitment to self-care. The third step is to assess the source and severity of moral distress along with one's readiness to act. Finally, the fourth step involves acting and working towards sustaining positive change. Formulaic or step-wise approaches to a complex problem are sometimes criticized, but the presentation of solutions to moral distress in an understandable and accessible way is an important step in making moral distress something that is explicitly acknowledged and addressed in the workplace.

NURSING ETHICS

Bioethics is a broad field of inquiry that can relate to a variety of health care professionals and activities. However, there is agreement that nursing as a profession requires a separate field of study to examine the ethical norms, unique relationships, and sphere of nursing practice. Nursing roles are diverse in terms of responsibility, breadth, and type of everyday practice, The diversity of roles include any number of aspects, such as provision of direct client care in an institutional, community, ambulatory, or home-care setting; supervision and management;

public health and health promotion; education and welfare; multidisciplinary and independent work; and advanced practice roles, such as the nurse practitioner or nurse clinician. As the profession of nursing evolves and the scope of nursing practice grows, so do the ethical challenges and the need for reflecting upon and examining these challenges.

Nursing ethics may be defined as the examination of the norms, values, and principles found in nursing practice (Yeo et al., 2010). It focuses on the distinctive relationships found within nursing practice—such as the nurse–client relationship, the nurse–nurse relationship, and the nurse–physician relationship—and the resulting moral commitments that nurses have to others within these relationships and others (Keatings & Smith, 2010; Storch et al., 2004; Yeo et al., 2010). Because nursing is situated within a relational context, it is considered by some as a "moral practice" (Gastmans, Dierekx de Casterle, & Schotsmans, 1998, p. 46).

Nursing ethics is both a field of inquiry into the norms and values in the nursing profession and a reference to the body of literature in which nursing scholars discuss, interpret, analyze, and apply these ethical norms and values. Such discussions are important to the evolution and advancement of the nursing profession, as evidenced by the existence and growth of nursing journals such as *Nursing Ethics* and *Nursing Philosophy*.

ETHICAL THEORIES

As noted, there are no magical solutions or easy algorithms for solving ethical dilemmas. However, systematic approaches can help us decide what is right and wrong. These are known as **ethical theories.** A rich body of theories exists as approaches to sorting through complex ethical challenges. However, the focus here is on two specific types of theories: the consequentialist, or teleological, and the deontological, or non-teleological theories.

Consequentialist theories put forth that when deciding between possible actions, the most important moral obligation is to maximize the positive consequences and minimize the negative consequences (Thomas & Waluchow, 2002). This theory, of course, requires knowledge of both the good and the negative consequences of an action. Consequentialist theories also involve reaching agreement among diverse people regarding what are positive and negative consequences. Finally, it must also be possible to prospectively evaluate and measure the goodness of actions.

Utilitarian theories, the most commonly cited type of consequentialist theories, assess the moral rightness of actions based on how much happiness they might produce. From a utilitarian perspective, deciding upon alternatives is simple and formulaic, involving three distinct steps. First, the consequences of each possible alternative must be estimated. Second, the balance of happiness and unhappiness must be calculated and compared to their alternatives. As a third step, the alternative estimated to produce the most happiness for the greatest number of people should be chosen (Yeo et al., 2010). This apparently simple formula results in three difficulties. First, one can never be sure of the consequences of any action as one is always predicting into an unsure future. Second, what one person may consider a good consequence may not be evaluated as a good outcome by another reasonable person. Third, how do we measure good consequences or happiness?

Deontological theories posit that an action's inherent rightness never lies in its consequences but in its very adherence to a duty. Moral obligation involves determining one's moral duties or imperatives and acting consistently, according to those duties (Yeo et al., 2010). Immanuel Kant (1724–1804) is one of the most well-known deontologists. According to Kant, the rightness of an action is never dependent on the consequences that might result from an action. Rather, an action is justified if it can meet Kant's categorical imperative, which gives no credence to possible consequences whatsoever. This imperative, as Kant describes it, compels a person to choose an action that can be universalized to all similar situations; that is, it becomes a morally binding rule for action (Yeo et al., 2010). Kant would ask us to imagine that every time a similar situation arose, we would decree it so that everyone would always act in accordance with the duty we recognize and the subsequent action prescribed. If we could conceive that the subsequent action can be universalized then it is the action we must take, in accordance with our duty.

Two difficulties are evident when we consider deontological theories. First, we are often not clear on what our duties are. As nurses, we might have a number of duties: to the client, to the institution that employs us, to our colleagues and profession, and to society. Moreover, we have moral duties not only in our work lives but in our personal, social, and family lives, which leads to the second difficulty. When we have conflicting duties, deontological theories offer little guidance on how to move forward and decide which duty should override.

When evaluating whether an action is ethical, the consequentialist always looks at what might happen as a result of an action. In other words, the consequentialist uses a forward-looking perspective. Meanwhile, the deontologist does not look at what might happen as a result of the action, instead using a backward-looking approach. Deontologists have little concern for the consequences of an action, only the duty lying behind it, which they must be able to articulate.

CRITICAL THINKING

Andrew is a nurse practitioner in a busy urban teaching hospital. While on his lunch break in a very crowded and busy cafeteria, he overhears his colleagues at the next table talking loudly about a particularly difficult client and family. Knowing that he is familiar with the client, his colleagues call him over to join the discussion. Andrew faces a difficult choice. Should he join the discussion with his colleagues, risking his own moral integrity and knowing that they may be easily overheard? Or should he tell his colleagues that he will not join them and that they have a professional obligation not to discuss clients and families in public places?

Sometimes, consequentialists and deontologists may agree on the moral rightness of an alternative; however, their justification for choosing the particular alternative might be markedly different. Consider the example in the Critical Thinking feature.

If we use a deontological theory to decide which action Andrew should take, we would consider the duty that we have to protect our clients' confidentiality and not discuss their cases in elevators or in cafeterias. We should refrain from doing so not out of consideration of the consequences but because we must adhere to this duty. The consequentialist might agree with this decision, but would, however, offer different reasons for not talking about clients outside of the clinical setting. The consequentialist would examine the consequences, both good and bad, of talking about clients at the cafeteria table and make a decision based on which alternative would produce the most happiness and the least unhappiness—likely ceasing the conversation. Although the deontologist and the consequentialist might agree on the preferred action in this case, they would be motivated by different factors.

PRINCIPLISM

In the 1970s general moral philosophy and medical ethics had not yet met. Much work in academic philosophy examined ethical theories, while the biomedical community focused on preventing harm and "doing good" for their clients. Little discussion of ethical principles occurred outside of individual professional codes of conduct, which were discipline-specific and not well suited to approaching complex and emerging ethical challenges. At that time a set of basic ethical principles

were articulated and formulated into a framework that is commonly referred to as **principlism** (Beauchamp & Childress, 1994). This framework for considering ethical issues includes the following guiding principles: (1) respect for autonomy, (2) beneficence, (3) nonmaleficence, and (4) justice.

Autonomy refers to the ability to self-govern and to have control over decision making concerning one's own life. **Beneficence** requires that we consider and act in the best interests of others. **Nonmaleficence** refers to the requirement that we avoid doing harm to others. Finally, **justice** is a broad principle encompassing the notion of fair distribution of benefits, resources, and risks (Beauchamp & DeGrazia, 2004).

Principlism is widely used in biomedical and health care ethics curricula as a framework for approaching ethical dilemmas. Many students in health care professions find this approach appealing because they can relate to the principles, drawn from traditional professional values, which are found in health professions, such as medicine and nursing.

Each of the ethical theories we have discussed help to answer the question, What action should I take? These theories also effectively focus the ethical issue on *action*, which may be motivated by certain factors and may be intended to abide by specific duties or to produce desired consequences. The most important consideration of these theories is the action that results from contemplation of one or more of the ethical theories.

FEMINIST ETHICS

Feminist ethics arose when scholars and philosophers recognized that, often, it is not enough to turn to a set of principles, duties, or rights when trying to resolve moral and ethical dilemmas. Moral dilemmas necessarily involve human relationships, which are inherently contextual, based on imbalances of power and involving complex understandings of priorities, stakes, and risks. The approach to moral dilemmas found in feminist ethics is affected by a perspective of the world that acknowledges the importance and influence of gender. Feminists such as Carol Gilligan posit that the differences in the social experiences and the relationships of men and women affect our moral development. In a social structure that has been traditionally male dominated, the experiences and lives of women and men are markedly different. Females, as a gender, have traditionally been oppressed and dominated within social systems (Liaschenko & Peter, 2003).

Feminism in ethics proposes that we examine ethical issues while keeping in mind conventional patterns of "discrimination, exploitation and dominance" (Sherwin, 1992, p. 4). Feminist ethics comprises a variety of approaches that are beyond the scope of this chapter. However, the common foundation of these approaches is the acknowledgment that moral dilemmas necessarily involve relationships between people at a variety of levels and within a variety of contexts. These relationships may involve power differences, politics, perceptions of imbalances of power, and diverse moral orientations, all of which may be grounded in gender. In challenging traditional approaches to ethical issues, feminist ethics strives to uncover and make explicit alternative approaches to ethical problems that openly address and incorporate considerations of these patterns and contexts (Liaschenko & Peter, 2003; Wolf, 1994).

FOUNDATIONS FOR ETHICAL CARE IN CANADA

Canada, unlike the United States, does not have a formalized bill of rights for clients. The U.S. Patient's Bill of Rights was formulated in 1973, by the American Hospital Association, with the most recent revisions made in 1992. The aim of the document is to articulate the rights and responsibilities of clients and their families, health care professionals, and the institutions in which they deliver care (American Hospital Association, 1992).

In Canada approaches to care are embedded in the Canadian Charter of Rights and Freedoms, a document that outlines the rights and freedoms of all citizens living in Canada. The Charter outlines particular civil, legal, social, and political rights of Canadian citizens and embodies a set of principles through articulation of an agreement on these rights. It is important, however, to note that the Charter does not explicitly identify health as a right or discuss health as a concept to which equality applies (Robinson Vollman, & Potter, 2006).

Particularly relevant to health care are two sections of the Charter: Sections 7 and 15(1). Section 7 outlines the legal rights of Canadians to life, liberty, and the security of people: Everyone has the right to life, liberty and security of the person and the right not to be deprived thereof except in accordance with the principles of fundamental justice. (Canadian Charter of Rights and Freedoms, 1982, Section 7).

Section 15(1) outlines the equality rights of every Canadian citizen, to equality before and under the law as well as equal protection and benefit of the law, and reads as follows:

Every individual is equal before and under the law and has the right to the equal protection and equal benefit of the law without discrimination and, in particular, without discrimination based on race, national or ethnic origin, colour, religion, sex, age, or mental or physical disability. (*Canadian Charter of Rights and Freedoms,* 1982, Section 15[1]).

The emphasis on equality of people and equality of treatment of people is also embedded in another key document that guides health care in Canada, the Canada Health Act (CHA), a federal legislation for publicly funded health care insurance, which received Royal Assent in 1984. The CHA outlines specific principles that all provincial and territorial governments must abide by in the delivery of health care, as each province and territory develops, administers, and finances health care services, along with the federal contribution, the Canada Health Transfer (CHT). The CHA's five program criteria, or principles, are shown in Table 20-1.

CODES OF ETHICS IN NURSING

A professional code of ethics is not part of health law or statutory law, nor is it a set of rules. Instead, it is a code to which professionals must adhere as part of their responsibility and duty.

Professional codes of ethics define expectations of a profession. They are usually defined and shaped by members of that profession and provide guidelines and values to adhere to and to promote, in creating an ethical, accountable practice.

In 1953 the International Council of Nurses (ICN) published a code of ethics that was rewritten in 1973: The ICN Code for Nurses—Ethical Concepts Applied to Nursing and most recently revised in 2005 (ICN, 2006). The ICN Code of Ethics situates the ethical responsibilities of nurses in a framework that includes a number of relationships in which nurses participate, including "nurses and people," "nurses and practice," "nurses and the profession," and "nurses and co-workers" (ICN, 2006).

In its early days the Canadian Nurses Association (CNA) adopted the ICN Code of Ethics. Then in 1978, the CNA decided to have its own unique code of ethics for nurses in Canada. After several drafts, the Code of Ethics for Nursing was published in 1985, and has been revised as necessary, with the most recently published version in 2008 (CNA, 2008a).

The first section of the newest revision of the CNA Code of Ethics situates the ethical expectation of nurses practising in Canada around seven primary values or responsibilities. According to the CNA, these are key to the practice of nursing: providing safe, compassionate, competent, and ethical care; promoting health and well-being; promoting and respecting informed decision making; preserving dignity; maintaining privacy and confidentiality; promoting justice; and being accountable. Within each of these values, explanatory responsibility statements outline specific practices, behaviours, and

TABLE 20-1	PRINCIPLES OF THE CANADA HEALTH ACT
1. Public administration	Health care services must be delivered by a nonprofit, publicly administered agency.
2. Comprehensiveness	All "medically necessary" services of physicians and hospitals are provided.
3. Universality	All permanent residents of a province or territory, no matter where they live, are entitled to be insured by the publicly funded system.
4. Portability	For Canadians who move or travel within Canada or travel outside of Canada, insured services must be maintained.
5. Accessibility	All Canadians should have reasonable access to hospital and physician services, regardless of their geographic location, age, income, status, or gender.

Source: *The Canada Health Act: Overview and Options.* Health Canada.

expectations (CNA, 2008). The second section of the CNA Code of Ethics outlines "ethical endeavours" (p. 3) that nurses can undertake to address specific situations of social inequity. The focus in this section is on the role of the nurse in addressing broader issues of social justice that have an effect on the health state of individuals, groups, and populations.

A professional code of ethics doesn't guarantee that all involved in the profession will act ethically. It is a guideline and an explicit but general statement of expectations. It does not prescribe particular actions of behaviour in specific circumstances.

Alongside a code of ethics, nurses have their own values, which may evoke strong personal responses to ethical dilemmas. **Values** are personal beliefs about the truth of ideals, standards, principles, objects, and behaviours that give meaning and direction to life. Our values arise from our familial, cultural, religious, and educational experiences and can change over time as we develop our moral selves and, in doing so, become more autonomous.

The challenge of being part of a profession with a moral engagement and obligation is that we may encounter situations in which our values conflict with the values of a client, an institution, or a professional situation. Whereas much of the study of ethics deals with the values, wishes, and rights of others, as professionals, we must also focus on our own values and how they may have an effect upon our reactions, behaviours, and beliefs in professional practice. It is impossible to simply turn off our own values as we engage in our work. Instead we must take

steps to acknowledge our own values and to be able to recognize situations in which we are conflicted.

In the Critical Thinking feature, Clarissa has critically examined her own values and understands that, in this case, they conflict with her ethical obligation to provide quality nursing care. In the best interests of the clients, other health care professionals, and for the sake of June's own moral integrity, Clarissa should not be forced to take part in a procedure for which she has such strong conflicting personal beliefs (Yeo et al., 2010).

She may request to change her assignment today and move to another operating room. However, this reassignment must be done in such a way that it does not abandon or significantly disadvantage the clients. The CNA Code of Ethics clearly states that if a nurse is asked to provide care that conflicts with the nurse's personal values "the nurse must provide safe, compassionate, competent and ethical care until alternative care arrangements are in place to meet the person's desires or wishes" (CNA, 2008a, p. 19). So, Marc may move Clarissa to another area under two conditions. First, Marc and Clarissa must find another registered nurse who has the relevant and necessary skills and experience to take Clarissa's assignment and provide competent care. Second, they must ensure that the clients are not abandoned in the interim. Once these two conditions are met, Clarissa can safely and ethically take another assignment. At a later time, it would be worthwhile for Marc and Clarissa to have a discussion and for Clarissa to reflect on her own reasons, beliefs, and goals related to working in this area.

CRITICAL THINKING

Clarissa is an operating room (OR) nurse and has worked in this hospital for six years. Recently the hospital amalgamated with another institution, and the result is a great deal of changing roles and responsibilities in the OR. Clarissa has found that her day-to-day job has markedly changed as she has been asked to take part in new procedures. Today, she arrives for her shift and sees that she has been assigned to Operating Room C, in the day surgery area, an area in which she has not yet worked. When she scans the list of today's procedures, she notices a number of therapeutic abortions. Clarissa is very upset. Her personal belief is that abortion is wrong, and based on her religious and cultural beliefs, she does not consider abortion as a viable or moral option for any woman. She has never been asked to assist in a therapeutic abortion procedure, and she is worried about her ability to do her job and provide thorough, empathetic, and effective care. Additionally, she feels that she would be betraying herself and her religious beliefs by assisting with such a procedure. Clarissa approaches Marc, the operating room manager, explains her moral dilemma and requests to be removed from this assignment.

As the nurse manager, how should Marc respond? Should he honour Clarissa's request, or should he insist that Clarissa cover her assignment and fulfill her duties?

PROFESSIONAL DILEMMAS

There is no end to the kinds of ethical challenges that nurses will face in their careers on a daily basis. In this section, we will examine four specific ethical issues arising in nursing practice: consent and autonomy, resource allocation, end-of-life care, and truth telling.

CONSENT AND AUTONOMY

The issue of informed consent has been addressed and discussed extensively in the ethics and nursing literature. The provision of an informed consent is embedded within the notion of autonomy and allowing people the right to make informed, voluntary choices regarding their person and their care. The Code of Ethics for Registered Nurses in Canada outlines 11 specific responsibilities of registered nurses in regard to clients' choices.

These responsibilities involve respecting the informed decision-making capabilities of those in their care, allowing the subsequent expression of each client's health needs—as well as a recognition of power differentials between health care professionals and clients, and the freedom of the client to choose to involve their family or community in decision making (CNA, 2008a). Autonomy and respect are the underlying values in this section of the Code.

To act autonomously one needs information about the choices as well as the freedom to act. Informed consent, like autonomy, can be considered to have two important elements: the element of voluntariness and the element of cognition, or the ability of someone to understand the choice and aspects of the choice (Appelbaum, Lidz, & Meisel, 1987; Yeo et al., 2010). For example, if preoperative clients receive full information regarding an optional research study they are eligible to participate in, and they are then encouraged to provide their consent by the surgeon who will be operating on them in the morning, these clients may feel implicit *coercion* to participate in the research. Alternatively, consider the client who is provided with written information on two procedures, each with similar benefits and risks, and is asked to choose which procedure is preferred. The written information is left at the client's bedside. This information is written in high-level language and has been given to a client who has limited literacy skills. The client may have been given the freedom to choose between the two procedures but cannot make a fully *informed* decision, due to lack of understanding about the procedure. Thus, an informed consent necessarily implies that the client not only understands the choices, their risks, benefits, and alternatives but also has the ability to make a voluntary choice, free of coercion, influence, or pressure. Ontario's Health Care Consent Act states that consent is valid only if it is informed and voluntary, and it has not been obtained by misrepresentation, misinformation, or coercion (Health Care Consent Act, 1996).

A variety of issues within consent are debatable. For example, how much information is required to be informed? Who is the best person to provide consent? What about people with limited or fluctuating capacity? How is competence or capacity assessed? These are a few of the specific issues pertaining to consent.

For nurses, the key elements in facilitating the provision of informed consent are respect for autonomy and support for people when they seek information. Nurses can contribute to the maintenance of autonomy through informed consent by building trusting relationships with clients; providing current, complete information; ensuring understanding; respecting clients' wishes even though they may differ from the nurse's own wishes; providing opportunities for clients to make choices; respecting prior wishes communicated by an advance

CRITICAL THINKING

Ralph is a 78-year-old man being admitted for coronary bypass surgery. The night before surgery, the surgeon visits him to obtain his informed consent. They have a quick and friendly meeting, and the surgeon leaves the room with a signed consent form on the chart.

Later that night, as the nurse does rounds, Ralph pulls her aside and expresses his trepidation at the upcoming surgery. He states that the surgeon told him that he might die, although he can't remember the "numbers" the surgeon used. He also asks her if he might get an "infection and die" or a "big stroke and never wake up." He says that he isn't exactly sure what the surgical team will be doing but thinks that they'll be opening his heart up and "unplugging something or other." Finally, he tells her he didn't want to bother the surgeon with his worries and questions, as he seemed so busy.

Ralph goes on to tell her that at his appointments at the surgeon's office, he was too overwhelmed to understand or listen properly and depended on his son to speak for him and agree to anything. His son is out of town, returning tomorrow to be at the hospital after the surgery. Finally, Ralph says that he doesn't want the surgery if it is risky; he would rather live as he has been. He is visibly shaky, highly anxious, and unsettled.

What should the nurse do?

Should she provide comfort, some clarification of the procedure, perhaps a sleeping aid, and leave it at that?

Should she call the surgeon and have Ralph re-informed?

Do you think Ralph provided a voluntary, informed consent, earlier with the surgeon? Why or why not?

directive or a substitute decision maker; and including relevant stakeholders in decision-making processes.

Nurses cannot provide care without the informed consent of the client (CNA, 2008a). Doing so may constitute battery or harm to the client. Thus, any physical touch, even a slight or minor touch, done without the consent of another person may legally constitute battery (Keatings & Smith, 2010). All people have the right to provide consent for any kind of touch, be it a physical treatment or intervention, a nursing action, a medication administration, or a procedure. Although some actions such as surgeries, medical procedures, and therapies require a formal, written consent process, consent for actions such as a bed bath or a dressing change may be negotiated through less formal mechanisms. By asking the client if a nursing action is acceptable and having the client simply express agreement or expose the dressing for the nurse, usually implies consent and is, in most cases, sufficient.

Consent, although binding for the health care professional, is dynamic. That is, a client's consent is required before initiating any kind of procedure or action. However, it must be noted that because consent is a dynamic and contextual concept, clients may change their mind or withdraw their consent at any time. Clients who pro-

vide an informed consent for surgery in the morning may, upon awakening, have an additional question or clarification or may have changed their mind about the procedure. This change of status or withdrawal of consent must be respected. Similarly, if a client allows a dressing change to be done, but then, due to pain or fatigue or any other reason, decides not to have the dressing changed, this decision must be respected; the dressing change must be delayed until the client provides consent.

RESOURCE ALLOCATION

Emily and the team have a difficult decision, but not an uncommon one. Frequently, decisions are made that provide for one client while simultaneously denying another client. Every day in busy emergency rooms and overcrowded intensive care units (ICUs), these kinds of decisions are made by triage nurses and nurse managers, who must allocate a position on a waiting list or an ICU bed to one client among many who are waiting. In allocating the emergency room time or the ICU bed to one client, however, they place others further down on a waiting list or deny others access to a necessary ICU bed. These kinds of decisions may be life-and-death decisions, or they may be simply perceived as inconvenient, frustrating, or unfair.

CRITICAL THINKING

Emily, a nurse clinician, works on a hectic transplant ward. Often she finds herself caring for transplant candidates for long periods of time while they await their transplant. Over these periods of time, she gets to know the clients, their families, and their lives quite well, and she develops what she feels are strong therapeutic relationships. Tonight, a call comes to the unit informing them a liver is available that is a match for two of their critically ill clients awaiting an organ transplant. The decision regarding who is to receive the organ is left up to Emily and her multidisciplinary team. They must make a decision quickly. The first client, George, is a 46-year-old architect with congenital liver disease that has caused his liver to fail. George has a wife and two young children. He has been waiting eight months for a liver. The second client, Thomas, is a 53-year-old single lawyer. His liver disease resulted from excessive alcohol consumption. He has been waiting ten months for a liver.

The team members must make a decision but are having difficulty with this task since both clients are an ideal match and have similarities in wait time, degree of urgency, and prognosis. Because Emily knows both clients quite well, she is asked who she feels should receive the organ. Before she answers, she realizes that, in her own view, she relates on a personal level much more to George because she also has young children. She also is conscious of the fact that she feels George is a more worthy candidate than Thomas. She realizes that she may have difficulty preventing her own personal views, values, and beliefs from taking over her decision-making process. She is puzzled, though, because she is unsure of what other criteria can be used to separate the two candidates.

Should Emily voice her distress and indecisiveness?

What criteria would you consider to be important in decision making in this case?

Is there a way to be fair to both clients in this case?

Resource allocation is an important issue to address because all health care systems operate with limited or scarce resources and, unless sensible constraints are placed on those resources, their sustainability is questionable. Decisions regarding resource constraints give rise to many challenging ethical issues. In Canada, health care administrators and politicians are in a period of examining and evaluating the sustainability of our health care system. Discussions of reform focus on how to allocate resources in such a way that avoids morally arbitrary decision making but attempts to both meet society's expectations and encompass its values.

The allocation of resources is frequently a concern and responsibility of nurses. Nurse managers may find that they are forced to make staffing and retention decisions within the context and constraints of shrinking budgets. Staff nurses in hospitals undergoing cutbacks may find that their units are poorly staffed on weekends and nights and that their client assignment is markedly more difficult on those shifts. Operating room procedures may be cancelled due to nursing or support staff shortages or because of a lack of nursing staff in the recovery or intensive care area for postoperative care. Clients often find that some of their direct physical care is being provided by other health care team members, such

as unregulated care providers (UCPs) or licensed practical nurses (LPNs). They may also find that their linens are no longer changed daily and that, upon discharge, only a limited amount of home care is available. All these examples are situations that involve the allocation or distribution of human and practical resources, including programs and services.

In health care, we usually discuss three levels of resource allocation. **Macro-allocation** decisions are made by governments at all levels. **Meso-allocation** decisions are those made at the institutional or program level. Finally, **micro-allocation** refers to decisions made at the bedside, regarding individual clients. All three levels are obviously linked, with each having a trickle-down effect on the others.

By virtue of the work nurses do, they often experience the end result of institutional or organizational policy changes related to resource allocation decisions. Cutbacks in nursing staff have a direct effect on client care. Additionally, cutbacks affect the remaining nurses who then need to deliver care to more clients with fewer staff. Often nurses find themselves advocating for the best interests of their clients, armed with the knowledge that a particular client or group of clients need increased accessibility to a particular resource. Nurses also are the ones who often experience the frustration, anger, and dissatisfaction of clients who may perceive that, as a result of cutbacks or constraints on the system, they are receiving less care than they would like, are forced to do more things for themselves, or are waiting for services that are difficult to access.

There is no framework for working through ethical issues related to the allocation of resources. Health care practitioners tend to contemplate these issues within the broad sphere of justice, with particular relevance to theories of distributive justice. In keeping with the Canadian Charter of Rights and Freedoms, certain features are considered irrelevant to resource allocation decision making; these include religion, ability, social status, race, or sexual orientation. Criteria such as medical need, prognosis, risk, and benefit are felt to be morally relevant and objective criteria for decision making. However, even using criteria that appear to be objective and relevant can still result in ethical dilemmas and ambiguity. We may also have situations in which medical need, prognosis, and benefit may be similar—as Emily's case, in the Critical Thinking feature, on page 417, demonstrates. In these cases, how do we favour one client over another? What kinds of criteria do we use to resolve this very practical dilemma?

Daniels addresses these thorny dilemmas as he identifies four difficult-to-resolve issues in resource allocation (Daniels, 1994):

1. The fair chances versus best outcomes problem. Should we always try to favour providing access to those with the best chance of a positive outcome over giving every possible client an opportunity to access resources?
2. The priorities problem. Should we give the most ill or disabled clients the priority to access resources?

CRITICAL THINKING

Patrick is a 25-year-old man with an acquired brain injury from a motor vehicle accident at age 19 that left him paralyzed and unable to care for himself. He was also severely burned in the accident. Patrick lives in a long-term care institution, requiring 24-hour complete care. He has been plagued with serious and painful complications, including severe infections and persistent bedsores. He is completely and likely permanently respirator-dependent and must frequently undergo painful treatments.

Previous to his injury, Patrick had been awarded a full university scholarship for football. His family and girlfriend visit once weekly. His football buddies visit once a month, but their times together are short and difficult for everyone. He looks forward to their visits but is depressed because the visits are infrequent and awkward. Last month he told his girlfriend she should move on with her life. She is planning to take a job overseas and will leave in two months. His parents are busy caring for his two younger siblings, and they have had difficulty coping with having their son in this state. Family counselling has been ongoing but unproductive; and at Patrick's request, it was discontinued. He says he stopped the counselling so that his parents "would not have to go through this anymore."

Patrick is becoming more withdrawn and quiet. On her daily rounds the nurse practitioner always takes time to speak with Patrick. She has noted that Patrick has asked vaguely, numerous times, about dying and assistance with dying. She decides to address this issue directly with Patrick; when she does, he appears to be relieved. He smiles and thanks her for bringing it up so directly.

Patrick goes on to say that he has a clear and accurate awareness of his future prognosis and that he considers it to be very bleak. He feels that he is a burden to his family and that he has no desire to continue his life as it is and will be. He states that he is at peace with his decision and that he has told his parents, who, although devastated, can abide by his decision.

He asks the nurse practitioner to talk to the team about discontinuing the respirator. She tells Patrick that she cannot support assisted suicide because it is illegal in Canada. Patrick says to her in response, "You wouldn't be assisting my suicide. You would simply be abiding by the wishes of a fully competent and informed client to have a particular treatment discontinued. After all, you have done other things I have requested. This is no different!"

Is this a case of abiding by the wishes of a competent client or is it an example of assisted suicide?

If you were the nurse practitioner, how would you respond to Patrick?

3. The aggregation problem. Should we favour the situation in which we can provide moderate benefits to a larger number of people over the situation in which we can provide more significant benefits to very few?

4. The democracy problem. Should we focus on the process by which decisions are made and rely on the fact that if we adhere to the democratic process we will come up with fair outcomes?

Although Daniels's work was published more than a decade ago, these kinds of unresolved ethical dilemmas in resource allocation persist. With the increasing costs and capabilities of new technologies, an aging population, competing priorities at all levels of government, and increasingly knowledgeable and empowered clients, these kinds of allocation issues will surely continue to be one of the most prevailing challenges for modern health care systems.

END-OF-LIFE ISSUES

End-of-life issues are extensively examined in nursing and ethics. Nurses are often the key multidisciplinary team members who can and do provide care and support throughout the entire dying process. By virtue of this intense involvement, nurses are often the ones who are engaged in the decision-making processes and the conversations and discussions about the end of life with clients and their families.

Many ethical dilemmas arise when considering death and dying. Davis and Aroskar (1983) classify three types of ethical dilemmas at the end of life: possible interventions by health professionals (i.e., resuscitation, prolonged ventilation, withdrawal of food or fluids); possible interventions by those close to the client (i.e., hastening death by various means, determining futility); and possible interventions by the client (i.e., suicide, request for assistance with suicide, use of advance directives, or refusal of interventions). This collection of ethical dilemmas, although not exhaustive, does include many important and frequent issues that arise in end-of-life care.

The need and desire for extensive examination of the dying process is a recent one. As recent as a few decades ago, dying was a more private and family process, often occurring at home and without the proliferation of assistive technologies that now function to keep dying people alive. Now, the capacity of technology to sustain life and delay death has increased, in many places becoming the norm. By virtue of this increased technological capacity, the locus of control for matters of living and dying has been transferred to specialists, and the traditional site of dying has moved from the home to the institution.

In response to these changes, two specific issues have emerged and have sparked much of the ongoing discussion and debate on end-of-life issues. The first issue is quality of life. Although it is a highly subjective and imprecise term, at the end of life, having **quality of life** may mean having some control over the process and one's final days. The other issue that leads directly from quality of life is the issue of power and control regarding decision making at the end of life.

We each have our own ideas and wishes regarding our eventual death. Many people would like to die in a place and manner of their choosing, with as much comfort and peace as possible. Overarching these ideas and wishes is the desire to have control over elements of a process that for most of us is outside of our control.

As technology became more and more a part of the dying process, a new vocabulary has developed as part of the discussions of death. One highly contentious term is **medical futility,** defined as "a medical treatment that is seen to be non-beneficial because it is believed to offer no reasonable hope of recovery or improvement of the client's condition" (CNA, 2001). This term evolved from the discussions on the high cost of technology used to keep alive the people who often had poor quality of life or little hope of a meaningful recovery. The term was met with resistance from many because it defined meaningfulness using the term *utility*. For many, the use of this term implied that the measure of a worthwhile or meaningful life was limited to the degree of utility a person could contribute instead of a more holistic and subjective measure of when life is meaningful and when it has lost meaning. For others, it was a contentious term as it was felt that when a treatment was deemed to be futile, it compels one to always ask, "Futile as compared to…?" (Truong, Brett, & Frader, 2004). Futility, it was felt, should be considered in subjective and humane terms by the person most affected by the dying process—the client. For many, the term *medical futility* emphasizes the inappropriate focus on the economic impact of intervening in the dying process. For many, simply providing some care, even to a client in a grave situation with a very poor prognosis, is not futile because it serves to keep the body functioning, albeit at a suboptimal level (Collier & Haliburton, 2011).

Resuscitation via cardiopulmonary resuscitation (CPR), medication, and ventilation is a common method of attempting to prolong life. Traditionally, when a person has a cardiac arrest or a respiratory arrest, the response is to initiate measures to take over the functions of the heart and lungs and, in doing so, to save the person's life and prevent death. However, clients and their families, together with their health care providers, often decide that a *do-not-resuscitate* order is most appropriate and desired in the particular situation. Resuscitation is sometimes perceived as too invasive, unlikely to result in appreciable improvement in condition, or likely to lead to more serious complications or distress. Specifically, resuscitation, in some cases, may lead to increased pain, discomfort, and suffering and may only serve to prolong the dying process (CNA, 1995). A new document, for the public, published jointly by the Canadian Nurses' Association, the Canadian Medical Association, the Canadian Healthcare Association and the Catholic Health Association of Canada emphasizes that CPR is not appropriate in all situations (n.d.). Furthermore, it goes on to emphasize that decision making about CPR is very difficult and that there are a number of issues to consider prior to making decisions about resuscitation for oneself or a loved one.

The Canadian Nurses Association's Joint Statement on Resuscitative Interventions (1995) outlines important classifications regarding the efficacy of CPR in restoring function to individual people. The statement notes four categories of clients when considering whether CPR is a realistic or humane option: those who are likely to benefit from CPR, those for whom benefit is uncertain, those for whom benefit is unlikely, and those who most certainly will not benefit. This policy statement notes there is no obligation to provide or offer non-beneficial or futile treatment, which in some cases may include CPR. The futility or benefit of CPR must be "determined with reference to the person's own subjective judgement about his or her overall well-being" (p. 3).

Importantly, the CNA Joint Statement notes that the decision to withhold resuscitation by no means implies that other treatments, supportive care, or elements of palliative care should or will be withheld. It also notes the importance of communication and education of health care recipients, family members and significant others, and health care providers.

A decision to withhold resuscitation should include the client and the client's family and significant others, as noted by the client and the health care team. Key elements in the establishment of a DNR order are the clarity of roles and responsibilities, inclusion of all stakeholders, open discussions, and regular opportunities to revisit the discussion as the situation changes.

Although only physicians can write do not resuscitate (DNR) orders in Canada, nurses, because of practice and roles, are often the health care practitioners most affected by such an order. Nurses are often present at the death of a client, and their roles, responsibilities, and feelings about their roles are affected by a DNR policy. Nurse leaders must take responsibility and be an active part of educating staff on the health care setting or unit's DNR policy and its application in everyday practice. Often nurses must also assume a role in educating and discussing options for DNR status with families and clients. Although this responsibility is not clearly a nursing or medical role, every team member must be able to be open, approachable, and well informed about options and implications of resuscitation status for each person.

Many people at the end of life may not be able to voice their own wishes regarding the dying process. Nevertheless, they may have previously discussed their wishes with another person or documented their wishes as part of a living will. **Living wills** are documents voluntarily signed by clients that specify the type of care they desire if and when they are in a terminal state and cannot sign a consent form or convey this information verbally. Living wills can outline a client's wishes regarding specific interventions that may prolong life, such as CPR, artificial ventilation, and administration of medication, dialysis, or surgery. Now more commonly referred to as **advance directives,** these types of documents provide for two specific provisions. First, their existence aims to ensure that the wishes of a previously competent person are carried out when that person is no longer able to speak for him or herself. Second, an advance directive allows for the appointment of a specific person, a substitute decision maker, who can help to carry out those wishes and ensure that they are followed (Singer, 1993). Across the country, these documents may look very different. Additionally, the adherence to these kinds of documents may vary from one setting to another. Unfortunately, unforeseen circumstances and lack of education, awareness, and information can all contribute to difficulty, hesitation, or unwillingness to identify and carry out the wishes of an advance directive.

During the dying process, nurses may be confronted with issues around easing the suffering of the dying person or facilitating the dying process. These actions may be formally requested by a client or a family member, or they may be intimated through gestures, words, or implications. **Euthanasia** is defined as "a deliberate act undertaken by one person with the intention of ending the life of another person to relieve that person's suffering where the act is the cause of death" (Special Senate Committee on Euthanasia and Assisted Suicide, 1995). Examples of euthanasia may include discontinuation of respiratory assistance in a person who is ventilator-dependent, administration of a high dose of narcotic analgesia causing respiratory failure, or withdrawal of food and fluids. Euthanasia may be classified as either voluntary, involuntary, or nonvoluntary, depending on the person's competence, awareness, and known or voiced wishes (Lavery, Dickens, Boyle, & Singer, 1997).

Additionally, euthanasia is classified by some as either **passive euthanasia,** in which treatment may be ceased or withheld, and the person is thereby made more vulnerable to the underlying processes that cause death; or **active euthanasia,** in which body processes necessary to sustain life are actively interfered with or interrupted (Battin, 1994). Although these terms may provide a practical distinction, many believe that no moral or ethical distinction exists between these classifications. There is an active and ongoing debate on the following considerations: (1) which classification is felt to be morally acceptable, (2) whether withdrawal of treatment can be considered as morally similar or as humane as withholding of treatment, and (3) whether passive euthanasia is morally and practically inhumane. **Assisted suicide** is defined as "the act of intentionally killing oneself with the assistance of another who deliberately provides the knowledge, means, or both" (Special Senate Committee on Euthanasia and Assisted Suicide, 1995). An example of assisted suicide is the person who requests information on how much of a narcotic is necessary for an overdose and seeks to have enough of a stockpile of such medication on hand.

In Canada euthanasia and physician-assisted suicide are illegal under the Criminal Code of Canada, regardless of the client or person's wishes (Criminal Code of Canada, 1985, Part VIII). However, as noted, nurses may play an important role in the dying process for many clients.

The CNA Code of Ethics states that nurses have an obligation to assist people to achieve their optimal level of well-being in all states: health, illness, injury, or in the dying process (CNA, 2008a). The CNA position statement on providing nursing care at the end of life articulates the roles of the nurse at the end of life as advocacy and promotion of a "dignified and peaceful death" (CNA, 2008). These roles are carried out by ensuring that clients have access to and understanding of current treatments, alternatives, and options, and by facilitating informed choice and the expression of clients' needs, wishes, and beliefs regarding the dying process (CNA, 2008b).

TRUTH TELLING

In everyday life we encounter situations in which it is easier to not tell the entire truth, in order to avoid hurting others' feelings, causing unnecessary harm to others, or being chastised. However, the nature of the relationships that we have in everyday life differs from the nature of the relationships that we have in clinical settings. As clinicians, we have a **fiduciary obligation** to those for whom we provide care. A fiduciary obligation was originally a legal term to describe the responsibility of those entrusted to place the best interests of others above their own personal interests. By upholding the principles of beneficence (i.e., by acting in another's best interests) and nonmaleficence (i.e., by avoiding harm to another), a fiduciary relationship is one built on trust, conviction, and care. Part of this fiduciary duty is the obligation and expectation that nurses will be truthful and explicit in their communication with clients.

Traditionally, the physician has assumed the role of the clinician who provides important or difficult information to clients, such as diagnoses or prognoses. However, with the expanding roles of the nurse and the increased use of advance practice nurses in health care settings, nurses are more likely to be responsible for taking part in communicating difficult messages to clients and their families. Even in more traditional or hierarchical health care settings, although physicians may still be the ones

who deliver difficult news, clients often approach nurses to clarify, interpret, or advise. As a result of the physical proximity and intimate nature of nursing work, clients may turn to their nurses when they are unsure, worried, or confused. Nurses may find themselves being asked to reiterate or explain, and to offer advice or elucidation. In these types of situations, nurses need to be truthful, even in challenging circumstances or when discussing difficult or tragic outcomes and possibilities. Clients require accurate and honest information to make informed decisions about their health and well-being.

In some circumstances, truth telling can be especially difficult: situations of uncertainty, situations in which truth telling may be felt to be a potential source of harm to the client, or incidences of medical or nursing error (Hebert, Hoffmaster, Glass, & Singer, 1997). In these cases, the truth may be avoided in order to act beneficently, to avoid harm (i.e., nonmaleficence), or to avoid damage to the client–nurse relationship. Truth telling by all clinicians in these cases may be easier said than done, but in the long run, being honest helps to reduce resentment, increase trust, and strengthen clients' faith in the integrity of the health care team and the care they receive.

Some of the strategies that nurses may employ when they impart difficult news to clients include ensuring that clients and families have access to accurate, relevant, and complete information at levels they can comprehend; providing resources, supports, and follow-up services; supporting clients in their decision making; and educating clients not only on specific issues but also on their rights and the options and alternatives available to them. The Canadian Nurses Association Code of Ethics (2008a) reinforces these strategies. The Code of Ethics does not explicitly address truth telling in the section Providing Safe, Compassionate, Competent and Ethical Care. However, it does specify that nurses should "take all necessary actions to prevent or minimize harm resulting from an adverse event. They work with others to reduce the potential for future risks and preventable harms" (CNA, 2008a, p. 9). Furthermore, the Code of Ethics states that "nurses build trustworthy relationships as the foundation of meaningful communication, recognizing that building these relationships requires a conscious effort" (p. 8). Finally, honesty as a virtue in nursing is referred to explicitly in the section on Ethical Considerations with Nursing Students. It states that "all nurses and nursing students treat each other with respect and honesty" (p. 50).

The importance of **veracity,** the obligation to tell the truth, cannot be overemphasized. In a health care setting, the power imbalance created by knowledge can be overwhelming and intimidating for clients and can contribute to clients' feelings of powerlessness, confusion, and distrust. Nurses must aim to carry out their

CRITICAL THINKING

A na is a 28-year-old single woman, who has a history of depressive episodes and two unsuccessful suicide attempts. She lives with her parents and is with them in the outpatient unit today, undergoing a final test for her general symptoms of malaise, body aches, and night sweats.

While Ana is dressing, the physician and the nurse manager take her parents aside to speak to them. They tell the parents that Ana has Hodgkin's lymphoma, a malignant cancer that, in Ana's case, will require fairly aggressive and prompt radiation therapy and chemotherapy. The therapy and preparations can begin in two days.

Her parents are very upset and ask the physician and nurse manager not to tell Ana about her diagnosis. They feel that it would be best if they tell her and initiate treatment at some point later on. For now, they would like the physician to tell Ana that there is nothing serious. They inform the physician that Ana is very dependent on them and has been spiralling downwards into her recurrent depression. They are worried that news of the diagnosis would further upset her, and she would be unable to cope or make good decisions.

Furthermore, they are celebrating their 30th wedding anniversary by going on a 20-day cruise and are leaving next week. They have never been away together, having been caregivers for Ana in addition to working full-time. It is too late to get a refund from cancelling their trip. They would like to wait until they return to tell Ana about her diagnosis and begin treatment. While they are away, she will be staying with her brother, with whom she is not particularly close. Her parents are worried that Ana will not have adequate supports to deal with the diagnosis while they are away.

What should Ana be told, and why?

Who should make decisions regarding Ana's care and treatment?

What should be the role of the health care professionals involved in this case?

---

interactions in all aspects of the care they provide with integrity, honesty, and a commitment to the process of building trusting relationships over time.

LEADERSHIP ROLES AND CHALLENGES IN ETHICS

Today, nurses have many unique and rewarding opportunities to assume leadership roles in areas of ethics in a variety of settings, including hospitals, organizations, and academic institutions. Nurses may serve as members of clinical or research ethics committees in hospitals, private organizations, and academic institutions. Clinical ethics committees serve a number of purposes within health care settings, including a resource and consultation role, promotion and dissemination of research and education, and participating in policy development (Chidwick, Faith, Godkin, & Hardingham, 2004). Research ethics committees review and approve proposed and ongoing research to ensure that it meets with the guidelines for ethical research in Canada, which are outlined in the 2010 Tri-Council Policy Statement by the Canadian Institutes of Health Research, the Natural Sciences and Engineering Research Council of Canada, and the Social Sciences and Humanities Research Council of Canada. Aiming for representation from a variety of professions and groups on ethics committees ensures that no one group or perspective will take precedence in decision-making and deliberative processes.

Most hospitals have bioethicists on staff who serve in a variety of ways. They provide guidance, support, and advice for staff, clients, and families who face ethical challenges. The role of the bioethicist can be filled by a nurse with a completed graduate degree in bioethics. Interdisciplinary centres across Canada offer various graduate programs to equip nurses, physicians, and other health care professionals to assume leadership positions in ethics. Such centres include the Joint Centre for Bioethics at the University of Toronto, the W. Maurice Young Centre for Applied Ethics at the University of British Columbia, the John Dossetor Health Ethics Centre at the

University of Alberta, and the Department of Bioethics at Dalhousie University. A nurse with clinical expertise alongside graduate knowledge in bioethics may be an effective bioethicist and may also serve in a leadership or mentorship position for other nurses.

Leadership in terms of ethics may well be less formal, however. Nurse leaders or managers who encourage an ethical environment may also become mentors in their own practice. Encouraging open discussion of situations and issues that staff find challenging, distressing, or worrisome can lead to a more ethical environment in nursing units. In some environments nurses are afraid to speak up because they are worried that they will not be supported if they do or they are hesitant to discuss ethical issues for fear of reprisal. Instead, nursing leaders should facilitate and nurture an environment in which nurses are supported, listened to, and considered valuable stakeholders in ethical issues.

From a practical perspective, such an environment can be achieved iteratively, through a number of relatively accessible and creative endeavours. One suggestion is to have open case conferences over lunch in which nursing staff can bring forward ethical issues from their daily practice and discuss them in a safe, confidential, and supportive environment. Another suggestion is to address ethical issues using a prospective model. Instead of allowing situations to develop over time, becoming more complex and complicated, it is always advisable to open up discussion about particular issues early and to reopen discussions on as required. Additionally, a good ethical leader can also recognize situations that may be causing distress to clinicians and should have an open-door policy for confidential discussions of such situations. This approach encourages discussion and a level of comfort which may translate to a more ethically sensitive and effective group of clinicians.

Consistently involving clients and their families in discussions and decision making sets a clear example of ethical practice. Another way to prevent one group or one discipline's perspective from dominating decision-making processes is to involve a multidisciplinary team and provides opportunities for all disciplines and team members to have a voice. These kinds of practices can be instituted by nurse leaders and enforced through local norms and policies.

Being involved in policy-making is one way that nurses and nurse leaders can help to create an ethical work environment. For example, if an institution were considering developing a policy for discontinuation of food and fluids for palliative clients, nurses and nurse leaders from that unit should be involved in the discussion and formation of such a policy. They could also advocate for the inclusion of laypeople who may have been involved in a similar situation with a family member or friend.

Finally, if a nurse leader conducts decision making in a unilateral or paternalistic way, this sets a tone for others to think that their contribution and perspective is unimportant. Nurse leaders may create an ethical environment by simply carrying out their day-to-day decision making by involving staff with a stake in those decisions, carrying out such processes in an open and transparent way, and allowing for discussion and debate over decisions without reprisal. One way to create an ethical environment might be to adapt an ethical decision-making model into the day-to-day decision-making processes of a unit, clinic, institution, or organization.

TWO MODELS FOR ETHICAL DECISION MAKING

Although ethical theories may be limited in their scope and the degree to which they can be applied in the real world—and ethical theories alone provide little guidance for actual decision making—they do provide perspectives into approaches to ethical analysis and reasoning. Furthermore, few of us can confidently say that we are consistently true deontologists or true consequentialists in all aspects of our lives and in every ethical decision-making process. Different ethical problems within a variety of contexts and with unique players often require different approaches.

So how can nurses approach ethical problems? Models for ethical decision making may not help to illuminate the right answer to a problem, but they can provide direction and guidance for a systematic approach to ethical problems (Rodney, 1991). Table 20-2 provides a comparative account of two ethical decision-making models. McDonald provides a conceptual framework for approaching ethical problems (McDonald, 2001). He notes that this framework is not a recipe for finding solutions to ethical problems, but a guide for approaching problems. His framework emphasizes examining problems from all possible perspectives and considering contexts and subtexts, while ensuring that discussion and resolution is inclusive of all involved people. McDonald acknowledges that, even with a decision-making framework and the involvement of committed ethical people, it may not be possible to reach what is considered a perfect solution. It is most important to be able to learn and grow as a result of this process. Ethical decision making, if we take McDonald's model further, is not something that can be done on a sporadic basis or in isolation. It must be done regularly and vigorously as part of a team and carried out with compassion and care in a mutually supportive environment (McDonald, 2001). Rodney (1991) adapts Curtin's model of ethical decision making

TABLE 20-2	COMPARISON OF TWO ETHICAL DECISION-MAKING MODELS

A Framework for Ethical Decision Making

(Adapted from McDonald, 2001)

1. **Identify the problem and collect as much information as you can.** The key at this stage is twofold: first, be alert to ethical situations within your everyday practice. Second, be aware of what you know and what you do not know regarding the situation. It is necessary to gather as much information and as many alternative interpretations as possible, keeping in mind that there may be time constraints in real-life practice situations. Present the case with the facts you have collected and try to focus on the decision(s) that need to be made. As always, be aware of three elements: the specific and dynamic context of the situations, any potential conflicts of interest for any involved stakeholders, and your own stake and position in the process and potential outcomes.

2. **Specify potentially feasible alternatives.** State the possible alternatives for decision making, considering both direct and indirect consequences for all potentially affected persons.

3. **Use your own ethical resources to help decide what is morally relevant for each alternative.** At this stage, you likely have a number of ethical resources that you can use to help you decide between possible alternatives. These may include the stated ethical principles of your community, profession, or institution; moral mentors and trusted colleagues; policies, contexts, or relationships; formal case conferences; an ethicist; or an ethics committee.

4. **Propose and test possible resolutions.** Find the alternative resolution that you believe to be the best option, and ask yourself a number of questions: What would have to change to get me to alter the choice of this alternative? Would a good person or clinician do this? What if everyone in a similar situation did the same? Will implementing this decision have a negative impact on anyone or any trust relationships?

5. **Finally, make your choice.** Live with it and learn from it.

Source: Adapted from McDonald, M. (2001). Canadian governance of health research involving human subjects: Is anyone minding the store? *Health Law Journal,* 9: 1–21.

An Ethical Decision-Making Model for Critical Care Nursing

(Adapted from Rodney, 1991)

1. **Gather background information.** The priority is gathering relevant information in order to define and describe the problem.

2. **Identify whether the problem is an ethical issue.** Through gathering relevant information, determine whether this problem is an ethical issue, as opposed to a practical, legal, or professional issue. If you determine that it is an ethical problem, then use an ethical theory to try to articulate rights, duties, principles, moral obligations, or roles.

3. **Identify key stakeholders.** In addition to identifying and articulating the problem, identify the key players; that is, anyone who might be affected by this ethical issue or who has a stake in the outcome. Concepts such as responsibility, authority, professional roles, personal relationships, competence, conflicting rights, or conflicts of interest may be relevant.

4. **Identify possible courses of action.** As you identify possibilities for action, consequences must also be considered.

5. **Reconcile the facts of the case with relevant principles.** Consider alternatives in terms of their inherent value, relative to the principles that you identify as important to the case.

6. **Resolution.** Try to achieve consensus in decision making, keeping in mind that constraints may emerge, due to professional obligations, legal requirements, or social expectations. These constraints should be made explicit throughout the process.

Source: Adapted from Rodney, P. A. (1991). Dealing with ethical problems: An ethical decision-making model for critical care nurses. *Canadian Critical Care Nursing Journal,* 8(2): 8–10.

to critical care nursing and the ethical challenges arising in this area. This model, although notably more concise, provides a straightforward approach to ethical decision making that can be applied in a variety of settings.

One important point to note is that most models of ethical decision making incorporate, in some way, a consideration of one's own values and beliefs, which is an important step that is often difficult to articulate or explicitly describe. Our personal values and feelings about issues are based in our own experiences, religions, cultures, and families, and thus, they cannot simply be put aside while we struggle with a value-laden problem in practice. We should not use ethical problems as opportunities to either further or promote our own personal beliefs or values to others, but as part of the initial phases of decision making we are responsible for examining our own feelings and personal values if they are relevant to a particular case or concept.

KEY CONCEPTS

- Ethics is the branch of philosophy that concerns the distinction between right and wrong.

- A personal philosophy stems from an individual's beliefs and values. This personal philosophy will influence an individual's philosophy of nursing.

- Two ethical theories are consequentialism and deontology.

- Ethical principles and rules include beneficence, nonmaleficence, justice, and respect for autonomy.

- Ethics committees provide guidance for decision making about ethical dilemmas that arise in health care settings.

- Values clarification is an important step in the decision-making process.

- Two helpful tools are the framework for ethical decision making and the ethical decision-making model for critical care nursing.

- Today's nurses face numerous ethical issues and moral dilemmas.

- Nurse leaders who are dedicated to ethical principles can influence organizational ethics.

KEY TERMS

active euthanasia	fiduciary obligation
advance directives	justice
assisted suicide	living will
autonomy	macro-allocation
beneficence	medical futility
bioethics	meso-allocation
consequentialist theories	micro-allocation
deontological theories	moral distress
ethical dilemma	morality
ethical theories	nonmaleficence
ethics	nursing ethics

euthanasia	passive euthanasia
principlism	utilitarian theories
professional code of ethics	values
quality of life	veracity

REVIEW QUESTIONS

1. Mrs. Green rides the elevator to the third floor where her husband is a client. While on the elevator, Mrs. Green hears two nurses talking about Mr. Green. They are discussing the potential prognosis and whether he should be told. The nurses are violating which of the following ethical principles?
   A. autonomy
   B. confidentiality
   C. beneficence
   D. nonmaleficence

2. When evaluating whether an action is ethical, which of the following approaches will the consequentialist use?
   A. forward-looking approach
   B. backward-looking approach
   C. consequentialist approach
   D. duty-oriented approach

3. Which of the following principles is not included in the framework for considering ethical issues?
   A. principlism
   B. beneficence
   C. nonmaleficence
   D. justice

REVIEW ACTIVITIES

1. Review the Critical Thinking features in this chapter. As you are doing so, try to advocate from the perspective of each different person. For example, in the end-of-life Critical Thinking feature, page 418, examine and discuss the case from the perspective of Patrick, the nurse manager, and Patrick's family.

2. Examine a case from your own day-to-day practice. Use the ethical theories presented here to work through possible alternatives. Reflect on the effectiveness of the theories as you apply them to real-life cases.

3. Examine the Critical Thinking features found in the chapter. Using McDonald's Framework for Ethical Decision Making, work through the features using the information provided. Identify when you would have required more information, if it were a real-life case.

EXPLORING THE WEB

Read about codes of ethics from various nursing bodies:

- International Council of Nurses: *http://www.icn.ch/about-icn/code-of-ethics-for-nurses/code-of-ethics-for-nurses.html*

- Canadian Nurses Association: *http://www.cna-aiic.ca/CNA/practice/ethics/code/default_e.aspx*

- College of Nurses of Ontario: *http://www.cno.org/docs/prac/41034_Ethics.pdf*

Learn more about Canadian organizations dedicated to ethics:

- Canadian Bioethics Society: *http://www.bioethics.ca/index-ang.html*

- Alberta Provincial Health Ethics Network: *http://www.phen.ab.ca/*

Visit these university-based academic/clinical ethics centres:

- University of Toronto Joint Centre for Bioethics: *http://www.jointcentreforbioethics.ca/index.shtml*

- John Dossetor Health Ethics Centre, University of Alberta: *http://www.ualberta.ca/~bioethic/*

- W. Maurice Young Centre for Applied Ethics, University of British Columbia: *http://www.ethics.ubc.ca/*

- Department of Bioethics, Dalhousie University: *http://bioethics.medicine.dal.ca/*

Other useful links for exploration and learning:

- Canadian Medical Association Journal Bioethics for Clinicians series: *http://www.cmaj.ca/cgi/collection/bioethics_for_clinicians_series*

- Bioethics Resources on the Web (National Institutes of Health): *http://bioethics.od.nih.gov/*

A comprehensive list of links by subject, provided by the Provincial Health Ethics Network, Alberta: *http://www.phen.ab.ca/netlinks/*

REFERENCES

American Association of Critical Care Nurses. (2006). *The 4A's to rise above moral distress.* Aliso Viejo, CA: Author.

American Hospital Association. (1992). *A patient's bill of rights.* Chicago: Author.

Appelbaum, P. S., Lidz, C. W., & Meisel, A. (1987). *Informed consent: Legal theory and clinical practice.* New York: Oxford University Press.

Battin, M. (1994). *The least worst death: Essays in bioethics on the end of life.* New York: Oxford University Press.

Beauchamp, T. L., & Childress, J. F. (1994). *Principles of biomedical ethics* (4th ed.). New York: Oxford University Press.

Beauchamp, T. L., & DeGrazia, D. (2004). Principles and principlism. In G. Khushf (Ed.), *Handbook of bioethics* (pp. 55–74). Dordrecht: Kluwer Academic.

Beauchamp, T. L., & Walters, L. (1999). *Contemporary issues in bioethics.* Belmont, CA: Wadsworth.

Boetzkes, S., & Waluchow, W. J. (2000). *Readings in health care ethics.* Peterborough: Broadview.

Burkhardt, M. A., & Nathaniel, A. K. (2002). *Ethics and issues in contemporary nursing* (2nd ed.). New York: Delmar Thompson.

Canadian Institutes of Health Research, Natural Sciences and Engineering Research Council of Canada, and Social Sciences and Humanities Research Council of Canada. (2010). *Tri-council policy statement: Ethical conduct for research involving humans.* Ottawa: Author.

Canadian Nurses Association. (1995). *Joint statement on resuscitative interventions.* Ottawa: Author.

Canadian Nurses Association. (2001). *Futility presents many challenges for nurses. Ethics in practice series paper.* Ottawa: Author.

Canadian Nurses Association. (2008a). *Code of ethics for registered nurses.* Ottawa: Author.

Canadian Nurses Association. (2008b). *Position statement: Providing nursing care at the end of life.* Ottawa: Author.

Canadian Nurses Association, Canadian Medical Association, Canadian Healthcare Association, and Catholic Health Association of Canada (n.d.). *Making Decisions about CPR: Cardiopulmonary Resuscitation.* Ottawa: Author.

Chidwick, P., Faith, K., Godkin, D., & Hardingham, L. (2004). Clinical education of ethicists: The role of a clinical ethics fellowship. *BMC Medical Ethics, 5*(6). Retrieved from http://www.biomedcentral.com/1472-6939/5/6

Collier, C., & Haliburton, R. (2011). Bioethics in Canada: A philosophical introduction. Toronto: Canadian Scholars Press.

Criminal Code of Canada (RS 1985, c. C-46) *Part VIII: Offences against the person and reputation.* Retrieved from http://laws.justice.gc.ca/en/C-46/

Daniels, N. (1994). Four unsolved rationing problems: A challenge. *Hastings Center Report, 24*(4), 27–29.

Davis, A. J., & Aroskar, M. A. (1983). *Ethical dilemmas and nursing practice* (2nd ed.). Norwalk, CT: Appleton, Century, Crofts.

Gastmans, C., Dierekx de Casterle, B., & Schotsmans, P. (1998). Nursing considered as moral practice: A philosophical-ethical interpretation of nursing. *Kennedy Institute of Ethics Journal, 8*(1), 43–69.

Health Canada (2005). *Canada Health Act: Overview.* Retrieved from http://www.hc-sc.gc.ca/hcs-sss/medi-assur/overview-apercu/index_e.html

Health Care Consent Act. (1996). S.O. 1996, c. 2. Schedule A.

Hebert, P. C., Hoffmaster, B., Glass, K. C., & Singer, P. A. (1997). Bioethics for clinicians: 7. Truth telling. *Canadian Medical Association Journal*, 156(2), 225–228.

International Council of Nurses. (2006). *The ICN Code of ethics for nurses.* Geneva: Author.

Jameton, A. (1984). *Nursing practice: The ethical issues.* Upper Saddle River, NJ: Prentice-Hall.

Jameton, A. (1993). Dilemmas of moral distress: Moral responsibility and nursing practice. *AWHONN Clinical Issues*, 3(4), 542–551.

Keatings, M., & Smith, O. B. (2010). *Ethical and legal issues in Canadian nursing* (3rd ed.). Toronto: Mosby Elsevier Ltd.

Lavery, J. V., Dickens, B. M., Boyle, J. M., & Singer, P. A. (1997). Bioethics for clinicians: 11. Euthanasia and assisted suicide. *Canadian Medical Association Journal*, 156(10), 1405–1408.

Liaschenko, J., & Peter, E. (2003). Feminist ethics. In V. Tschudin (Ed.), *Approaches to ethics: Nursing beyond boundaries* (pp. 33–44). New York: Butterworth.

McDonald, M. (2001). Canadian governance of health research involving human subjects: Is anyone minding the store? *Health Law Journal*, 9, 1–21.

Robinson Vollman, A., & Potter, P. A. (2006). The Canadian health care delivery system. In J. C. Ross-Kerr & M. J. Wood (Eds.). *Canadian fundamentals of nursing* (3rd ed., pp. 18–34). Toronto: Mosby Elsevier Ltd.

Rodney, P. A. (1991). Dealing with ethical problems: An ethical decision-making model for critical care nurses. *Canadian Critical Care Nursing Journal*, 8(2), 8–10.

Sherwin, S. (1992). *No longer patient: Feminist ethics & health care.* Philadelphia: Temple University Press.

Singer, P. A. (1993). *Living will.* Toronto: University of Toronto Joint Centre for Bioethics.

Special Senate Committee on Euthanasia and Assisted Suicide. (1995). *Of life and death.* Ottawa: Supply and Services Canada. [cat no YC2-351/1-OIE]

Storch, J. L., Rodney, P., Starzomski, R. (2004). *Toward a moral horizon: Nursing ethics for leadership and practice.* Toronto: Pearson Education Canada.

Thomas, J., & Waluchow, W. J. (2002). *Well and good: A case study approach to biomedical ethics.* Peterborough: Broadview Press.

Truong, R. D., Brett, A. S., & Frader, J. (2004) The problem with futility. In F. Baylis, J. Downie, B. Hoffmaster, & S. Sherwin (Eds.), *Health care ethics in Canada* (pp. 504–513). Toronto: Harcourt Brace.

Wolf, S. M. (1994). Shifting paradigms in bioethics and health law: The rise of a new pragmatism. *American Journal of Law and Medicine*, 20(4), 395–415.

Yeo, M., Moorhouse, A., Khan, P., & Rodney, P. (Eds.). (2010). *Concepts and cases in nursing ethics* (3rd ed.). Peterborough: Broadview Press.

SUGGESTED READINGS

Baylis, F., Downie, J., Hoffmaster, B., & Sherwin, S. (1995). *Health care ethics in Canada.* Toronto: Harcourt Brace Canada.

Benner, P. A., Tanner, C. A., & Chesla, C. A. (1996). *Expertise in nursing practice: Caring, clinical judgment and ethics.* New York: Springer.

Birnie, L. H., & Rodriguez, S. (1994). *Uncommon will: The death and life of Sue Rodriguez.* Toronto: Macmillan.

Butts, J. B., & Rich, K. L. (2005). *Nursing ethics: Across the curriculum and into practice.* Sudbury, MA: Jones and Bartlett.

Johnstone, M.-J. (1999). *Bioethics: A nursing perspective* (3rd ed.). Philadelphia: Harcourt Saunders.

Kikuchi, J. F. (2005). Commentary on the CNA code of ethics. *Canadian Nurse*, 101(8), 16–18.

Kluge, E.-H. W. (2005). *Readings in biomedical ethics: A Canadian focus* (3rd ed.). Toronto: Pearson Prentice Hall.

Kuhl, D. (2002). *What dying people want: Lessons for living from people who are dying.* New York: Public Affairs.

McKinley, S., Rodney, P., Storch, J., & McAlpine, H. (2004). The role of ethics in nursing. *Nursing BC*, 36(1), 12–16.

Parsons, A. H., & Parsons, P. H. (1992). *Health care ethics.* Toronto: Wall & Emerson.

Storch, J. L. (2007). Enduring values in changing times: The CAN Codes of Ethics. *Canadian Nurse*, 103(4), 29–33, 37.

Tschudin, V. (2003). *Ethics in nursing: The caring relationship* (3rd ed.). New York: Butterworth-Heinemann.

CHAPTER ENDNOTES

1. Aristotle, *Nicomachean Ethics,* as cited in Burkhardt, M. A., & Nathaniel, A. K. (2002). Ethics and issues in contemporary nursing (2nd ed.). New York: Delmar Thompson.

CHAPTER 21

Collective Bargaining

Janice Tazbir, RN, MS, CCRN
Adapted by Heather Crawford, BScN, MEd, CHE

Giving nurses a voice with power is our role and our continuing goal. We are the Canadian Federation of Nurses Unions. (Canadian Federation of Nurses Unions, 2007)

OBJECTIVES

The purpose of this chapter is to enable the reader to

- review the history of collective bargaining;
- discuss collective action models and associated terminology;
- identify the steps involved in union certification;
- discuss professionalism in the context of unionization; and
- list the pros and cons of collective bargaining.

Ken Faught/GetStock.com

You are a new nurse on an internal medicine unit. When you have your meal break, you decide to sit in the conference room with the rest of the nurses. Two nurses are having a discussion. Sally is a registered nurse with 15 years of experience, and she says, "I'm really tired of assignments that don't allow me to spend any time talking to my patients." Rose, a registered nurse with four years' experience asks, "Have you taken your concerns to our manager?" Sally responds, "Of course. I point out the number and complexity of the patients, but she says we need to cope." Rose says, "I wonder if we would have better success with these issues if we discussed them as a group, and made some suggestions to improve our satisfaction."

What are your thoughts about this situation?

What are some of the choices the nurses have?

Historically, nurses were perceived as hardworking, submissive women who did what they were told. The scope of nursing has changed so dramatically that today's nurses cannot afford to have a submissive image and do only what they are told. Clients, their illnesses, and their families are more complex than ever. Nurses are educated to advocate for their clients and themselves. Clinical situations arise in which nurses must voice their opinions and stand up for what is best for clients. To be effective in today's world, nurses must understand the tools available to them to deal with problems.

Managers must also understand the interrelationship of unionization and management, the legislation that exists related to employment practices, and the impact of both on health care. Managers need to recognize the interconnectedness of organization, worker, work life balance, and personal points of view. If they can do this, they will be able to understand how managers and workers can work together cooperatively regardless of unionization.

Collective action, or simply acting as a group with a single voice, is one method of dealing with problems. **Collective bargaining** refers to the practice of employees bargaining as a collective group with management on matters such as wages, work practices, work environment, and other benefits.

This chapter discusses different types of collective action models and also includes information concerning unionization, and professionalism in the context of unionization.

HISTORY OF NURSING UNIONIZATION IN CANADA

The Canadian Federation of Nurses Unions (CFNU) celebrated its 25th anniversary in 2003. Kathleen Connors provided an exceptional summary of the history of nursing unionization in Canada. A synopsis of the information she provided follows[*].

In 1975, the then prime minister, Pierre Elliott Trudeau, announced wage and price controls in order to prevent further inflation. Shortly thereafter, Canada experienced a 42-day postal strike, which led to the federal cabinet overturning one of the first major decisions by the Anti-Inflation Board when it allowed the postal workers a 20 percent pay increase. At that time, nurses from across the country participated in a collective bargaining conference, an informal meeting that allowed senior staff of Canadian unions to share information, knowledge, and strategies. At that time, it was recognized that there was no national voice to speak on behalf of nurses, particularly in response to Trudeau's wage and price controls.

In 1978, the Canadian Nurses Association (the nurses' professional association) drafted a code of ethics, which, among other things, implied that it would be unethical for nurses to strike in Canada. Again, nurses were reminded of the importance of having a national voice for unionized nurses. At the next collective bargaining conference, nurses' unions set up a committee to examine potential structures, terms of reference, and constitutional language for a national voice. The leadership for this endeavour was provided by the Saskatchewan Union of Nurses, the Newfoundland and Labrador Nurses Union, and the Prince Edward Island Nurses Union. The founding convention was held in April 1981, and on May 1, 1981, the National Federation of Nurses Unions was created to represent unionized nurses at the national level. In 1999, the name was changed to the Canadian Federation of Nurses Unions (CFNU).

In 1987 the CFNU established a full-time office and a full-time president's position in Ottawa. The organization's focus was initially on negotiated contracts, grievances, and other labour relations issues;

---

[*] Canadian Federation of Nurses Unions, "CFNU Celebrates its 25th Anniversary." Retrieved from http://www.nursesunions.ca/cms/updir/2006-05-30-CFNU_25_years_-_history.pdf, September 1, 2006.

however, the health care system and social justice concerns soon became important issues for nurses. As a result, the Manitoba Nurses Union brought a resolution to the 1982 Special Convention that the Canadian Federation of Nurses Unions should join the Canadian Health Coalition to champion medicare and other social justice issues, which then became the focus for CFNU.

Additional provincial nursing unions gradually joined the national collective, which led to the Canadian government recognizing that CFNU was a strong and realistic voice for nurses. The British Columbia Nursing Union became a member in 1994, followed by the Staff Nurses Association of Alberta (SNAA), which affiliated in 1985. The United Nurses of Alberta affiliated in 1999, two years after amalgamating with the SNAA. In 2000, the Saskatchewan Union of Nurses, the Nova Scotia Nurses Union, and the Prince Edward Island Nurses Union reaffiliated. In November 2000, the Ontario Nurses Association became a member. The only provincial union not a member is the Fédération des Infirmiers et Infirmières du Québec (FIIQ), which does attend board meetings and conventions as an observer.

The Saskatchewan Nurses Union has a long history of firsts. In 1974, it became the first nursing union to form in Canada. In 1996, it was the first nursing union to affiliate with a provincial federation of labour, the Saskatchewan Federation of Labour. In 1997, it was the first nursing union to join the Canadian Labour Congress (CLC), and was followed by the British Columbia Nurses Union and the Manitoba Nurses Union, which joined the CLC in 1999.

A constitutional change was required for the Canadian Federation of Nurses Unions and its member organizations to affiliate with the Canadian Labour Congress, which occurred in 1997, at the CFNU convention in Vancouver. In January 1998, the CFNU became a member of the CLC, with a seat on the CLC's executive committee. The CLC membership provided the CFNU with support for collective bargaining in such areas as occupational health and safety, pensions, and other benefits.

The British Columbia Nurses Union president was an invited speaker to the Canadian Nursing Advisory Committee, which, in 2002, released its report confirming a national nursing shortage. CFNU continues to have strong advocacy efforts. It meets with premiers, participates in discussion panels, and holds press conferences. In addition, it publishes position papers regarding national nursing issues in order to keep health care on the first ministers' agendas.[1]

CFNU also represents the 25,000 student nurses who are members of the Canadian Nursing Students' Association.

COLLECTIVE ACTION MODELS

The Canadian Federation of Nurses Unions states that its main purpose is "protecting the health of patients and our public health system, promoting nurses and the nursing profession at the national level—and doing it effectively."[2]

One of the main purposes of collective action is to advance the profession of nursing (Underwood, 1997). Many nurses belong to numerous collectives, including specialty nursing organizations, church organizations, special interest clubs, and community groups. The reason most people belong to these organizations is to better themselves and their communities or to promote and support the special interests of a group. Two types of nursing collective action are discussed in this chapter: workplace advocacy and collective bargaining. Shared governance, another type of collective action, is discussed in Chapter 13.

WORKPLACE ADVOCACY

Workplace advocacy refers to activities nurses undertake to address problems in their everyday workplace setting. It is probably the most common type of collective action in nursing. An example of workplace advocacy is forming a committee to address problems, devise alternatives to achieve optimal care, and invent new ways to implement change. A supportive management will view workplace advocacy as a way to strengthen staff and promote teamwork. If the management is authoritative, however, workplace advocacy may not be encouraged, because it may be perceived as a threat to management and its policies.

COLLECTIVE BARGAINING

In collective bargaining, the group is bargaining with management for what the group desires. If the group cannot achieve its desires through informal collective bargaining with management, the group may decide to use a collective bargaining agent to form a union.

FACTORS INFLUENCING NURSES TO UNIONIZE

In general, nurses who are content in their workplace do not unionize (Hart, 1998). It is usually when nurses feel powerless that they initiate attempts to unionize. Other motivations to unionize include the following: (1) the desire to eliminate discrimination and favouritism, to increase an individual's power, or to increase input into organizational decision making; (2) the need to comply with a requirement of being employed in the organization; and (3) the belief that client outcomes and quality of care will be improved (Marquis & Huston, 2012). Research by Seago and Ash (2002) shows that a positive relationship between client outcomes and registered nurse unions extends beyond wages and numbers of hours and involves staff stability, collaboration with physicians, autonomy, and increased participation in practice decisions. Nurses are also motivated to join unions when they feel the need to communicate concerns and complaints to management without fear of reprisal. Many nurses believe that they need a collective voice so that management will hear them and changes will be instituted.

Common issues for collective bargaining include better working conditions including wages, staffing levels, health and safety, improved client care (quality), and job security (Canadian Federation of Nurses Unions). Many nurse managers believe it is best to deal quickly and effectively with issues as they arise. In this way they can avoid collective bargaining, which usually entails an increase in costs to the hospital and limitations being placed on managers. See Figure 21-1 to assist in understanding collective bargaining by nurses.

Unions

A **union** is a formal and legal group that works through a collective bargaining agent to formally present desires to management, that is, through the legal context of labour legislation. The Canada Labour Code regulates and sets standards for government employees and inter-provincial

enterprises; however, each province establishes its own labour legislation. As a result, Canada has both federal and provincial labour relations systems. Because the procedures for collective bargaining are different across the provinces and territories, nurses are able to strike in some jurisdictions, but not in others.

Table 21-1 lists some collective action terminology, which is useful in understanding the collective bargaining process.

CRITICAL THINKING

Name two collective groups to which you belong. What are these collective groups able to accomplish as a whole? Are these collective groups more effective and stronger than you are, as an individual, in these interest areas? What are the downsides of belonging to a collective group?

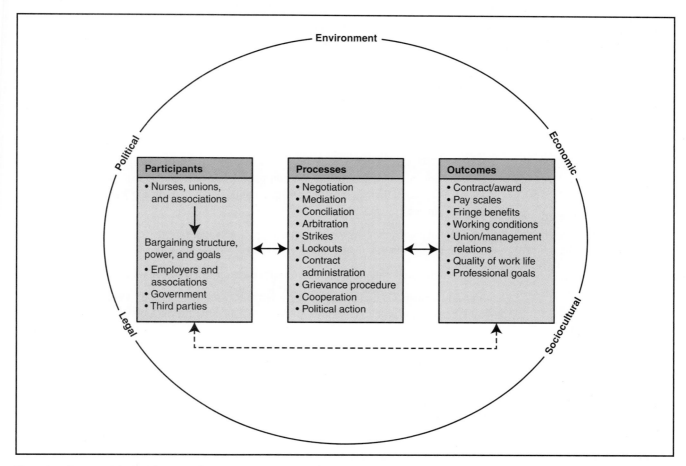

Figure 21-1 Framework for Understanding Collective Bargaining by Nurses

Source: From Judith M. Hibberd & Donna Lynn Smith, *Nursing Leadership and Management in Canada,* 3rd edition (Figure 29 and page 671). Copyright © 2006 Elsevier Canada, a division of Reed Elsevier Canada, Ltd. All rights reserved. Reprinted by Permission of Elsevier Canada, 2011.

TABLE 21-1	COLLECTIVE BARGAINING TERMINOLOGY

Term	Definition
Agency shop	Synonymous with *open shop*. Employees are not required to join the union but may join it.
Arbitration	The last step in a dispute. A non-partial third party will make the final decision. Arbitration may be voluntary or imposed by the government.
Collective agreement	A set of guidelines and rules voted and agreed upon by union members and agreed upon by representatives of management. The collective agreement, also known as a contract, states the rights and responsibilities of managers and union members and guides work practices, wages, and other benefits.
Collective bargaining	The practice of employees, as a collective, bargaining with management in reference to wages, work practices, and other benefits.
Collective bargaining agent	An agent who works with employees to formalize collective bargaining through unionization.
Fact finding	Fact finding is used in labour management disputes or grievances that involve government-owned companies. It is the process in which the claims of labour and management are reviewed. In the private sector, fact finding is usually performed by a board of inquiry.
Grievance	A formal complaint or a dispute between management and a union member regarding the interpretation, application, or alleged violation of the terms of the collective agreement.
Grievance proceedings	A formal process by which a union member files a grievance to seek a settlement that is agreeable to both sides. The steps usually include (1) communication of the grievance to management, (2) mediation with a union representative and a member of management, and possibly (3) arbitration. The dispute may be settled at any step.
Lockout	An act in which management closes a place of business for the purpose of forcing employees to accept management's terms.
Mediation	A step in the grievance process in which a non-partial third party meets with management and the union to assist them in reaching an agreement. The third party, the mediator, has no actual power in decision making.
Strike	An act in which union members withhold their supply of labour for the purpose of forcing management to accept the union's terms.
Supervisor	A person with the authority to (1) impart corrective action and (2) delegate to an employee.
Union	A formal and legal group that brings forth desires to management through a collective bargaining agent and within the context of the provincial or territorial legislation.
Union dues	Money required of all union employees to support the union and its functions.
Union shop	A place of employment in which all employees are required to join the union and pay dues. *Union shop* is synonymous with the term *closed shop*.
Whistle-blowing	Whistle-blowing is the act in which an individual discloses information regarding the violation of a law, rule, or regulation, or a substantial and specific danger to public health or safety.
Work-to-rule	A job action taken to challenge terms of the contract, such as refusal to work overtime or refusal to attend meetings.

CRITICAL THINKING

Y ou are a nurse working at an institution in which there is limited flexibility in the scheduling. You want to institute self-scheduling, with the staff nurses responsible for making and maintaining the schedule. Make a plan to present this idea to the manager. How will you elicit the support of other nurses? Now put yourself in the role of the manager. How would you respond to this request?

CRITICAL THINKING

Y ou are a nurse working on a busy internal medicine unit. The union contract expired six months ago, and there has just been a strike vote. The union received an 80 percent mandate to strike.

One of the union's main issues is wages. However, the issue of greater concern to you is vacation and paid time-off provisions. In addition, you would like to see more dollars provided for an education allowance. The union is focused more on wages. You have never attended a union meeting. What is your role to ensure that the local union executive knows what the real issues are for nurses? What advice would you give to this nurse? Have you ever attended your union's meetings?

WHISTLE-BLOWING

One of the ethical dilemmas faced by individuals working in the health care field is the potential conflict between loyalty to their employers, colleagues, and professional standards and a duty to protect their clients against incompetent, illegal, or unethical behaviour. When these conflicts arise, they are challenging in both ethical and practical terms for the individual. Nurses are often aware of errors that have been made, or actions that have been taken against an individual, but they are hesitant to speak to the individuals directly involved or to a supervisor for fear of reprisal.

In the Report of the Review and Implementation Committee for the Report of the Manitoba Pediatric Cardiac Surgery Inquest in May 2001, **whistle-blowing** was defined as "the unauthorized internal or external disclosure of information concerning a harmful act that a superior or a colleague has committed, is allowing to occur, or is contemplating" (Provincial Court of Manitoba, 2001, p. 479). In 2005 Manitoba introduced whistle-blowing legislation that required health care workers to report any "critical incidents" that affect the care of clients. The new law protected workers from being disciplined or penalized for coming forward. The Regional Health Authorities Amendment and Manitoba Evidence Amendment Act "requires the reporting of critical incidents that may happen during the provision of health services and help health care providers participate fully and openly in an investigation of a critical incident."[3]

Disclosing misconduct within an organization is usually less damaging than leaking information to external sources. Because studies suggest that whistle-blowers pay a high price in terms of their careers and personal lives, stronger legal protection will help protect individuals who legitimately and reasonably disclose wrongdoings. In addition, greater accountability can be demanded from leaders and the organizations that retaliate against justified complaints and reports. Ideally, organizations will develop policies and strategies to minimize the need for individuals to report on illegal behaviour or other wrongdoings.

In November 2005, the Liberal government enacted Bill C-11, the Disclosure Protection legislation commonly known as "whistleblower" legislation. This act established a procedure for the disclosure of wrongdoings in the public sector, including the protection of persons who disclose the wrongdoings. The bill was introduced in response to the sponsorship scandal.[4]

THE PROCESS OF UNIONIZATION

The process of choosing a collective bargaining unit and negotiating a contract may take from three months to three years. A **collective bargaining agent** is a union representative who works with employees to formalize collective bargaining through unionization. One of the primary organizing strategies to promote union membership, as suggested by Murray (2001), is identification of issues critical to nurses: for example, such as the amount of change in the health care system, human resource shortages, and reengineering. Several formal steps are required to legally form a union. See Table 21-2 for the steps involved in organizing a collective bargaining unit in Ontario.

TABLE 21-2	STEPS IN ORGANIZING A COLLECTIVE BARGAINING UNIT IN ONTARIO

Bring together a group of nurses supportive of collective bargaining.

Arrange a meeting with a representative of the provincial nurses association to discuss organizing.

Assess the feasibility of an organizing campaign at your facility.

Conduct the necessary research, such as the needs and/or complaints of the employees, to develop a plan of action.

Establish an organizing committee and subcommittees to facilitate organizing.

Union representatives will meet with the employees and discuss the process with them.

Complete and submit a union membership card to the union.

The Ontario Labour Relations Act states that if at least 40 percent of the employees sign union membership cards, then an application for certification to the Ontario Labour Relations Board (OLRB) can be submitted.

The OLRB holds a secret vote at the workplace one week after applying for certification.

If 50 percent plus one of the employees who cast a ballot vote in favour of the union, the union is successful.

The union is then certified to represent the employee group, or bargaining unit.

The process of initiating contract negotiations for the first collective agreement is started.

Your decision is private, and the law protects the secrecy of the card signer and the vote. Your employer doesn't know you signed a membership card. A Labour Board officer conducts the vote.

Sources: Adapted from Flanagan, L. (1991). How the bargaining process works. *American Nurse, 23*(9), 11–12; Ontario Nurses Association. Retrieved from http://www.ona.org/join_ona/how_do_i_organize_my_workplace.html

TABLE 21-3	THE MANAGER'S ROLE DURING INITIATION OF UNIONIZATION

Know the law; make sure the rights of the nurses as well as the rights of management are clearly understood.

Act clearly within the law, no matter what the organization delegates to you as a manager.

Find out the reasons the nurses want collective action.

Discuss and deal with the nurses and the problems directly and effectively.

THE MANAGER'S ROLE

Registered nurses have the legal authority to participate in collective bargaining in the majority of health care facilities in the country. It is important to maintain an open mind and develop collegial relationships with the potential union steward and the union membership. Equally important, listen to problems and concerns, investigate them promptly, and suggest solutions.

When a manager is flexible, fair, and open to suggestions, the chances that nurses will want to unionize may be reduced. Table 21-3 lists some ways managers can respond during a drive for unionization.

THE EMPLOYEE'S ROLE

Nurses desiring to choose a collective bargaining agent must ensure they carefully follow the laws pertaining to unionization. Carefully choose the collective bargaining agent, such as the Ontario Nurses Association or the British Columbia Nurses Union. Research the agent and learn how nurses will be supported and where and how the union dues are spent. Talk to nurses in union settings to see how their contract is structured and whether collective bargaining has helped with the issues that led them to unionize in the first place. See Table 21-4 for a synopsis of the role of nurses during unionization.

CASE STUDY 21-1

You are a nurse working in a cardiac catheterization laboratory. You notice that a certain physician routinely performs cardiac catheterizations on clients who are in their early 40s and who have no risk factors for cardiac history. The catheterizations are always negative for disease. You love your job but are troubled by this practice. You are fearful that clients will have complications. When you ask the physician why these procedures are performed on clients who do not appear to need this testing, his response is, "You don't worry about what I do; these procedures keep us all employed with healthy paycheques." You discuss this situation with your nursing manager who says, "Just do your job and let the doctor decide what is best for his clients."

You decide that whistle-blowing is your next action. What is your first step? Should you notify your manager of your whistle-blowing? What policies exist in your facility to guide the nurse when the nurse finds unprofessional activities?

TABLE 21-4	THE NURSE'S ROLE DURING INITIATION OF UNIONIZATION

Know your legal rights and the rights of the manager.

Act clearly within the law at all times.

If a manager acts unlawfully, such as firing an employee for organizing, report it to the labour relations board in your province or territory.

Keep all nurses informed by holding regular meetings close to the hospital.

Set meeting times conveniently around shift changes and assist with child care during meetings.

STRIKING

Many nurses are morally opposed to unions because they believe if they are members of a union, they may be forced to strike. In reality, a collective bargaining agent cannot make the decision to strike. The decision to strike is made only if the majority of union members decide to do so. Provisions guarantee the continuation of adequate client care by requiring the union (in consultation with the organization) to provide sufficient nurses to care for the clients who were unable to be discharged to an alternate facility.

The manager should not lose sight of the fact that eventually the strike will be over! Maintain amicable, professional relationships during the strike so that client care is not compromised and the work environment does not become poisoned. Although a strike may occur, unions are responsible and allow enough staff to work to provide essential service.

NURSING ASSOCIATIONS

The **Canadian Nurses Association (CNA)** is a federation of 11 provincial and territorial nursing associations and colleges, representing more than 143,843 Canadian registered nurses.[5] It is the national professional voice of registered nurses and represents Canadian nursing to other organizations and to government nationally and internationally. The CNA advances the practice and profession of nursing to improve health outcomes and strengthen Canada's publicly funded not-for-profit health system.[6] It is not considered a union. However, in 1944, the Canadian Nurses Association approved the principle of collective bargaining for nurses.

The **Canadian Federation of Nurses Unions (CFNU)** is the body that promotes nurses and the nursing

CRITICAL THINKING

You are a nurse working in a hospital that is a union shop. Nurses are concerned about unsafe staffing and being assigned to units with client populations they are not properly trained to care for. The collective bargaining agent for the union has met with management concerning these issues, but nothing has been resolved. According to the rumours, these working conditions could be an issue when it is time to negotiate a new contract. Nurses may decide to strike as a result of this issue not being resolved.

What issues make people consider striking? What is your provincial or territorial association's stance on striking? What steps can be taken to avoid a strike?

profession at the national level. The CFNU pressures the federal government to recognize the professional skills and knowledge that nurses bring to their jobs.[7] In addition, it is the national voice for nurses at the Canadian Labour Congress. Each of the provincial nurses unions, with the exception of Québec, is a member of the CFNU.

In October of 2008 Health Canada approved a proposal by the Canadian Federation of Nurses Unions to implement nine pilot projects designed to increase the retention and recruitment of nurses across the country. In November 2009 a tenth pilot project based in Nunavut was approved. Together, the pilots are known as Research to Action: Applied Workplace Solutions for Nurses. These pilots involve innovative strategies that bring research to action, including programs that address staffing ratios to enhance the quality of client care, systems to offer support to new nursing graduates, and opportunities for education and professional development. A national steering committee helps oversee the implementation of the project; there are two representatives from each pilot project and representation from the CFNU and its national partners— the Canadian Nurses Association, the Canadian Healthcare Association, and the Dietitians of Canada.[8]

The ten pilot projects were completed by the end of 2010, and the national evaluation process concluded in March 2011. At the time of this writing, the results had not been published. The projects documented that changes in the nursing workplace can improve retention and recruitment rates. The results included a 10 percent reduction in overtime, absenteeism, and turnover costs and a 147 percent increase in the number of nurses reporting a high level of leadership and support.[9]

The American Nurses Association (ANA) represents 2.6 million registered nurses in the United States through its 54 constituent state and territorial associations. The ANA's mission is to work for the improvement of health standards and availability of health care services for all people, to foster high standards for nursing, to stimulate and promote the professional development of nurses, and to advance their economic and general welfare (ANA, n.d.). The National Labor Relations Board recognizes the ANA as a collective bargaining agent. The ANA's dual role of being both a professional organization and a collective bargaining agent causes controversy. Some nurses believe that unionization is not professional and that the ANA cannot truly support nursing as a profession if it is also a collective bargaining agent. Because nurse managers are excluded from union membership, many nurse managers believe they have been left outside the organization that is supposed to represent all of nursing. Other nurse managers do not feel this separation (The Role of Collective Bargaining and Unions, 1998).

The ANA represents the interests of nurses in collective bargaining, advances the nursing profession by fostering high standards for nursing practice, and lobbies U.S. Congress and regulatory agencies on health care

LITERATURE APPLICATION

Citation: Raso, R. (2010). Establishing healthy union relationships and the "best" unit in the hospital. *Nursing Management,* 41(8): 56.

Discussion: This is a brief question and answer article related to establishing healthy union relationships and the "best" unit in the hospital.

Implications for Practice: Principles of a healthy work environment are a good place to start to guide the discussions related to any type of workforce relationship. Choosing the right staff with the right competencies to meet client needs is essential. In addition, you need to build good working relationships—up, down, and sideways. Unit goals should be established, shared, and communicated frequently and clearly. Give and receive feedback often. Be clear on what you expect. Celebrate accomplishments and recognize staff individually and collectively. Focus on client safety and quality in a healthy practice environment. Relationship-building is important. Know the collective-bargaining agreement or contract and consistently follow it.

issues affecting nurses and the general public. The ANA initiates many policies involving health care reform. It also publishes its position on issues ranging from whistleblowing to patients' rights. The ANA recently launched a major campaign to mobilize nurses to address the staffing crisis, to educate and gain support from the public, and to develop and implement initiatives designed to resolve the crisis (United American Nurses, 2001).

PROFESSIONALISM AND UNIONIZATION

Requirements for a vocation to be considered a profession include (1) a long period of specialized education, (2) a service orientation, and (3) the ability to be autonomous (Jacox, 1980). Jacox (1980) defines autonomy as a characteristic of a profession in which the members of that profession are self-regulating and have control of their functions in the work situation. Nurses agree that specialized education and a service orientation are necessary to become a nurse, but many nurses disagree on the concept of autonomy. This disagreement is the central argument that divides nurses with regard to whether it is professional to be part of a union.

REAL WORLD INTERVIEW

I believe it is professional to be in a union because you have more opportunities to stand up for your clients and your own nursing practice. Having worked in both a union and a non-union environment, I think being in a union allows you to speak your mind without fear of losing job security. They can't dismiss you for just any reason. There are grievance proceedings. In a non-union environment, if they don't like you or what you say, they can punish you. But I've also seen the downside of unions. An example is when a contract comes out. The more senior union nursing staff wants to hold out from agreeing on a contract that does not address all of our concerns while the junior union nursing staff want to agree on the first contract that is presented. Holding out for what you want is why there is arbitration. The junior nurses don't realize the power of the bargaining unit in nursing. I think most nurses don't realize what we as nurses can accomplish if we stick together.

Susan Zielinski, RN
Staff Nurse

REAL WORLD INTERVIEW

I don't think it's any less professional for a physician to be in a union than any other health care provider. Doctors agree to try to help people. In return, physicians should be able to charge for that service and provide the best care they know how to deliver. Doctors should be able to bargain for better conditions and autonomy like the rest of society. More and more, the governing decision is not so much the client care as what is cost-effective. Doctors are not making those decisions and that's inherently wrong. As more and more of the medical structure become corporate, the workers, which doctors have become, need a means of negotiating with their employers.

Jonathan Fisher, MD
Surgical Resident

Many nurses believe that for nursing to be considered a profession, nurses must exercise autonomy and, like most professionals, work out issues themselves. Many argue that issues cannot be resolved without unionization. The debate about whether it is professional to be a part of a nurse's union has plagued nursing since the inception of nursing unions.

PHYSICIAN UNIONIZATION

In many provinces student physicians are members of unions. Upon graduation, the physicians become members of provincial or territorial medical associations. These associations negotiate with provincial governments to represent the political, clinical, and economic interests of the medical profession. The Canadian Medical Association consults with the provinces on issues of fee and benefit schedule comparisons and negotiation strategies, but does not function as a union.

UNIONIZATION OF UNIVERSITY PROFESSORS

The unionization of kindergarten through twelfth-grade teachers is well established in Canada. Now, an increasing number of professors at postsecondary institutions are choosing to unionize. Again, wages and work environment have motivated university professors to join unions. As the average age of university faculty increases and fewer people show interest in teaching, unions may be able to protect professors from becoming overburdened and to financially reward those who enter teaching at the university level.

MANAGING IN A UNION ENVIRONMENT

Managers must work with the union to manage within the rules and context of contract agreements. In some ways managing after a union is in place is less difficult because of the explicit language in most union contracts. Such measures as corrective actions and rules concerning allowed absences are agreed upon, voted on, and written in the contract.

GRIEVANCES

When a union member disputes management's interpretation or application of the terms of the contract, or collective agreement, this formal complaint is called a **grievance.** All union contracts specify the steps in grievance proceedings.

Grievance proceedings usually start with an employee who believes a wrongdoing has occurred on the part of management. Next, the member talks with a union representative, who helps the employee judge whether the act or condition actually justifies a formal complaint. The union representative uses knowledge of the contract, knowledge of labour legislation, and personal judgment to assist the employee. Next, the union member and the union representative meet with the manager to voice the grievance. At this point, the conflict may be resolved. If the conflict is not resolved, the next step may be to appeal management's decision and mediate with a higher level manager. Grievance proceedings may differ from union to union.

PROS AND CONS OF COLLECTIVE BARGAINING

Nurses make a personal decision whether to support collective bargaining in the form of a union. Table 21-5 summarizes the pros and cons of collective bargaining.

TABLE 21-5	PROS AND CONS OF UNIONIZATION

Pros	Cons
The contract guides standards.	There is reduced allowance for individuality.
Members are able to be a part of the decision-making process.	Other union members may outvote your decisions.
All union members and management must conform to the terms of the contract without exception.	All union members and management must conform to the terms of the contract without exception.
A process can be instituted to question a manager's authority if a member feels something was done unjustly. More people are involved in the process.	Disputes are not handled with an individual and management only; there is less room for personal judgment.
Union dues are required to make the union work for you.	Union dues must be paid even if individuals do not support unionization.
Unions give a collective voice for employees.	Employee may not agree with the collective voice.
Employees are able to voice concerns to management without fear of reprisal.	Unions may be perceived by some as not professional.

REAL WORLD INTERVIEW

The union affects my role as manager in many ways. There are so many pros and cons with it. I get frustrated as a manager when I feel like I cannot use my judgment because it may contradict the contract. For example, an employee lost a grandparent who was essentially this employee's parent, but I couldn't give this employee time off because it was not technically a parent who died. The contract also doesn't allow me to really commend employees who work hard and do their best every day. The hard-working person's pay and benefits are exactly the same as a mediocre employee. My hands are tied.

If you violate the contract, it becomes a time-consuming project for me as the manager. For example, if I had chosen to give the person time off for the grandparent who died, I would have grievances from other people because I did not give them time off for their grandparent's death. I would have to document what I did and why and would ultimately lose the grievance and have to find a way to compensate the other people for not giving them time off. I come from a pro-union family, and I understand how unions can protect employees. In general, it is good for employees to have somebody who is on their side and who treats all as equals. It's hard for me to imagine that there are managers who mistreat their employees in other institutions.

Ann Marie O'Connor, RN
Unit Manager

KEY CONCEPTS

■ Nursing collective bargaining has existed in Canada since 1946.

■ Workplace advocacy is a collective action model that is more informal and encompasses the everyday creativity and problem solving that occur in nursing.

■ Collective bargaining through unionization is a collective action model that is formal and legally based. It uses a written contract to guide nursing and workplace issues.

■ Nurses who are unhappy in the workplace because of issues such as wages and poor staffing often attempt to unionize to rectify workplace problems. Nurses who are not managers have the legal right to unionize. Employees and managers must be aware of the specific steps that must be taken during the initiation of unionization.

■ The Canadian Nurses Association is a professional organization that represents the country's entire registered nurse population. Unlike the American Nurses Association, the CNA does *not* have a dual role of being a professional organization and a collective bargaining agent for nursing. The CNA is politically active and lobbies on issues affecting nursing and the general public.

■ The Canadian Federation of Nurses Unions promotes nurses and nursing at the national level.

■ Other professionals who do not have a tradition of unionization are opting to unionize. Physicians and university professors are joining unions for the same reasons that some nurses have chosen to join unions: to improve their wages and working conditions.

KEY TERMS

Canadian Federation of Nurses
  Unions (CFNU)
Canadian Nurses Association
  (CNA)
collective action
collective bargaining

collective bargaining
  agent
grievance
unions
whistle-blowing
workplace advocacy

REVIEW QUESTIONS

1. A manager should do which of the following if nurses are attempting to unionize?
   A. Nothing; most often the union attempt fails.
   B. Do not hire any registered nurses who are pro-union.
   C. Learn the reason nurses want collective action.
   D. Fire the nurse instigating unionization.

2. Which of the following best defines workplace advocacy?
   A. a management-defined solution for the workplace
   B. holding managers and nurses accountable
   C. a formal structure that is voted on
   D. activities nurses undertake to address problems in the workplace

3. Which of the following is *not* a common reason why nurses unionize?
   A. client care issues
   B. wages
   C. staffing issues
   D. being content in the workplace

REVIEW ACTIVITIES

1. You are a new graduate nurse and have begun working on a medical unit. The nurse manager explains that the unit uses workplace advocacy. What is workplace advocacy? How will it affect your functioning as a registered nurse on the unit?

2. You are hired in a hospital that is a union shop. How does unionization differ from other collective action models, such as workplace advocacy? Give three examples of how unionization differs from workplace advocacy.

3. You are a graduate nurse, and you found out you passed the CRNE examination. As a registered nurse, you are represented by the British Columbia Nurses Union. What is the mission of the BCNU? Is the BCNU active in politics?

EXPLORING THE WEB

What sites would you recommend to someone inquiring about collective bargaining?

- *http://www.hrsdc.gc.ca/eng/labour/labour_relations/info_analysis/index.shtml*

Go to the site for the Canadian Federation of Nurses Unions and find your provincial nursing union. What did you learn about your provincial nursing union?

- *http://www.nursesunions.ca/*

What site would you access to find out the history of collective bargaining?

- *http://www.nursesunions.ca/*

- *http://www.ona.org/faq/index.html#union_his*

- *http://www.law-faqs.org/wiki/index.php/Main_Page*

Go to the site for the British Columbia Nurses Union: *http://www.bcnu.org/*. Click on the What's New link and read some articles, then click on the Campaigns/Issues link to access the Practice Issues page. What did you learn about nursing and current events?

REFERENCES

American Nurses Association. (n.d.). *Mission statement.* Retrieved from http://www.nursingworld.org/FunctionalMenuCategories/AboutANA.aspx

Canadian Federation of Nurses Unions. (2007). *About us.* Retrieved from http://www.nursesunions.ca/about-us

Flanagan, L. (1991). How the bargaining process works. *American Nurse, 23*(9), 11–12.

Hart, C. (1998). The state of the unions. *Nursing Times, 94*(15), 36–37.

Hibberd, J., & Smith, D. L. (2006). *Nursing leadership and management in Canada* (3rd ed.). Toronto: Elsevier Canada, a division of Harcourt Canada Ltd.

Jacox, A. (1980). Collective action: The basis for professionalism. *Supervisor Nurse, 11*(9), 22–24.

Junor, J. (1998). What roles do unions have in preparing nursing leaders to effective change for the future? *Concern, 27*(1), 18–19.

Kalist, D. E. (2002). The gender earnings gap in the RN labour market. *Nursing Economics, 20*(4), 155–162.

Marquis, B. L., & Huston, C. J. (2012). *Leadership roles and management functions in nursing: Theory and application* (7th ed.). Philadelphia: Lippincott, Williams and Wilkins.

Murray, M. K. (2001). The new economy and new union organizing strategies: Union wins in healthcare. *Journal of Nursing Administration, 31*(7/8), 339–343.

Raso, R. (2010). Establishing healthy union relationships and the "best" unit in the hospital. *Nursing Management, 41*(8), 56.

Provincial Court of Manitoba. (2001). *Report of the Review and Implementation Committee for the Report of the Manitoba Pediatric Surgery Inquest.* Winnipeg: Government of Manitoba.

Seago, J. A., & Ash, M. (2002). Registered nurse unions and patient outcomes. *Journal of Nursing Administration, 32*(3), 143–151.

The role of collective bargaining and unions in advancing the profession of nursing. (1998). *Nursing Trends & Issues, 3*(2), 1–8.

Thinknursing!ca. (2010). *Research to action: Applied workplace solutions for nurses.* Ottawa: Canadian Federation of Nurses Unions. Retrieved from http://www.thinknursing.ca/rta

Underwood, P. (1997). Nurses need collective action to "build" profession. *Michigan Nurse, 70*(10), 3.

United American Nurses (UAN) mobilizes nurses on staffing crisis. (2001). *American Journal of Nursing, 101*(1), 65.

SUGGESTED READINGS

Camfield, D. (2005). *An analysis of the hospital employees' union strike of 2004.* Unpublished manuscript.

Canadian Nurses Association. (2002). *Planning for the future: Nursing human resource projections.* Ottawa: Author.

Fitzpatrick, M. (2001). Collective bargaining: A vulnerability assessment. *Nursing Management, 32*(2), 40–42.

Forman, H., & Davis, G. A. (2002). The anatomy of a union campaign. *Journal of Nursing Administration, 32*(9), 444–447.

Forman, H., & Kraus, H. R. (2003). Decertification: Management's role when employees rethink unionization. *Journal of Nursing Administration, 33*(6), 313–316.

Forman, H., & Powell, T. A. (2003). Managing during an employee walkout. *Journal of Nursing Administration, 33*(9), 430–433.

Jamison, D. T., Frenk, J., & Knaul, F. (1998). International collective action in health: Objectives, functions and rationale. *Lancet,* 351(9101), 514–517.

Malott, M. (2005). From the front-line to the picket-line. *The Heart: Newsletter of the McGill School of Nursing Community/La Coeur: Communiqué de la communauté de l'École des sciences infirmières de McGill,* 24, 11.

Meier, E. (1999). Politically speaking. *ONS News,* 14(10), 13.

Meier, E. (2000). Is unionization the answer for nurses and nursing? *Nursing Economics,* 18(1), 36–38.

Melville, E. (1995). The history of industrial action in nursing. *Professional Nurse,* 11(2), 84–86.

Nurse staffing law may herald benchmarks. (1999). *Healthcare Benchmarks,* 6(120), 137–138.

Porter-O'Grady, T. (2001). Collective bargaining: The union as partner. *Nursing Management,* 32(6, Pt. 1), 30–32.

Seltzer, T. M. (2001). Collective bargaining: A wake-up call—part 2. *Nursing Management,* 32(4), 35–37, 48.

Tone, B. (1999, August 9). Pulled apart: Does unionizing serve the interests of the profession? *NurseWeek,* 1–5.

Trossman, S. (1998). Doctors increasingly are looking for the union label. *American Nurse,* 30(4), 19.

Walmsley, J. (1996). Collective action brought change. *Kaitiaki: Nursing New Zealand,* 9(1), 28.

CHAPTER ENDNOTES

1. Canadian Federation of Nurses Unions, "CFNU Celebrates its 25th Anniversary." Retrieved from http://www.nursesunions.ca/history

2. Canadian Federation of Nurses Unions, "About Us." Retrieved from http://www.nursesunions.ca/about-us

3. National Union of Public and General Employees, "Whistle-blower bill to protect Manitoba health workers." Retrieved from http://www.nupge.ca/news_2005/n16ma05a.htm

4. Government of Canada. "Bill C-11." Retrieved from http://www.parl.gc.ca/HousePublications/Publication.aspx?doc=C-11&Language=E&parl=38&pub=bill&ses=1/

5. Canadian Nurses Association, "What is the Canadian Nurses Association?" Retrieved from http://www.cna-aiic.ca/CNA/about/who/default_e.aspx

6. Ibid.

7. Canadian Federation of Nurses Unions, "About Us." Retrieved from http://www.nursesunions.ca/about-us

8. Canadian Federation of Nurses Unions. (2010). *Research to action: Applied workplace solutions for nurses.* Retrieved from http://www.thinkingnursing.ca/rta

9. Canadian Federation of Nurses Unions. (2011). *Nurses call on the provincial premiers to find pan-Canadian solutions to public health care. A united front will be needed to engage the federal government.* Retrieved from http://www.nursesunions.ca/news/nurses-call-premiers-find-pan-canadian-solutions-public-health-care-united-front-will-be-needed

CHAPTER 22

Career Planning and Development: Creating Your Path to the Future

Janice Waddell, RN, PhD

*Learning without thought
is labour lost; thought
without learning is perilous.*
(Confucius)

OBJECTIVES

The purpose of this chapter is to enable a senior-level student to

- define career planning and development;

- describe the Donner-Wheeler Career Planning and Development Model (the Model);

- complete initial work in the five phases of the Model (Creating Your Career Vision, Completing Your Self-Assessment and Reality Check, Scanning Your Environment, Developing Your Strategic Career Plan, and Marketing Yourself) use the Model to choose a first job as a registered nurse; and

- identify resources to be used with the Model in preparing an application to graduate studies.

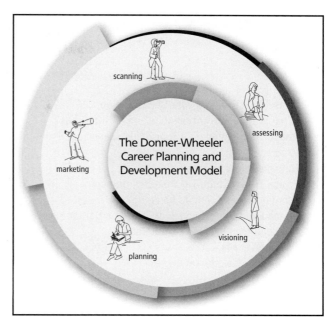

Figure 22-1 The Donner-Wheeler Career Planning and Development Model

Source: Donner, 2004. Copyright © 2007 donnerwheeler. All rights reserved.

Alya is entering the final year of her baccalaureate nursing program. She is very excited to be so close to her dream of becoming a registered nurse, but her excitement is accompanied by a sense of anxiety. She wants to ensure that she makes the best of her final year so that she is positioned for a nursing job that will help her advance toward her career goal of working with children and families in an acute care setting. She plans to stay in Canada, likely within her home province. Although some opportunities are available for fourth-year student practice experiences in acute care of children and families, due to the current health care environment, not all students who wish such a placement can be accommodated. Alya is asking such questions as, How can I plan my career now and in the future? How can I use my educational experiences in the coming year to help me progress toward my career goal—whether or not I am able to have a practice experience focused on children and families? How can I make sure that I choose the job that is right for me? How do I market myself? Where do I start? Who can help me?

The purpose of this chapter is to introduce the Donner-Wheeler Career Planning and Development Model (the Model) as a tool for career planning as you complete your nursing program and move to your first job as a registered nurse! The author of this chapter is a senior associate of donnerwheeler and has worked closely with Gail Donner, RN, PhD, and Mary Wheeler, RN, MEd, ACC, in the development and application of the Model to student nurses and new graduates. The Model can help you to achieve a sense of control over both your academic career and your professional practice career (see Figure 22-1).

You entered your nursing program with dreams, ideas, and hopes for your future career. The career planning and development model and process provides a guide to help you to achieve your dreams and to create new possibilities as you build your nursing career. In this chapter, you will learn about the importance of career planning and development as you consider and plan for completing your nursing education and the transition to the workplace. You will also learn how to use the five phases of the Model to develop your unique career goals and to guide your academic activities and your search for your first job as a registered nurse.

A career is what we choose as our profession, our path, or our life's work (Donner, 2009). You chose your path when you accepted your admission into your nursing program, and your nursing career began the day you attended your school of nursing orientation. You have now entered the final year(s) of your nursing education program. Your many classroom and practice experiences, as well as your exposure to broader professional activities, have shaped your sense of the kind of nurse you aspire to be and, perhaps, the type of nursing practice that interests you most. You are ready to take the wheel and navigate your career.

The five phases of the career planning and development model introduced in this chapter (see Table 22-1) prompt you to dedicate some time, thought, and reflection to both understanding and influencing the environment in which you complete the final years of your education and the environment in which you will assume your first

TABLE 22-1	THE DONNER-WHEELER CAREER PLANNING AND DEVELOPMENT MODEL ADAPTED FOR STUDENTS

Phase One: Creating Your Career Vision
What are the current realities and future trends?
Phase Two: Completing Your Self-Assessment and Reality Check
Who am I?
How do others see me?
Phase Three: Scanning Your Environment
What do I really want to be doing?
Phase Four: Developing Your Strategic Career Plan
How can I achieve my career goals?
Phase Five: Marketing Yourself
How can I best market myself?

nursing position. Through this process, you will create a vision of your career, assess your strengths and the areas that require further development, and develop a realistic plan to help you progress toward your career vision. Although marketing is a separate phase of the Model, you will also gain an awareness of the importance of marketing yourself throughout your work in all phases of the Model. Strategic and thoughtful marketing skills will help you to achieve your plan and progressively advance toward your career goals. In other words—this is all about you!

CREATING YOUR CAREER VISION

Your **career vision** describes where you want to go in your nursing career—it is a description of who and what you wish to become. Your career vision helps you describe the kind of nurse you wish to be and can also include where you hope to focus your nursing practice. Your career vision focuses on what is possible. It makes use of your resources and has the ability to harness and direct your energy. It is a personal statement of your hopes for your career; think of it as your career fantasy! As with any fantasy—think and dream big! Find a quiet spot and give yourself some time to think about your career vision. Pretend that you are leaving your home to go to your perfect nursing job. You can situate your vision one, two, or up to five years after your graduation.

Close your eyes and reflect on the following questions:

- Where are you living?
- Who and what is in your home that nurtures your ability to go to work with such positive anticipation?

- What do you most look forward to as you head into your perfect job each day?
- In what type of organization do you work?
- Describe the setting.
- Describe your colleagues.
- Describe your clients.
- How would your colleagues describe you?
- How would your clients describe you?
- What does your organization offer you that fosters your ability to be the best you can be each day?

Alya's career vision may look something like this:

I live in an urban location in my home province with my partner and two dogs. My partner is very supportive of my career and is an equal contributor in all areas of our lives. My two dogs are fun, loving, and always happy to see me! Each day when I head to work, I look forward to making a difference in the lives of children and their families. I work in an acute care pediatric teaching hospital in a downtown health setting. It is a bright and beautiful building. I am involved in direct care of children and families and serve as a resource to my colleagues. I work with an amazing interprofessional team of colleagues who is committed to providing a high quality of family-centred care. I feel confident in my practice, and my peers describe me as an expert pediatric nurse, a supportive member of the health care team and an effective formal and informal leader. I am recognized for my ability to work effectively with both families and colleagues. I feel a part of a team that values and respects my contributions—and I theirs. Eventually, I plan to pursue graduate studies to help me prepare to be an advanced practice family health nurse, and the organization in which I work supports advanced education both philosophically and financially.

If you envision a specific role, organization, location, that is great. If you envision many roles and possibilities for your ideal workplace, that too is great. More important than the *where* or the *what* in your vision, will be the *who*. Who are you as a nurse in your vision? What is important to you, and what do you value most? Are you amongst colleagues who share your values, and does the place in which you work allow you to live your values? Revisit your vision every few months—the where and what may change to reflect the dynamic and exciting nature of your nursing career. However, ensure that your reflection includes the most meaningful questions: Am I still having fun? Do I feel proud and have a sense of wonder? The answer to those questions will give the true measure of your career success.

Whatever your focus, your vision can provide you with a sense of purpose and a goal, and it can help you focus your learning and development in the coming year—and as you make the transition to the workplace. Your vision offers the foundation for your self-assessment, some cues to the type of work environment that will satisfy you, and ideas for selecting potential employment settings and developing interview questions.

By putting your career vision in writing, it becomes more accessible to you, and more real. Keep your written account in a place where you can see it often (likely your computer screen). During those times when you feel overwhelmed with the work you have to do to be successful in your academic and professional work, your career vision can be a reminder of why you are doing what you are doing, who you wish to be, and where you are going. It can also help you focus on making your activities fit with your vision. Sharing your vision allows others to support your efforts and help you keep on the path you have chosen.

At this point in your academic career, you might be quite confident that your vision will not change. However, you may have experiences in the coming year(s) that transform your vision. Career visions are not written in stone—if your vision changes, you simply revisit all, or the most relevant, phases of the Model to help you apply your work achievements in a different way and create new opportunities and directions. As noted earlier in the chapter, the Model is both a tool to use and a reflection of the dynamic nature of your present and future career.

Alya's vision can help her focus on developing key competencies that she needs to actualize her dream. Her vision directs her to develop confidence and competence in her knowledge, communication, leadership, interprofessional teamwork, family-centred care, and practice competencies. She can use this vision to engage in self-assessment and an environmental scan, which will ensure that she considers not only where she is now but also where she hopes to be in the future. Her vision also lets her see that if she doesn't obtain a practice placement in a children's and family health acute care setting,

she can still focus on competencies that she will need to achieve her vision: communication, family-centred care, developmental care, leadership, interprofessional care, expanding her knowledge base, and competencies that span her area of specialized practice.

YOUR SELF-ASSESSMENT AND REALITY CHECK

Your **self-assessment** is about looking inside yourself (Donner, 2009). You have completed a substantial portion of your nursing education and may feel, as many students do, that you are a different person now than when you entered nursing. You have likely learned a great deal about yourself through your classroom, practice experiences and your overall involvement in your program and profession. Your professional knowledge grows daily, and your identity as a nurse is shaped and influenced continuously. Values that you held at the time you began the program have helped you interpret and respond to your new learning and experiences—these values may also shift or change as a result of your professional development. Self-knowledge helps you create meaning in your learning and recognize opportunities for further development.

Most nursing curricula include the development of skills related to reflective analysis. At this point in your program, an asset in the career planning and development process is your ability to reflect on your experiences, their relevance to your professional growth, and how experiences can guide your future learning. The ability to reflect upon and articulate responses to the questions, who am I? and how would I describe myself? is a significant professional and personal strength. Who you are includes your beliefs, values, knowledge, professional competencies, and also your interests, accomplishments, and hopes for the future.

A thorough self-assessment takes dedicated time. You have gathered diverse and challenging experiences that have each contributed to your unique professional identity. After each new experience, return to your self-assessment and reflect on the contribution that experience has made to who you are as a nurse. Your most meaningful experiences, and those that have allowed you to live your values and beliefs most fully, offer guidance and direction as you work on the remaining phases of the Model. Equally informative are those experiences that were not positive or fulfilling. Reflecting on those experiences can also help you clarify your values and articulate your interests and priorities both for your learning and for your continued development as a nurse.

You have also accomplished many things over the course of your nursing education, both curricular and extracurricular. Remember to include these achievements in your self-assessment. Making note of your accomplishments helps you recognize your overall personal and professional growth and development. Ask yourself: If I could live my career vision today, in what ways will my strengths and accomplishments help me progress toward my vision? Confidence in your strengths paves the way for creativity and growth in your career.

Your self-assessment, together with your environmental scan, serves as the foundation of your career planning and development. Neither the self-assessment nor the scan is static. The dynamic nature of your nursing education experiences and your professional career will be reflected in these and all phases of the Model.

Once you have worked through your self-assessment, ask faculty members, nursing peers, preceptors, and other people involved in your life to give you feedback regarding your strengths, unique traits, and areas for development. This aspect of your self-assessment is called the **reality check.** Often the feedback you receive will highlight strengths and attributes that you have not recognized in yourself. More often than not, the reality check is an affirming process that enhances your confidence as you begin to market your competencies, unique attributes, and accomplishments.

Alya can use the self-assessment process to build on the values, interests, and beliefs she identified by examining her current strengths in relation to the strengths she needs to progress toward her vision and also the areas in which her need for development is greatest. By asking others who know her to assess her strengths and achievements during her curricular and extracurricular experiences, Alya will be able to expand and feel confident about her self-assessment. Alya will have a more in-depth understanding of the scope of nursing practice, the areas in which she needs to focus her learning in the coming year, and her potential employment options. She is ready for the next phase of the Model—scanning her environment.

SCANNING YOUR ENVIRONMENT

Scanning the environment is simply taking a good look around to determine how the world around you can help you develop and achieve your career vision and related goals. The process of scanning the environment, together with the knowledge and insight you gleaned from your career vision and self-assessment, provides information about potential opportunities for nursing practice. You will also form ideas of how you can, in the coming year, approach your classroom, practice, and broader professional experiences so that your academic endeavours are congruent with your personal career vision and goals. As

a senior-level student, your scan needs to include information about what is happening outside your academic institution, including current issues within the health care sector and the nursing profession, particularly focusing on your area of interest. You had the opportunity to complete your fundamental practice experiences across diverse settings. You have also had exposure to faculty members with a range of expertise in areas of nursing scholarship and practice. Early and ongoing experiences and contacts serve as the foundation of your environmental scan.

Extending your scan to include awareness of health care issues and trends at national and international levels is important as you contemplate potential opportunities for your first job. Knowing the realities and potentials of the current health care environment can enhance your insight regarding what is "out there" for you and the factors you need to consider as you seek your first nursing position. You can also use data from your scan to further inform your self-assessment, particularly in terms of focusing your learning within classroom and nursing practice courses and keeping abreast of information that you need for entry to practice. Furthermore, what you learn from your scan can help you prepare for an interview and develop the questions you want to ask potential employers. While doing your scan consider the following questions:

- What are the key issues in health care today?
- What are some of the important social and health issues that relate to my areas of professional practice and my location? Nationally? Internationally?
- What are significant nursing issues in my local area, as well as nationally and internationally, that may influence my chosen practice area—and my career more broadly?
- What are global health and social issues?

Like all phases of the Model, scanning is not a one-time activity, but rather a continuous process. You will scan throughout your career to keep on top of current and future opportunities related to your career goals. Sources for your scan can include faculty members, course readings and assignments, professional journals, professional organizations, nursing practice settings, preceptors, the Internet, news media, social media, friends, and your fellow students.

If you are interested in a particular practice setting—in terms of a potential practice placement or future employment—a significant aspect of your scan can involve researching the mission, philosophy, professional practice model, and mandate of an organization overall and of the nursing department specifically. If you can, obtain the job descriptions of positions in your area of interest. By identifying key professional competencies required of the position, you will inform both your self-assessment and your academic and future career planning.

CRITICAL THINKING

Alya has a particular interest in working with children and families in an acute care setting. The third year of her nursing program focused on community health; so she has current knowledge and information related to many health and social issues faced by families within the community context. She will need to explore these issues with acute care health settings in mind—as well as related nursing issues and scopes of practice. Taking some time to review recent publications in the area of family and children's health care will help Alya become informed about the nature of practice, models of care, and current issues in the care of children and families.

Alya's scan can include the faculty members within her school of nursing. One or more faculty members have practice and research expertise in the area of family and children's health, and can serve as excellent resources and mentors! Scanning the acute care health organizations that have a pediatrics department and obtaining nursing job descriptions can provide Alya with valuable information regarding the professional competencies she needs to work in this area of practice.

Alya can also access resources in her provincial professional nursing organization, perhaps including an interest group that focuses on family and children's health.

Alya would like to make sure that she knows as much as possible about the role of a children's and family health nurse so that she can take advantage of learning opportunities, and create new ones, related to her career interest over the coming year.

What are other key sources of information for Alya's environmental scan? What key questions can guide her scan? How can she use her scan to develop a learning plan that would also help her develop competencies related to her career goal?

Your scan will inform and be influenced by your work in all other phases of the Model. It is always a work in progress!

CREATING YOUR STRATEGIC CAREER PLAN

A **strategic career plan** requires you to take the knowledge and skills you have developed in creating learning plans and client care plans and apply this to *your* nursing career. The main difference is that you are doing this for yourself—not to fulfill course requirements, client needs, or the expectations of others. It is your unique and personal action guide.

Like plans you are accustomed to, your strategic career plan should include your vision statement, related career goals, action steps, resources, timelines, and indicators of success. Setting both short- and long-term goals allows you to make realistic and achievable progress toward your vision. Your career vision, self-assessment, and environmental scan, will provide you with the data you need to develop your plan. Your vision shows where you are headed; your assessment has helped you to articulate your strengths, your unique attributes, and the areas you

would like to further develop; and your scan prompted you to identify opportunities and realities related to your areas of interest. Use all of this information to guide you in deciding what you need to do to meet the short- and long-term goals related to your career vision. Your plan transforms your vision from fantasy to reality.

If you are ready to begin your search for the right job, your strategic career plan can focus on the short- and long-term goals related to your ideal job. See Table 22-2 for Alya's strategic career plan.

MARKETING YOURSELF

Marketing means being able to communicate your strengths, interests, and goals with confidence and clarity. You have actually been marketing yourself as a nursing student and future registered nurse throughout your program. In each encounter you have had with clients, nurses, faculty members, and other health care professionals over the course of your nursing education, you have conveyed who and what you are. Perhaps, until now, your marketing has been unintentional. As you complete your nursing education and make plans for your transition to the workplace you need to be intentional in how

TABLE 22-2	**EXAMPLE OF A STRATEGIC CAREER PLAN**

Alya's Strategic Career Plan could look like this:

Alya's Vision: I live in an urban location in my home province with my partner and two dogs. My partner is very supportive of my career and is an equal contributor in all areas of our lives. My two dogs are fun, loving, and always happy to see me! Each day when I head to work, I look forward to making a difference in the lives of children and their families. I work with an amazing interprofessional team of colleagues who is committed to providing a high quality of family-centred care. I work in an acute care pediatric teaching hospital in a downtown health setting. It is a bright and beautiful building. I am involved in direct care of children and families and serve as a resource to my colleagues. I feel confident in my practice and my peers describe me as an expert pediatric nurse, a supportive member of the health care team and an effective formal and informal leader. I am recognized for my ability to work effectively with both families and colleagues. I feel a part of a team that values and respects my contributions—and I theirs. Eventually, I plan to pursue graduate studies to help me prepare to be an advanced practice family health nurse, and the organization in which I work supports advanced education both philosophically and financially.

Career Goal: At the end of my undergraduate nursing education program, I will have the necessary professional competencies to work as a staff nurse and effective interprofessional team member on a pediatric unit in an acute care hospital.

Action Steps—Fall 2011	**Timeline**	**Resources**	**Indicators of Success**
1. Obtain job descriptions of a pediatric staff nurse position and the models of care from three acute care teaching hospitals	September 5, 2011	Hospital websites Human resources departments Nursing education departments	I have copies of three pediatric staff nurse job descriptions and descriptions of their models of care
2. Using the job descriptions, revise my self-assessment to identify existing strengths and areas I need to work on this term to work toward competencies related to pediatric nursing and my current placement setting	September 15, 2011	Job Descriptions of pediatric staff nurse positions, information re: my current practice placement expectations and requirements, previous nursing practice evaluations, and self-assessment	My self-assessment is up-to-date and reflects my strengths and areas for development related to my current placement setting and pediatric job descriptions or models of care
3. Meet with my faculty advisor to review my self-assessment and my career vision so that I can develop learning goals that fit with both my practice setting and my career goal	September 20, 2011	Knowledge of current practice placement expectations and requirements, self-assessment related to practice setting and pediatric staff nurse job description, practice course expectations	I will have a draft learning plan that focuses on learning goals that allow me to develop competencies that prepare me to practice competently in my practice setting and progress toward my career goal

(Continued)

TABLE 22-2	EXAMPLE OF A STRATEGIC CAREER PLAN (CONTINUED)

Action Steps—Fall 2011	Timeline	Resources	Indicators of Success
4. Schedule regular meetings with my mentors to help me focus on my career vision and goals for this term	September 30, 2011	Mentors*	I have regularly scheduled meetings with both of my mentors
5. Join the provincial professional nursing association pediatric nurse interest group	October 30, 2011	Organization website	I am a member of the interest group
6. Attend one pediatric nursing interest group meeting in the fall and winter	End of fall term and end of winter term	Interest group meeting schedule	I will have attended one meeting in the fall and one meeting in the winter
7. Meet with child and family health nurse practitioner mentor to explore option of shadowing a pediatric nurse for a couple of shifts over the holiday break in December	November 15, 2011	Mentor*	I will have arranged a shadowing experience for the holiday break

*See upcoming Marketing Section under Personal Resources for a discussion related to Mentors

you communicate your values, strengths, and identity as a nurse.

Marketing yourself is much easier when your approach genuinely reflects your values, your communication style, and is true to your abilities. The work you have done in your self-assessment will be very helpful because you have already taken the time to consider and articulate your values, strengths, areas for continued development, and your unique attributes. You have the information to engage in informed and intentional self-marketing.

This phase of the Model will help you develop self-marketing strategies that are effective in helping you take advantage of and create career opportunities of significance to you. You use both personal and written resources in your marketing activities. The interview process is a significant marketing strategy as well.

PERSONAL RESOURCES

The most important personal resource you have is YOU! Knowing and having the ability to articulate who you

are, your career vision, and your career goals is your best marketing strategy. A second personal resource can be a mentor. A **mentor** is a person you admire and wish to emulate. A mentor is also someone who takes a personal and professional interest in your career. This individual may practise in your area of interest or exemplify what you believe is the nurse you wish to become. Either way, a mentor can provide you with guidance, support, and opportunities to help you transform your career vision to reality. You can also have more than one mentor: many students and new graduates have a number of individuals who play significant roles in their professional development. A mentor is more than a professional role model; being a mentor is an active role that requires time and commitment on behalf of the mentor and yourself. If you have someone in mind, don't hesitate to formally ask this person to be your mentor. Don't leave it to chance or assume that the person whom you would like to have as your mentor is aware of your feelings. It is an honour to be asked to mentor someone, and people who are able

LITERATURE APPLICATION

Citation: Waddell, J. (2005). Choosing the right graduate program. *Canadian Nurse,* 101(5), 30–31.

Waddell, J., Donner, G. J., & Wheeler, M. M. (2004). *Building your nursing career: A guide for students* (3rd ed.). Toronto: Elsevier Canada.

Discussion: Like any other career decision, the choice to pursue graduate studies need to be informed, responsive to the unique needs of the individual, and congruent with one's career goals. Many excellent graduate programs are offered within and outside of Canada. Finding the right program can be a daunting and sometimes overwhelming task for an undergraduate student. Waddell, together with Donner and Wheeler, describes how students can use the Donner-Wheeler Career Planning and Development Model to plan for their application to graduate studies and position themselves to be successful in achieving admission to graduate programs that fit with their career goals. The authors describe how both beginning and graduating students can approach each of the five phases of the Model (creating your career vision, completing your self-assessment and reality check, scanning your environment, developing your strategic career plan, and marketing yourself), with a particular focus on preparing a winning application for graduate studies. The suggested activities can be initiated at any level of nursing education but have particular relevance to students in final years of their program.

Implications for Students: Engaging in graduate studies is a significant personal and financial investment. Graduate education provides nurses with the opportunity to have a dedicated focus on their area of practice and research interest and expertise. The career planning and development model provides a structure and process to guide students in their exploration and assessment of graduate programs with the goal of choosing the program that will best allow them to achieve their career goals. The broader implication is that active involvement in the career planning process can help nursing students, at any point in their academic and professional practice career, take control of their progress toward both short- and long-term career goals in their pursuit of their career vision.

---

to assume the role benefit as much from the relationship as the mentee. Mentors take their role seriously, and a person who accepts to be your mentor will be making a commitment to you and to your career. Make sure you are in a position to make a commitment to actively work on your career with your mentor.

A third personal resource is **networking** activities. You may already be involved in student organizations, the work of your school of nursing, professional nursing organizations, and your personal and professional communities. If so, you have already benefited from networking and can use your career vision, self-assessment, and scan to continue your professional involvement with a focus on your career vision and goals. However, if you have not been actively involved in extracurricular activities within and outside your education program, it is never too late to start!

Use your environmental scan to learn of opportunities to become involved in professional activities that fit with your interests, areas for development, and overall career goals. Strategic networking can help you identify professional organizations that have interest groups dedicated to a wide range of practice specialties. Involvement in professional groups creates opportunities for you to

meet with nurses who practise in areas of interest to you—and for you to market your interests and strengths. You can also speak with new graduates who work in your areas of interest. New graduates offer helpful advice, particularly to help you prepare for your entry to the workforce. Your mentor can guide you in research related to networking opportunities and can often open doors for you as you move toward the world of professional nursing practice.

A final note regarding personal marketing resources: Be mindful of how you market yourself through social media sources such as Facebook, Twitter, and blogs. Ensure that your telephone voicemail message and your email messages are appropriate for a professional. Don't forget to monitor your personal conversations in public spaces where you may be in the company of health care professionals, clients and their families, faculty members, or the general public—all of whom may be your colleagues or clients now or in the future.

Alya has been an active member of her school of nursing since the first year of her program. She was often the spokesperson of her class when the students wished to give the school feedback regarding the curriculum, school resources, policies, and other matters.

In the second year of her program, she became an active member of the Canadian Nursing Students' Association (CNSA) and was able to travel to CNSA regional and national conferences to represent the school and her student colleagues.

In her third year, Alya was elected to president of the Nursing Course Union at her university. As a result of her involvement in each of these roles, Alya developed excellent skills in leadership, lobbying, organization, and negotiation. She also was able to work with her faculty and get to know them in ways that would be difficult if she had only been exposed to them in the classroom or practice setting. The faculty were also able to observe Alya's growth in her leadership role and to learn of her career aspirations.

Alya asked two faculty members to be her mentors. One mentor exemplified the type of professional to which Alya aspired. This mentor not only had a strong professional presence by being active in a wide range of professional organizations but also was student-centred and knowledgeable. This person introduced Alya to professional organizations that focused on the advancement of the profession at local, national, and international levels. Her second mentor was a faculty member who was a nurse practitioner in child and family health. This individual helped Alya to access professional organizations relevant to her area of interest and opened the door to many opportunities for her to meet new graduates and experienced nurses practising child and family health in acute care settings. Networking within and external to her school of nursing helped her affirm that she was heading in the right direction and to clarify and refine her strengths and career vision. After each experience she can return to phases of the Model to update and review her progress toward her vision. In her fourth year, she plans to join the provincial professional organization's pediatric nurse interest group and the local chapter of Sigma Theta Tau International.

Do not worry if, to date, you have not been active in your nursing program, or your school, college, university or nursing community. You can begin to become actively involved in one or all of these realms of nursing at any time. With your up-to-date vision, self-assessment, and environmental scan, you have what you need to strategically engage in academic and professional activities that will help you progress toward your career goals.

WRITTEN RESOURCES

Written marketing strategies include your résumé, cover letter, and business card. Because your résumé is generally the first opportunity a prospective employer has to see who you are and what you may be able to contribute to the organization, it is your most valuable written self-marketing strategy. A **résumé** is a brief summary of your background, education, and your nursing and related experiences. Generally, a résumé should not be longer than two pages, so it needs to contain concise information that clearly identifies your career objective, your strengths, accomplishments, and experiences that have contributed to your professional development. Cross-referencing your vision, self-assessment and your résumé on an ongoing basis will ensure that your résumé is current and relevant.

A résumé should be honest and easy to read. There is no one perfect résumé style. However, an effective résumé has the following qualities: (1) attracts the employer's interest; (2) identifies the applicant's career objective, education, work experience, and other professional activities that are relevant to the position being applied for; (3) creates a favourable first impression about you and your abilities; (4) conveys that you are someone who is a good fit for the position and the organization; and (5) is visually appealing.

If you have worked through the phases of the Model, you have completed the most difficult aspects of résumé development. Creating a customized résumé to fit the job you are applying for should be a breeze! It is helpful to keep a generic résumé on hand that includes all your education, nursing practice and work experiences, and extracurricular activities. You can then draw from this comprehensive résumé to create customized versions for specific positions.

Although there are two types of résumés—the chronological résumé and the functional résumé—the latter format is better suited to students and new graduates. In the functional résumé, you list your education, employment experiences, and clinical practice experiences in reverse chronological order.

Three unique aspects of a new graduate's résumé are (1) the brief summary of the nursing practice experience; (2) the list of selected practice experiences, outcome competencies, and accomplishments; and (3) documentation of past working experiences, including summer employment. Select practice experiences that are most pertinent to the position you are applying for. Limit the list of your selected nursing practice placements to one or two, choosing only those experiences with responsibilities, accomplishments, and competencies that relate directly to the nursing position you are applying for.

Your résumé should include the following headings:

- Career Objective
- Education
- Selected Practice Placements—with descriptions of outcome, professional competencies, and accomplishments *or*
- Summary of Practice Accomplishments per Year (for third and fourth year)
- Professional Activities
  - Curricular
  - Extracurricular

- Honours and Awards
- Professional Memberships
- Professional Development
- Employment
  - Focus on professional competencies related to the position you are applying for
- Volunteer and Community Activities

This may seem like a lot of information, but if you are concise and use action-oriented words you will be able to include all this information on two pages, allowing for margins of at least 2.5 centimetre (one inch) and adequate white space. Don't be alarmed if you don't have anything to put in some of the categories. Create your generic résumé with all the headings. Gaps in your résumé can help you plan for short- and long-term activities that fit with your career vision and contribute to the development of a comprehensive and impressive résumé. If you have a heading that remains incomplete, do not include it in your résumé, but keep working at it.

Students often find the most difficult task of writing a résumé is describing what they have accomplished using action verbs and phrases with meaning. Weigh your choice of words. Remember, you have the attention of recruiters for an average of 30 seconds only as they review your résumé. Use meaningful phrases, such as *organizational ability, ability to adapt to change, self-directed, excellent problem-solving ability, lifelong learner, and active and contributing team member,* when one word does not fully express a complete thought. When writing your résumé, keep in mind that it is not boasting to write about your strengths and accomplishments. If you do not write about your strengths, you may not have the opportunity to obtain an interview. See Table 22-3 for a summary of action verbs for résumé preparation.

Make sure to use a spell checker and then have someone else review your résumé for any spelling or grammatical errors. When printing a résumé for a nursing position, it is best to use white, ivory, or pale grey paper of good quality. Use a printer that prints clearly and darkly. Choose a legible, professional font, such as Times New Roman or Arial. See Figure 22-2 for Alya's résumé.

Accompany your résumé with a one-page cover letter written on personal letterhead paper. The cover letter has three components. The introduction states the position to which you are applying and where you learned of the position. The second paragraph briefly and broadly highlights your professional strengths related to the position. The final component indicates your interest in participating in an interview and your contact information. Use personal language and focus on what you can do for the unit and organization. See Figure 22-3 for Alya's cover letter.

ELECTRONIC RÉSUMÉS

Many hiring managers and recruiters prefer to receive résumés by email. Electronic résumés can be formatted as a Microsoft Word file, a text file, or a PDF file (Bookey-Bassett, 2004). If employers request an electronic résumé, be sure to send it in the requested format, or check with them if you are unsure which format they prefer. You need to be able to send your résumé via email so that the recipient can read the résumé, regardless of the software the recipient is using. There are several ways to create an electronic résumé, including writing the résumé using

TABLE 22-3	LIST OF ACTION VERBS FOR RÉSUMÉ			
accomplished	delivered	identified	operated	reorganized
achieved	demonstrated	increased	organized	revamped
administered	designed	initiated	oversaw	revised
analyzed	developed	innovated	performed	simplified
approved	directed	instituted	planned	solved
built	earned	launched	proposed	streamlined
communicated	eliminated	listed	provided	supervised
completed	established	maintained	purchased	taught
conceived	evaluated	managed	redesigned	terminated
conducted	expanded	mastered	reduced	trained
contributed	explored	motivated	reengineered	transformed
coordinated	generated	negotiated	reinforced	utilized
created				

Alya Surname
123 City Street, City
Province, Postal Code
Phone, Email

CAREER OBJECTIVE:

To contribute as an interprofessional health team member to holistic, comprehensive, developmental and family-centred nursing care in a tertiary acute pediatric setting. To further my professional development in the care of acutely ill children and families.

EDUCATION:

2003–2007   University Name, BScN
- Expected date of completion April 2007.

AWARDS AND ACHIEVEMENTS:

2004–2006	Dean's List Standing (first, second, and third year of BScN)
May 2006	Induction to Sigma Theta Tau Nursing Honour Society
May 2006	Royal Bank Community Services Award
Jan. 2005	Induction to Golden Key Honour Society
May 2004	Scholarship for Advocacy and Dedication

PROFESSIONAL EXPERIENCE:

Nursing Practice Experience—BScN Program

Selected Family-Centred Care Practice Experiences

Jan. 2005–April 2006   Maternal Infant Program
- Provided family-centred education regarding pain management options; prenatal care via parent groups and individual meetings for parents expecting multiples and singletons; care and counselling to young mothers, through the MIP Young Mothers Program.

Sept. 2004–Dec. 2004   Healthy Babies Healthy Children
- In collaboration with a public health nurse, conducted follow-up phone calls within the first 24 to 48 hours post-delivery to new mothers. Assessment of mother and infant conducted over the phone, with the option for additional home visit to mother and child. Pre- and postnatal home visits to provide education regarding issues, such as general infant well-being and safety. Neonatal physical assessment provided in home. Developed competence in the provision of family-centred care within the community context.
- Co-facilitation of high-risk parenting program aimed at empowering parents and interprofessional education related to parenting styles, child development, behaviour, discipline, nutrition, and stress.

Other Nursing Practice Experiences—BScN Program

Sept. 2005–Dec. 2005:	"Name of Hospital" Hospital Medical Oncology
Jan. 2004–May 2004:	"Name of Hospital" Nephrology/Medicine
Sept. 2003–Dec. 2003:	"Name of Hospital" Alternate Level of Care Unit

LEADERSHIP ACTIVITIES:

Jan. 2005–Current: Collaborative Nursing Degree Program Evaluation Committee
- Elected student member of a faculty/placement partner/student committee to evaluate implementation and outcomes of Collaborative Degree Program. Active participation in the initiation of formal evaluation processes and data analysis.

Figure 22-2 Alya's Résumé

May 2002 Current: University Nursing Course Union
- Two terms as president, one term as past-president (current)
- Represented collaborative program students on student council, under the nursing division, to coordinate social, political, and educational events. Liaison between the student body and administration.

Sept. 2003–May 2005:   University Academic Student Council-Student Member
- Student voting member on the academic council, to represent the student vote in such matters as curriculum changes and program entrance requirements.

EMPLOYMENT EXPERIENCES:

May–Aug. 2004–2006:   "Name" Retirement Centre—Personal Care Assistant Summer Employment
- Worked collaboratively with health profession team to provide individualized, developmental care to senior residents. Utilized positive and effective communication skills. Acknowledged for strengths in conveying compassion, sensitivity, and respect to residents and their families. Reliable and responsible; active member of the health care team.

COMMUNITY INVOLVEMENT: Sept. 2005–May 2006:   Volunteer with the Children's Wish Foundation.

REFERENCES: Available upon request.

Figure 22-2 Continued

Alya's cover letter for a new graduate position could be the following.

Alya Surname
123 City Street, City
Province, Postal Code
Phone and Email

Date
Name of Individual Noted on Job Posting

Title
Address

Dear "Name of Individual,"

I am writing in response to the advertisement posted in the Pediatric Nurse Interest Group April 2007 newsletter for a staff nurse position in the General Pediatric Medical Unit of your organization.

I will be graduating from my nursing baccalaureate program in May 2007. Over the course of my education, I have focused on the development of professional competencies relevant to the care of children experiencing acute illness and their families. I am committed to the concept and practice of developmental and family-centred care, a value that is strongly supported in your organization. I look forward to continuing my professional development in child and family health and, as a member of the interprofessional health care team, contributing to quality family-centred care within your program.

Figure 22-3 Alya's Cover Letter

My enclosed résumé details how my nursing practice placements and related educational experiences have prepared me to fulfill the requirements of your staff nurse position. I would appreciate the opportunity to discuss my potential contribution to your general pediatric medical unit program. I look forward to hearing from you. Thank you for your consideration.

Sincerely,
[Signature]

Alya Surname
Enclosure: Résumé

Figure 22-3 Continued

TABLE 22-4	CREATING AN ELECTRONIC RÉSUMÉ
Step 1	In the word processing program, set margins so that 16.25 centimetres (6.5 inches) of text are displayed. This amount of text is easily viewed by the majority of email programs.
Step 2	Write the résumé using an easy-to-read font in 12-point type, such as Arial or Times New Roman.
Step 3	Save the résumé as a text-only file with line breaks. Do not use the Tab key. Use the space bar instead. Format the text with left justification.
Step 4	Open this new file in a text editor, such as Microsoft Notepad.
Step 5	Review the résumé to see how the recipient will see it once it is transmitted via email. Pay careful attention to unsupported formats or those formats that your word processing program may not be able to read. You may have to add ASCII-supported characters, such as asterisks, to make the résumé easier to view. Proofread!
Step 6	Copy and paste the résumé in the body of a test email message. Send it back to yourself or to a friend who uses a different email program to see how the recipient views your résumé.
Step 7	When applying for a job electronically, a cover letter should also accompany your résumé. Rather than sending both the cover letter and the résumé in the text area, or as separate attachments, the preferred approach is to send the cover letter in the text portion of the email and attach the résumé.

Source: Adapted from Smith, Rebecca (1999). *Electronic Resumes and Online Networking.* Franklin Lakes, N.J.: Career Press, p. 72.

standard word processing software, such as Microsoft Word or Corel WordPerfect. For tips on creating an electronic résumé, see Table 22-4.

Type the résumé using word processing software and then save it in one of three formats: ASCII plain text (.txt), rich-text (.rtf), or as hypertext (.html). ASCII text files are the most common types of data files found on the Internet. This file type allows for simplicity in reading the text but does not allow any type of text format-ting, such as boldface characters, bullets, underlining, or italics. The recipient receives plain, clear text without any identifying marks, tabs, or visually appealing format-ting. If you want to highlight a specific area, you can use a character such as an asterisk (*).

It is important to use keywords when sending an electronic résumé. When recruiters are looking for someone with specific skills, they often perform a search using keywords such as *pediatric nurse practitioner* or *oncology registered nurse.* Be sure to use correct grammar, spelling, and punctuation.

BUSINESS CARDS

Business cards are a way to introduce yourself to others and provide them with your contact information in a professional manner. As you increase your networking activities at job fairs, conferences, and other professional forums, a business card is an important and often requested self-marketing tool. Student business cards can include your name, phone number, and email address (preferably your academic or student email address). Like your résumé and cover letter, your business card should be easy to read, printed on material that is neutral in colour and professional in appearance. You can have business cards made at stationery and business retail stores. You can also find many websites where you can create and print your own business card.

PREPARING FOR AN INTERVIEW

As you prepare for an interview, it is a good idea to scan the environment with a particular focus on the organization to which you are applying and on current issues and practices that are relevant to the position that you will be discussing in your interview. Information that you should research prior to the interview and that can be located on the organization's website includes the following:

- specific job description
- vision and mission statement of the organization
- vision and mission of the department of nursing
- professional practice model or theory adopted by the department of nursing

Also make sure that you are informed regarding the following details:

- type of interview you can expect (e.g., individual or panel, behavioural)
- time, date, and location—particularly if the organization has more than one site

Remember that the interview is a mutual discovery process. The organization needs to make sure that you are appropriate and prepared to fulfill the requirements of the job; you need to know that the organization is a place where you can both contribute and progress toward your career vision. Prepare some questions to ask based on your values, self-assessment, and career vision. Be ready to articulate how your skills, expertise, and accomplishments meet the position requirements. You can also anticipate the questions you may be asked (see Table 22-5) and prepare your answers to those questions. Remember to keep your responses concise and clear. It is a good idea to practise interviewing with a friend or your mentor.

TABLE 22-5	POTENTIAL INTERVIEW QUESTIONS

- Tell us about yourself, your background, your education, and your short- and long-term career goals.
- Where do you see yourself in five years?
- What words best describe you? How would your colleagues describe you? How will your references describe you?
- Describe a difficult work situation you have had to deal with. How did you handle it?
- What are your strengths? What do you see as your areas for development?
- Why do you want to work for this organization? Why do you want this job?
- Why should we hire you?
- How can you make a difference to this organization?
- What is your philosophy of nursing? What does nursing mean to you?
- Describe a situation that demonstrates your ability to adapt to changes at work.
- Describe the best advisor/faculty member/supervisor you have ever worked with. What made them the best?

Sources: From G.J. Donner & M.M. Wheeler, *Taking Control of Your Nursing Career,* 2nd edition (p. 84). Copyright © 2004 Elsevier Canada, a division of Reed Elsevier Canada, Ltd. All rights reserved. Reprinted with permission of Elsevier Canada, 2011.

On the day of the interview, plan your time well and expect to arrive early. Bring a copy of your résumé so that you can refer to it in the event that an interviewer poses specific questions related to its content. Be polite and respectful to everyone in the organization. Remember that you are marketing yourself to everyone you encounter during the interview process, including support personnel who are often your first contact.

You will also be offered the opportunity to ask questions of the interviewer, so be prepared with several questions that help you understand how the organization can support both your practice as a new graduate and your short- and long-term career goals. Feel free to write your questions down so that you don't forget them. If your questions have been answered do not feel that you have to ask a question that is not relevant to you. You can simply say that the questions that you had coming into the interview have been answered during the interview process. For samples of questions to ask during an interview, see Table 22-6.

A NOTE ABOUT REFERENCES

Your references play a key role in marketing your professional strengths to potential employers. Like your résumés, your choice of referees should be specific to the job you are applying for. Make sure that you contact your desired referees and ask if they would be willing to provide you with a positive reference. Provide your potential referee with an updated résumé and a description of the job for which you are asking them to serve as a reference. Let them know the date of your interview and when they may be contacted by the employer.

If, after the interview, you are interested in pursuing the position, offer the potential employer the names and contact information for the referees you have chosen for this position. Immediately following your interview, contact your chosen referees to let them know how the interview went, and if there are any areas that you would like them to focus on in their discussion with the employment agency. Referees are often interested in whether you were successful in your interview and if you accepted the position. Send a written note offering thanks for serving as your reference and updating them on the outcome.

You are on your way! You can now use The Donner-Wheeler Career Planning and Development Model to orchestrate the final years of your program and create the path to your future—Enjoy!

TABLE 22-6	SAMPLE QUESTIONS TO ASK DURING AN INTERVIEW

- What type of orientation would I receive?
- How can I prepare myself to be a successful member of the nursing team?
- What resources will I have access to during my orientation?
- What are the ongoing opportunities for professional development?
- What other health care providers work on this team/service/program? What is the skill mix?
- What do you think will be the major challenges of this position?
- How are the working hours scheduled?
- How would you describe the ideal candidate for this position?
- How are preceptors assigned?
- How long would I work with a preceptor?
- What are the next steps in the hiring process?
- When will the hiring decision be made?

Sources: Adapted from G.J. Donner & M.M. Wheeler, *Taking Control of Your Nursing* Career, 2nd edition (p. 85). Copyright © 2004 Elsevier Canada, a division of Reed Elsevier Canada, Ltd. All rights reserved. Reprinted with permission of Elsevier Canada, 2011.

KEY CONCEPTS

- Career planning and development can begin at any point in your academic or professional practice career.

- The Donner-Wheeler Career Planning and Development Model (the Model) offers students and registered nurses a structure and process to take control of their career.

- Career development is not a one-time activity and does not need to follow a step-by-step process. You can move back and forth among the phases as you gather more experiences and learn more about yourself and your wishes for your career.

- The Model can be used to help you prepare for specific goals, such as applying to graduate programs and choosing your first job.

- Your career vision is your guide for reflection and action.

- A strategic career plan is your blueprint for action.

- You market yourself with every professional encounter.

- Information and insights gathered from your work in each phase of the Model informs your résumé and helps you to prepare for interviews.

- The interview is a mutual process of discovery—you are an active participant in the interview.

- You don't have to be a registered nurse to have a business card. A business card is a professional means of communication, particularly during your networking activities.

- A mentor can guide your career development and open doors for you.

KEY TERMS

career vision
marketing
mentor
networking
reality check

résumé
scanning the
  environment
self-assessment
strategic career plan

REVIEW ACTIVITIES

1. Write your career vision in narrative form, answering all of the questions on pages 444–445 in as much detail as possible.

2. With your career vision in mind, begin your self-assessment. Identify three key values, three related strengths, and three areas that you need to develop further to actualize your vision.

3. Based on your career vision and self-assessment, develop a short-term career goal that you can work on in the next six months.

4. After reviewing the work you have accomplished in the previous three activities, develop four interview questions that, when answered, will help you determine whether the position will be congruent with your values and help you meet your career goals.

5. List three qualities you would like in a mentor.

6. Identify one potential mentor.

REVIEW QUESTIONS

1. Which of the following is the best response to the interview question, What are your strengths?
   A. "I have many. Where do you want me to begin?"
   B. "My professional and therapeutic communication skills have been acknowledged as strong."
   C. "I think I am well liked and get along with everyone."
   D. "Well, I am just a new nurse without many strengths right now, but I am enthusiastic and a fast learner."

2. Which of the following components are absolutely necessary to include in a résumé?
   A. Identifying information, career objective, formal education, educational experiences, employment experiences, and professional and community involvement.
   B. Identifying information, employment experiences, education, professional organizations, and awards and honours.
   C. Identifying information, employment experiences, education, professional organizations, and references.
   D. Identifying information, employment experiences, education, and professional organizations.

3. When creating an electronic résumé, which of the following is essential?
   A. setting margins so that 17.5 centimetres (7 inches) of text are displayed in a word processing program
   B. using a type font in 12 point, such as Arial or Times New Roman
   C. saving the résumé using the right justification format
   D. using the bold and underline function in the résumé as a way of highlighting information

4. What is the primary function of a cover letter?
   A. to entice the prospective employer to become interested enough to read the résumé
   B. to have a letter to include with your résumé
   C. to include references not listed on a résumé
   D. to reiterate all that is on your résumé

REFERENCES

Bookey-Bassett, S. (2004). Marketing yourself. In G. J. Donner & M. M. Wheeler (Eds.), *Taking control of your nursing career* (pp. 63–90). Toronto: Elsevier.

Donner, G. J. (2004). Taking control of your nursing career: The future is now. In G. J. Donner & M. M. Wheeler (Eds.), *Taking control of your nursing career* (pp. 3–11). Toronto: Elsevier.

Donner, G. J., & Wheeler, M. M. (Eds.). (1994). *Taking control of your nursing career*. Toronto: Elsevier.

Donner, G. J., & Wheeler, M. M. (Eds.). (2009). *Taking control of your nursing career*. Toronto: Elsevier.

Smith, R. (1999). *Electronic résumés and online networking*. Franklin Lakes, NJ: Career Press.

Waddell, J. (2005). Choosing the right graduate program. *Canadian Nurse, 101*(5), 30–31.

Waddell, J., Donner, G. J., & Wheeler, M. M. (2009). *Building your nursing career: A guide for students* (3rd ed.). Toronto: Elsevier.

SUGGESTED READINGS

Bolles, R. N. (2003). What color is your parachute? A practical manual for job-hunters and career changers. Berkeley, CA: Ten Speed Press.

Stovall, P., & Teddlie, J. (1993). Student guide to bias-free career planning: Opening all options. Columbus, OH: Career, Education, and Training Associates.

Wickman, F., & Sjodin, T. (1997). Mentoring: A success guide for mentors and protégés. Chicago: Irwin.

Something unforeseen and magnificent is happening. Health care, having in our time entered its dark night of the soul, shows signs of emerging, transformed. (Barbara Dossey & Larry Dossey)

CANADIAN REGISTERED NURSE EXAMINATION

Each provincial or territorial nursing regulatory body in Canada is responsible for ensuring that the individuals it registers as nurses meet an acceptable level of competence before beginning to practise.

The level of competence of registered nurses in all provinces and territories except Québec is measured, in part, by the Canadian Registered Nurse Examination (CRNE). The Canadian Nurses Association (CNA) develops and maintains the CRNE through its testing company, Assessment Strategies Inc., and in collaboration with the regulatory authorities. The provincial and territorial nursing regulatory authorities administer the exam and determine eligibility to write it.

The purpose of the CRNE is to protect the public by ensuring that entry-level registered nurses possess the competencies required to practise safely and effectively.

EXAMINATION LENGTH AND FORMAT

The RN Exam consists of approximately 200 multiple choice questions.

ITEM PRESENTATION

The multiple-choice questions are presented either as case-based or independent questions. Case-based questions are presented as a set of three to five questions associated with a brief health care scenario. Independent questions each contain the information necessary to answer the questions.

The Canadian Registered Nurse Examination Prep Guide (2010) indicates that there are 148 competencies that make up the content domain for the CRNE. Each question on the CRNE is linked to one of these competencies. The framework and definitions of the four competency categories are relevant to the June 2010–May 2015 exam. Some of the competencies lend themselves to one or more categories, so they should be viewed as an organizing mechanism only.

CRNE PREPARATION TOOLS

The CNA, the developer and owner of the CRNE, offers two official tools to assist candidates studying for the exam. These two tools, the Canadian Registered Nurse Exam Prep Guide and the LeaRN™ CRNE Readiness Test, complement each other to help candidates prepare for the CRNE.

CANADIAN REGISTERED NURSE EXAM (CRNE) PREP GUIDE[1]

The CRNE Prep Guide is a study guide in print format with an accompanying CD-ROM. Available in either English or French, the prep guide offers 200 multiple-choice practice questions. The CD-ROM allows students to study questions by format or by content category, with an additional 50 questions. This affords the student the opportunity to receive immediate feedback, create a performance profile and focus on competencies where you need practice.

The guide also provides the following tools:

1. answers and explanations to help you learn;
2. a performance profile to identify your strengths and weaknesses; and
3. valuable test-taking strategies and study tips.

You may purchase the CRNE Prep Guide from your school bookstore or from the CNA Bookstore at sales@cna-aiic.ca or by calling 1-800-385-5881. CNA's prep guide price is $74.95 plus taxes and shipping and handling.

LEARN CRNE READINESS TEST[2]

The LeaRN CRNE Readiness Test is the first of a series of tools and resources trademarked under the title LeaRN, which will be offered by the Canadian Nurses Association. These resources are provided to assist nurses to meet the requirements to be registered as RNs in Canada, and to integrate into the Canadian health care system.

The LeaRN CRNE Readiness Test will help to assess readiness to take the Canadian Registered Nurse Examination (CRNE). The CRNE is part of the registration requirements for nurses in all provinces or territories in Canada, with the exception of Québec. For additional information on the Québec exam, visit the website of Ordre des infirmières et infirmiers du Québec (www.oiiq.org).

COMPETENCY FRAMEWORK[3]

A framework was developed to identify and organize the competencies the CRNE should assess. The resulting framework reflects a primary health care nursing model. The framework and definitions of the four framework categories are presented below. The number of competencies in each category is indicated in parentheses following the category name. The number of competencies in each category does not necessarily reflect the importance of each area of competency in the practice of nursing.

PROFESSIONAL PRACTICE (28 COMPETENCIES)

Each nurse is accountable for safe, competent, and ethical nursing practice. Professional practice occurs within the context of the CNA Code of Ethics for Registered Nurses (2008) and provincial or territorial standards of practice and legislation. Nurses are expected to demonstrate professional conduct as reflected by attitudes, beliefs, and values espoused in the Code of Ethics for Registered Nurses. Professional practice in nursing involves the demonstration of teamwork, leadership attributes, basic management skills, advocacy, and political awareness. Leadership attributes, such as vision, knowledge, initiative, integrity, confidence, communication, and innovation, are necessary for the advancement of nursing practice, the nursing profession, and health care delivery systems. Entry-level management skills involve

the ability to work within an organization using appropriate resources to achieve the organization's mission and vision. Professional practice includes awareness of the need for, and the ability to ensure, continued professional development. Professional development involves the capacity to perform self-assessments, seek feedback, and plan self-directed learning activities that foster professional growth. Nurses are expected to know how to locate and use results of research findings to inform and build an evidence-based practice.

NURSE-CLIENT PARTNERSHIP (14 COMPETENCIES)

The nurse-client partnership focuses on the therapeutic use of self, communication skills, nursing knowledge and collaboration to achieve the client's identified health goals. This partnership is a purposeful, goal-directed relationship between nurse and client that is directed at advancing the best interest and health outcome of clients.

HEALTH AND WELLNESS (27 COMPETENCIES)

Nursing competencies in this category are focused on recognizing and valuing health and wellness. This category encompasses health promotion, illness and injury prevention, and the implementation of community or societal approaches. Practice is guided by the principles of primary health care. Nurses work in partnership with communities to influence the determinants of health, with the goal of enabling people to increase control over their health and to improve their health. Nurses partner with individuals to develop personal skills, create supportive environments for health, strengthen community action, reorient health services, and build healthy public policy. Practice reflects changes in cultural composition, demographics, health trends, and economic factors (e.g., an aging population and globalization).

CHANGES IN HEALTH (79 COMPETENCIES)

Nursing competencies in this category involve care across the lifespan for the person experiencing alterations in health that require acute, chronic, rehabilitative, or palliative care. Such care may be delivered across a range of institutional and community settings. Essential aspects of nursing involve critical thinking, problem solving, and decision making in providing care. Using current knowledge, nurses collaborate with the person and other health professionals to identify health priorities. In responding to and managing health issues, the aim of nursing is to promote maximal independence and to maintain optimal quality of life or ensure that individuals at the end of life experience a peaceful death.

Canadian Practical Nurse Registration Examination

Licensed practical nurses write a national exam, called the Canadian Practical Nurse Registration Examination (CPNRE). Starting in January 2012, the CPNRE will consist of 180–200 objective multiple-choice questions. There is one Test Book that is written over a four-hour period.

The Canadian Practical Nurse (PN) Exam Prep Guide will help you to prepare to write the Canadian Practical Nurse Registration Exam. The Prep Guide will enable you to become familiar with the format of the actual examination and provide you with information on the content of the exam. It contains a full length Practice Exam which will help you to review and integrate the concepts you have learned in your program of study. It will help you to assess your skill in applying that knowledge. After you have completed the exam, you can create your Performance Profile to identify your strengths and weaknesses. To purchase the Prep Guide, you can obtain it at your school bookstore or by calling 1-888-562-5561. The cost is $74.95 plus tax.

Two predictor tests are available. Each predictor test comprises 100 multiple-choice questions, matching the Blueprint for the Canadian Practical Nurse Registration Examination.[4] Predictor Test 1 and Predictor Test 2 have completely different sets of questions, but are similar in difficulty. Both tests contain case-based and independent questions. Each test is available in both French and English, and students can switch freely between languages while taking the test.

The test comes equipped with a timer to simulate an actual examination environment. However, you can continue taking the test after time has "been called." If, for some reason, you have to stop the test before completing it, you will be able to return to the test later, provided you have not yet submitted your answers. Once you have completed the test and submitted your answers, you will be presented with your results. You will not be able to re-enter the test; however, if you log in again at any time after completing the test, you will be able to view the results page. The results will also be available for printing by using the link that will be sent to you by email.

The predictor tests are most useful when taken under test-like conditions. You should adhere to the time limits (2.5 hours for each test), and not use any notes or textbooks when taking the tests. The prediction of readiness to take the CPNRE will only be meaningful and useful if you follow these instructions and complete the predictor tests without any assistance. The predictor tests are designed to help you focus your future studying and to help you gauge your readiness for the CPNRE. If you require a practice test, it is recommended that you consider the Canadian PN Exam Prep Guide.

See the Canadian Practical Nurse Registration Examination Blueprint for 2012–2016 for important information related to the competencies candidates will be measured against. This can be found at http://www.cpnre.ca/examblueprint_e.asp.

Endnotes

1. "Canadian Registered Nurse Exam (CRNE) Prep Guide." Retrieved from http://www.cna-nurses.ca/CNA/nursing/rnexam/preptools/default_e.aspx

2. "LeaRN CRNE Readiness Test." Retrieved from http://www.cna-nurses.ca/CNA/nursing/rnexam/preptools/learn/default_e.aspx

3. Retrieved from http://www.cna-nurses.ca/CNA/nursing/rnexam/competencies/default_e.aspx

4. "Format of the Test." Retrieved from http://cpnre.ca/predictor_format_e.asp

ABBREVIATIONS

AAHP	American Association of Health Plans
AC	Accreditation Canada
ACHHR	Advisory Committee on Health Human Resources
ACEN	Academy of Canadian Executive Nurses
AHRQ	Agency for Healthcare Research and Quality
AHS	Aboriginal Head Start
AIDS	Acquired Immune Deficiency Syndrome
ALOS	average length of stay
ALS	amyotrophic lateral sclerosis
AMA	American Medical Association
AMI	Acute Myocardial Infarction
ANA	American Nurses Association
ANCC	American Nurses Credentialing Center
ARDS	acute respiratory distress syndrome
ASA	acetylsalicylic acid
BCNU	British Columbia Nurses Union
BSN	bachelor of science in nursing
CACCN	Canadian Association of Critical Care Nurses
CADTH	Canadian Agency for Drugs and Technologies in Health
CARP	Canadian Association for the Fifty-Plus
CASN	Canadian Association of Schools of Nursing
CCHL	Canadian College of Health Leaders
CCOHS	Canadian Centre for Occupational Health and Safety
CCS	Canadian Cancer Society
CCU	coronary care unit
CDSMP	Chronic Disease Self-Management Program
CEO	chief executive officer
CERN	Conseil Européen pour la Recherche Nucléaire (European Laboratory for Particle Physics)
CEU	continuing education unit
CFNU	Canadian Federation of Nurses Unions
CHA	Canada Health Act
CHA	Canadian Healthcare Association
CHC	Community Health Centre
CHE	Certified Health Executive
CHPCA	Canadian Hospice Palliative Care Association
CHSRF	Canadian Health Services Research Foundation
CHST	Canada Health and Social Transfer
CIHI	Canadian Institute for Health Information
CIHR	Canadian Institutes of Health Research
CINAHL	Cumulative Index to Nursing and Allied Health Literature
CIPS	Canadian Information Processing Society
CIS	clinical information system
CLC	Canadian Labour Congress
CMA	Canadian Medical Association
CMG	case mix group
CNA	Canadian Nurses Association
CNAC	Canadian Nursing Advisory Committee
CNIA	Canadian Nurses Informatics Association
CNSA	Canadian Nursing Students' Association

COACH	Canadian Organization for Advancement of Computers in Health
CPHA	Canadian Public Health Association
CPHI	Canadian Population Health Initiative
CPR	cardiopulmonary resuscitation
CPNRE	Canadian Practical Nurse Registration Examination
CQI	continuous quality improvement
CRNE	Canadian Registered Nurse Examination
DER-CA	Diabetes Education Resource for Children and Adolescents
DM	disease management
DNR	Do not resuscitate
DRG	diagnosis-related group
EBP	evidence-based practice
ECE	early childhood education
ED	emergency department
EHR	electronic health record
EI	emotional intelligence
EMT	emergency medical technician
ENIAC	Electronic Numerical Integrator and Computer
EPC	evidence-based practice centre
ERG	existence-relatedness-growth theory (Alderfer, 1969)
EXTRA	Executive Training for Research Application
FASD	Fetal Alcohol Spectrum Disorder
FIIQ	Fédération des Infirmiers et Infirmié res du Québec
FLAT	Factual, Legible, Accurate, Timely
FTE	full-time equivalent
GDP	gross domestic product
GRADE	Grading of Recommendations, Assessments, Development and Evaluation
HEAL	Health Action Lobby
HIV	human immunodeficiency virus
HPI	Human Poverty Index
ICFASD	Interdepartmental Committee on Fetal Alcohol Spectrum Disorder
ICN	International Council of Nurses
ICU	intensive care unit
IMCN	intermediate care nursery
IOM	Institute of Medicine
ISMP Canada	Institute for Safe Medication Practices Canada
JCAHO	Joint Commission on Accreditation of Healthcare Organizations
KTE	Knowledge Transfer and Exchange
LHINs	Local Health Integration Networks
LOS	length of stay
LPI	leadership practices inventory
LPN	licensed practical nurse
MDGs	Millennium Development Goals
MEDLARS	Medical Literature Analysis and Retrieval System
MeSH	Medical Subject Headings
MIS	management information systems
MLOA	maternity leave of absence
MOHLTC	[Ontario] Ministry of Health and Long-Term Care
MRI	Magnetic Resonance Imaging
MS-HUG	Microsoft Healthcare Users Group
MSN	master's degree in nursing
NCSBN	National Council of State Boards of Nursing
NGC	National Guideline Clearinghouse
NHPPD	nursing hours per patient day

NHSRU	Nursing Health Services Research Unit
NICU	Neonatal Intensive Care Unit
NLM	National Library of Medicine
NNA	national nursing association
NWIG-AMIA	Nursing Working Informatics Group of the American Medical Informatics Association
OACHA	Ontario Advisory Committee on HIV/AIDS
OECD	Organisation for Economic Co-operation and Development
OHIH	Office of Health and the Information Highway
OLRB	Ontario Labour Relations Board
OR	operating room
P3s	public–private partnerships
PAHO	Pan American Health Organization
PBMA	program budgeting and marginal analysis
PC	personal computer
PCS	patient classification system
PDCA	Plan-Do-Check-Act
PDSA	Plan-Do-Study-Act
PERT	Program Evaluation and Review Technique
P-F-A	purpose-focus-approach
PFI	public finance initiative
PHAC	Public Health Agency of Canada
PHC	Primary Health Care
PHIPA	Personal Health Information Protection Act
PI	performance improvement
PIPEDA	Personal Information Protection and Electronic Documents Act
POSDCORB	planning, organizing, supervising, directing, coordinating, reporting, and budgeting
PRP	Participative Resolution Program
QA	quality assurance
QI	quality improvement
RIW	resource intensity weight
RN	registered nurse
RNABC	Registered Nurses Association of British Columbia
RNAO	Registered Nurses Association of Ontario
ROPs	Required Organizational Practices
RPN	registered practical nurse
RPN	registered psychiatric nurse
SARS	Severe Acute Respiratory Syndrome
SPAN	Staff Planning Action Network
SRNA	Saskatchewan Registered Nurses Association
SWOT	strengths, weaknesses, opportunities, threats
TB	tuberculosis
TQM	total quality management
UC	ubiquitous computing
UCP	unregulated care provider
UNA	United Nurses of Alberta
URL	uniform resource locator
UTI	urinary tract infection
VR	virtual reality
WHO	World Health Organization
WWW	World Wide Web

GLOSSARY

accommodating Satisfying the needs of others, sometimes at the expense of self. (p. 135)

accountability Liability for actions. (pp. 48, 248)

accounting An activity that nurse managers engage in to record and report financial transactions and data. (p. 209)

achievement Accomplishment of goals through effort. (p. 319)

active euthanasia A deliberate act in which body processes necessary to sustain life are actively interfered with or interrupted. (p. 422)

activities of daily living Tasks related to toileting, bathing, grooming, dressing, feeding, mobility, and verbal and written personal communication. (p. 108)

adjourning The fifth and final stage of group development, in which the group has met its objectives and the primary focus is closure activities and the termination of team relationships. (p. 194)

administrative principles General principles of management that are relevant to any organization. (p. 164)

advance directives Documents whose purpose is twofold: to ensure that a person's wishes are carried out when that person is no longer able to communicate, and to appoint a specific person, a substitute decision maker, to ensure those wishes are carried out. (p. 422)

affiliation Associations and relationships with others. (p. 319)

altruism The unselfish concern for the welfare of others. (p. 45)

anticipatory grief Grief that starts when one receives bad news; it is felt by both client and family and is an expression of loss, lost dreams, and anticipation of a downhill trajectory of illness and approaching death. (p. 400)

assault A threat of touching another in an offensive manner without that person's permission. (p. 377)

assisted suicide The act of intentionally killing oneself with the assistance of another who deliberately provides the knowledge, means, or both (Special Senate Committee on Euthanasia and Assisted Suicide, 1995). (p. 423)

attending Active listening to gain an understanding of the client's message. (p. 132)

auditory Pertaining to hearing. (p. 127)

authority A person's right to delegate, based on the provincial or territorial nursing scope of practice, and based on that person also receiving official power from an agency to delegate. (p. 249)

autocratic leadership A centralized decision-making style with the leader making decisions and using power to command and control others. (p. 173)

autonomy The ability to self-govern and to have control over decision making concerning one's own life. (p. 414)

avoiding Retreating. (p. 135)

balanced scorecard Documentation tool providing a snapshot image of pertinent information and activity reflecting a point in time. (p. 209)

battery The touching of another person without that person's consent. (p. 377)

benchmarking The continual and collaborative discipline of measuring and comparing the results of key work processes with those of the best performers. (pp. 225, 335)

beneficence Considering and acting in the best interests of others. (p. 414)

best research evidence Methodologically sound, clinically relevant research on the effectiveness and safety of nursing interventions, the accuracy and precision of nursing assessment measures, the power of prognostic markers, the strength of causal relationships, the cost-effectiveness of nursing interventions, and the meaning of illness to client experiences. (p. 64)

bioethics Ethical inquiry in response to new technologies, choices, and concerns in matters of maintaining and intervening in the lives of human beings, such as health care, research, and the environment; sometimes this is referred to as health care ethics or biomedical ethics. (p. 412)

blended payment schemes A payment method that combines both capitation and salary models; for example, a physician might receive both a salary and an incentive based on services provided over and above the core services. (p. 52)

bureaucratic organization Hierarchy with clear superior-subordinate communication and relations, based on positional authority, in which orders from the top are transmitted down through the organization via a clear chain of command. (p. 164)

Canadian Federation of Nurses Unions (CFNU) The organization for Canada's nursing unions that promotes nurses and the nursing profession at the national level. (p. 437)

Canadian Nurses Association (CNA) The professional organization representing the nation's entire registered nurse population. (p. 437)

capital budget The accounting of the purchases of major new or replacement equipment. (p. 208)

capitation Payment of a fixed dollar amount, per person, for the provision of health services to a client population for a specified period of time (e.g., one month). (p. 52)

case-costing A method for operationalizing activity-based costing (ABC). (p. 56)

care delivery model A method of organizing the work of caring for clients. (p. 222)

career vision A description developed in phase three of the Donner-Wheeler Career Planning and Development Model, in which individuals express where they want to go in their career—essentially a description of who and what a person wishes to become. (p. 446)

case management A strategy to improve client care and reduce costs through coordination of care. (p. 240)

case mix groups (CMGs) A Canadian client classification system used to group and describe types of clients discharged from acute-care hospitals. (p. 224)

change To make something different from what it was. (p. 292)

change agent An individual who is responsible for implementation of a change project. (p. 299)

chaplain A member of the health team responsible for spiritual and religious care. Chaplains are most often trained and ordained in their own faith, but act in a multi-faith capacity to provide spiritual and religious care for all; chaplains are in health care, the military, and corrections facilities. (p. 400)

civil law A body of rules and legal principles that govern relations, rights, and obligations among individuals, corporations, or other institutions. (p. 375)

clarifying Restating, rephrasing, or questioning a message to help make its meaning clear. (p. 132)

client acuity A measure of nursing workload that is generated for each client. (p. 224)

client-centred care A care delivery model in which care and services are brought to the client. (p. 170)

client-focused clinical information system A system in which automation supports client care processes; typical applications include order entry, results reporting, clinical documentation, care planning, and clinical pathways. (p. 90)

clinical information system (CIS) A collection of software programs and associated hardware that supports the entry, retrieval, update, and analysis of client care information and associated clinical information related to client care. (p. 90)

clinical ladder A promotional model that acknowledges that staff members have varying skill sets based on their education and experience; therefore, depending on skills and experience, staff members may be rewarded differently and carry differing responsibilities for client care and the governance and professional practice of the work unit. (p. 280)

clinical pathway A care management tool that outlines the expected clinical course and outcomes for a specific client type. (p. 240)

clinical practice guidelines Evidence-based statements of best practice in the prevention, diagnosis, or management of a given symptom, disease, or condition for individual clients. (p. 240)

collaborating Resolving conflict so that both parties are satisfied. (p. 135)

collective action A method of dealing with problems by acting as a group with a single voice. (p. 431)

collective bargaining The practice of employees negotiating as a collective group with management in reference to wages, work practice, and other benefits. (p. 431)

collective bargaining agent An individual who works with employees to formalize collective bargaining though unionization. (p. 435)

committee A work group with a specific task or goal to accomplish. (p. 192)

common law The body of law that develops from precedents set by judicial decisions that, over time, have the force of law, as distinguished from legislative enactments. (p. 373)

Community Health Centres (CHCs) Nonprofit organizations that provide primary health and health promotion programs for individuals, families, and communities. (p. 113)

competing Engaging in rivalry to meet a goal. (p. 135)

compromising Finding a middle-ground solution where each party makes a concession. (p. 135)

computer literacy The knowledge and understanding of computers combined with the ability to use them effectively. (p. 94)

conflict Disagreement about something of importance to each person involved. (p. 301)

confronting Working jointly with others to resolve a problem or conflict. (p. 132)

connection power The extent to which nurses are connected with others having power. (p. 315)

consensus The situation in which all group members agree to live with and support a decision, regardless of whether they totally agree. (p. 364)

consequentialist theories Views that state—when one is deciding between possible actions—the most important moral obligation is to maximize the positive consequences and to minimize the negative consequences; also known as teleological theories. (p. 413)

consideration A focus on the employee with an emphasis on relating to and getting along with people. (p. 174)

constitution A set of basic laws that specify the powers of the various segments of the government and how these segments relate to each other. (p. 373)

construction budget The accounting of expenditures when renovation or new structures are planned. (p. 209)

contingency theory The view that acknowledges that other factors in the environment influence outcomes as much as leadership style, and that leader effectiveness is contingent upon or depends upon something other than the leader's behaviour. (p. 175)

continuous quality improvement (CQI) A systematic process used to improve outcomes based on customers' needs. (p. 328)

contract law Rules that regulate certain transactions between individuals and/or legal entities, such as businesses. (p. 375)

cost centres Departmental subsections or units used for the tracking of financial data. (p. 213)

critical thinking A mode of thinking in which the quality of thinking is improved by skilfully taking charge of the structures inherent in thinking and imposing intellectual standards upon them. (p. 349)

cyclical scheduling A process by which the nurse manager generates a schedule for a specified number of weeks at a time. This schedule repeats itself at the end of the cycle. (p. 232)

data capture Collection and entry of data into a computer system. (p. 91)

decision making The cognitive process leading to the selection of a course of action among alternatives, and the behaviour exhibited in making a selection from alternatives and implementing a course of action. (p. 352)

delegation Transferring to a competent individual the authority to perform a selected nursing task in a selected situation. (p. 248)

delivery The method used to provide health care to the public. (p. 51)

Delphi technique A process that groups employ to arrive at a decision, though group members never meet face to face; questionnaires are distributed for opinions, and the responses are then summarized and disseminated to group members until consensus is achieved. (p. 364)

democratic leadership Style in which participation is encouraged and authority is delegated to others. (p. 173)

deontological theories Views that posit that an action's inherent rightness never lies in its consequences but in its very adherence to duty; also known as non-teleological theories. (p. 413)

departmental clinical information system A system that meets the operational needs of a particular department, such as the laboratory, radiology, pharmacy, health records, or finance. (p. 90)

determinants of health Social and environmental factors that strongly affect the health of a population. (p. 108)

direct care The provision of hands-on care to clients. (p. 223)

disease management Systematic, population-based approach to identify persons at risk, intervene with a specific program of care, and measure clinical and other outcomes. (p. 21)

economics The study of how scarce resources are allocated among their possible uses. (p. 44)

egoism The tendency to be self-centred or to consider only oneself and one's own interests. (p. 45)

electronic health record (EHR) The electronic record that includes all information about an individual's lifetime health status and health care; it replaces the paper medical record as the primary source of information for health care for meeting all clinical, legal, and administrative requirements. (p. 90)

emotional intelligence The ability both to recognize the meaning of emotions and their relationships and to reason and solve problems on the basis of emotions. (p. 170)

empathy Having a compassionate understanding for others. (p. 403)

employee-centred leadership Style with a focus on the human needs of subordinates. (p. 173)

empowerment Process by which we facilitate the participation of others in decision making and take action within an environment where there is an equitable distribution of power. (p. 317)

enterprise risk management (ERM) A comprehensive process that is used to evaluate all risk exposures confronting an organization.

episodic care unit A unit that treats clients for defined episodes of care; examples include dialysis or ambulatory care units. (p. 227)

ethical dilemma A situation in which the best course of action is often not clear, and strong ethical reasons exist to support each position. (p. 412)

ethical theories Systematic approaches that can help one decide what is right and wrong. (p. 413)

ethics The doctrine that the general welfare of society is the proper goal of an individual's actions rather than egoism; a way of understanding and reflecting upon social morality that encompasses moral issues, norms, and practices. (pp. 45, 411)

euthanasia "A deliberate act undertaken by one person with the intention of ending the life of another person to relieve that person's suffering where the act is the cause of death" (Special Senate Committee on Euthanasia and Assisted Suicide, 1995). (p. 422)

evidence-based care Care based on state-of-the-art science reports and recognized by nursing, medical, health care institutions, and health care policymakers. It is a process approach to collecting, reviewing, interpreting, critiquing, and evaluating research and other relevant literature for direct application to client care. (p. 63)

evidence-based medicine The integration of individual clinical medical experience with external clinical evidence using a systematic research approach. (p. 63)

evidence-based nursing practice The conscientious, explicit, and judicious use of theory-derived, research-based information in making decisions about care delivery to individuals or groups of individuals, and in consideration of individual needs and preferences (Ingersoll, 2000, p. 152). (p. 65)

evidence-based practice The conscientious, explicit, and judicious use of current best evidence in making decisions about the care of individual clients (Sackett et al., 1996, p. 71). (p. 63)

expert power Power derived from the knowledge and skills nurses possess. (p. 314)

false imprisonment The intentional restraint of individuals who are incorrectly led to believe they cannot leave a place. (p. 379)

fee-for-service A funding method in which physicians are paid separately for each service they provide. (p. 50)

feedback A new message that is generated by the receiver in response to the original message from the sender. (p. 127)

fiduciary obligation The responsibility to be truthful and explicit in communications with clients. (p. 423)

financing The method by which health care is paid for. (p. 50)

focus groups Small groups of individuals selected because of a common characteristic (e.g., a specific client population, clients in day surgery, new diabetics) and who are invited to meet in a group and respond to questions about a topic in which they are expected to have an interest or expertise. (p. 263)

formal leadership Within an organization, the position of authority or the sanctioned role that connotes influence. (p. 169)

forming The first stage of group development, in which several critical phases begin: the expectation phase, the interaction phase, and the boundary formation phase. (p. 193)

full-time equivalent (FTE) Measure of the work commitment of a full-time employee. (p. 222)

functional health status The ability to care for oneself and meet one's human needs. (p. 108)

functional nursing A care delivery model that divides the nursing work into functional units that are then assigned to one of the team members. (p. 236)

funding The method by which the provincial and territorial health plans pay the provider of care. (p. 50)

Good Samaritan laws Laws that have been enacted to protect the health care professional from legal liability for actions rendered in an emergency when the professional is giving service without pay. (p. 382)

grapevine An informal communication channel through which information moves quickly and is often inaccurate. (p. 131)

grievance A formal complaint in which a union member disputes management's interpretation or application of the terms of the contract, or collective agreement. (p. 440)

group A collection of individuals who are in an interdependent relationship with one another. (p. 196)

group development The five stages that a group normally progresses through as it reaches maturity: forming, storming, norming, performing, and adjourning. (p. 193)

Hawthorne effect The phenomenon of being observed or studied, which results in changes in behaviour. (p. 165)

health-based allocation model (HBAM) A new, made-in-Ontario, funding methodology that is based on direct measures of health status and takes into account both population and provider-based factors. (p. 56)

health promotion The process of enabling people to increase control over their health and to improve their health. (p. 108)

health-related quality of life Those aspects of life that are influenced either positively or negatively by one's health status and health risk factors. (p. 108)

health risk factors Modifiable and non-modifiable variables that increase or decrease the probability of illness or death; synonymous with determinants of health. (p. 108)

health status The level of well-being of an individual, family, group, population, or community; the sum of existing health risk factors, level of wellness, existing diseases, functional health status, and quality of life. (p. 108)

horizontal integration A health care system that contains several organizations of one type, such as hospitals. (p. 21)

human relations movement A movement that espouses the individual worker as the source of control, motivation, and productivity in organizations. (p. 165)

indirect care Time spent on activities that are client related but do not involve hands-on client care. (p. 223)

indirect costs Costs not explicitly related to client care, including utility costs and salaries of those who are not involved in direct client care. (p. 331)

informal leader An individual who demonstrates leadership outside the scope of a formal leadership role or as a member of a group, rather than the head or leader of the group. (p. 169)

information communication Interoperability of systems and linkages for exchange of data across disparate systems. (p. 92)

information power The authority held by a person who shares knowledge that is both accurate and useful. (p. 315)

initiating structure A type of leadership behaviour that involves an emphasis on the work to be done and a focus on the task and production. (p. 174)

inpatient unit A hospital unit that is able to provide care to clients 24 hours a day, 7 days a week. (p. 227)

instrumental activities of daily living (IADLs) Tasks related to food preparation and shopping; cleaning; laundry; home maintenance; verbal, written, and electronic communications; financial management; and transportation, along with activities to meet social and support needs, manage health care needs, access community services and resources, and meet spiritual needs. (p. 108)

integrated delivery system A network of health care organizations that provides a coordinated continuum of service to a defined population and is willing to be held clinically and fiscally accountable for the outcomes and the health status of the population served. Networks include hospitals, nursing homes, schools, public health departments, and social and community health organizations. (p. 14)

interpersonal communication Communication between individuals. (p. 130)

interprofessional team A group composed of members with a variety of clinical expertise. (p. 192)

intrapersonal communication Self-talk. (p. 130)

job-centred leaders Individuals whose leadership style focuses on schedules, cost, and efficiency, with less attention to developing work groups and high-performance goals. (p. 173)

justice A broad principle encompassing the notion of fair distribution of benefits, resources, and risks. (p. 414)

kinesthetic Sense of awareness of movement of voluntary muscles. (p. 127)

knowledge workers Those involved in serving others through their specialized understanding of information. (p. 168)

laissez-faire leadership A passive and permissive style in which the leader defers decision making. (p. 173)

leader-member relations Feelings and attitudes of followers regarding acceptance, trust, and the credibility of the leader. (p. 175)

leadership The process of influence whereby the person in charge influences others toward goal achievement. (p. 168)

LEADS in a Caring Environment framework A capibilities framework which defines the knowledge, skills, and attitudes a leader needs to exhibit in order to successfully contribute to an effective and efficient Canadian health system. (p. 31)

legitimate power The influence derived from the position a nurse holds in a group; it indicates the nurse's degree of authority. (pp. 314)

living will A document voluntarily signed by clients that specifies the type of care they desire if and when they are in a terminal state and are unable to either sign a consent form or convey this information verbally. (p. 378, 422)

macro-allocation Resource allocation decisions that are made by governments at all levels. (p. 419)

maintenance or hygiene factors (Herzberg) Elements such as salary, job security, working conditions, status, quality of supervision, and relationships with others that prevent job dissatisfaction. (p. 167)

malpractice The wrongful conduct in the discharge of professional duties or failure to meet the standards of care for the profession, which results in harm to another individual entrusted to the professional's care. (p. 386)

management The process of coordinating actions and allocating resources to achieve organizational goals. (p. 161)

management process The function of planning, organizing, coordinating, and controlling. (p. 161)

marketing In the fifth and final phase of the Donner-Wheeler Career Planning and Development Model, the ability to communicate one's strengths, interests, and goals with confidence and clarity. (p. 449)

medical futility A medical treatment that is seen to be non-beneficial because it is believed to offer no reasonable hope of recovery or improvement of the client's condition. (p. 421)

MEDLARS (Medical Literature Analysis and Retrieval System) The computerized system of databases and databanks offered by the National Library of Medicine. (p. 99)

mentor A person who takes a personal and professional interest in your career and exemplifies the nurse you wish to become. (p. 451)

meso-allocation Resource allocation decisions that are made at the institutional or program level. (p. 419)

message A series of verbal and nonverbal stimuli that originate with a sender and are taken in by a receiver. (p. 127)

micro-allocation Resource allocation decisions that are made at the bedside, regarding individual clients. (p. 419)

mission statement A formal expression of the purpose or reason for existence of the organization. (p. 269)

modular team nursing A team nursing care delivery system that divides a geographical space into modules of clients with each module having a team of staff led by an RN to care for them. (p. 236)

moral distress The result when ethical dilemmas are not acknowledged or effectively dealt with; when communication between team members, clients, and families is ineffective; or when professionals feel isolated or unsupported in their approach to solving such dilemmas. (p. 412)

morality Beliefs or traditions about what is determined to be right or wrong in terms of conduct toward ourselves and others. (p. 412)

motivation The incentive that influences our choices and creates direction, intensity, and persistence in our behaviour. (p. 165)

motivation factors (Herzberg) Elements such as achievement, recognition, responsibility, advancement, and the opportunity for development that contribute to job satisfaction. (p. 167)

multi-faith Usually refers to inclusiveness of world religions, including Judaism, Islam, Buddhism, Hinduism, Christianity, and others; often confused with the term *ecumenical*, which pertains to multi-denominational Christianity. (p. 399)

negligence Failure to provide the care a reasonable person would ordinarily provide in a similar situation. (p. 376)

networking The continuous process of initiating and maintaining professional relationships through communication and information sharing. (p. 452)

nominal group technique A group decision-making technique comprised of four stages: members (1) write out their ideas to an issue or question posed; (2) present ideas to the group; (3) discuss ideas to clarify and evaluate; and (4) vote privately. (p. 364)

nonmaleficence The principle of doing no harm. (p. 414)

non-unit producing Refers to indirect care activities that support the work of the direct care providers. (p. 223)

nonverbal communication Aspects of communication that are outside what is spoken. (p. 128)

norming The third stage of group development, in which people have a general understanding of the issues at hand and how to progress toward solving them. Positions in the group are established, and members have a sense both of belonging and of setting goals to meet expectations. (p. 193)

nursing ethics The examination of the norms, values, and principles found in nursing practice. (p. 413)

nursing hours per patient day (NHPPD) Standard measure that quantifies the nursing time available to each client by the available nursing staff. (p. 223)

operating budget The accounting of the income and expenses associated with day-to-day activity within a department or organization. (p. 208)

organizational change An alteration of an organization's culture, structure, technology, physical setting, or human resources. (p. 292)

organization evidence Information about an organization's capacity to execute tasks. (p. 68)

outcome elements of quality The end products of quality care that review the status of clients as a result of health care. Outcome elements ask the question, Is the client better as a result of health care? (p. 28)

palliative care A philosophy of care for those with a life-threatening or life-limiting illness. Clients receiving palliative care most often benefit from a spiritual assessment and care. (p. 398)

passive euthanasia A deliberate act in which treatment is ceased or withheld, and the person is thereby made more vulnerable to the underlying processes that cause death. (p. 422)

pastoral care This term originated from the church which provided compassionate care from one member to another. In health care, this term has been replaced by Spiritual Care which is more inclusive of all—those with religious affiliations, and those without. (p. 391)

payer A third-party reimburser, typically an insurance company or a government agency. (p. 44)

performance improvement (PI) A structured system for creating organization-wide participation and partnership in planning and implementing continuous improvement methods to understand and meet or exceed customer needs and expectations. (p. 326)

performing The fourth stage of group development, in which people understand their roles and work interdependently on the work needed to achieve the group's objectives. (p. 194)

personal change An alteration made voluntarily for one's own reasons, usually for self-improvement. (p. 292)

philosophy of an organization A value statement of the principles and beliefs that direct the organization's behaviour. (p. 269)

political evidence Information that gives a sense of how various stakeholders may respond to policies; for example, the barriers or facilitators that may have to be managed. (p. 68)

political voice The stated views of individuals supporting or opposing an issue. (p. 151)

politics The process by which people use a variety of methods to achieve their goals. (p. 144)

population-based nursing practice The practice of nursing in which the focus of care is to improve the health status of vulnerable or at-risk population groups within the community; this involves health promotion and disease prevention interventions across the health continuum. (p. 113)

population health An approach to health care that focuses on the determinants of health in order to help reduce inequities among different groups, particularly the people who are the most vulnerable; a concept that the population, or a community, as a whole has a particular state of health. (pp. 8, 107)

position power The degree of formal authority and influence associated with a leader. (p. 175)

power The ability to create, acquire, and use resources to achieve one's goals. (p. 312)

power of attorney A legal document executed by an individual (the principal) granting another person (the agent) the right to perform certain activities in the principal's name. (p. 379)

primary health care Services that emphasize the promotion of health and the prevention of illness or disability. (p. 13)

primary nursing A care delivery model that clearly delineates the responsibility and accountability of the RN and places the RN as the primary provider of nursing care to clients. (p. 237)

principlism A framework for considering ethical issues that includes four guiding principles: respect for autonomy, beneficence, nonmaleficence, and justice. (p. 414)

problem solving An active process that starts with a problem and ends with a solution. (p. 351)

process elements of quality The nursing and health care interventions that must be in place to deliver quality, including managing the health care process, using clinical practice guidelines and standards for nursing and medical interventions, and administering medications. (p. 28)

professional change The alteration made in an individual's position or job such as obtaining education or credentials. (p. 292)

professional codes of ethics The guidelines and values that members of a profession adhere to and promote in creating an ethical, accountable practice; this is usually defined and shaped by members of the profession. (p. 415)

program budgeting and marginal analysis (PMBA) A mechanism that can link physicians to organizational decision-making processes. (p. 54)

public communication Direction of a message to an audience or group of people with a common interest. (p. 130)

public health system A system of health care that is responsible for helping to protect people from injury and disease and for helping people stay healthy. (p. 12)

public law A general classification of law, generally consisting of both constitutional and criminal law; it defines a citizen's relationship with government. (p. 373)

quality assurance (QA) An inspection approach to ensure that minimum standards of care exist in health care institutions, primarily hospitals. (p. 326)

quality of life (1) The level of satisfaction one has with the actual conditions of one's life, including satisfaction with socioeconomic status, education, occupation, home, family life, recreation, and the ability to enjoy life, freedom, and independence; at the end of life, having some control over the process and one's final days. (2) An individual's perception of daily well-being; quality of life often changes during the course of illness. Spiritual Care seeks to assist and improve the ill person's experience in the moment. (p. 108)

reality check The feedback, received from people involved in one's life, regarding one's strengths, unique traits, and areas for development. The reality check is part of self-assessment, the second phase of the Donner-Wheeler Career Planning and Development Model. (p. 448)

receiver One who takes in a message and analyzes it. (p. 127)

reengineering Turning an organization upside down and inside out through fundamental rethinking and radical redesign of processes to achieve dramatic improvements in critical performance. (p. 262)

referent power Authority derived from the degree to which others respect and like an individual, group, or organization. (p. 314)

reflective thinking Watching or observing ourselves as we perform a task or make a decision about a certain situation, followed by thinking about what we have done, and how we could have done it better. (p. 351)

regionalization An integrated health care delivery system that is structured by geographic areas. (p. 14)

religious care Often provided by chaplaincy and pastoral care teams, religious care seeks to provide for faith needs by ritual, practice and faith community. (p. 393)

resources The people, money, facilities, technology, rights to properties and services, and technologies that are used to fulfill a function or achieve an end. (p. 144)

resource intensity weights (RIWs) Developed by the Canadian Institute for Health Information (CIHI), this relative resource methodology estimates a hospital's inpatient-specific costs for both acute care and day procedure care. (p. 224)

responding Verbal and nonverbal acknowledgment of a sender's message. (p. 132)

responsibility Reliability, dependability, and the obligation to accomplish work. (p. 249)

résumé Brief summary of your background, training, and experience as well as your qualifications for a position. (p. 453)

revenue Income generated through a variety of means (e.g., billable client services, investments, and donations to the organization). (p. 214)

reward/coercive power The authority to reward or punish others, as well as the ability to instill fear in others by influencing them to change their behaviour; resentment is often the result of withholding rewards or achieving a goal by causing fear. (p. 314)

risk adjustment The process of statistically altering client data to reflect significant client variables. (p. 23)

scanning the environment The first phase of the Donner-Wheeler Career Planning and Development Model, in which individuals take a good look around to determine how the world around them can help to both develop and achieve their career goals. (p. 448)

self-assessment The second phase of the Donner-Wheeler Career Planning and Development Model, in which individuals look inside themselves to create meaning in their learning and to recognize opportunities for future development. (p. 447)

self-scheduling A process in which staff on a unit collectively decide and implement the monthly work schedule. (p. 232)

sender One who initiates the message or communication (p. 127)

sentinel event An unexpected occurrence involving death or serious physical or psychological injury to a client. (p. 335)

shared governance A situation in which nurses and managers work together to define their roles and expected outcomes, holding everyone accountable for their role and expected outcomes. (p. 278)

situational leadership A framework that maintains that there is no one best leadership style, but rather that effective leadership lies in matching the appropriate leadership style to the individual's or group's level of motivation and task-relevant readiness. (p. 282)

skill mix The percentage of one type of staff to the total staff complement. (p. 226)

sources of power Combination of conscious and unconscious factors that allow an individual to influence others to think or act in a certain way. (p. 314)

spiritual care Care that seeks to provide energy, support, and strength as a coping mechanism during illness; it is individual and may include religious care. (p. 391)

staffing pattern A plan that articulates how many and what kind of staff are needed, by shift and day, to staff a unit or department. (p. 226)

stakeholder A provider, employer, customer, or client who may have an interest in, and may seek to influence, the decisions and actions of an organization. (p. 263)

stakeholders Vested interest groups. (p. 144)

stakeholder assessment A systematic consideration of all potential stakeholders to ensure that the needs of each of these stakeholders are incorporated in the planning phase. (p. 263)

storage Physical location of data in an electronic health record (EHR) system. (p. 92)

storming The second stage of group development, in which people begin to feel more comfortable with each other and differences among the group members may become apparent, leading to tension and conflicts. (p. 193)

strategic career plan A personalized action plan, developed in the fourth phase of the Donner-Wheeler Career Planning and Development Model, to help meet the short- and long-term goals of a career vision. (p. 449)

strategic plan The sum total or outcome of the processes by which an organization engages in environmental analysis, goal formulation, and strategy development with the purpose of organizational growth and renewal. (p. 262)

strategic planning A process that is designed to achieve goals in dynamic, competitive environments through the allocation of resources. (p. 262)

structure elements of quality The structure elements that must be in place in a health care system or health care unit to deliver quality health care, including a well-constructed hospital, quality client care standards, quality staffing policies, environmental standards. (p. 28)

substitutes for leadership Variables that may influence or have an effect on followers to the same extent as the leader's behaviour. (p. 175)

SWOT analysis A tool that is frequently used to conduct environmental assessments. SWOT stands for Strengths, Weaknesses, Opportunities, and Threats. (p. 262)

system An interdependent group of items, people, or processes with a common purpose. (p. 330)

task structure The degree to which work is defined by specific procedures, explicit directions, and measurable goals. (p. 175)

team Small number of people with complementary skills who are committed to a common purpose, performance goals, and approach for which they hold themselves accountable (Katzenbach & Smith, 1993). (p. 192)

team nursing Care delivery model that assigns staff to teams that then are responsible for a group of clients. (p. 236)

Theory X The view that in bureaucratic organizations employees prefer security, direction, and minimal responsibility; coercion, threats, or punishment are necessary because people do not like the work to be done. (p. 168)

Theory Y The view that in the context of the right conditions, people enjoy their work, can show self-control and discipline, are able to contribute creatively, and are motivated by ties to the group, the organization, and the work itself; the belief that people are intrinsically motivated by their work. (p. 168)

Theory Z The view of collective decision making and a focus on long-term employment that involves slower promotions and less direct supervision. (p. 168)

tort A civil wrong committed by one person against another, such that some injury or damage is caused to either person or property. (p. 376)

total pain An expression used to describe the discomfort that arises from the accumulation of physical, emotional, and spiritual distress. (p. 400)

total patient care A care delivery model in which nurses are responsible for the total care of their client assignment during the shift they are working. (p. 235)

transactional leader A traditional manager concerned with day-to-day operations. (p. 177)

transformational leader An individual who is committed to a vision that empowers others. (p. 177)

ubiquitous computing (UC) A term coined by Mark Weiser of Xerox PARC to describe the phase of computing in which there are many computers to one person. (p. 95)

union A formal, legal group that works through a collective bargaining agent and within the legal context of labour legislation to bring forth workers' requests to management. (p. 433)

unit producing Refers to direct care activities. (p. 223)

utilitarian theories The most commonly cited type of consequentialist theories; they assess the moral rightness of actions based on how much happiness they might produce. (p. 413)

values The boundaries an organization will have while pursuing its vision. (p. 270)

veracity The obligation to tell the truth. (p. 423)

verbal communication The aspect of communication that relies on spoken words to convey a message. (p. 128)

vertical integration The linking of different stages of health care that are delivered by one agency. (p. 21)

vision A statement that provides a clear picture of what the future will look like for an organization. (p. 270)

visual Pertaining to seeing. (p. 127)

voting block Group that represents the same political position or perspective. (p. 151)

vulnerable population groups Sub-groups of a community that are powerless, marginalized, or disenfranchised, and are experiencing health disparities. (p. 109)

whistle-blowing An act in which an individual discloses information concerning a harmful act that a superior or colleague has committed, is allowing to occur, or is contemplating; or discloses information concerning a violation of a law, rule, or regulation, or a substantial and specific danger to public health or safety. (p. 435)

workload measurement system System for distinguishing among different clients based on their acuity, functional ability, or resource needs. (p. 223)

workplace advocacy Activities nurses undertake to address problems in their everyday workplace setting. (p. 432)

INDEX

Note: Page numbers preceded by "F" and "T" refer to figures and tables.

A

Aboriginal Health Centres, 116
Accommodating, 135, 302–303
Accord on Health Care Renewal, 4
Accountability-based care delivery, 284
Accountability, 48–50, 248–49, F49
    consumer demand for, 152–53
    and power, 314–16
Accreditation, 21–22
    patient safety goals, 24
    Qmentum Standards, 24
    regulatory requirements, 335
Achievement, 319
Active euthanasia, 422
Activities of daily living (ADLs), 30
Activity-based costing, 56
Adams, D.F., 23
Adams, I., 45
Adjourning, 194
Administrative principles, 164
Advance directives, 422
Adverse events, 261
Advocacy, and nurses, 151–52
Affiliation, 319
Aging population, 126
Agnes, M., 45
AIDS, 57
Aiken, L.H., 170, 179, 233, 261, 353, 354
Al-Assaf, A.F., 330
Aldarrab, A., T333, T334, T336
Alexander, R., 62, 95
Alfaro-LeFevre, R., 349–50, 366
Allen, D.W., 172
Alma Ata Declaration, 13, 107
Alspach, J., 280
Altruism, health care as, 45
American Hospital Association, 415
American Nurses Association
        (ANA), 88, 438
Anderson, Margaret M., 291
Anderson, R.A., 179
Androwich, Ida M., 43, 260
Androwich O'Malley, Amy, 260
Anger, 133–34, 400
Anticipatory grief, 400
Anti-Inflation Board, 431
Appelbaum, P.S., 417
ARPAnet, 97

Articles
    full-text, locating, 99
Assault, 377
ASSET model, T397
Assignment making, 249
Assisted suicide, 423
Attending, 132
Auditory (channel of communication), 127–28
Authority, 249
Autocratic decision process, 202
Autocratic leadership, 173
Autonomy, 414, 417–18
Avoiding, 135, 302
Ayers, D.L., 295

B

Baggs, J.G., 35
Bailey, J.T., 356
Baker, G.R., 27, 261, T26
Balanced scorecard, 209
Ball, M.J., 87
Barnard, C., 164
Bass, B., 177
Battery, 377
Battin, M., 422
Beauchamp, T.L., 412, 414
Belcher, A., 396
Bellack, J.P., 349
Benchmarking, 225, 335
Beneficence, 414
Benefit hours, 222, F223
Benner, P., 34, 176, 280, 354
Benner's novice to expert, 280–82
Bennis, W., 169, 172, 177, 182, 196, 296, 297, 300
Bernat, Anne L., 221, 263
Berners-Lee, Timothy, 97
Best research evidence, 64
Bill 8, Ontario, 50
Bioethics, 412
Biological variations, cultural delegation, 257
Blake, R.R., 174
Blended payments, physician remuneration, 52
Block funding, 4
Block, P., 352, 353, 356
Blue Cross, 50, 329
Blythe, J., 168
Boetzkes, S., 412
Bonney, E., T26
Bookey-Bassett, S., 454
Bookmarks, 98

Bothamley, J., 316
Bradford, L.P., 194
Brown, A.D., 48, 326
Brown, L.D., 147
Bruch, H., 161
Budget development, 214–17
    expenses, 214–15
    human resources and, 215–16
    revenue, 214
    staffing, 216–17
    supplies, 215
Budget(s)
    accounting, 209
    approval and monitoring, 217–19
    balanced scorecard, 209, F210, F211
    cost centres, 213
    demographic information, 212
    development, 214–17
    history, 214
    overview, 209, 212
    preparation, 212–13
    regulatory influences, 212–13
    service goals, 213–14
    strategic plans, 213
    types of, 208–209
Bureaucratic organization, 163
Burkhardt, M.A., 411
Burns, J.M., 177, 196
Bushy, A., 298
Business cards, 458
Byers, S.A., 5

C
Cain, Sister Kathleen, 372
Caldwell, C., 337
Campbell, B., 355
Canada Health Act (1984), 4, 51, 56, 148, 374, T416
Canada Health Infoway, 93
Canada Health and Social Transfer (CHST), 4
Canada Health Transfer (CHT), 5, 415
Canada Labour Code, 375, 473
Canada's Association for the Fifty-Plus (CARP), 150
Canadian Adverse Events Study, The, 4, 24, 27–28, 261
Canadian Agency for Drugs and Technologies in Health (CADTH), 65, 78, 99
Canadian Centre for Occupational Health and Safety (CCOHS), 375
Canadian Charter of Rights and Freedoms, 373, 415, 420
Canadian College of Health Leaders, 30–31
Canadian Constitution (1982), 373
Canadian Federation of Nurses Unions (CFNU), 225, 431, 437
Canadian Healthcare Association (CHA), 152

Canadian Health Services Research Foundation (CHSRF), 24, 76, 78
Canadian Hospice Palliative Care Association (CHPCA), 317, 404
Canadian Institute for Health Information (CIHI), 5, 52, 64, 89, 113, 224, 238
Canadian Institutes of Health Research (CIHR), 78
Canadian Labour Congress (CLC), 432
Canadian Medical Association (CMA), 152, 240, 317
Canadian Nurses Association (CNA), 87, 88, 90, 150, 152, 160, 248, 261, 317, 355, 380, 392, 412, 415, 437
Canadian Nursing Advisory Committee (CNAC), 225, 352, 432
Canadian Nursing Students' Association (CNSA), 432, 453
Canadian Population Health Initiative (CPHI), 9, 78
Canadian Public Health Association (CPHA), 13, T14
Canadian Registered Nurse Examination, 247
Capital budget, 208–209
Capitation, physician remuneration, 52
Care delivery management tools, 238–42
    case management, 240–42
    case mix groups (CMGs), 238
    clinical pathways, 240, T241
    clinical practice guidelines, 240
    resource intensity weights (RIWs), 238
Care delivery model, 235
    client-centred collaborative practice, 238
    functional nursing, T236
    primary nursing, F237–38
    team nursing, 236–37, F237
    total patient care, 235–36
Career planning
    career vision, 446–47
    interview, preparation for, 458–59, T458, T459
    marketing yourself, 449–58
    scanning your environment, 448–49
    self-assessment/reality check, 447–48
    strategic career plan, 449, T450–51
Care maps, *see* Clinical pathways
Carman, J.M., 356
Carroll-Johnson, R., 35
Carruthers, Chris, 262
Case-costing, 56
Case management, 240–42
Case mix groups (CMGs), 224, 238
Cawthorpe, D., 364
Chang, C., 44
Change, 292–93
    chaos theory, 294
    and conflict management, 307

Change (*Continued*)
  emerging theories of, 294–96
    Havelock's Six-Step Change Model, 294, T295
    learning organization theory, 294–95
    Lewin's Force-Field Model, 294, T295
    Lippitt's Phases of Change, 294, T295
    resistance to, 298
    responses to, 298–99
    Rogers' Diffusion of Innovation Theory, 294, T295
    traditional theories of, 294, T295
    types of, 292–93
Change agent, 299–301
  strategies, 300–301
Change process, 296–97
  assessment, 296
  change strategies, 297, T298
  evaluation of change, 297
  planning, 296–97
  stabilization of, 297
  steps in, 296–97
Chaplain, 402
Charismatic theory, 176–77
Chester, S., 50
Chidwick, P., 424
Chronic disease/injury prevention, 12
Chronic Disease Self-Management Program (CDSMP), 21
CINAHL (Cumulative Index to Nursing and Allied Health Literature), 97
Civil Code of Quebec, 382
Civil law, 375–80
  intentional torts, 377
  non-intentional torts, 376–77
  tort law, 376–77
Clarifying, 132
Clarke, D.M., 401
Cleland, V., 354, 356
Client acuity, 224
Client-centred care, 238
Client-focused care, 178, 201
Client-focused clinical information system, 90
Clinical information, 90–93
Clinical information system (CIS), 90
Clinical ladder, 280
Clinical pathways, 240, F241
Clinical practice council, 278
Clinical practice guidelines, 240
CNA Code of Ethics, 249, 357, 380, 415–16, 423
CNA's Joint Statement on Resuscitative Interventions, 422
Code of Ethics for Registered Nurses in Canada, 417
Coercive power, 314

Collaborating, 135, T303
Collaboration, 304
Collective action, 432
Collective bargaining, 432
  pros and cons, T440
  terminology, T434
  unionization process, 432–33, 435, 439–40
Collective bargaining agent, 435
College of Nurses of Ontario, 247, 304, 374
Colorado Differentiated Nursing Practice Model, 282, F283
Commission on the Future of Health Care in Canada, 374, *see also* Romanow Report
Committee, 192–93
Common law, 373
Communication
  anger, 133–34
  barriers to, 133–35, T135
  channels, 127–28
  with clients/families, 137–38
  cultural delegation, 255
  culture and, 133
  diagonal, 131
  downward, 131
  gender and, 133
  lateral, 130
  levels of, 130–31
  mentor/prodigy, 138–39
  process, 127
  upward, 131
Communication skills, 131–33, T132
Community Health Centres (CHCs), 18, 113
Community health nurses, 113
Competency, 280
Competing, 135, 303, T303
Compromising, 135, 304, T303
Computer literacy, 94
Computers, 86
Computing
  modern developments, 94–97
  trends in, 94–97
  ubiquitous, 95
  virtual reality, 95–97
Conflict, 135, 301
  Guide for the Assessment of, F306–308
  management and change, 307
  process, 302
  sources of, 301, T302
  types of, 301–302
Conflict resolution, 302–305, T303
  leadership and management roles, 305
  negotiation strategies, F305
  strategies for facilitating, 304–305
Confronting, 132–33, 304

Confucius, 444
Conger, J., 176, 182
Connection power, T315
Connors, Kathleen, 431
Consensus, 364
Consent, 417–18
    informed, 377–78
Consequentialist theories, 413
Consideration, 174
Constitution, 373
Constitution Act (1867), 4
Constitutional law, 373–74
Construction budget, 209
Consultative decision process, 202
Consumer alliances, 151–52, T152
Consumer demands, 152–53
Content motivation theories, 166
Contingency theory, 175
Continuous quality improvement (CQI), 326
    participation, 329–30
Contract law, 375–76
Coordinating council, 255
Co-payments, 51
Correnti, D., 354
Cost-benefit analysis, 118
Cost centres, 213
Covey, S.R., 166, 269
Coxcomb diagram, 2, F3
Criminal Code of Canada, 374, 423
Critical thinking, 349–50
Crosby, P.B., 325
Crowe, Cathy, 114
Cultural care, 399
    leadership roles, 402
    multiculturalism, 399
Culture
    and delegation, 255–57
    organizational, 356
Cyclical scheduling, 232

D
Daft, R.L., 162, 163, 164
Danford, Leanne, 201
Daniels, N., 420
Data
    collection programs, 118
    illustration, 338, F339, F340
    time series, 338, F339
Data capture, 91–92
Davis, A.J., 421
Decision making, 351–52
    caution vs. courage, 353
    client choice and rights, 356–57
    competence, 355

dependency vs. autonomy, 353
    effective, limitations to, 365
    extrinsic factors, 356–60
    factors influencing, 353–60
    knowledge and experience, 354–55
    legislation and regulation, 357
    maintenance vs. greatness, 352
    nurses' role in client, 366
    nursing and, 352–53
    organizational climate and culture, 356
    personal perception and preference, 354
    self-confidence, 355–56
    steps in process of, 357–60
    strategies to improve, 366
    stress, 356
    use of technology, 366
Decision making, group, 360–65
    consensus, 364
    consensus building, 364
    Delphi technique, 364
    ethical, 425–27, T427
    groupthink, 364–65
    nominal technique, 364
    techniques of, 364–65
Decision-making process
    clinical application, 358–59
    decision tree, 359
    Gantt chart, 359–60
    grid sample, F359
    management application, 359
    steps in, 358
Delegated decision process, 202
Delegation, 247
    assignment making, 249
    authority, 249
    biological variations, 257
    communication, 256
    considerations in, F252
    defined, 248
    direct vs. indirect, 251–52
    environmental control, 257
    five rights of, 251, T253
    inappropriate, 253–54
    responsibilities of health team members, 249–51
    space, 256
    suggestions for RNs or LPNs, T250
    time, 256–57
    transcultural, 255–57
    underdelegation, 252–53
Delivery, 51
Delivery function of health care system, 51
Delphi technique, 364
Deming, W.E., 325
Democratic leadership, 173

Demoralization, 400–401
Deontological theories, 413
Departmental clinical information system, 90
Depression, 400–401
Determinants of health, 113
Devlin, R.A., 52
Dewey, John, 350
Diagnosis and Treatment of Existing Health
    Problems, 5, T6
DiCenso, A., 63, 64, 67
Direct care, 223
Disappointment, 400–401
Disease management, 21
Disempowerment, 316–17
Doctors, *see* Physician(s)
Dolamo, B.L., 395
Donabedian, A., 28
Donaghy, M.E., 351
Donatelle, R., 12
Donner, G., 447, F445, T458
Do Not Resuscitate (DNR) Orders, 378–79
Doran, D.A., 356
Doucette, E., 168
Dreyfus, S.E., 280
Drucker, P.F., 180, 272, 326, 328
Drummond, M.F., 30
Dunham, J., 169, 177
Dunham-Taylor, J., 171, 177
Dwyer, D.W., 355

E
Ebola, 57
Economics, *see* Health care, economics and
Education council, 278
Egoism, 45
Electronic communication, 128–29
Electronic health record (EHR), 90–93
    confidentiality, 92
    data capture, 91–92
    privacy, 92
    security, 92
    storage, 92
Ellis, J.R., 249
Elser, R., 218
Emergency Medical Aid Act (Alta), 382
Emotional intelligence (EI), 171
Empathy, 403
Employee-centred leadership, 173
Empowerment, 316–17
    media, role of, 317
    personal, plan for, 317
End-of-life issues, 421–23
Enterprise risk management (ERM), 343–44
Environmental control, cultural delegation, 257

Episodic care unit, 227
Esmail, N., 6, 45
Estabrooks, C., 66
Ethical care
    foundations for in Canada, 415
Ethical decision making, 425–27, T426
Ethical dilemma, 412
Ethical theories, 413–15
Ethics, 40, 411–12
    code of, for RNs, 415–16
    consent, 417–18
    end-of-life issues, 421–23
    feminist, 414–15
    leadership roles/challenges, 424–25
    nursing, 412–13
    principlism, 414
    professional dilemmas, 417–24
    quality of life, 421
    resource allocation, 418–21
    resuscitation, 421
    truth telling, 423–24
Euthanasia, 422–23
Evans, D., 354
Evidence-based care, 65
Evidence-based decisions
    knowledge-transfer, 78–79
    policy, 78–79
Evidence-based medicine, 63
Evidence-based nursing practice, 65
Evidence-based practice
    attributes of, 66–67
    five steps, T71–72
    history of, 63–64
    importance of, 64–66
    levels of evidence, 76–77
    misconceptions about, 67
    research terminology, T72–76
    United States, 65
Expert power, 314, T315

F
Factor system, 224
Fagin, C., 146
Fagin, C.M., 169
False imprisonment, 379–80
Fayol, H., 161, 164
Fear, 400
Federal Commissioner of Health Care, T31
Federal-Provincial Fiscal Arrangements and
    Established Programs Financing Act, 4
Feedback, 127, 249
Fee-for-service (FFS), 50
Fiduciary obligation, 423
Fielder, F., 174

Fielder's contingency theory, 175
Fielding, John, 198
Fiesta, S., 377
Final Gifts (1992), 399
Financing health care reform
    co-payments, 51
    user fees, 51
First Nations, health delivery by, 2, 56–57
Fisher, M., 247
Flanagan, L., T436
Flower, J., 294
Focus groups, 263
Follet, Mary Parker, 161
Fooks, C., 35
Formal leadership, 169
Forming, 193
Frederickson, Pat, 143, 147, 155
Full-time equivalent (FTE), 359, F222–23
    needed to staff episodic care unit, 227–30
Functional health status, 108
Functional nursing, 236
Funding, 50
    function of health care system, 50
    health reform, 52–56

G
Galloway, L., F326, F327
Gantt chart, 335, 359–60, F336, F363
Gastmans, C., 413
Gebbie, K.M., 147
Gelinas, L.S., 171
General and Industrial Management
        (Fayol), 161
George, V., 178
Gift, R.G., 335
Gilbreth, F., 163
Gilbreth, L., 163
Girvan, J., 171
Glasziou, P., 76
Goals, planning, 268
Goddard, M., 11
Goleman, D., 170
Gonzalez, Virginia, 21
Good Samaritan Act (2006) (Ontario), 382
Good Samaritan law, 382
Grade working groups, 77
Grapevine, 131
Graphical depictions of data, 338, F339, F340
Greenberg, J., 315, 317
Grievance, 440
Griffiths, M., 396
Grohar-Murray, M.E., 127, 212, 256
Group roles, 194–95
    functional vs. divisional members, 194–95

Groups
    decision making and, 360–65
    effective concepts, 195–98
    five stages of development, 193–95, T194
    types of, 193–95
Groupthink, 364–65
Guillory, W.A., 391
Guilt, 400
Gulick, L., 161

H
Hagbaghery, M.A., 355
Hales, C.P., 161
Hammond, J.S., 365
Harrison, A., 54
Hart, C., 432
Havelock, R.G., 294
Havelock's Six-Step Change Model, 294, T295
Havens, D.S., 261, 317
Haviley, Corinne, 207
Hawthorne effect, 165
Health-based allocation model (HBAM), 56
Health Canada, 329
Health care
    accreditation, 21–23, T22–23
    altruism, 45
    approaches to, 8–21
    economics and, 44–45
    evidence-based practice, 23–28
    finance reform, 51–52
    funding for, 4
    need for determined by provider, 45
    nursing role, 34–35
    organization of, 4–5
    practice variations, 23–28
    principles of, 4
    recent changes in, 30–31, T31
    2004 reform, 5
    right to, 45–48
    stakeholders, 144–47
    strategies influencing, 33–36, T33–34
    trends in, 33–34
Health Care Consent Act (1996) (Ontario), 377,
        417
Health care costs, 45–57
    accountability for, 48–50, F50, T49
    reform of, 51–57
    traditional perspective on, 51–57
Health care economics, 44
Health care networks, 21
Health care professionals, 5, T7
    nurses, *see* Nurse(s)
    workplace communication, 136
Health care services, 5, T6

Health care system
  delivery function, 51
  financing, 50
  functions of, 50–51, F54
  funding function, 50–51
  reports on, 48
Health Council of Canada (HCC), 21
Health delivery reform
  First Nations, 57
  public/private partnerships, 57
Health emergencies, 12
Health Outcomes for Better Information and Care
    (HOBIC), 65, 66
Health promotion, 5, 12, 108, T6
Health-related quality of life, 108
Health risk factors, 108
Health Services Restructuring Commission, 15
Health status, 108
Henke, D., 401
Hersey and Blanchard's situational theory,
    175–76
Hersey, R.E., 282–83
Hibberd, J.M., 50–51, 316, 380
Hierarchy of needs (Maslow), 166, F167, F395
Hiltzik, M., 95
Hofstede, G., 356
Holistic care, T394
Horizontal integration, 21
Hospital insurance, 4
House, R.H., 176
Houser, J., 178
Houston, Karen, 324
Huber, D., 202, 357
Hughes, R.L., 166
Human relations, T165
  movement, 165
  social facilitation, 165
Human services
  and cultural heritage, 148
  politics/demographic change, 148, 150
  politics and economics, 147–48
  population aging, 148, 150

I
Iacocca, Lee, 176
Incongruent responses, 134
Indirect care, 223
Indirect costs, 59, 208, 331
Infant mortality rate, 11
Informal leadership, 169
Informal organization, 164
Informatics nurse
  clinical information system interface, 93–94
Informatics, see Nursing Informatics

Information communication, 92
Information power, T315
Information presentation, 93
Information processing, 92
Initiating structure, 175
Inpatient unit, 217, 227
Institute of Medicine Committee on Health Care
    Quality Reports, 25
Instrumental activities of daily living (IADCs), 108
Integrated delivery system(s), 14
International Classification of Functioning
    Disability & Health (ICIDH-2), 108
International conferences, 13
International Council of Nurses (ICN), 415
Internet, 97–101
  evaluating information from, 99–101
  links and bookmarks, 98
  power and, 316
  professional/consumer resources, 98–99
  use in clinical practice, 97
Interpersonal communication, 130–31
Interprofessional nursing practice, 35–36
Interprofessional team, 192
Interviews, 263
  preparation for, 458–59, T458, T459
Intrapersonal communication, 130
Iron, K., F210

J
Jacox, A., 439
Jakarta Declaration, 108, 117
Jameton, A., 412
Jarvis, C., 364–65
Job-centred leaders, 173
Johnson, Dorothy, 279
Johnson, I., T117
Jones, C., 391
Jones, K., 147
Jones, R.A.P., 359
Joos, I., 89
Joseph, D.H., 354, 355
Juran, J., 326
Justice, 414

K
Kant, Immanuel, 413
Kanter, K.M., 261
Kaplan, R., 209
Katz, D., 162
Keatings, M., 341, 373, 375, 376, 377, 378, 386, 412,
    413, 418
Keenan, J., 353
Kelly, Patricia, 1
Kerr, S., 176

Kiley, G., 395
Kinesthetic (channel of communication), 128
Kingma, M., 375
Kirby Report, 9, 48
Kirkpatrick, S.A., 170
Kissane, D.W., 401
Knowledge Transfer and Exchange (KTE), 78
Knowledge workers, 168, 180
Kohn, L., 25
Kotter, J., 169
Kouri, D., 15
Kouzes, J.M., 178, 179
Kouzes and Posner's practice, 178
Kramer, M., 170, 179
Kraus, S., 169–70

L
Lacoursiere, R.B., 193, T194
Laissez-faire leadership, 173
Lalonde, Marc, 8
Lalonde Report, 8
Langfield-Smith, K., 356
Langley, G.J., 325, 330, 331
Lapp, J., 298
Laswell, H.D., 127
Laurent, Diana, 21
Lavery, J.V., 422
Law
    civil, 375–80
    public, 373–75
    sources of, 373
Lazarus, R.S., 355–56
Leach, L.S., 159, 177–78
Leader-member relations, 175
Leadership, 168–69
    behavioural approaches to, 173–74
    characteristics, 169–70
    contemporary approaches, 176–78
    contingency approaches to, 175–76
    emotional intelligence, 170
    in ethics, 402
    Fielder's Contingency theory, 175
    future directors, 179–83
    generational, 181–82
    Hersey and Blanchard's situational theory,
        175–76
    Kouzes and Posner's practice, 178
    learning and growing, 392
    management theories, 162–65, T164–65
    management vs., 169
    for modelling spiritual/cultural care, 402
    motivation theories of, 165–68, T166
    New, The, 180–81
    nursing, T403

Olympic vision, 169
organizational change, 171
path-goal theory, 176
quality of, 171
responsibilities, 168
substitutes for leadership, 176
theories of, 172–78
Leadership Practices Inventory (LPI), 179
LEADS in Caring environment framework,
        31, T32
Leape, L.L., 23
Learning organization theory, 294–95
Leatt, P., 15, 171
Leddy, S., 148
Lee, X.Q., 401
Legitimate power, 314, T315
Lentsch Schoon, Patricia M., 106
LeStorti, A., 351
Lewicki, R.J., 304
Lewin, K., 173, 196, T295
Lewin's Force-Field Model, 294, T295
Lewis, S., 15, 18, 19
Liability, 385–86, T386
Liaschenko, J., 414–15
Licensed practical nurse, responsibilities of, 251
Life expectancy at birth, 11, 44
Links, Internet, 98
Lippitt, R., 173
Lippitt's Phases of Change, 294
Literature resources, 99
    full-text articles, 99
Little-Stoetzel, Sharon, 348
Living will, 378, F379
Local culture, 399
Local Health Integration Networks (LHINs),
        15, 89
Loneliness, 400
Lord Acton, 316
Lorig, Kate, 21
Love, A., 401

M
MacDonald, C., 353
Machiavelli, 319
MacIvor, H., 373
Macro-allocation, 419
Maddox, P., 25
Maintenance (hygiene) factors, 167
Malpractice, 386
Management, 161–62
    administration principles, 164
    bureaucratic theory, 163, T164
    classical viewpoint, 163
    Hawthorne studies, T165

Management (*Continued*)
 informal organization, 164
 nursing leadership and, 182–83
Management council, 254–55
Management focus, 161
Management process, 161–62
 POSDCORB, 161
Managerial roles, 162
Managerial work, 168
Manager, time in roles, 162
Manthey, M., 169, 171, 182
Marchildon, G.P., 56–57
Marketing, 449
Marketing plan, 268
Marquis, B.L., 161, 182, 200, 261, 296, 297, 299,
  302, 304, 305, 355, 358, 432
Marthaler, Maureen T., 246
Martin, Judith W., 372
Maslow, A., 166
Mason, D., 146
Mayo, E., 165
McCall, M.W.Jr., 161, 169
McCloskey, J.C., 169
McClure, M., 170
McDonald, M., 425, 426
McGillis Hall, L., 30, 179, 225, 233
McGregor, D., 168, 196
McGregor, Rita, 143
McGregor's Theory X and Theory Y, 167–68
McLaughlin, Mary, 324
McNeese-Smith, D., 177–78
Mears, T., 196
Medical futility, 421
Medicare, 45
MEDLARS (Medical Literature Analysis and
  Retrieval System), 99
MEDLINE, 97, 99–100
MEDLINEplus, 97–98
Meighan, M., 171
Mentor, 451
Mentoring, 138–39
Meso-allocation, 419
Message, 127
Micro-allocation, 419
Miller, Terry W., 143, 311
Milstead, J.A., 146
MIS Guidelines, 56
Mission statement, 269
Moats Kennedy, M., 182
Modular team nursing, 236
Molloy, W., 378
Moorhead, G., 173
Moral distress, 412
Morality, 411–12

Motivation, 165
 factors, 167
Motivation theories, 165–68, T166
 Maslow's hierarchy of needs, F167, T166
 Theory X and Y (McGregor's), 167–68
 Theory Z (Ouchi), 168, T166
 two-factor theory (Hertzberg), T166–67
Multi-faith, 399
Murphy, M., 170
Murray, M.K., 435

N
Nagle, Dr. Lynn, 91
Narayanasamy, A., 391
National Council for Excellence in Critical
  Thinking Instruction, 349
National Council of State Boards of Nursing,
  248, 251
National Labour Relations Board, 438
National Library of Medicine, 98, 99
 MEDLARS, 99
Needs, spiritual
 comfort, 399
 creativity, 400
 hope, 400
 legacy, 400
 reminiscence, 400
 spiritual, 399
Negligence, 376
Negotiating, 304
Nelson, E., 285
Nelson, R., 89
Networking, 452
New Age, 86
Nicoll, L.H., 85, 99
Nightingale, Florence, 2, 33, 44, 45, 65, 107, 222,
  235, 247, 395, F3
Nightingale model of nursing, 2
Nominal group technique, 364
Nonmaleficence, 414
Non-unit producing, 223
Nonverbal communication, 128
Norming, 193–94
Northouse, P., 169, 176
Norton, D., 337
Nosek, Laura J., 43
Nurse autonomy, 353
Nurse manager, responsibilities of, 250
Nurse perceptor, 140
Nurse(s)
 assessment, spiritual/cultural, 395–97,
  T396
 client advocates, 133
 co-workers, 136

credibility, 154–55
marketing yourself, 449–51
new graduates' responsibilities, 250
Olympic vision, 169
political activist, as, 150–51
political influence, 146, 151, 153
politics/stakeholders and, 145–46
proficient, 282
references, career, 459
responsibilities of, 250–51
skillful communication, 382
spiritual practices, 403–404
staffing outcomes, 233–35
striking, 437
subordinates and, 136
workplace advocacy, 432
Nursing
    codes of ethics in, 415–16
    decision making, 352–53
    leadership, T403
    mentoring, 138–39
    military roots, 171
    politics of advocacy and, 151
    productivity/utilization, 163
    role-playing, 139
    and spirituality, 391–92
    team, see Team nursing
Nursing Act (1991) (Ontario), 375
Nursing associations, 437–39
Nursing Best Practice Guidelines, 65
Nursing ethics, 412–13
Nursing Health Services Research Unit (NHSRU),
    65, 79
Nursing hours per patient day (NHPPD), F223
Nursing informatics, 86, T87
    career opportunities, 90
    certification in, 89–90
    education in, 88–89
    formal programs, 88–89
    informal education, 89
    specialty of, 87–88
Nursing leadership, see also Leadership
    outcomes, 178–79
Nursing and Outcomes Project, 65
Nursing practice
    doctor's orders, 382
    enterprise risk management programs, 385–86
    government inquiries, 380–81
    legal protections, 380–86
    Sinclair Inquiry, T381
Nursing unionization, 431–32
    collective action models, 432–35
    collective bargaining, 432–33
    factors influencing unions, 432–33

O
Objectives, planning, 268
O'Brien-Pallas, Linda, 65, 163, 223, 225
Occupation Health and Safety Act (Ontario), 375
O'Connell, B., 151
Ogilvie, Marcy, 304
Olsen-Chavarriaga, D., 377
O'Neill, M.L., 56
Operating budget, 208
O'Reilly, P., 352, 354
Organisation for Economic Co-operation and
    Development (OECD), 45, F47, T46
Organization
    mission statement, 269
    philosophy, 269–70
    values, 270–71
    vision, 270
Organizational change, 292–93
Organizational communication, 131
Organizational structure, 271–76
    centralized vs. decentralized, 272–73
    division of labour, 273–75
    flat vs. tall, 272
    geographic area labour division, 276
    home health care agencies, T274
    hospitals, T274
    labour division by program, 276
    matrix structure, 272
    pharmaceutical companies, T274
    primary nursing, 276
    regional health authorities, T274
    reporting relationships, 275
    roles and responsibilities, 275
    types of, 272
Organization evidence, 68
Ottawa Charter, 107, 108
Ouchi, W., 168
Outcome elements of quality, 28

P
Palliative care, 404–405
Pan-American Health Organization (PAHO), 107
Pan-Canadian Public Health Network, 12
Pardue, S., 354
Participative Resolution Program (PRP), 304
Passive euthanasia, 422
Pastoral care, 391
Path-goal theory, 176
Patient classification system, see Workload
    measurement systems
Paul, R., 349–50
Payer, for health care services, 44–45
Performance improvement (PI), 326, 335
Performing, 194

Personal change, 292
Personal Health Information Protection Act
(Ontario) (PHIPA), 380
Personal Information Protection Act (BC,
Alta), 380
Personal Information Protection and Electronic
Documents Act (Canada) (PIPEDA), 30,
357, 380
Personalities, difficult
strategies for coping with, T195
Personal resources, 451–53
mentoring, 451–52
networking, 452
Pesut, D.J., 351
Petterson, E.F., 391
Pew Health Professions Commission, 349
P-F-A Assessment, 97–100
Philosophy, 269–70
core beliefs, 269, T270
Philosophy of an organization, 269
Physician remuneration, 52–54
Physician(s), 6
unionization, 439
workplace communication, 136–37
Physician services, 4
Pillai, R., 168
Pinkerton, S., 35
Plan Do Study Act cycle, 331, F332
Polifko-Harris, Karin, 191
Political evidence, 68
Political voices, 151
Politics, 144
Poole, V., 133, 256
Population assessment
needs, T117
Population-based health care initiatives, 109,
T110–12
Population-based needs assessment, T117
Population-based nursing practice, 113
Population health, 8–12, 107–109, F11
Porter-O'Grady, T., 58, 168, 171, 278, 284, 301–302
POSDCORB, 161
Position power, 175
Potter, P., 127, 133, 137
Power, 285
accountability, 314
connection, T315
definitions of, 312–14
expert, 314, T315
information, T315
legitimate, 314, T315
limits of information and, 317
Machiavelli on, 319
personal orientation and Internet, 316

referent, 314, T315
reward and coercive, 314–15, T315
sources of, 314–16
Power of Attorney, 378
Practical Nurses Canada (PNCanada), 403
Precede-Proceed Model, 117
Priest, A., 25, 192
Primary health care (PHC), 13–14, 107–108
guiding principles, 13
Primary Health Care Transition Fund, 13
Primary nursing, 237–38, 276
model, 131, F237
Principlism, 414
Privacy Act (1983) (Canada), 30, 380
Privacy legislation, 30
Privatization of health delivery, 56–57
Problem solving, 351
skills, 202–203
Process, 330
elements of quality, 28
motivation theories, 166
Professional change, 292
Professional codes of ethics, 415–16
Professional development, 280
Professional practice
accountability-based care delivery, 284
Benner's novice to expert, 280–82
clinical practice council, 278
competency and professional
development, 280
coordinating council, 255
education council, 278
management council, 254–55
process of, 282–84
quality council, 278
research council, 278–79
shared governance, F278
situational leadership, 282–84
structure of, 278–82
Program budgeting and marginal analysis
(PBMA), 54–55
Program planning/evaluation, 117–18
Proselytize, 398
Prototype system, 224–25
Provinces, health care initiatives, T110–13
Provost, K., 147
Public communication, 130
Public health, 12–13
nurses, 113
service delivery, T12
system, 12
Public Health Agency of Canada (PHAC), 12
health care institutions, T111
Public Hospitals Act (Ontario), 376

Public law, 373–75
 constitutional law, 373–74
 criminal law, 374
 statutory law, 374–75

Q

Quality assurance (QA), 326
 continuous quality improvement, 326, T328
 history of, 325–28
 performance improvement, 326
 total quality management, 326–28
Quality compass, 285, F287
Quality council, 278
Quality health care, T29
 Donabedian's framework, 28
 3M Health Care Quality Team Awards, 30
 outcome measurement, 30
 performance measures, T29
Quality improvement
 balanced scorecard, 335–37
 based on data, 330
 benchmarking, 335
 client satisfaction data, 337–38
 continuous process, 330
 enterprise risk management (ERM), 343–44
 flow diagrams for, 331, F334
 focus methodology, 331–35
 Gantt chart, 359–60, F336, F363
 general principles of, 328–29
 health care customers, 325
 health care work process, 330–31
 implications for client care, 331
 methodologies for, 331–38
 organizational structure, 342
 outcomes monitoring, 343
 Plan Do Study Act cycle, 331, F332
 regulatory requirement, 335
 sentinel events, 335
 storyboard, 337
 system improvement, 343
 using data, 338
Quality of life, 108, 405, 421
Quality outcomes, 284–85
Quebec Charter of Human Rights and Freedoms, 382
Questionnaires, 263

R

Raphael, D., 8, 9
Reality check, 447–48
Real-time, 86
Receiver, 127
Reengineering, 262

Referent (charismatic) power, 314, T315
Reflective thinking, 350–51
Regionalization, 14–15, T15–18
Registered nurses, see Nurse(s)
Registered Nurses Association of Ontario (RNAO), 65, 153, 160, 375
Regulated Health Professions Act (1991) (Ontario), 357, 375, 376
Rehabilitation, T6
Religion, 392
 beliefs, 397–98
 faith, 398
 needs, 397–99
 and spirituality, F394–95
Religious care, see Spiritual care
Reports on health care system
 federal and provincial, 48
Research council, 278–79
Resource allocation, 418–21
Resource intensity weights (RIWs), 56, 224, 238
Resources, 144
Responding, 132
Responsibility, 249
 health team members, 249–51
 licensed practical nurse, 251
 new graduate, 250
 nurse manager, 250
 registered nurse, 250
 unregulated care provider (UCP), 251
Résumé, 453–54, F454
 electronic, 454, 457, T457
Revenue, 214
Reverby, S., 58
Reward and coercive power, 314–15, T315
Right to health care, 45–48
Risk adjustment, 23–24
RN Delegation Decision-Making Framework, 248
RNs, see Nurse(s)
Robbins, S., 262, 292, 293
Robinson Vollman, A., 415
Rodger, Dr. Ginette L., 181
Rodney, P.A., 425, T426
Roesch, P., T270
Roethlisberger, J.F., 165
Rogers, C.M., 294
Rogers' Diffusion of Innovations Theory, 294, T295
Romanow Report, 14, 48, 146
Romanow, Roy, 374
Rondeau, K.V., 325
Ross, A., 201
Ross-Kerr, J., 45
Ruthman, Jacklyn L., 125

S

Sackett, D.L., 63
Salary, physician remuneration, 52
Salovey, P., 170
Satinsky, M.A., 241
Scanning the environment, 448–49
Scheduling, 230–32
    client needs, 230
    cyclical, 232
    impact on client care, 232
    self-scheduling, 232, T233
    staff experience, 230–31
    weekend program, 231, F232
Scientific literature, 68
Scientific management, 163, T164
Scott, J.G., 170, 353
Scriven, M., 349, 350
Seeman, N., 326
Self-assessment, 447–48
Self-confidence, 355–56
Self-scheduling, 232, T233
    boundaries of, 232
Sellers, K.F., 260, 280
Semancik, M., 90
Sender, 127
Senge, P.M., 196, 262, 295, 296
Sentinel event, 335
Shared governance, 253
Shared Leadership Concept Program (SLCP), 178
Shein, E., 356
Sherwin, S., 414
Shortell, S.M., 14, 33, 272, 273, 276
Shortt, S.E.D., 48, 49, T49
Silber, M.B., 298
Simms, L.M., 2, 130
Sinclair, C.M., 381
Sinclair, D., 15
Sinclair Inquiry, T381
Singer, P.A., 422, 423
Situational leadership, 282–84
Skill mix, 226
Smith, P.M., 171
Smith, R., 457
Snow, J.L., 178
Social media, 129–30
Somerville, M., 1
Soukup, F.M., 34
Sources of power, 314–16
Space, cultural delegation, 256
Spence Laschinger, H., 168
Spiritual care, 391
    compassionate care, 395
    domains, 404
    end-of-life care, 404–405, F405

    hierarchy (Maslow's), 395
    holistic, 394
    leadership roles, 402
    religious roots, examples, 395
    working with team, 402
Spirituality, 391–92
    abuse, 401–402
    assessment education, 395–97
    distressors, 400
    ethical concerns, 405
    models of, F394–95
    and nursing, 391–92
    religious needs, 397–99
Staffing
    benefit hours, 222, F223
    client outcomes, 233, 235
    core concepts, 222–23
    evaluating effectiveness, 233, 235
    models of care delivery, 235–38
    needs, determining, 222–25
    nurse outcomes, 233–35
    nursing hours per patient day (NHPPD), F223
    resource and FTEs, 222–23, F222, F223
    scheduling, 230–31
    weekend program, 231, F232
    worked hours, 222, F223
    workload measurement systems, 223–24
Staffing pattern, 225, 226
    benchmarking, 225
    considerations in developing, 225–26
    determining FTEs needed, 227
    establishing, 226
    financial implications, 232
    historical information, 226
    inpatient unit, 227
    new options for, 231–32
    regulatory requirements, 225
    staff support, 226
    worksheet, F228–29
Stakeholder(s), 144, 263
    assessment, 175
    and health care, 144–47
Stark, J., 372, 390–407
Stichler, J.F., 278
Stodgill, R.M., 170
Storage, 92
Storch, J.L., 411, 412, 413
Stordeur, S., 171
Storming, 193
Strategic career plan, 449
Strategic planning, 261–68
    advisory panel, 263
    community and stakeholder assessment, 263
    definition, 262

environmental assessment, 262–63
focus groups and interviews, 263
Framework, F264
goals and objectives, 268
marketing plan, 268
organization mission, 267–68
purpose, 262
questionnaires, 263
review of literature, 267
steps, 262, T268
surveys, 263
SWOT analysis, 262–63, F267
Strategic Service Plan, F264
Structure elements of quality, 28
Styles, M.M., 87
Substitute Decisions Act (1992) (Ontario), 377
Substitutes for leadership, 176
Sullivan, E., 294, 301, 303, 364
Sunnak, A., 18
Surveys, 263
SWOT analysis, 262–63, F267
System, 330
Systematic reviews, 70

T

Tanner, C.A., 354
Tanyi, R.A., 391
Tappen, R.M., 194, 294, 301
Task structure, 175
Taylor, Frederick, 163
Tazbir, Janice, 430
Team building, creating environment for, 198
Team evaluation checklist, T199
Team meetings, effective, 200
Team nursing, 236–37, F237
    modular nursing, 236
Team process, 193–94, T194
    group roles, 193–94
Teams, *see also* Groups
    defined, 192
    groups vs., T196–97
    guidelines, 196–98, F197
    problem-solving skills, 202–203
    successful relationships, 203–204
    theories of, 196
Teamwork, client care unit, 199–200
Teekman, B., 350
Theory X (McGregor's), 168
Theory Y (McGregor's), 168
Theory Z (Ouchi), 168
Thomas, J., 413
Tichy, N., 177
Time, cultural delegation, 256–57
Tomey, A., 366

Tort, 376
Tort law
    Do Not Resuscitate (DNR) Orders, 378–79
    false imprisonment, 379–80
    informed consent, 377–78
    intentional torts, 377
    non-intentional torts, 376–77
    privacy, right to, 380
Total pain, 400
Total patient care, 235–36
Total quality management (TQM), 326–28
Tranmer, J., 353
Transactional leader, 177
Transformational leader, 177
Transformational leadership theory, 177–78
Trofino, J., 177
Trudeau, Pierre Elliott, 431
Tuckman, B.W., 193
Two-factor theory, T166–67
    maintenance (hygiene) factors, 167
    motivation factors, 167

U

Ubiquitous computing, 95
Udod, S.A., 64, 67
Underwood, P., 432
Unionization
    in Canada, 431–32
    initiation of, T436
    physician, 439
    process of, 435–37
    professionalism and, 439
    pros and cons of, T440
    university professors, 439–40
Union(s), 433
    environment, 440
    grievances, 440
United Nations Human Development Index, 11
United Nation's Human Poverty Index (HPI), 11
Unit producing, 223
University professors, 439–40
Unregulated care provider(s) (UCPs), 250
    responsibilities of, 251
Upshur, R.E., 77
Urban ethnic diversity, 399
Useem, M., 365
User fees, 51–52
U.S. National Guideline Clearinghouse (NGC), 99
U.S. Patient's Bill of Rights, 415
Utilitarian theories, 413

V

Values, 270–71, 416
Vasile, G., 285

Veracity, 423
Verbal communication, 128
Vertical integration, 21
Virtual reality, 95–96
Vision, 250
Visual (channel of communication), 127
Volunteer Services Act (NS), 382
Voting block, 151
Vroom, V.H., 360
Vulnerable population groups, 109

W
Waddell, J., 444
Wade, G.H., 353
Wagner, C.M., 294
Walton, Nancy, 410
Watts, J., 95
Weatherill, S., 57
Weekend program, 231, F232
Wein, S., 401
Weiser, M., 94, 95
Wennberg, J., 23
Wesorick, B., 270
Wheatley, M.J., 180
Wheeler, M., 452, 458, 459
Whistle-blowing, 435
Williams, Brian, 262
Williams, R.P., 146
Wolf, G., 177
Wolf, S.M., 415
Wolper, I.F., 24

Wordsworth, H., 391
Workload measurement systems, 223–24
    client acuity, 224
    factor system, 224
    prototype system, 224–25
    utilization of classification system data, 225
Workplace advocacy, 432
Workplace communication, 136
    coworkers, 136
    subordinates, 136
    superiors, 136
World Health Organization (WHO), 13,
        107, 108
    goals, 120
    health care initiatives, T110
    health definition, 120
    ICIDH-2, 108
World Wide Web, *see* Internet
Wren, D., 163
Wright, L., 392

Y
Yeo, M., 412, 413, 416, 417
Yoder-Wise, P.S., 218
Yogo, Y., 128
Young, S., 177
Yukl, G., 161, 162, 168

Z
Zalenik, K.A., 169
Zander, K., 241